Handbook of Adaptive Designs in Pharmaceutical and Clinical Development

Handbook of Adaptive Designs in Pharmaceutical and Clinical Development

Edited by
Annpey Pong
Shein-Chung Chow

CRC Press
Taylor & Francis Group
Boca Raton London New York

CRC Press is an imprint of the
Taylor & Francis Group an **informa** business
A CHAPMAN & HALL BOOK

CRC Press
Taylor & Francis Group
6000 Broken Sound Parkway NW, Suite 300
Boca Raton, FL 33487-2742

Printed in the United States of America on acid-free paper
10 9 8 7 6 5 4 3 2 1

International Standard Book Number: 978-1-4398-1016-3 (Hardback)

Library of Congress Cataloging-in-Publication Data

Handbook of adaptive designs in pharmaceutical and clinical development / edited by Annpey Pong, Shein-Chung Chow.
p. ; cm.
Includes bibliographical references and index.
ISBN 978-1-4398-1016-3 (hardcover : alk. paper)
1. Clinical trials--Handbooks, manuals, etc. 2. Drugs--Research--Methodology--Handbooks, manuals, etc. I. Pong, Annpey. II. Chow, Shein-Chung, 1955-
[DNLM: 1. Clinical Trials as Topic--methods. 2. Research Design. 3. Statistics as Topic--methods. QV 771]

R853.C55H355 2011
615.5072'4--dc22 2010037121

Visit the Taylor & Francis Web site at
http://www.taylorandfrancis.com

and the CRC Press Web site at
http://www.crcpress.com

Contents

Preface

In recent years, as motivated by the U.S. Food and Drug Administration (FDA) *Critical Path Initiative*, the use of innovative adaptive design methods in clinical trials has attracted much attention from clinical investigators and regulatory agencies. Pharmaceutical Research Manufacturer Association (PhRMA) Working Group on Adaptive Design defines an adaptive design as a clinical trial design that uses accumulating data to decide how to modify aspects of the study as it continues, without undermining the validity and integrity of the trial. Adaptive designs are attractive to clinical scientists for several reasons. First, it does reflect medical practice in the real world. Second, it is ethical with respect to both efficacy and safety (toxicity) of the test treatment under investigation. Third, it provides an opportunity for a flexible and an efficient study design in the early phase of clinical development. However, there are some major obstacles when applying adaptive design methods in clinical development. These obstacles include (i) operational biases are inevitable to avoid, (ii) it is difficult to preserve the overall Type I error when many adaptations are applied, (iii) statistical methods and software packages are not well established, (iv) current infrastructure and clinical trial processes may not be ready for implementation of adaptive design methods in clinical trials, and (v) little regulatory guidelines or guidances are available.

The purpose of this book is to provide a comprehensive and unified presentation of the principles and methodologies (up-to-date) in adaptive design and analysis with respect to modifications (changes or adaptations) made to trial procedures and/or statistical methods based on accrued data of on-going clinical trials. In addition, this book is intended to give a well-balanced summary of current regulatory perspectives in this area. It is our goal to provide a complete, comprehensive, and updated reference book in the area of adaptive design and analysis in clinical research.

Chapter 1 gives an overview for the use of adaptive design methods in clinical trials. Chapter 2 provides fundamental theory behind adaptive trial design for the unplanned design change with blind data. Chapter 3 focuses on the application of the Bayesian approach in adaptive designs. The impact of potential population shift due to protocol amendments is studied in Chapter 4. Statistical methods from group sequential design to adaptive designs are reviewed in Chapter 5. Sample-size calculation for classical design is summarized in Chapter 6, while methodologies for flexible sample-size reestimation and adaptive interim analysis are discussed in Chapters 7 and 8, respectively. In Chapters 9 through 11, basic philosophy and methodology of dose finding and statistical methods for classical and adaptive dose finding trials are explored. Chapters 12 and 13 discuss statistical methods and issues that are commonly encountered when applying Phase I/II and Phase II/III seamless adaptive designs in clinical development, respectively. The sample-size estimation/allocation for multiple (two) stage seamless adaptive trial designs is studied in Chapter 14. Chapters 15 through 18 deal with various types of adaptive designs including adaptive randomization trial (Chapter 15), hypotheses-adaptive design (Chapter 16), treatment-adaptive designs (Chapter 17), and predictive biomarker diagnostics for new drug development (Chapter 18). Chapter 19 provides some insight regarding clinical strategies for endpoint selection in translational research. Chapters 20 through 21 provide useful information regarding infrastructure and independent data monitoring committee when implementing adaptive design methods in clinical trials. Chapter 22 provides an overview of the enrichment process in targeted clinical trials for personalized medicine. Applications of adaptive designs utilizing genomic or genetic information are given in Chapter 23. Chapter 24 provides detailed information regarding adaptive clinical trial simulation, which is often considered a useful tool for evaluation of the performances of the adaptive design methods applied. The issue regarding the efficiency of adaptive design is discussed in Chapter 25. Some case studies are presented in Chapter 26. Chapter 27 concludes the book with standard operating procedures for good adaptive practices.

We sincerely express our thanks to all of the contributors that made this book possible. They are the opinion leaders in the area of clinical research at the pharmaceutical industry, academia, or regulatory agencies. Their knowledge and experience will provide complete, comprehensive, and updated information to the readers who are involved or interested in the area of adaptive design and analysis in clinical research.

From Taylor & Francis, we would like to thank David Grubbs and Sunil Nair for providing us the opportunity to edit this book. We would like to thank colleagues from Merck Research Laboratories and the Department of Biostatistics and Bioinformatics and Duke Clinical Research Institute (DCRI) of Duke University School of Medicine for their constant support during the preparation of this book. In addition, we wish to express our gratitude to the following individuals for their encouragement and support: Roberts Califf, MD; Ralph Corey, MD; and John McHutchison, MD of Duke Clinical Research Institute and Duke University Medical Center; Greg Campbell, PhD of the U.S. FDA; and many friends from the academia, the pharmaceutical industry, and regulatory agencies.

Finally, we are solely responsible for the contents and errors of this book. Any comments and suggestions will be very much appreciated.

Annpey Pong
Shein-Chung Chow

Editors

Annpey Pong, PhD, is currently a manager at the Department of Biostatistics and Research Decision Sciences, Merck Research Laboratories, Rahway, New Jersey. Dr. Pong is the Associate Editor of the *Journal of Biopharmaceutical Statistics*, as well as the Guest Editor of the special issues on "Adaptive Design and Analysis in Clinical Development" (2004), "Recent Development of Adaptive Design in Clinical Trials" (2007), and the Organizer and Section Chair for "Recent Development of Design and Analysis in Clinical Trials" in the 17th Annual ICSA Applied Statistics Symposium (2008). Dr. Pong is the author or co-author of numerous publications in the field of pharmaceutical research. Dr. Pong received a BS in mathematics from Providence University, Taiwan, an MS in biostatistics from the University of Michigan–Ann Arbor, another MS in mathematics from Eastern Michigan University–Ypsilanti, and a PhD in statistics from Temple University–Philadelphia, Pennsylvania.

Shein-Chung Chow, PhD, is currently a professor at the Department of Biostatistics and Bioinformatics, Duke University School of Medicine, Durham, North Carolina, and a professor of clinical sciences, Duke–National University of Singapore Graduate Medical School, Singapore. Dr. Chow is currently the Editor-in-Chief of the *Journal of Biopharmaceutical Statistics*. He was elected Fellow of the American Statistical Association in 1995 and became a member of the International Statistical Institute in 1999. Dr. Chow is the author or co-author of over 200 methodology papers and 18 books, which include *Design and Analysis of Bioavailability and Bioequivalence Studies* (Marcel Dekker, 1992); *Sample Size Calculations in Clinical Research* (Marcel Dekker, 2003); *Encyclopedia of Biopharmaceutical Statistics* (Marcel Dekker, 2000); *Adaptive Design Methods in Clinical Trials* (Taylor & Francis, 2006); *Translational Medicine* (Taylor & Francis, 2008); and *Design and Analysis of Clinical Trials* (John Wiley & Sons, 1998). Dr. Chow received his BS in mathematics from National Taiwan University, Taiwan, and his PhD in statistics from the University of Wisconsin–Madison.

Contributors

Kwangmi Ahn
Department of Public Health Sciences
Pennsylvania State College of Medicine
Hershey, Pennsylvania

Arthur Berg
Department of Public Health Sciences
Pennsylvania State College of Medicine
Hershey, Pennsylvania

Rahul Bhattacharya
Department of Statistics
West Bengal State University
Barasat, Kolkata, India

Atanu Biswas
Applied Statistics Unit
Indian Statistical Institute
Kolkata, India

Björn Bornkamp
Department of Statistics
TU Dortmund University
Dortmund, Germany

Frank Bretz
Statistical Methodology
Integrated Information Sciences
Novartis Pharma AG
Basel, Switzerland

Carl-Fredrik Burman
Statistics and Informatics
AstraZeneca R&D
Mölndal, Sweden

Bill Byrom
Perceptive Informatics
Nottingham, United Kingdom

Mark Chang
Biostatistics and Data Management
AMAG Pharmaceuticals Inc.
Lexington, Massachusetts

George Y. H. Chi
Statistical Science
J&J Global Development Organization
Raritan, New Jersey

Shein-Chung Chow
Department of Biostatistics and Bioinformatics
Duke University School of Medicine
Durham, North Carolina

Christy Chuang-Stein
Statistical Research and Consulting Center
Pfizer, Inc.
Kalamazoo, Michigan

Lu Cui
Biostatistics
Eisai Inc.
Woodcliff Lake, New Jersey

Kiranmoy Das
Department of Statistics
Pennsylvania State University
University Park, Pennsylvania

Vladimir Dragalin
Center for Statistics in Drug Development
Quintiles Innovation
Morrisville, North Carolina

Tim Friede
Abteilung Medizinische Statistik
Universitätsmedizin Göttingen
Göttingen, Germany

Paul Gallo
Novartis Pharmaceuticals
East Hanover, New Jersey

Yonghong Gao
Division of Biostatistics/CDRH
U. S. Food and Drug Administration
Rockville, Maryland

Gerhard Hommel
Institut für Medizinische Biometrie, Epidemiologie und Informatik
Universitätsmedizin Mainz
Mainz, Germany

Christopher Jennison
Department of Mathematical Sciences
University of Bath
Bath, United Kingdom

Qi Jiang
Global Biostatistics & Epidemiology
Amgen, Inc.
Thousand Oaks, California

Simon Kirby
Statistical Research and Consulting Center
Pfizer, Inc.
Sandwich, Kent, United Kingdom

Shiowjen Lee
Office of Biostatistics and Epidemiology/CBER
U.S. Food and Drug Administration
Rockville, Maryland

Jiahan Li
Department of Statistics
Pennsylvania State University
University Park, Pennsylvania

Ning Li
Department of Regulatory and Medical Policy, China
Sanofi-aventis
Bridgewater, New Jersey

Yao Li
Department of Statistics
West Virginia University
Morgantown, West Virginia

Jen-Pei Liu
Division of Biometry
Department of Agronomy
Institute of Epidemiology
National Taiwan University
Taipei, Taiwan, Republic of China

and

Division of Biostatistics and Bioinformatics
Institute of Population Health Sciences
National Health Research Institutes
Zhunan, Taiwan, Republic of China

Qing Liu
Statistical Science
J&J Global Development Organization
Raritan, New Jersey

Qingshu Lu
Department of Statistics and Finance
University of Science and Technology of China
Anhui, People's Republic of China

Jiangtao Luo
Department of Mathematics
University of Florida
Gainesville, Florida

and

Department of Public Health Sciences
Pennsylvania State College of Medicine
Hershey, Pennsylvania

Jeff Maca
Statistical Methodology Group
Novartis Pharmaceuticals
East Hanover, New Jersey

Damian McEntegart
Perceptive Informatics
Nottingham, United Kingdom

Frank Miller
Statistics and Informatics
AstraZeneca R&D
Södertälje, Sweden

Graham Nicholls
Perceptive Informatics
Nottingham, United Kingdom

José Pinheiro
Statistical Methodology
Integrated Information Sciences
Novartis Pharmaceuticals
East Hanover, New Jersey

Annpey Pong
Department of BARDS
Merck Research Laboratories
Rahway, New Jersey

William Rosenberger
Department of Statistics
George Mason University
Fairfax, Virginia

Richard Simon
Biometric Research Branch
National Cancer Institute
Bethesda, Maryland

Steven Snapinn
Department of Global Biostatistics & Epidemiology
Amgen, Inc.
Thousand Oaks, California

Nigel Stallard
Warwick Medical School
The University of Warwick
Coventry, United Kingdom

Naitee Ting
Department of Biometrics and Data Management
Boehringer-Ingelheim Pharmaceuticals, Inc.
Ridgefield, Connecticut

Siu Keung Tse
Department of Management Sciences
City University of Hong Kong
Hong Kong, People's Republic of China

Bruce W. Turnbull
Department of Statistical Science
Cornell University,
Ithaca, New York

Marc Vandemeulebroecke
Translational Sciences Biostatistics
Integrated Information Sciences
Novartis Pharma AG
Basel, Switzerland

Zhong Wang
Department of Public Health Sciences
Pennsylvania State College of Medicine
Hershey, Pennsylvania

Gernot Wassmer
University of Cologne
Cologne, Germany

and

ADDPLAN GmbH
Cologne, Germany

Kiat Wee Wong
Statistics and Informatics
AstraZeneca R&D
Södertälje, Sweden

Rongling Wu
Department of Public Health Sciences
Pennsylvania State College of Medicine
Hershey, Pennsylvania

and

Department of Statistics
Pennsylvania State University
University Park, Pennsylvania

and

Department of Biotechnology
Beijing Forestry University
Beijing, People's Republic of China

Xiaoru Wu
Department of Statistics
Columbia University
New York City, New York

Guosheng Yin
Department of Statistics and Actuarial Science
The University of Hong Kong
Hong Kong, People's Republic of China

Ying Yuan
Department of Biostatistics
M. D. Anderson Cancer Center
The University of Texas
Houston, Texas

Lanju Zhang
MedImmune LLC
Gaithersberg, Maryland

1

Overview of Adaptive Design Methods in Clinical Trials

Annpey Pong
Merck Research Laboratories

Shein-Chung Chow
Duke University School of Medicine

1.1 Introduction

In the past several decades, as pointed out by Woodcock (2005), increasing spending of biomedical research does not reflect an increase in the success rate of pharmaceutical/clinical research and development. The low success rate of pharmaceutical development could be due to (i) a diminished margin for improvement that escalates the level of difficulty in proving drug benefits, (ii) genomics and other new science have not yet reached their full potential, (iii) mergers and other business arrangements have decreased candidates, (iv) easy targets are the focus as chronic diseases are harder to study, (v) failure rates have not improved, and (vi) rapidly escalating costs and complexity decreases willingness/ability to bring many candidates forward into the clinic (Woodcock 2005). As a result, the U.S. Food and Drug Administration (FDA) kicked off a *Critical Path Initiative* to assist the sponsors in identifying the scientific challenges underlying the medical product pipeline problems. In 2006, the FDA released a *Critical Path Opportunities List* that calls for advancing innovative trial designs by using prior experience or accumulated information in trial design. Many researchers interpret it as the encouragement of using innovative adaptive design methods in clinical trials, while some researchers believe it is the recommendation for using the Bayesian approach. The purpose of adaptive design methods in clinical trials is to provide the flexibility to the investigator for identifying best (optimal) clinical benefit of the test treatment under study in a timely and efficient fashion without undermining the validity and integrity of the intended study.

The concept of adaptive design can be traced back to the 1970s when adaptive (play-the-winner) randomization and a class of designs for sequential clinical trials were introduced (Wei 1978). As a result, most adaptive design methods in clinical research and development are referred to as adaptive randomization (see, e.g., Efron 1971; Lachin 1988; Atkinson and Donev 1992; Rosenberger et al. 2001; Hardwick and Stout 2002; Rosenberger and Lachin 2002), group sequential designs with the flexibility for stopping a trial early due to safety, futility, and/or efficacy (see, e.g., Lan and DeMets 1987; Wang and Tsiatis 1987; Lehmacher and Wassmer 1999; Posch and Bauer 1999; Liu, Proschan, and Pledger 2002), and sample size reestimation at interim for achieving the desired statistical power (see, e.g., Cui, Hung, and Wang 1999; Chung-Stein et al. 2006; Chow, Shao, and Wang 2007). The use of adaptive design methods for modifying the trial procedures and/or statistical procedures of on-going clinical trials based on accrued data has been practiced for years in clinical research and development. Adaptive design methods in clinical research are very attractive to clinical scientists for several reasons. First, it reflects medical practice in real world. Second, it is ethical with respect to both efficacy and safety (toxicity) of the test treatment under investigation. Third, it is not only flexible, but also efficient in the early phase of clinical development. However, it is a concern whether the p-value or confidence interval regarding the treatment effect obtained after the modification is correct or reliable. In addition, it is also a concern that the use of adaptive design methods in a clinical trial may lead to a totally different trial that is unable to address scientific/medical questions that the trial is intended to answer.

In recent years, the potential use of adaptive design methods in clinical trials have attracted much attention. For example, the Pharmaceutical Research and Manufacturers of America (PhRMA) and Biotechnology Industry Organization (BIO) have established adaptive design working groups and proposed/published white papers regarding strategies, methodologies, and implementations for regulatory consideration (see, e.g., Gallo et al. 2006; Chang 2007a). However, there are no universal agreement in terms of definition, methodologies, applications, and implementations. In addition, many journals have also published special issues on adaptive design for evaluating the potential use of adaptive trial design methods in clinical research and development. These scientific journals include, but are not limited to, *Biometrics* (Vol. 62, No. 3), *Statistics in Medicine* (Vol. 25, No. 19), *Journal of Biopharmaceutical Statistics* (Vol. 15, No. 4 and Vol. 17, No. 6), *Biometrical Journal* (Vol. 48, No. 4), and *Pharmaceutical Statistics* (Vol. 5, No. 2). In addition, many professional conferences/meetings have devoted special sessions for discussion of the feasibility, applicability, efficiency, validity, and integrity of the potential use of the innovative adaptive design methods in clinical trials in the past several years. For example, the FDA/Industry Statistics Workshop has offered adaptive sessions and workshops from industrial, academic, and regulatory perspectives consecutively between 2006 and 2009. More details regarding the use of adaptive design methods in clinical trials can be found in the books by Chow and Chang (2006) and Chang (2007a).

The purpose of this handbook is not only to provide a comprehensive summarization of the issues that are commonly encountered when applying/implementing the adaptive design methods in clinical trials, but also to include recently development such as the role of the independent data safety monitoring board and sample size estimation/allocation, justification, and adjustment when implementing a much more complicated adaptive design in clinical trials. In the next section, commonly employed adaptations and the resultant adaptive designs are briefly described. Also included in this section are regulatory and statistical perspectives regarding the use of adaptive design methods in clinical trials. The impact of protocol amendments, challenges of *by design* adaptations, and obstacles of retrospective adaptations when applying adaptive design methods in clinical trials are described in Section 1.3. Some trial examples and strategies for clinical development are discussed in Sections 1.4 and 1.5, respectively. The aim and scope of the book are given in the last section.

1.2 What is Adaptive Design?

It is not uncommon to modify trial procedures and/or statistical methods during the conduct of clinical trials based on the review of accrued data at interim. The purpose is not only to efficiently identify clinical benefits of the test treatment under investigation, but also to increase the probability of success for the intended clinical trial. Trial procedures are referred to as the eligibility criteria, study dose, treatment duration, study endpoints, laboratory testing procedures, diagnostic procedures, criteria for evaluability, and assessment of clinical responses. Statistical methods include a randomization scheme, study design selection, study objectives/hypotheses, sample size calculation, data monitoring and interim analysis, statistical analysis plan (SAP), and/or methods for data analysis. In this chapter, we will refer to the adaptations (changes or modifications) made to the trial and/or statistical procedures as the adaptive design methods. Thus, an adaptive design is defined as a design that allows adaptations to trial and/or statistical procedures of the trial after its initiation without undermining the validity and integrity of the trial (Chow, Chang, and Pong 2005). In one of their publications, with the emphasis of the feature by design adaptations only (rather than ad hoc adaptations), the PhRMA Working Group on Adaptive Design refers to an adaptive design as a clinical trial design that uses accumulating data to decide on how to modify aspects of the study as it continues, without undermining the validity and integrity of the trial (Gallo et al. 2006). The FDA defines an adaptive design as a study that includes a *prospectively* planned opportunity for modification of one or more specified aspects of the study design and hypotheses based on analysis of data (usually interim data) from subjects in the study (FDA, 2010). In many cases, an adaptive design is also known as a flexible design (EMEA 2002, 2006).

1.2.1 Adaptations

An adaptation is referred to as a modification or a change made to trial procedures and/or statistical methods during the conduct of a clinical trial. By definition, adaptations that are commonly employed in clinical trials can be classified into the categories of prospective adaptation, concurrent (or ad hoc) adaptation, and retrospective adaptation. Prospective adaptations include, but are not limited to, adaptive randomization, stopping a trial early due to safety, futility, or efficacy at interim analysis, dropping the losers (or inferior treatment groups), sample size reestimation, and so on. Thus, prospective adaptations are usually referred to by design adaptations as described in the PhRMA white paper (Gallo et al. 2006). Concurrent adaptations are usually referred to as any ad hoc modifications or changes made as the trial continues. Concurrent adaptations include, but are not limited to, modifications in inclusion/exclusion criteria, evaluability criteria, dose/regimen and treatment duration, changes in hypotheses and/or study endpoints, and so on. Retrospective adaptations are usually referred to as modifications and/or changes made to a SAP prior to database lock or unblinding of treatment codes. In practice, prospective, ad hoc, and retrospective adaptations are implemented by study protocols, protocol amendments, and statistical analysis plans with regulatory reviewer's consensus, respectively.

1.2.2 Type of Adaptive Designs

Based on the adaptations employed, commonly considered adaptive designs in clinical trials include, but are not limited to: (i) an adaptive randomization design, (ii) a group sequential design, (iii) an N-adjustable (or flexible sample size reestimation) design, (iv) a drop-the-loser (or pick-the-winner) design, (v) an adaptive dose finding design, (vi) a biomarker-adaptive design, (vii) an adaptive treatment-switching design, (viii) a adaptive-hypothesis design, (ix) an adaptive seamless (e.g., phase I/II or phase II/III) trial design, and (x) a multiple-adaptive design. These adaptive designs are all briefly described below.

1.2.2.1 Adaptive Randomization Design

An adaptive randomization design allows modification of randomization schedules based on varied and/or unequal probabilities of treatment assignment in order to increase the probability of success. As a result, an adaptive randomization design is sometimes referred to as a play-the-winner design since it will increase the probability of success. Commonly applied adaptive randomization procedures include treatment-adaptive randomization (Efron 1971; Lachin 1988), covariate-adaptive randomization, and response-adaptive randomization (Rosenberger et al. 2001; Hardwick and Stout 2002).

Although an adaptive randomization design could increase the probability of success, it may not be feasible for a large trial or a trial with a relatively longer treatment duration because the randomization of a given subject depends on the response of the previous subject. A large trial or a trial with a relatively longer treatment duration utilizing adaptive randomization design will take a much longer time to complete. Besides, a randomization schedule may not be available prior to the conduct of the study. Moreover, statistical inference on treatment effect is often difficult to obtain due to the complexity of the randomization scheme. In practice, a statistical test is often difficult to obtain—if not impossible—due to complicated probability structure as the result of adaptive randomization, which has also limited the potential use of adaptive randomization design in practice.

1.2.2.2 Group Sequential Design

A group sequential design allows for prematurely stopping a trial due to safety, futility/efficacy, or both with options of additional adaptations based on results of interim analysis. Many researchers refer to a group sequential design as a typical adaptive design because some adaptations may be applied after the review of interim results of the study such as stopping the trial early due to safety, efficacy and/or futility. In practice, various stopping boundaries based on different boundary functions for controlling an overall type I error rate are available in the literature (see, e.g., Lan and DeMets 1987; Wang and Tsiatis 1987; Jennison and Turnbull 2000, 2005; Rosenberger et al. 2001; Chow and Chang 2006). In recent years, the concept of two-stage adaptive design has led to the development of the adaptive group sequential design (e.g., Cui, Hung, and Wang 1999; Posch and Bauer 1999; Lehmacher and Wassmer 1999; Liu, Proschan, and Pledger 2002).

It should be noted that when additional adaptations such as adaptive randomization, dropping the losers, and/or adding additional treatment arms (in addition to the commonly considered adaptations) are applied to a typical group sequential design after the review of the interim results, the resultant group sequential design is usually referred to as an adaptive group sequential design. In this case, the standard methods for the typical group sequential design may not be appropriate. In addition, it may not be able to control the overall type I error rate at the desired level of 5% if (i) there are additional adaptations (e.g., changes in hypotheses and/or study endpoints), and/or (ii) there is a shift in target patient population due to additional adaptations or protocol amendments.

1.2.2.3 Flexible Sample Size Reestimation Design

A flexible sample size reestimation (or N-adjustable) design allows for sample size adjustment or reestimation based on the observed data at interim. Sample size adjustment or reestimation could be done in either a blinding or unblinding fashion based on the criteria of treatment effect-size, variability, conditional power, and/or reproducibility probability (see, e.g., Proschan and Hunsberger 1995; Cui, Hung, and Wang 1999; Posch and Bauer 1999; Liu and Chi 2001; Friede and Kieser 2004; Chung-Stein et al. 2006; Chow, Shao, and Wang 2007). Sample size reestimation suffers from the same disadvantage as the original power analysis for sample size calculation prior to the conduct of the study because it is performed by treating *estimates* of the study parameters, which are obtained based on data observed at interim, as true values.

In practice, it is not a good clinical/statistical practice to start with a small number and then perform sample size reestimation (adjustment) at interim by ignoring the clinically meaningful difference that one wishes to detect for the intended clinical trial. It should be noted that the observed difference at interim based on a small number of subjects may not be of statistically significance (i.e., it may be observed by chance alone). In addition, there is variation associated with the observed difference that is an estimate of the true difference. Thus, standard methods for sample size reestimation based on the observed difference with a limited number of subjects may be biased and misleading. To overcome these problems in practice, a sensitivity analysis (with respect to variation associated with the observed results at interim) for sample size reestimation design is recommended.

1.2.2.4 Drop-the-Losers Design

A drop-the-losers design allows dropping the inferior treatment groups. This design also allows adding additional (promising) arms. A drop-the-losers design is useful in the early phase of clinical development especially when there are uncertainties regarding the dose levels (Bauer and Kieser 1999; Brannath, Koening, and Bauer 2003; Posch et al. 2005; Sampson and Sill 2005). The selection criteria (including the selection of initial dose, the increment of the dose, and the dose range) and decision rules play important roles for this design. Dose groups that are dropped may contain valuable information regarding dose response of the treatment under study. Typically, drop-the-losers design is a two-stage design. At the end of the first stage, the inferior arms will be dropped based on some prespecified criteria. The winners will then proceed to the next stage. In practice, the study is often powered for achieving a desired power at the end of the second stage (or at the end of the study). In other words, there may not be any statistical power for the analysis at the end of the first stage for dropping the losers (or picking up the winners).

In practice, it is not uncommon to drop the losers or pick up the winners based on so-called *precision analysis* (see, e.g., Chow, Shao, and Wang 2007). The precision approach is an approach based on the confidence level for achieving *statistical significance*. In other words, the decision will be made (i.e., to drop the losers) if the confidence level for observing a statistical significance (i.e., the observed difference is not by chance alone or it is reproducible with the prespecified confidence level) exceeds a prespecified confidence level. Note that in a drop-the-losers design, a general principle is to drop the inferior treatment groups or add promising treatment arms but at the same time it is suggested that the control group be retained for a fair and reliable comparison at the end of the study. It should be noted that dose groups that are dropped may contain valuable information regarding dose response of the treatment under study. In practice, it is also suggested that subjects who are assigned in the inferior dose groups should be switched to the better dose group for ethical consideration. Treatment switching in a drop-the-losers design could complicate statistical evaluation in the dose selection process. Note that some clinical scientists prefer the term *pick-the-winners* rather than drop-the-losers.

1.2.2.5 Adaptive Dose Finding Design

The purpose of an adaptive dose finding (e.g., escalation) design is multifold, which includes (i) the identification whether there is a dose response, (ii) the determination of the minimum effective dose (MED) and/or the maximum tolerable dose (MTD), (iii) the characterization of dose response curve, and (iv) the study of dose ranging. The information obtained from an adaptive dose finding experiment is often used to determine the dose level for the next phase of clinical development (see, e.g., Bauer and Rohmel 1995; Whitehead 1997; Zhang, Sargent, and Mandrekar 2006). For adaptive dose finding design, the method of continual reassessment method (CRM) in conjunction with the Bayesian approach is usually considered (O'Quigley, Pepe, and Fisher 1990; O'Quigley and Shen 1996; Chang and Chow 2005). Mugno, Zhus, and Rosenberger (2004) introduced a nonparametric adaptive urn design approach for estimating a dose-response curve. For more details regarding PhRMA's proposed statistical methods, the reader should consult with a special issue recently published in the *Journal of Biopharmaceutical Statistics* (Vol. 17, No. 6).

Note that according to the ICH E4 guideline on *Dose-Response Information to Support Drug Registration*, there are several types of dose-finding (response) designs, which are (i) randomized parallel dose-response designs, (ii) crossover dose-response design, (iii) forced titration design (dose-escalation design), and (iv) optimal titration design (placebo-controlled titration to endpoint). Some commonly asked questions for an adaptive dose finding design include, but are not limited to (i) how to select the initial dose, (ii) how to select the dose range under study, (iii) how to achieve statistical significance with a desired power with a limit number of subjects, (iv) what are selection criteria and decision rules if one would like to make a decision based on safety, tolerability, efficacy, and/or pharmacokinetic information, and (v) what is the probability of achieving the optimal dose. In practice, a clinical trial simulation and/or sensitivity analysis is often recommended to evaluate or address the above questions.

1.2.2.6 Biomarker-Adaptive Design

A biomarker-adaptive design allows for adaptations based on the response of biomarkers such as genomic markers. An adaptive biomarker design involves biomarker qualification and standard, optimal screening design, and model selection and validation. It should be noted that there is a gap between identifying biomarkers associated with clinical outcomes and establishing a predictive model between relevant biomarkers and clinical outcomes in clinical development. For example, correlation between a biomarker and true clinical endpoint makes a prognostic marker. However, correlation between a biomarker and true clinical endpoint does not make a predictive biomarker. *A prognostic biomarker* informs the clinical outcomes, independent of treatment. They provide information about the natural course of the disease in individuals who have or have not received the treatment under study. Prognostic markers can be used to separate good- and poor-prognosis patients at the time of diagnosis. *A predictive biomarker* informs the treatment effect on the clinical endpoint (Chang 2007a).

A biomarker-adaptive design can be used to (i) select right patient population (e.g., enrichment process for selection of a better target patient population that has led to the research of target clinical trials), (ii) identify nature's course of disease, (iii) early detection of disease, and (iv) help in developing personalized medicine (see, e.g., Charkravarty 2005; Wang, O'Neill, and Hung 2007; Chang 2007a).

1.2.2.7 Adaptive Treatment-Switching Design

An adaptive treatment-switching design allows the investigator to switch a patient's treatment from an initial assignment to an alternative treatment if there is evidence in a lack of efficacy or safety of the initial treatment (e.g., Branson and Whitehead 2002; Shao, Chang, and Chow 2005). In cancer clinical trials, estimation of survival is a challenge when treatment-switching has occurred in some patients. A high percentage of subjects who switched due to disease progression could lead to a change in hypotheses to be tested. In this case, sample size adjustment for achieving a desired power is necessary.

1.2.2.8 Adaptive-Hypotheses Design

An adaptive-hypotheses design allows modification or change in hypotheses based on interim analysis results (Hommel 2001). Adaptive-hypotheses designs are often considered before a database lock and/or prior to data unblinding, which are implemented by the development of SAP. Typical examples include the switch from a superiority hypothesis to a noninferiority hypothesis and the switch between the primary study endpoint and the secondary endpoints. The purpose in switching from a superiority hypothesis to a noninferiority hypothesis is to increase the probability of the success of the clinical trial. A typical approach is to first establish noninferiority and then test for superiority. In this way, we do not have to pay for statistical penalty due to the principle of closed testing procedure. The idea of switching the primary study endpoints and the secondary endpoints is also to increase the probability of success for clinical development. In practice, it is not uncommon to observe positive results in the secondary endpoint while failing to demonstrate clinical benefit for the primary endpoints. In this case, there is a strong desire to switch the primary endpoints and the secondary endpoints whenever it is scientifically, clinically, and regulatory justifiable.

It should be noted that, for the switch from a superiority hypothesis to a noninferiority hypothesis, the selection of noninferiority margin is critical, which has an impact on sample size adjustment for achieving the desired power. According to the ICH guideline, the selected noninferiority margin should be both clinical and statistical justifiable (ICH 2000; Chow and Shao 2006). For a switch between the primary endpoint and the secondary endpoint, it has been a tremendous debit for controlling the overall type I error rate at the 5% level of significance. As an alternative, switch from the primary endpoint to either a *co-primary* endpoint or a *composite* endpoint. However, the optimal allocation of the alpha spending function has raised another statistical/clinical/regulatory concern.

1.2.2.9 Adaptive Seamless Trial Design

An adaptive seamless trial design is a program that addresses within single trial objectives that are normally achieved through separate trials of clinical development. The design would use data from patients enrolled before and after the adaptation in the final analysis (Kelly, Stallard, and Todd 2005; Maca et al. 2006; Chow and Chang 2008). Commonly considered are an adaptive seamless Phase I/II design in early clinical development and Phase II/III in late phase clinical development.

An adaptive seamless phase II/III design is a two-stage design consisting of a learning or exploratory stage (phase IIb) and a confirmatory stage (phase III). A typical approach is to power the study for the phase III confirmatory phase and obtain valuable information with certain assurance using confidence interval approach at the phase II learning stage. Its validity and efficiency, however, has been challenged (Tsiatis and Mehta 2003). Moreover, it is not clear how to perform a combined analysis if the study objectives (or endpoints) are similar but different at different phases (Chow, Lu, and Tse 2007; Chow and Tu 2008). More research regarding sample size estimation/allocation and statistical analysis for seamless adaptive designs with different study objectives and/or study endpoints for various data types (e.g., continuous, binary, and time-to-event) is needed.

1.2.2.10 Multiple-Adaptive Design

Finally, a multiple-adaptive design is any combinations of the above adaptive designs. These commonly considered designs might include (i) the combination of adaptive group sequential design, drop-the-losers design, and adaptive seamless trial design, and (ii) adaptive dose-escalation design with adaptive randomization (Chow and Chang 2006). Since statistical inference for a multiple-adaptation design is often difficult in practice, it is suggested that a clinical trial simulation be conducted to evaluate the performance of the resultant multiple adaptive design at the planning stage.

When applying a multiple adaptive design, some frequently asked questions include (i) how to avoid/control potential operational biases that may be introduced due to various adaptations that apply to the trial, (ii) how to control the overall Type I error rate at the 5%, (iii) how to determine the required sample size for achieving the study objectives with the desired power, and (iv) how to maintain the quality, validity, and integrity of the trial. The trade-off between the flexibility/efficiency and scientific validity/integrity need to be carefully evaluated before a multiple-adaptive design is implemented in clinical trials.

1.2.3 Regulatory/Statistical Perspectives

From a regulatory point of view, the use of adaptive design methods based on accrued data in clinical trials may introduce operational bias such as selection, method of evaluation, early withdrawal, and modification of treatment. Consequently, it may not be able to preserve the overall type I error rate at the prespecified level of significance. In addition, p-values may not be correct and the corresponding confidence intervals for the treatment effect may not be reliable. Moreover, it may result in a totally different trial that is unable to address the medical questions that original study intended to answer. Li (2006) also indicated that commonly seen adaptations that have an impact on the type I error rate include but are not limited to (i) sample size adjustment at interim, (ii) sample size allocation to treatments, (iii) delete, add, or change treatment arms, (iv) shift in target patient population such as changes in inclusion/exclusion criteria, (v) change in statistical test strategy, (vi) change in study endpoints; and (vii) change in study objectives such as the switch from a superiority trial to a noninferiority trial. As a result, it is difficult to interpret the clinically meaningful effect size for the treatments under study (see also, Quinlan, Gallo, and Krams 2006).

From a statistical point of view, major (or significant) adaptations to trial and/or statistical procedures could (i) introduce bias/variation to data collection, (ii) result in a shift in location and scale of the target patient population, and (iii) lead to inconsistency between hypotheses to be tested and the corresponding statistical tests. These concerns will not only have an impact on the accuracy and reliability of statistical inference drawn on the treatment effect, but also present challenges to biostatisticians for development of appropriate statistical methodology for an unbiased and fair assessment of the treatment effect.

Note that although the flexibility of modifying study parameters is very attractive to clinical scientists, several regulatory questions/concerns arise. First, what level of modifications to the trial procedures and/or statistical procedures would be acceptable to the regulatory authorities? Second, what are the regulatory requirements and standards for review and approval process of clinical data obtained from adaptive clinical trials with different levels of modifications to trial procedures and/or statistical procedures of on-going clinical trials? Third, has the clinical trial become totally different after the modifications to the trial procedures and/or statistical procedures for addressing the study objectives of the originally planned clinical trial? These concerns should be addressed by the regulatory authorities before the adaptive design methods can be widely accepted in clinical research and development.

1.3 Impact, Challenges, and Obstacles

1.3.1 Impact of Protocol Amendments

In practice, for a given clinical trial, it is not uncommon to have three to five protocol amendments after the initiation of the clinical trial. One of the major impacts of many protocol amendments is that the target patient population may have been shifted during the process, which may have resulted in a totally different target patient population at the end of the trial. A typical example is the case when significant modifications are applied to inclusion/exclusion criteria of the study protocol. As a result, the resultant actual patient population following certain modifications to the trial procedures is a *moving* target patient population rather than a fixed target patient population. As indicated in Chow and Chang (2006), the impact of protocol amendments on statistical inference due to a shift in target patient population (moving target patient population) can be studied through a model that links the moving population means with some covariates (Chow and Shao 2005). Chow and Shao (2005) derived statistical inference for the original target patient population for simple cases.

1.3.2 Challenges in *By Design* Adaptations

In clinical trials, commonly employed prospective (by design) adaptations include stopping the trial early due to safety, futility, and/or efficacy, sample size reestimation (adaptive group sequential design), dropping the losers (adaptive dose finding design), and combining two separate trials into a single trial (adaptive seamless design). These designs are typical multiple-stage designs with different adaptations. In this section, major challenges in analysis and design are described. Recommendations and future development for resolution are provided whenever possible.

The major difference between a classic multiple-stage design and an adaptive multiple-stage design is that an adaptive design allows adaptations after the review of interim analysis results. These *by design* adaptations include sample size adjustment (reassessment or reestimation), stopping the trials due to safety, efficacy/futility, or dropping the losers (picking the winners). Note that commonly considered adaptive group sequential design, adaptive dose finding design, and adaptive seamless trial design are special cases of multiple-stage designs with different adaptations. In this section, we will discuss major challenges in design (e.g., sample size calculation) and analysis (controlling Type I error rate under moving target patient population) of an adaptive multiple-stage design with K–1 interim analyses.

A multiple-stage adaptive group sequential design is very attractive to sponsors in clinical development. However, major (or significant) adaptations such as modification of doses and/or change in study endpoints may introduce bias/variation to data collection as the trial continues. To account for these (expected and/or unexpected) biases/variation, statistical tests are necessary adjusted to maintain the overall type I error and the related sample size calculation formulas have to be modified for achieving the desired power. In addition, the impact on statistical inference is not negligible if the target patient population has been shifted due to major or significant adaptations and/or protocol amendments. This has presented challenges to biostatisticians in clinical research when applying a multiple-stage adaptive design. In practice it is worthy to pursue the following specific directions that (i) derive valid statistical test procedures for adaptive group sequential designs assuming model, which relates the data from different interim analyses, (ii) derive valid statistical test procedures for adaptive group sequential designs assuming the random-deviation model, (iii) derive valid Bayesian methods for adaptive group sequential designs, and (iv) derive sample size calculation formulas for various situations. Tsiatis and

Mehta (2003) showed that there exists an optimal (i.e., uniformly more powerful) design for any class of sequential design with a specified error spending function. It should be noted that adaptive designs do not require, in general, a fixed error spending function. One of the major challenges for an adaptive group sequential design is that the overall type I error rate may be inflated when there is a shift in target patient population (see, e.g., Feng, Shao, and Chow 2007).

For adaptive dose finding design, Chang and Chow's method can be improved by following specific directions (i) study the relative merits and disadvantages of their method under various adaptive methods, (ii) examine the performance of an alternative method by forming the utility first with different weights to the response levels and then modeling the utility, and (iii) derive sample size calculation formulas for various situations. An adaptive seamless Phase II/III design is a two-stage design that consists of two phases; namely, a learning (or exploratory) phase and a confirmatory phase. One of the major challenges for designs of this kind is that different study endpoints are often considered at different stages for achieving different study objectives. In this case, the standard statistical methodology for assessment of treatment effect and for sample size calculation cannot be applied.

Note that, for a two-stage adaptive design, the method by Chang (2007b) can be applied. However, Chang's method, like other stagewise combination methods, is valid under the assumption of constancy of the target patient populations, study objectives, and study endpoints at different stages.

1.3.3 Obstacles of Retrospective Adaptations

In practice, retrospective adaptations such as adaptive-hypotheses may be encountered prior to database lock (or unblinding) and implemented through the development of SAP. To illustrate the impact of retrospective adaptations, we first consider the situation where switching hypotheses between a superiority hypothesis and a noninferiority hypothesis. For a promising test drug, the sponsor would prefer an aggressive approach for planning a superiority study. The study is usually powered to compare the promising test drug with an active control agent.

However, the collected data may not support superiority. Instead of declaring the failure of the superiority trial, the sponsor may switch from testing superiority to testing the following noninferiority hypotheses. The margin is carefully chosen to ensure that the treatment of the test drug is larger than the placebo effect and, thus, declaring noninferiority to the active control agent means that the test drug is superior to the placebo effect. The switch from a superiority hypothesis to a noninferiority hypothesis will certainly increase the probability of success of the trial because the study objective has been modified to establish noninferiority rather than showing superiority. This type of switching hypotheses is recommended provided that the impact of the switch on statistical issues and inference (e.g., appropriate statistical methods) on the assessment of treatment effect is well justified.

1.4 Some Examples

In this section, we will present some examples for adaptive trial designs, which have been implemented in practice (see, e.g., Chow and Chang 2008). These trial examples include (1) an adaptive dose-escalation design for early phase cancer trials, (2) a multiple-stage adaptive design for Non-Hodgkin's Lymphoma (NHL) trial, (3) a Phase IV drop-the-losers adaptive design for multiple myeloma (MM) trial, (4) a two-stage seamless Phase I/II adaptive trial design for hepatitis C virus (HCV) trial, and (5) a biomarker-adaptive design for targeted clinical trials.

Example 1: Adaptive Dose-Escalation Design for Early Phase Cancer Trials

In a phase I cancer trial, suppose that the primary objective is to identify the maximum tolerated dose (MTD) for a new test drug. Based on the animal studies, it is estimated that the toxicity (dose limiting toxicity (DLT) rate) is 1% for the starting dose 25 mg/m^2 (1/10 of the lethal dose). The DLT rate at MTD is

TABLE 1.1 Summary of Simulation Results for the Designs

Method	True MTD	Mean Predicted MTD	Mean No. Patients	Mean No. DLTs
3 + 3 TER	100	86.7	14.9	2.8
CRM	100	99.2	13.4	2.8
3 + 3 TER	150	125	19.4	2.9
CRM	150	141	15.5	2.5
3 + 3 TER	200	169	22.4	2.8
CRM	200	186	16.8	2.2

Source: Chow, S. C. and Chang M., *Orphanet Journal of Rare Diseases*, 3, 1–13, 2008.

defined as 0.25 and the MTD is estimated to be 150 mg/m^2. A typical approach is to consider so-called 3 + 3 traditional escalation rule (TER). On the other hand, an adaptive type approach is to apply the CRM in conjunction with a Bayesian approach. We can compare the 3 + 3 TER approach and the Bayesian CRM adaptive method through simulations. A logistic toxicity model is chosen for the simulations. The dose interval sequence is chosen to be the customized dose increment sequence (increment factors = 2, 1.67, 1.33, 1.33, 1.33, 1.33, 1.33, 1.33, 1.33). The evaluations of the escalation designs are based on the criteria of safety, accuracy, and efficiency. Simulation results for all three methods in three different MTD scenarios are summarized in Table 1.1.

In this example, it can be seen that if the true MTD is 150 mg/m^2 the TER approach underestimates MTD (125 mg/m^2), while the Baysian CRM adaptive method also slightly underestimates the MTD (141 mg/m^2). The average number of patients required are 19.4 and 15.5 for the TER approach and the Bayesian CRM adaptive method, respectively. From a safety perspective, the average number of DLTs are 2.9 and 2.5 per trial for the TER approach and the Bayesian CRM, respectively. As a result, the Bayesian CRM adaptive method is preferable. More details regarding Bayesian CRM adaptive method and adaptive dose finding can be found in Chang and Chow (2005) and Chow and Chang (2006), respectively.

Example 2: Multiple-Stage Adaptive Design for NHL Trial

A Phase III two parallel group NHL trial was designed with three analyses. The primary endpoint is progression-free survival (PFS), the secondary endpoints are (i) overall response rate (ORR) including complete and partial response, and (ii) complete response rate (CRR). The estimated median PFS is 7.8 months and 10 months for the control and test groups, respectively. Assume a uniform enrollment with an accrual period of 9 months and a total study duration of 23 months. The estimated ORR is 16% for the control group and 45% for the test group. The classic design with a fixed sample size of 375 subjects per group will allow for detecting a three month difference in median PFS with 82% power at a one-sided significance level of $\alpha = 0.025$. The first interim analysis will be conducted on the first 125 patients/group (or total $N_1 = 250$) based on ORR. The objective of the first interim analysis is to modify the randomization. Specifically, if the difference in ORR (test-control), $\Delta_{ORR} > 0$, the enrollment will continue. If $\Delta_{ORR} \leq 0$, then the enrollment will stop. If the enrollment is terminated prematurely, there will be one final analysis for efficacy based on PFS and possible efficacy claimed on the secondary endpoints. If the enrollment continues, there will be a second interim analysis based on PFS. The second interim analysis could lead to either claim efficacy or futility, or continue to the next stage with possible sample size reestimation. The final analysis of PFS. When the primary endpoint (PFS) is significant, the analyses for the secondary endpoints will be performed for the potential claim on the secondary endpoints. During the interim analyses, the patient enrollment will not stop.

Example 3: Drop-the-Losers Adaptive Design for Multiple Myeloma Trial

For phase IV study, the adaptive design can also work well. For example, an oncology drug had been on the market for a year, physicians used the drug with different combinations for treating patients with MM.

TABLE 1.2 Simulation Results of Phase IV Drop-the-Losers Design

Interim Sample Size Per Group	Final Sample Size Per Group	Probability of Identifying the Optimal Arm
25	50	80.3%
50	100	91.3%

Source: Chow, S. C. and Chang, M., *Orphanet Journal of Rare Diseases*, 3, 1–13, 2008.

Note: Response rate for the five arms: 0.4, 0.45, 0.45, 0.5, and 0.6.

However, there was a strong desire to know what combination would be the best for the patient. Many physicians have their own experiences, no one has convincing data. Therefore, the sponsor is planned a trial to investigate the optimal combination for the drug. In this scenario, we can use a much smaller sample size than phase III trials because the issue is focused on the type-I control as the drug is approved. The issue is that given a minimum clinically meaningful difference (e.g., two weeks in survival), what is the probability the trial will be able to identify the optimal combination. Again this can be done through simulations, the strategy is to start with about five combinations, drop inferior arms, and calculate the probability of selecting the best arm under different combinations of sample size at the interim and final stages. In this adaptive design, we will drop two arms based on the observed response rate; that is, the two arms with the lowest observed response rates will be dropped at interim analysis and the other three arms will be carried forward to the second stage. The characteristics of the design are presented in Table 1.2 for different sample sizes.

Given the response rate 0.4, 0.45, 0.45, 0.5, and 0.6 for the five arms and 91% power, if a traditional design is used, there will be nine multiple comparisons (adjusted $\alpha = 0.0055$ using the Bonferroni method). The required sample size for the traditional design is 209 per group or a total of 1045 subjects comparing a total of 500 subjects for the adaptive trial (250 at the first stage and 150 at the second stage). In the case when the null hypothesis is true (the response rates are the same for all the arms), it doesn't matter what arm is chosen as the optimal.

Example 4: Two-Stage Seamless Phase I/II Adaptive Design for HCV Trial

A pharmaceutical company is interested in conducting a clinical trial utilizing a two-stage seamless adaptive design for evaluation of safety, tolerability, and efficacy of a test treatment as compared to a standard care treatment for treating subjects with HCV genotype 1 infection. The proposed adaptive trial design consists of two stages of dose selection and efficacy confirmation. The primary efficacy endpoint is the incidence of sustained virologic response (SVR), defined as an undetectable HCV RNA level (< 10 IU/mL) at 24 weeks after treatment is complete (Study Week 72). This assessment will be made when the last subject in Stage 2 has completed the study week 72 evaluation. In stages 1 and 2, the incidence of the following primary efficacy variables of (i) rapid virologic response (RVR) (i.e., undetectable HCV RNA level at study week 4), (ii) early virologic response (EVR) (i.e., ≥ 2-log10 reduction in HCV RNA level at study week 12 compared with the baseline level), (iii) end-of-treatment response (EOT) (i.e., undetectable HCV RNA level at study week 48) and (iv) SVR (i.e., undetectable HCV RNA level at study week 72: 24 weeks after treatment is complete).

Stage 1 is a four-arm randomized evaluation of three dose levels of continuous subcutaneous (SC) delivery of the test treatment compared with PegIntron (standard care) given as once weekly SC injections. All subjects will receive oral weight-based ribavirin. After all Stage 1 subjects have completed study week 12, an interim analysis will be performed. The interim analysis will provide information to enable selection of an active dose of the test treatment based on safety/tolerability, outcomes, and early indications of efficacy to proceed to testing for noninferiority compared with standard of care in Stage 2 (see Figure 1.1). Depending upon individual response data for safety and efficacy, Stage 1 subjects will

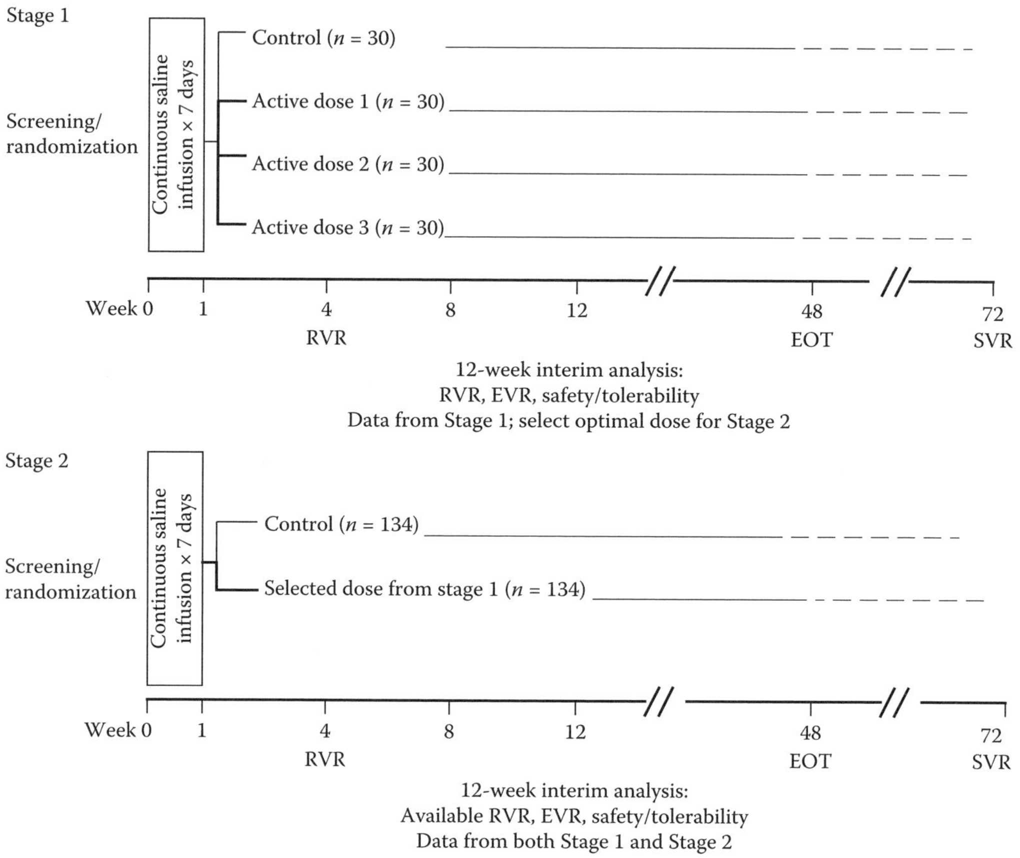

FIGURE 1.1 Diagram of study design.

continue with their randomization assignments for the full planned 48 weeks of therapy, with a final follow up evaluation at study week 72. Stage 2 will be a noninferiority comparison of a selected dose and the same PegIntron active-control regimen used in stage 1, both again given with oral ribavirin, for up to 48 weeks of therapy, with a final follow-up evaluation at study week 72. A second interim analysis of all available safety/tolerability, outcomes, and efficacy data from Stage 1 to Stage 2 will be performed when all Stage 2 subjects have completed study week 12. Depending upon individual response data for safety and efficacy, stage 2 subjects will receive the full planned 48 weeks of treatment, with final follow-up at study week 72.

For power analysis for sample size estimation, a total study enrollment of 388 subjects will be required (120 subjects or 30 subjects per arm for Stage 1 and 268 subjects or 134 subjects per arm for Stage 2) to account for a probable dropout rate of 15% as well as two planned interim analyses using the O'Brien—Fleming method. Stage 1 will enroll a total of 120 subjects divided equally among the four treatment arms to gather sufficient data to select an active dose of the test treatment to proceed to testing in stage 2. Stage 2 will enroll an additional cohort of 268 subjects divided equally between its two treatment arms to provide a sufficient number of subjects to evaluate noninferiority of continuous interferon delivery to standard-of-care interferon therapy, for an overall total of 306 subjects enrolled in Stage 1 and Stage 2 combined. Therefore, accounting for 15% attrition in each stage, we expect that 164 subjects from the selected dose arms (30 from Stage 1 plus 134 additional subjects enrolled in Stage 2) and 164 subjects from the PegIntron active-control arms (30 from Stage 1 plus an additional 134 subjects enrolled in Stage 2) will need to be enrolled to meet the study objective of achieving an

80% power for establishing noninferiority (with a noninferiority margin of 15%) at the overall Type I error rate of 5%.

Note that the above two-stage seamless trial design is a combination of group sequential design, drop-the-losers design, and seamless adaptive Phase I/II design utilizing precision analysis (i.e., confidence interval approach) for decision making on dose selection at the first stage. If we apply adaptive randomization for the second stage, the study design would be even more complicated. From a regulatory point of view, it is important to ensure that (i) no operational biases are introduced during the conduct of the trial, and (ii) the overall type I error rate is well controlled at the 5% level, when utilizing adaptive design methods in clinical trials.

Example 5: Targeted Clinical Trials—Biomarker-Adaptive Trial Design

This design is often considered for identifying patients who are most likely to respond to the test treatment under study through some validated diagnostic tests of biomarkers such as genomic markers. This process is referred to as the enrichment process in clinical trials, which has led to the concept of targeted clinical trials (Liu and Chow 2008). As indicated by many researchers (e.g., Simon and Maitournam 2004; Maitournam and Simon 2005; Varmus 2006; Dalton and Friend 2006; Casciano and Woodcock 2006), the disease targets at the molecular level can be identified after completion of the Human Genome Project (HGP). As a result, the importance of diagnostic tests for identification of molecular targets increases as more targeted clinical trials will be conducted for the individualized treatment of patients (*personalized medicine*). For example, based on the risk of distant recurrence determined by a 21-gene Oncotype DXf0d2 breast cancer assay, patients with a recurrence score of 11–25 in the Trial Assigning Individualized Options for Treatment (TAILORx) trial sponsored by the United States National Cancer Institute (NCI) are randomly assigned to receive either adjuvant chemotherapy and hormonal therapy or adjuvant hormonal therapy alone (Sprarano et al. 2006).

Despite different technical platforms employed in the diagnostic devices for molecular targets used in the trial, the assay falls in the category of the *in vitro* diagnostic multivariate index assays (IVDMIA; FDA 2006) based on the selected differentially expressed genes for detection of the patients with the molecular targets. In addition, to reduce the variation, the IVDMIAs do not usually use all genes during the development stage. Therefore, identification of the differentially expressed genes between different groups of patients is the key to the accuracy and reliability of the devices for molecular targets. Once the differentially expressed are identified, the next task is to search for an optimal representation or algorithm that provides the best discrimination ability between the patients with molecular targets and those without the targets. The current validation procedure for diagnostic device is for the assay based on one analyte. However, the IVDMIAs are, in fact, the parallel assays based on the intensities of multiple analytes. As a result, the current approach to assay validation for one analyte may not be appropriate or inadequate for validation of IVDMIAs.

With respect to the enrichment design for the targeted clinical trials, patients with positive diagnosis for the molecular targets are randomized to receive the test drug or the control. However, because no IVDMIA can provide the perfectly correct diagnosis, some patients with positive diagnosis may not actually have the molecular targets. Consequently, the treatment effect of the test drug for the patients with targets is underestimated. On the other hand, estimation of the treatment effect based on the data from the targeted clinical trials needs to take into consideration the variability associated with the estimates of accuracy of the IVDMIA, such as positive-predictive value and false-positive rates obtained from the clinical effectiveness trials of the IVDMIA.

In general, there are three classes of targeted clinical trials. The first type is to evaluate the efficacy and safety of targeted treatment for the patients with molecular targets. Herceptin clinical trials belong to this class. The second type of targeted clinical trials is to select the best treatment regimen for the patients based on the results of some tests for prognosis of clinical outcomes. The last type of the targeted clinical trials is to investigate the correlation of the treatment effect with variations of the molecular targets. Because the objectives of different targeted clinical trials are different, the

FDA Drug-Diagnostic Co-Development Concept Paper (FDA 2005) proposed three different designs to meet different objectives of targeted clinical trials. These three designs are given in Figures 1.2 through 1.4.

Design A is the enrichment design (Chow and Liu 2004) in which the only patients tested positively for identification of molecular targets are randomized either to receive the test drug or the concurrent control. The enrichment design is usually employed when there is a high degree of certainty that the drug response occurs only in the patients tested positively for the molecular targets and the mechanism of pathological pathways is clearly understood. Most of the Herceptin phase III clinical trials used the enrichment design. However, as pointed out in the FDA Concept Paper, the description of test sensitivity and specificity will not be possible using this type of design without drug and placebo data in the patients testing negative for the molecular targets. Design B is a stratified, randomized design and stratification factor is the results of the test for the molecular targets. In other words, the patients are stratified into two groups depending upon whether the diagnostic test is either positive or negative. Then a separate randomization is independently performed within each group to receive the test drug or concurrent control. The information of the test results for the molecular targets in Design C is primarily used as a covariate and is not involved with randomization. Sometimes, only a part of the patients are tested for the molecular targets. Design C is useful when the association of the treatment effect of the drug with the results of the diagnostic test needs to be further explored.

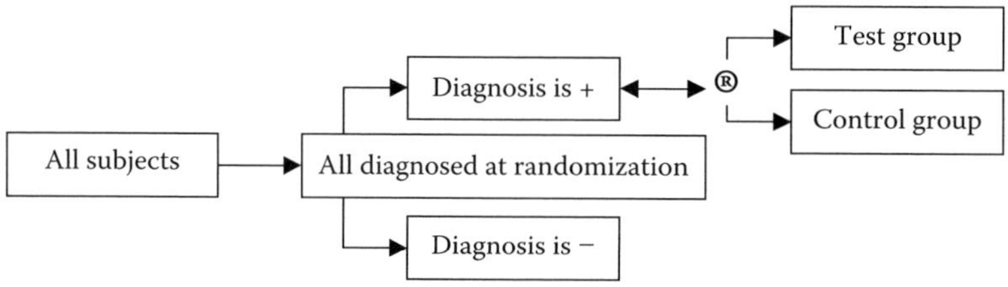

FIGURE 1.2 Design A for targeted clinical trials.

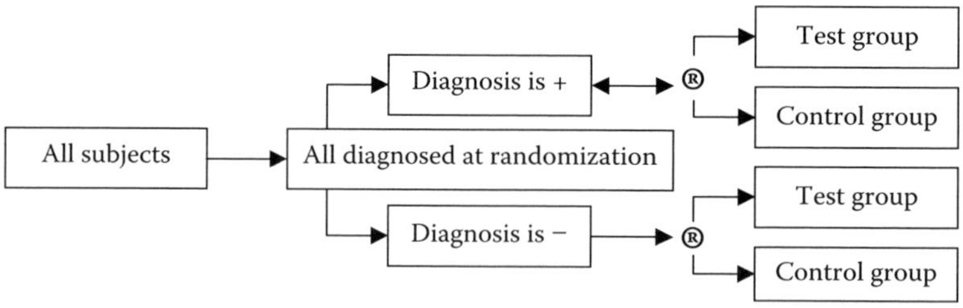

FIGURE 1.3 Design B for targeted clinical trials.

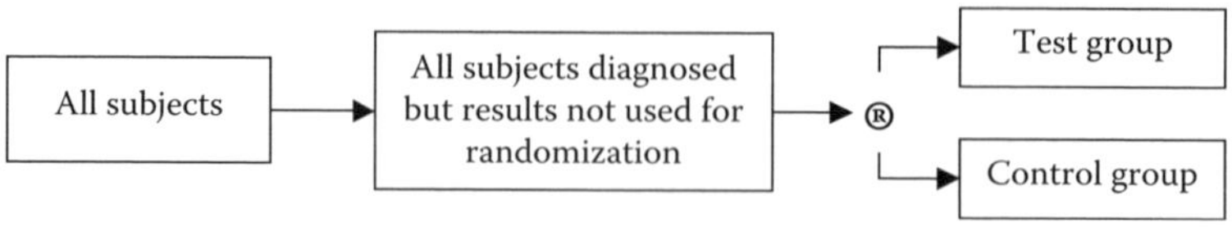

FIGURE 1.4 Design C for targeted clinical trials.

1.5 Strategies for Clinical Development

1.5.1 Adaptive Design Strategies

Clinical development of a new drug product is a lengthy and costly process, which includes phases I to III clinical development (prior to regulatory review and approval) and phase IV clinical development (postapproval). For life-threatening diseases or diseases with unmet medical need (rare diseases), this lengthy clinical development process is not acceptable. Thus, the use of adaptive design methods in clinical trials is called for. The purpose is to shorten the development process (speed) without compromising the safety and efficacy of the drug product under investigation (validity) by maximizing the power for identifying the best clinical benefit of drug products under investigation with a limited number of subjects (efficacy). As a result, many adaptive design methods are developed for archiving the ultimate goals of validity, efficiency, and speed in clinical development. However, in practice it should be noted that many other important factors beyond statistical components may have an impact on the development process. These factors include, but are not limited to, patient enrollment, treatment durations, and time required for regulatory review/approval.

Commonly considered strategies for the use of adaptive design methods in clinical development include, but are not limited to, adaptive dose finding, adaptive seamless Phase I/II in early clinical development, and adaptive seamless Phase II/III in late phase clinical development. These strategies help in not only shortening the development time in a more efficient way but also increasing the probability of success in clinical development. As an example, let us consider the development of a new drug product for a rare disease of MM with unmet medical need. A traditional approach is to conduct a typical Phase I study for identifying the MTD, which is often considered as the optimal dose for the late phase of clinical development. In practice, there are several options that we can run for this study with several doses or dose schedules. For example, this trial can be run with parallel dose groups or sequentially with the test drug as a single or add-on agent. The traditional approach will not be able to provide the entire spectrum of the dose response of the test drug. On the other hand, if we consider an adaptive approach, it allows us to use more options at the beginning and drop some of the arms (options) if they are either too toxic or ineffective (activity too low or requires very high dose that makes the treatment very costly—biologic product may be very costly). In addition, since the treatment arms are often correlated, the information such as DLT from different arms can be synchronized using methods such as Bayesian hierarchical model (see, e.g., Chang and Chow 2005).

Similar approaches can be used for Phase II trials, Phase I/II, or Phase II/III seamless design. In this approach, the interim endpoint may be a marker such as response rate or time to disease progression. Some of the inferior arms can be dropped at interim. If some of the arms are promising, we can apply different randomization schemes to assign more patients to the superior arms (play-the-winner). In this case, not only will the total cost not increase, but also we will increase the chance of success because the increase of sample size for the superior treatment arms are most promising. In addition, the schedules for the trial are similar because the total number of patients remains unchanged. This adaptive design strategy can be applied to Phase III trials, but with much less arms. For Phase IV studies, the adaptive design can also be applied. However, the situation is different because the drug has been approved during the Phase IV clinical development. The focus of Phase IV clinical development will be on safety rather than on efficacy.

1.5.2 Controversial Issues

As indicated earlier, although the use of adaptive design methods in clinical trials is motivated by its flexibility and efficiency, many researchers are not convinced and still challenge its validity and integrity (Tsiatis and Mehta 2003). As a result, many discussions are around the flexibility, efficiency, validity, and integrity. When implementing an adaptive design in a clinical trial, Li (2006) suggests a couple of principles: adaptation should not alter trial conduct, and type I error should be preserved and must be followed when implementing the adaptive design methods in clinical trials. Following these principles, some basic considerations such as dose/dose regimen, study endpoints, treatment duration, and logistics should be carefully evaluated for feasibility (Quinlan, Gallo, and Krams 2006). To maintain the validity and integrity of an adaptive design with complicated adaptations, it is strongly suggested that an independent data monitoring committee (IDMC) should be established. In practice, IDMC has been widely used in group sequential design with adaptations of stopping a trial early and sample size reestimation. The role and responsibility of an IDMC for a clinical trial using adaptive design should be clearly defined. IDMC usually convey very limited information to investigators or sponsors about treatment effects, procedural conventions, and statistical methods with recommendations in order to maintain the validity and integrity of the study.

When applying adaptive design methods in clinical trials, it is suggested that the feasibility of certain adaptations such as changes in study endpoints/hypotheses be carefully evaluated to prevent any possible misuse and abuse of the adaptive design methods. For a complicated multiple adaptive design, it is strongly recommended that an IDMC established to ensure the integrity of the study. It should also be noted that clinical trial simulation does provide *a* solution not *the* solution for a complicated multiple adaptive design. In practice, "how to validate the assumed predictive model for clinical trial simulation?" is a major challenge to both investigators and biostatisticians.

As the result of the 2006 FDA/PhRMA (Gallo et al. 2006) Workshop on adaptive design held in Washington DC, the FDA has decided to slow the escalating momentum behind adaptive clinical trial designs to allow time to craft better working definitions of the new models and build a better base before moving forward. As a result, it is suggested that effort should be directed to current issues such as the impact of protocol amendments, challenges in by design adaptations, and obstacles of retrospective adaptations as described in the previous sections. Note that a draft guidance entitled Guidance for Industry—Adaptive Design Clinical Trials for Drugs and Biologics has been developed and is currently being distributed for comments (FDA, 2010). In this draft guidance, the FDA classifies adaptive designs as either *well understood designs* or *less well understood designs* depending upon the nature of adaptations either blinded or unblinded. In practice, however, most of the adaptive designs considered are less well understood designs. As a result, one of the major challenges is the development of appropriate statistical methods under the less well understood designs for valid statistical inference of the test treatment under investigation. This needs further research.

In summary, from a clinical point of view, adaptive design methods reflect real clinical practice in clinical development. Adaptive design methods are very attractive due to their flexibility and are very useful especially in early clinical development. From a statistical point of view, the use of adaptive methods in clinical trials makes current good statistics practice even more complicated. The validity for the use of adaptive design methods is not well established and fully understood. The impact of statistical inference on treatment effect should be carefully evaluated under the framework of moving target patient population as the result of protocol amendments. In practice, regulatory agencies may not realize that the adaptive design methods for review and approval of regulatory submissions have been employed for years without any scientific basis. Guidelines regarding the use of adaptive design methods must be advanced so that appropriate statistical methods and statistical software packages can be developed accordingly.

References

Atkinson, A. C., and Donev, A. N. (1992). *Optimum Experimental Designs*. New York: Oxford University Press.

Bauer, P., and Kieser, M. (1999). Combining different phases in development of medical treatments within a single trial. *Statistics in Medicine*, 18:1833–48.

Bauer, P., and Rohmel, J. (1995). An adaptive method for establishing a dose-response relationship. *Statistics in Medicine*, 14:1595–1607.

Brannath, W., Koening, F., and Bauer, P. (2003). Improved repeated confidence bounds in trials with a maximal goal. *Biometrical Journal*, 45:311–24.

Branson, M., and Whitehead, W. (2002). Estimating a treatment effect in survival studies in which patients switch treatment. *Statistics in Medicine*, 21:2449–63.

Casciano, D. A., and Woodcock, J. (2006). Empowering microarrays in the regulatory setting. *Nature Biotechnology*, 24:1103.

Chang, M. (2007a). *Adaptive Design Theory and Implementation Using SAS and R*. New York: Chapman and Hall/CRC Press, Taylor & Francis.

Chang, M. (2007b). Adaptive design method based on sum of p-values. *Statistics in Medicine,* 26:2772–84.

Chang, M., and Chow, S. C. (2005). A hybrid Bayesian adaptive design for dose response trials. *Journal of Biopharmaceutical Statistics*, 15:667–91.

Charkravarty, A. (2005). Regulatory aspects in using surrogate markers in clinical trials. In *The Evaluation of Surrogate Endpoint,* eds. T. Burzykowski, G. Molenberghs, and M. Buyse. New York: Springer.

Chow, S. C., and Chang, M. (2006). *Adaptive Design Methods in Clinical Trials*. New York: Chapman and Hall/CRC Press, Taylor & Francis.

Chow, S. C., and Chang, M. (2008). Adaptive design methods in clinical trials—A review. *Orphanet Journal of Rare Diseases*, 3:1–13.

Chow, S. C., Chang, M., and Pong, A. (2005). Statistical consideration of adaptive methods in clinical development. *Journal of Biopharmaceutical Statistics*, 15:575–91.

Chow, S. C., and Liu, J. P. (2004). *Design and Analysis of Clinical Trials,* 2nd ed. New York: John Wiley & Sons.

Chow, S. C., Lu, Q., and Tse, S. K. (2007). Statistical analysis for two-stage adaptive design with different study points. *Journal of Biopharmaceutical Statistics*, 17:1163–76.

Chow, S. C., and Shao, J. (2005). Inference for clinical trials with some protocol amendments. *Journal of Biopharmaceutical Statistics*, 15:659–66.

Chow, S. C., and Shao, J. (2006). On margin and statistical test for noninferiority in active control trials. *Statistics in Medicine,* 25:1101–13.

Chow, S. C., Shao, J., and Wang, H. (2007). *Sample Size Calculation in Clinical Research,* 2nd ed. New York: Chapman and Hall/CRC Press, Taylor & Francis.

Chow, S. C., and Tu, Y. H. (2008). On two-stage seamless adaptive design in clinical trials. *Journal of Formosan Medical Association*, 107(2):S51–S59.

Chung-Stein, C., Anderson, K., Gallo, P., and Collins, S. (2006). Sample size reestimation: A review and recommendations. *Drug Information Journal*, 40:475–84.

Cui. L., Hung, H. M. J., and Wang, S. J. (1999). Modification of sample size in group sequential trials. *Biometrics*, 55:853–57.

Dalton, W. S., and Friend, S. H. (2006). Cancer biomarkers—An invitation to the table. *Science,* 312:1165–68.

Efron, B. (1971). Forcing a sequential experiment to be balanced. *Biometrika*, 58:403–17.

EMEA. (2002). Point to Consider on *Methodological Issues in Confirmatory Clinical Trials with Flexible Design and Analysis Plan*. The European Agency for the Evaluation of Medicinal Products Evaluation of Medicines for Human Use. CPMP/EWP/2459/02, London, UK.

EMEA. (2006). Reflection paper on *Methodological Issues in Confirmatory Clinical Trials with Flexible Design and Analysis Plan*. The European Agency for the Evaluation of Medicinal Products Evaluation of Medicines for Human Use. CPMP/EWP/2459/02, London, UK.

FDA. (2005). Draft concept paper on *Drug-Diagnostic Co-Development.* Rockville, MD: The U.S. Food and Drug Administration.

FDA. (2006). Draft Guidance on *In Vitro Diagnostic Multivariate Index Assays*. Rockville, MD: The U.S. Food and Drug Administration.

FDA. (2010). Guidance for *Industry—Adaptive Design Clinical Trials for Drugs and Biologics*. Rockville, MD: The U.S. Food and Drug Administration.

Feng, H., Shao, J., and Chow, S. C. (2007). Group sequential test for clinical trials with moving patient population. *Journal of Biopharmaceutical Statistics*, 17:1227–38.

Friede, T., and Kieser, M. (2004). Sample size recalculation for binary data in internal pilot study designs. *Pharmaceutical Statistics*, 3:269–79.

Gallo, P., Chuang-Stein, C., Dragalin, V., Gaydos, B., Krams, M., and Pinheiro, J. (2006). Adaptive design in clinical drug development—An executive summary of the PhRMA Working Group (with discussions). *Journal of Biopharmaceutical Statistics*, 16 (3): 275–83.

Hardwick, J. P., and Stout, Q. F. (2002). Optimal few-stage designs. *Journal of Statistical Planning and Inference*, 104:121–45.

Hommel, G. (2001). Adaptive modifications of hypotheses after an interim analysis. *Biometrical Journal*, 43:581–89.

ICH. (1994). International conference on harmonization tripartite guideline E4: Guideline on *Dose-Response Information to Support Drug Registration*. Rockville, MD: The U.S. Food & Drug Administration.

ICH. (2000). International Conference on Harmonization Guideline E10: Guidance on *Choice of Control Group and Related Design and Conduct Issues in Clinical Trials*. Rockville, MD: The U.S. Food and Drug Administration.

Jennison, C., and Turnbull, B. W. (2000). *Group Sequential Methods with Applications to Clinical Trials*. New York: Chapman and Hall.

Jennison, C., and Turnbull, B. W. (2005). Meta-analysis and adaptive group sequential design in the clinical development process. *Journal of Biopharmaceutical Statistics*, 15:537–58.

Kelly, P. J., Stallard, N., and Todd, S. (2005). An adaptive group sequential design for phase II/III clinical trials that select a single treatment from several. *Journal of Biopharmaceutical Statistics*, 15:641–58.

Lachin, J. M. (1988). Statistical properties of randomization in clinical trials. *Controlled Clinical Trials*, 9:289–311.

Lan, K. K. G., and DeMets, D. L. (1987). Group sequential procedures: Calendar versus information time. *Statistics in Medicine*, 8:1191–98.

Lehmacher, W., and Wassmer, G. (1999). Adaptive sample size calculations in group sequential trials. *Biometrics*, 55:1286–90

Li, N. (2006). Adaptive trial design—FDA statistical reviewer's view. *Presented at the CRT2006 Workshop with the FDA*, Arlington, Virginia, April 4, 2006.

Liu, J. P., and Chow, S. C. (2008). Statistical issues on the diagnostics multivariate index assay for targeted clinical trials. *Journal of Biopharmaceutical Statistics*, 18:167–82.

Liu, Q., and Chi, G. Y. H. (2001). On sample size and inference for two-stage adaptive designs. *Biometrics*, 57:172–77.

Liu, Q., Proschan, M. A., and Pledger, G. W. (2002). A unified theory of two-stage adaptive designs. *Journal of American Statistical Association*, 97:1034–41.

Maca, J., Bhattacharya, S., Dragalin, V., Gallo, P., and Krams, M. (2006). Adaptive seamless phase II/III designs—Background, operational aspects, and examples. *Drug Information Journal*, 40:463–74.

Maitournam, A., and Simon, R. (2005). On the efficiency of targeted clinical trials. *Statistics in Medicine*, 24:329–39.

Mugno, R., Zhus, W., and Rosenberger, W. F. (2004). Adaptive urn designs for estimating several percentiles of a dose response curve. *Statistics in Medicine*, 23:2137–50.

O'Quigley, J., Pepe, M., and Fisher, L. (1990). Continual reassessment method: A practical design for phase I clinical trial in cancer. *Biometrics*, 46:33–48.

O'Quigley, J., and Shen, L. (1996). Continual reassessment method: A likelihood approach. *Biometrics*, 52:673–84.

Posch, M., and Bauer, P. (1999). Adaptive two stage designs and the conditional error function. *Biometrical Journal*, 41:689–96.

Posch, M., Konig, F., Brannath, W., Dunger-Baldauf, C., and Bauer, P. (2005). Testing and estimation in flexible group sequential designs with adaptive treatment selection. *Statistics in Medicine*, 24:3697–3714.

Proschan, M. A., and Hunsberger, S. A. (1995). Designed extension of studies based on conditional power. *Biometrics*, 51:1315–24.

Quinlan, J. A., Gallo, P., and Krams, M. (2006). Implementing adaptive designs: Logistical and operational consideration. *Drug Information Journal*, 40:437–44.

Rosenberger, W. F., and Lachin, J. (2002). *Randomization in Clinical Trials*. New York: John Wiley and Sons.

Rosenberger, W. F., Stallard, N., Ivanova, A., Harper, C. N., and Ricks, M. L. (2001). Optimal adaptive designs for binary response trials. *Biometrics*, 57:909–13.

Sampson, A. R., and Sill, M. W. (2005). Drop-the-loser design: Normal case (with discussions). *Biometrical Journal*, 47:257–81.

Shao, J., Chang, M., and Chow, S. C. (2005). Statistical inference for cancer trials with treatment switching. *Statistics in Medicine*, 24:1783–90.

Simon, R., and Maitournam, A. (2004). Evaluating the efficiency of targeted designs for randomized clinical trials. *Clinical Cancer Research*, 10:6759–63.

Sprarano, J., Hayes, D., Dees, E., et al. (2006). Phase III randomized study of adjuvant combination chemotherapy and hormonal therapy vs. adjuvant hormonal therapy alone in women with previously resected axillary node-negative breast cancer with various levels of risk for recurrence (TAILORX Trial). http://www.cancer.gov/clinicaltrials/ECOG- PACCT-1. Accessed on June 5 2006.

Tsiatis, A. A., and Mehta, C. (2003). On the inefficiency of the adaptive design for monitoring clinical trials. *Biometrika*, 90:367–78.

Varmus, H. (2006). The new era in cancer research. *Science*, 312:1162–65.

Wang, S. J., O'Neill, R. T., and Hung, H. M. J. (2007). Approaches to evaluation of treatment effect in randomized clinical trials with genomic subset. *Pharmaceutical Statistics*, 6:227–44.

Wang, S. K., and Tsiatis, A. A. (1987). Approximately optimal one-parameter boundaries for a sequential trials. *Biometrics*, 43:193–200.

Wei, L. J. (1978). The adaptive biased-coin design for sequential experiments. *Annal of Statistics*, 9:92–100.

Whitehead, J. (1997). Bayesian decision procedures with application to dose-finding studies. *International Journal of Pharmaceutical Medicine,* 11:201–8.

Woodcock, J. (2005). DFA introduction comments: Clinical studies design and evaluation issues. *Clinical Trials*, 2:273–75.

Zhang, W., Sargent, D. J., and Mandrekar, S. (2006). An adaptive dose-finding design incorporating both toxicity and efficacy. *Statistics in Medicine*, 25:2365–83.

2

Fundamental Theory of Adaptive Designs with Unplanned Design Change in Clinical Trials with Blinded Data

Qing Liu and
George Y. H. Chi
J&J Global Development Organization

2.1 Background

Despite the tremendous progress and wide publicity of adaptive designs, many clinical trial planners avoid their prospective applications. There are a variety of reasons. The urban legend has always been that regulatory agencies discourage adaptive designs. In our observations of the pharmaceutical industry, we see two undocumented reasons. First and foremost, many trial planners are satisfied with the status quo of simple designs, which, in the eyes of many, represent a conservative approach. However, what is considered to be a "safe" approach often brings risks to patients, trial success, as well as financial sustainability of the sponsor. Ultimately, this leads to a high-attrition rate for drug development or deprives patients of the needed treatment early. The second reason is trial planners' over confidence, or lacking knowledge of the various explicit or implicit assumptions made for the trial design. In reality, clinical trials do not always operate according to overly optimistic assumptions made, but rather they are negatively impacted by circumstances that are often beyond the control of trial planners.

Whatever the actual stated or otherwise implied reasons are, trial planners are often confronted with external or trial related realities that force them to take corrective actions to modify on-going trials. Such actions seem supported by various regulatory documents (Section 2.4). For example, a recent U.S. Food and Drug Administration (FDA) guidance (2006) claims:

> When a DMC [data monitoring committee] is the only group reviewing unblinded interim data, trial organizers faced with compelling new information external to the trial may consider making changes in the ongoing trial without raising concerns that such changes might have been at least

> partly motivated by knowledge of the interim data and thereby endanger trial integrity. Sometimes accumulating data from within the trial (e.g., overall event rates) may suggest the need for modifications. (p. 5)

Motivated by an actual trial requiring a design change, a regulatory reviewer, who may be skeptical of such a sweeping claim, requested a sponsor to justify the design change to ensure a valid statistical inference. An extensive literature search fails to yield yet a single statistical article that broadly establishes the validity of the claim by the FDA guidance (2006).

In this article, we are concerned with comparative clinical trials where only blinded accumulating data are accessible to trial planners. The accumulating blinded data are closely monitored for checking the appropriateness of certain assumptions used in the original design. This process may trigger a design change. For this broad setting, we develop in Section 2.2 a general conditional theory to justify that an on-going trial can be executed later by a different design. In the Section 2.3, we provide an application to illustrate the conditional theory. In the Section 2.4, we lay out additional areas of research. We also point out various pitfalls that render any theoretical justification useless when blinding is compromised.

2.2 Conditional Theory

Blinded data reviews are often vaguely described, and subsequent design modifications are unplanned. It is difficult to know in advance those assumptions that may be inappropriate. Rather, the problem is often identified by experienced trial personnel once the accumulating data are properly reviewed. When the decision is made to ignore the problem, the trial proceeds according to the original design; otherwise, the design is modified to address only the problem at hand. To reflect this process adequately, we consider a general measure-theoretic framework, similar to the one used by Liu, Proschan, and Pledger (2002), and develop a conditional theory following the well-accepted *conditionality principle* (Cox and Hinkley, p. 38, 1974).

Let $(\Omega, \mathcal{F}, P)$ be a probability space. The blinded data are denoted by a sub-σ field $\mathcal{B}$ in $\mathcal{F}$. To incorporate settings where on-going trials are modified on the basis of external reasons, we further expand $\mathcal{B}$ to include all possible information external to the trial that may lead to design modifications. The process of blinded data reviews and subsequent design modifications implicitly defines a blinded adaptation rule τ by which a modified design is selected from potentially many designs upon a realization of the blinded data. It is assumed that the blinded adaptation rule τ is $\mathcal{B}$ measurable with a countable range, which is denoted by D. Following Liu, Proschan, and Pledger (2002), the measurability and countability assumptions are necessary on theoretical grounds to avoid pathological difficulties. For practical applications, these two assumptions impose absolutely no limit for τ to rule out any potential design modifications.

While this general formulation for design modifications is necessary to reflect the unplanned nature of the process, it could cause potential difficulties for inference. Following the *repeated sampling principle* (Cox and Hinkley, p. 45, 1974), the validity of an inference procedure is to be assessed in a long run of hypothetical replications. Thus an overall behavior, such as the type 1 error rate, of an inference procedure must take into account not only what has happened to the current trial but also what could have happened had the trial been repeated. For the problem at hand, only the decision of design modifications is known for the observed blinded data set, and the decisions for different realizations of the blinded data may not be known. The potential difficulties can be avoided following the *conditionality principle*, by which statistical analysis and interpretation of the results are made according to only the actual experiment conducted. To ensure that the type 1 error rate is controlled when evaluated in a long run of hypothetical replications, we require that a valid conditional inference is always performed for the actual experiment, regardless of the changes made. To develop this idea, let P_0 be a null probability measure, and we consider specifically the problem of testing against the null hypothesis H: $P = P_0$ in favor of some alternative hypothesis of interest. The conditional theory can be described in three hierarchical steps.

The first step starts with the basic formulation of the σ-field $\mathcal{B}$ and the blinded adaptation rule τ. For any design d in D, let $\mathcal{G}_d$ be a sub-σ field such that $\mathcal{B} \subset \mathcal{G}_d \subset \mathcal{F}$ and $\mathcal{G}_d \neq \mathcal{F}$. If the design d specifies a formal unblinded interim analysis, $\mathcal{G}_d$ is the σ field for the unblinded interim data; otherwise, $\mathcal{G}_d = \mathcal{B}$. Note that $\mathcal{G}_d = \mathcal{F}$ is not allowed as it would lead to post hoc analysis.

The second step consists of a conditional error function C_d and an unblinded adaptation rule ξ_d, which are defined over the sub-σ field $\mathcal{G}_d$. The conditional error function C_d is a $\mathcal{G}_d$ measurable real valued function such that $0 \leq C_d \leq 1$ and

$$E_H(C_d \,||\, \mathcal{B}) \leq \alpha, \tag{2.1}$$

where $\alpha \in (0, 1)$ is a given type 1 error rate common to all designs $d \in D$. The notation $E_H(\cdot||\mathcal{B})$ denotes the conditional expectation given $\mathcal{B}$ with respect to the probability measure P_0. Similar notations are used later without further clarifications. The unblinded adaptation rule ξ_d is $\mathcal{G}_d$ measurable with a countable range M_d. Similar to Liu, Proschan, and Pledger (2002), the unblinded adaptation rule ξ_d for $\tau = d$ selects further design modifications based on the unblinded interim data.

In the third step, a conditional test $T_{[d,m]}$ is specified for each $m \in M_d$, where m represents a set of further design modifications by ξ_d. The conditional test $T_{[d,m]}$ is a $\mathcal{F}$ measurable binary function, taking the value 1 for rejecting the null hypothesis H or the value 0 for not rejecting the null hypothesis H. It is required that

$$E_H(T_{[d,m]} \,||\, \mathcal{G}_d) \leq C_d. \tag{2.2}$$

That is, the size of the conditional test $T_{[d,m]}$ given $\mathcal{G}_d$ is not more than C_d. The theorem below establishes the validity of the conditional theory.

Theorem

i. *For any $d \in D$, let $T_{[d,\xi_d]} = \sum_{m \in M_d} I_{\{\xi_d = m\}} T_{[d,m]}$. Then $E_H(T_{[d,\xi_d]} \,||\, \mathcal{G}_d) \leq C_d$, and $E_H(T_{[d,\xi_d]} \,||\, \mathcal{B}) \leq \alpha$.*
ii. *Let $T_{[\tau,\xi_\tau]} = \sum_{d \in D} I_{\{\tau = d\}} T_{[d,\xi_d]}$. Then $E_H(T_{[\tau,\xi_\tau]} \,||\, \mathcal{B}) \leq \alpha$, and furthermore $E_H(T_{[\tau,\xi_\tau]}) \leq \alpha$.*

The proof of the theorem is given in the appendix.

It is worth noting that the conditional theory covers the adaptive design framework of Liu, Proschan, and Pledger (2002), for which $\mathcal{B}$ is simply the smallest σ field containing the sample space Ω and the empty set, and τ only select the prespecified adaptive design. While all existing adaptive designs based on combination tests in the literature are justified by the theory of Liu, Proschan, and Pledger (2002), the expansion of the theory presented in this article expands the scope of adaptive designs to include any traditional designs with blinded data access. In Liu, Proschan, and Pledger (2002), a sub-σ field of interim data and a prespecified conditional error function, but not the design changes that may be performed for different realizations of the interim data, are required to be specified in advance. With the expanded conditional theory, it almost seems that nothing regarding trial modifications needs to be specified. However, this is only true when a traditional trial design has already employed a conditional test procedure. We illustrate this in the next two sections.

2.3 Application

2.3.1 Trial Description

In this article, we are interested in the general setting where both blinded and unblinded data are used for trial modifications. The application is motivated by an actual trial. However, the description below as well as the numerical values used are totally fictional to create a more interesting illustration of the conditional theory; they do not reflect the actual design and conduct of the trial. In addition, the suggested possibility for increasing the total number of events and an additional interim analysis is not the decision made for the actual trial that is on-going at the time this article is written.

Consider a double-blind placebo-controlled phase 3 trial to demonstrate that a single daily dose of a new drug can reduce or delay the occurrence of events related to worsening of a disease condition. The trial was originally planned to perform a single test of treatment effect after the total number of events, say, 500, is reached. A total of 800 patients were enrolled. Based on default assumptions used by a computer software, it is projected that 500 events would be reached by October 31, 2008. The protocol specifies that the primary endpoint is the time to the occurrence of the event of interest. Patients who have not had the event by the time of reaching 500 events are censored. The log-rank test is specified in the protocol.

The trial started on January 15, 2007. Initial patient accrual was slow but 3 months later the accrual rate caught up with the original plan. The accrual target of 800 patients was reached on February 14, 2008, at the time the total number of events were 250. Around the time of closing patient accrual, there was a concern that the total 500 events may not be achievable by October 31, 2008. By September 7, 2008, only an additional 35 events were added. According to a plot of the Kaplan–Meyer curve of the blinded event times, it was projected that it would take another 2 years to reach the target of 500 events. This would be an unacceptable delay not only for completing the on-going trial but also for initiating subsequent trials of the clinical development program. Facing these difficulties, a consensus was reached by September 17, 2008 to perform a formal interim analysis with the number of events achieved by October 31, 2008. If an early efficacy boundary is crossed, the trial stops; otherwise, the trial continues with an additional 300 patients. A decision was also made to allow the appointed data monitoring committee (DMC) to decide at the interim analysis if the total number of events would be increased or an additional interim analysis would be performed.

2.3.2 Statistical Considerations

To implement these ideas, further statistical details are necessary. The sub-σ field $\mathcal{B}$ represents blinded data consisting of the blinded event times, which can be censored by noninformative calendar times. To specify a conditional error function, C_d, which satisfies the inequality in Equation 2.1, start with an efficacy boundary function so that the trial can stop early if the boundary is crossed by the log-rank statistic. There are additional statistical considerations for selecting the efficacy boundary function. First, the project statistician states that the effect size used to derive the total of 500 events is more conservative than what is expected, and therefore, would like to consider boundary function that is between the Pocock and O'Brien-Fleming boundary functions. The second consideration is the addition of a second formal interim analysis. This provides the DMC the flexibility to stop the trial at the second interim analysis if the boundary value at the first interim analysis is not, but almost, crossed. Even if the primary endpoint crosses the boundary at the first interim analysis, the trial may still continue for considerations of either secondary efficacy or safety endpoints (Liu and Anderson 2008). The third consideration is to avoid inferential difficulties of the Kim-DeMets family of *α-spending functions* $\{\alpha t^{\rho}: 0 < \alpha < 1, \rho > 0\}$, where $t \in [0, 1]$ represents information fractions. Specifically, the Kim-DeMets family does not permit a full ordering of the sample space, resulting sequential *p*-value values 1 for negative test statistics that are far away from $-\infty$ (Liu and Anderson 2008). These three considerations naturally lead to the choice of the Wang–Tsiatis family of *boundary functions* $\{A_d(\alpha)t^{\rho-1/2}: 0 < \alpha < 1, -\infty < \rho < \infty\}$, where $A_d(\alpha)$ is a constant for given d and α. It is well known that for $\rho = 1/2$, the Wang-Tsiatis family reduces to the Pocock family $\{A_d(\alpha): 0 < \alpha < 1\}$, and for $\rho = 0$, the O'Brien-Fleming family $\{A_d(\alpha)t^{-1/2}: 0 < \alpha < 1\}$. For the on-going trial, $\rho = .15$ is chosen for the in-between boundary function.

The database cutoffs for the two interim analyses are scheduled for October 31, 2008 and June 14, 2009. The boundary values for the two interim analyses as well as the final analysis depend on the information fractions $0 < t_{1d} < t_{2d} < 1$ of the two calendar dates, which are determined on October 31, 2008 at the first interim analysis. Let n_d be the total number of events for the final analysis, which is adjusted upward from the original total event number of 500 to account for the two interim analysis added. A procedure for calculating n_d using blinded data is given in Section 2.3.3. Let n_{1d} be the total number of events observed on October 31, 2008, and $\tilde{n}_{2d}$ be the total number of events estimated for June 14, 2009 based on the cumulative blinded data available on October 31, 2008. Then the information fractions are $t_{1d} = n_{1d}/n_d$ and $t_{2d} = \tilde{n}_{2d}/n_d$. Once t_{1d} and t_{2d} are determined, the coefficient $A_d(\alpha)$ can be calculated according to Equation 2.1 of Liu and Anderson (2008) without binding to any futility boundaries. Once the group sequential test is fully specified, the conditional error function C_d is calculated by the method of Müller and Schäfer (2001). As the process does not involve unblinded data, the conditional error function C_d is $\mathcal{G}_d$ measurable, or simply put, depends only on the accumulating data available from the first interim analysis.

It is known from the literature that even for normally distributed data a blinded sample size adjustment procedure may inflate the type 1 error rates. The pertinent question is, for the conditional error function C_d derived for the log-rank test via blinded data event times, whether the inequality $E_H(C_d \,||\, \mathcal{B}) \leq \alpha$ given in Equation 2.1, which is required by the conditional theory, is truly satisfied. For further clarification, write $C_d = C_d(Z_{1d})$ where Z_{1d} is the log-rank statistic of the first interim analysis. Following Müller and Schäfer (2001) or Liu, Proschan, and Pledger (2002), a functional form $C(\cdot)$ that is identical to $C_d(\cdot)$ satisfies the condition $E_H\{C(Z)\} = \alpha$ if Z follows a standard normal distribution. Thus $E_H\{C_d(Z_{1d}) \,||\, \mathcal{B}\} = \alpha$ is true if the conditional distribution of Z_{1d} given $\mathcal{B}$ follows exactly the standard normal distribution. Fortunately, the log-rank statistic is derived from a well-known conditional method (i.e., the Mantel–Haenszel method), by which the margins of a sequence of 2×2 tables, including the total number of events in each table, are held as fixed to eliminate unknown hazard rates of the control group (Collett, pp. 40–43, 1994). The log-rank statistic follows asymptotically a standard normal distribution, conditional on the blinded event times. Thus, $E_H\{C_d(Z_{1d}) \,||\, \mathcal{B}\} = \alpha$ is true asymptotically. The fact that the equation may not be exactly true is not because of the blinded adaptation process, but rather due to the nature of asymptotic approximation. If it is required for $C_d(Z_{1d})$ to satisfy strictly the inequality in Equation 2.1, the randomization distribution of Z_{1d} can be obtained following the actual randomization procedure used for the trial (Liu, Li, and Boyett 1997; Rosenberger and Lachin, pp. 98–99, 2002), and then transformed by the inverse of the cumulative distribution function of a standard normal distribution so that the resulting distribution is stochastically not larger than a standard normal distribution. Finally, the requirement in Equation 2.2 is easily satisfied (either asymptotically or exactly) for the log-rank test following the theory of Liu, Proschan, and Pledger (2002).

2.3.3 Calculation of n_d

As the modified design has two interim analyses, the total number of events n_d need to be increased so that the resulting group sequential design would maintain a required power $1 - \beta$ at a given effect size, where β is a Type 2 error rate. We propose an iterative method for calculating n_d using only blinded event times. In addition to the Wang–Tsiatis boundary function $A_d(\alpha)t^{\rho-1/2}$ with $\rho = .15$, we also consider the Kim-DeMets β-spending function βt^{η} for some $\eta > 0$ for a nonbinding futility boundary.

For the initial value $n_d = 500$, calculate the information fractions $t_{1d} = n_{1d}/n_d$ and $t_{2d} = \tilde{n}_{2d}/n_d$, which are then used to update the total number of events n_d using the nonbinding approach described by Liu and Anderson (2008). This updated n_d is then used to repeat the above steps. After several iterations, n_d converges to a value. The choice of η needs to reflect the need for stopping the trial for futility. If the probability of success is fairly high for a new treatment to be effective, then a large η, leading to a conservative futility boundary, should be selected; otherwise, a η value yielding larger futility probabilities should be chosen.

2.4 Discussion

We propose a general conditional theory and rigorous proof by which it is possible to make unplanned design changes to an on-going trial that starts with a fixed information design. For trials with time-to-event endpoints, we illustrate how the conditional theory can be applied to the log-rank test. From experience, the approach described in the Section 2.3 fits in well with many event-time driven cancer or cardiovascular trials, for which the sponsor is properly blinded to treatment assignments. Similar arguments as those given in Section 2.3.2 can also be made for applications with binary endpoints where Fisher's exact test or the Mantel–Haenszel test is prespecified in the protocol. It seems though that this approach can be adopted widely to handle a fairly common practice of making design changes through "protocol amendments" based on blinded data reviews. After all, this practice is supported recently by the FDA guidance (2006), which is quoted in Section 2.1. Earlier the International Conference on Harmonization guidance (ICH E9, 1998) states:

> One type of monitoring concerns … checking the appropriateness of design assumptions, etc. This type of monitoring does not require access to information on comparative treatment effects, nor unblinding of data, and therefore has no impact on type I error. (p. 49591)

This practice is reinforced further by the more recent reflection paper (2007) issued by the Committee for Medicinal Products for Human Use (CHMP 2007):

> Whenever possible, methods for blinded sample size reassessment that properly control the Type I error should be used. (p. 6)

Can a single illustration of the conditional theory given in Section 2.3 be extended to all clinical trial applications? Are there any pitfalls that require our cautions?

On a closer examination, however, it is evident that for applications with time-to-event endpoints or binary endpoints, conditional methods given blinded data (e.g., the log-rank test, Fisher's exact test or the Mantel–Haenszel test) are already available, making it a breeze to justify the requirement $E_H(C_d \| \mathcal{B}) \leq \alpha$ in Equation 2.1. In general, there is no readily available conditional test procedure for an application. For the ostensibly simple setting with normally distributed data, most blinded sample size procedures inflate the type 1 error rates. To rectify these problems, it seems that test procedures conditional on blinded data should be developed. An area of interest would be randomization tests, which are in fact conditional on blinded data. However, the presence of differential drop-outs between treatment groups (Edgington, pp. 358–359, 1995) or treatment effects on secondary efficacy or safety endpoints may raise concerns on the very foundation of randomization tests. For noninferiority trials, blinded sample size adjustment could substantially inflate the type 1 error rates (Friede and Kieser 2003). So far we are not aware of any randomization test procedure for noninferiority trials.

As innocuous as they may appear, blinded procedures in the literature may pose various risks to the integrity of clinical trials. Most literature, including regulatory documents; that is, ICH E9 (1998), the FDA guidance (2006), and the more recent CHMP reflection paper (CHMP 2007), provide extremely broad and unverifiable claims of validity, while overlooking the simple fact that blinding is only a procedural terminology in data management. Liu and Pledger (pp. 231–244, 2005) point out that while the data management procedural definition of blinding can be satisfied technically, it is fairly often and easy to unblind the data partially. Liu and Pledger (p. 235, 2005) documents that with the intention to cheat, a seemingly very innocent blinded sample size adjustment procedure can increase the type 1 error rate to 55% following an elementary analysis of variance (ANOVA) technique! In a recent paper (Ganju and Xing 2009), a referee suggests a pseudo-blinded procedure, which according to Hwang and Lan (p. 248, 2006) "should be considered tantamount to unblinding." Thus under the guise of blindness, abuse as such is even more likely. Interestingly enough, the authors fail to discuss this problem.

Hwang and Lan (pp. 248–249, 2006) provide a detailed account of yet another deleterious aspect of data monitoring:

> In principle, because data collection does not involve unblinding data, there should be no concern for bias introduction. In reality, however, this is not always the case. For example, certain aspects of the data, such as a typical AE [adverse event] or laboratory test, may associate with certain treatment but not with the others, would essentially reveal the treatment identity.

Hwang and Lan (pp. 248–249, 2006) forewarn that

> This problem is of particular concern when sophisticated computerized data monitoring browsing tools are available.

To further elaborate a mechanism of partially unblinding the data, Liu and Pledger (p. 235, 2005) describe that

> Another maneuver is to use a secondary variable that is differentially affected by the treatment of the study drug as compared with the control, e.g., the pseudo code based on ranks by the degree of a known side effect from within each randomization block would correlate with the true randomization.

A former colleague suggests that this risk to the integrity of clinical trials is ominous in the confirmative phase 3 trial setting as differential AE or laboratory test are often identified during early stages of a clinical development.

It is highly likely that there does not exist a single set of standard operating procedures (SOPs) by any organization, covering a broad area including clinical operations, biostatistics, programing, data management, and information technology, to prevent adequately from partially unblinding the data through a variety of schemes. This raises serious doubt on whether the type 1 error rates are controlled at all in practice for blinded trials. It seems that any level of worrisome inflation is possible. Thus the actual type 1 error rates for blinded trials are beyond anyone's guess. While it is understandable that these risks may not be identified by regulatory reviewers as many may have little practical clinical trial experience, it is a serious problem that authors of blinded procedures from organizations with a large number of historical and on-going trials, as well as journal reviewers, would be content with limiting the mathematical formulation in order to generate simulation studies with artificial levels of ignorable inflation, even though the formulation does not reflect the setup as well as the conduct of the actual trials.

In conclusion, we recommend restricting unplanned design modifications to settings where conditional methods are available. General design modifications via protocol amendments with blinded data should be avoided unless a valid conditional method is developed for the application at hand. There must also be rigorous SOPs in place and convincing evidence of impeccable enforcement that forestall any partial unblinding of the data. While it is necessary to plan a trial carefully in advance, it is also important to identify various potential issues that need to be resolved at formal interim analyses through prespecified adaptive designs.

Appendix

Proof of Theorem (i) Following the Adaptation Lemma of Liu, Proschan, and Pledger (2002),

$$E_H(T_{[d,\xi_d]} \,\|\, \mathcal{G}_d) = \sum_{m \in M_d} I_{\{\xi_d = m\}} E_H(T_{[d,m]} \,\|\, \mathcal{G}_d).$$

By the assumption given in Equation 2.2, the right side of the equation is not larger than $\Sigma_{m\in M_d} I_{\{\xi_d=m\}} \; C_d = C_d$. Thus $E_H(T_{[d,\xi_d]} \; || \; \mathcal{G}_d) \leq C_d$. Using double expectations, we have $E_H(T_{[d,\xi_d]} \,||\, \mathcal{B}) = E_H\{E_H(T_{[d,\xi_d]} \,||\, \mathcal{G}_d) \,||\, \mathcal{B}\} \leq E_H(C_d \,||\, \mathcal{B}) \leq \alpha$. (ii) Again, following the Adaptation Lemma of Liu, Proschan, and Pledger (2002),

$$E_H(T_{[\tau,\xi_\tau]} \,||\, \mathcal{B}) = \sum_{d\in D} I_{\{\tau=d\}} E_H(T_{[d,\xi_d]} \,||\, \mathcal{B}).$$

From (i), the right side of the equation is not larger than $\Sigma_{d\in D} \; I_{\{\tau=d\}} \; \alpha = \alpha$. Thus $E_H(T_{[\tau,\xi_\tau]} \; || \; \mathcal{B}) \leq \alpha$. Furthermore, $E_H(T_{[\tau,\xi_\tau]}) \leq \alpha$.

References

CHMP. (2007). On methodological issues in confirmatory clinical trials planned with an adaptive design. *CHMP/EWP/2459/02*.

Collett, D. (1994). *Modelling Survival Data in Medical Research*. London: Chapman & Hall.

Cox, D. R., and Hinkley, D. V. (1974). *Theoretical Statistics*. London: Chapman & Hall.

Edgington, E. S. (1995). *Randomization Tests*. New York: Marcel Dekker.

FDA. (2006). Guidance for clinical trial sponsors: Establishment and operation of clinical trial data monitoring committees. Rockville, MD: U.S. Food and Drug Administration. Available at http://www.fda.gov/downloads/RegulatoryInformation/Guidances/ucm127073.pdf

Friede, T., and Kieser, M. (2003). Blinded sample size reassessment in non-inferiority and equivalence trials. *Statistics in Medicine*, 22:995–1007.

Ganju, J., and Xing, B. (2009). Re-estimating the sample size of an on-going blinded trial based on the method of randomization block sums. *Statistics in Medicine*, 22:24–38.

Hwang, I. K., and Lan, G. K. K. (2006). Interim analysis and adaptive design in clinical trials. *Statistics in the Pharmaceutical Industry: Third Edition, Revised and Expanded*, ed. R. Buncher and J.-Y. Tsay. New York: Taylor & Francis.

ICH E9. (1998). Guidance on statistical principles for clinical trials. *Federal Register*, 63 (179): 49583–98.

Liu, Q., and Anderson, K. M. (2008). On adaptive extensions of group sequential trials for clinical investigations. *Journal of the American Statistical Association*, 103:1621–30.

Liu, Q., Li, Y., and Boyett, J. M. (1997). Controlling false positive rates in prognostic factor analyses with small samples. *Statistics in Medicine*, 16:2095–2101.

Liu, Q., and Pledger, G. W. (2005). Interim analysis and bias in clinical trials: The adaptive design perspective. *Statistics in the Pharmaceutical Industry: Third Edition, Revised and Expanded*, ed. R. Buncher and J.-Y. Tsay. New York: Taylor & Francis.

Liu, Q., Proschan, M. A., and Pledger, G. W. (2002). A unified theory of two-stage adaptive designs. *Journal of the American Statistical Association*, 97:1034–41.

Müller, H., and Schäfer, H. (2001). Adaptive group sequential designs for clinical trials: Combining the advantages of adaptive and of classical group sequential approaches. *Biometrics*, 57:886–91.

Rosenberger, W. F., and Lachin, J. M. (2002). *Randomization in Clinical Trials: Theory and Practice*. New York: John Wiley & Sons.

3

Bayesian Approach for Adaptive Design

Guosheng Yin
The University of Hong Kong

Ying Yuan
M.D. Anderson Cancer Center

3.1 Introduction

In the cancer drug development process, phase I clinical trials focus on identifying the maximum tolerated dose (MTD), which is typically defined as the dose with a toxicity probability closest to the target toxicity rate. Phase I clinical trials are critically important, as the determined MTD will be further investigated in the subsequent Phase II or Phase III trials. Misidentification of the MTD could result in an inconclusive trial, thereby wasting enormous resources, or a trial in which a substantial number of patients would be treated at excessively toxic doses. In addition, if a dose with low toxicity and negligible efficacy is inappropriately selected as the MTD, it may cause researchers to overlook a promising drug.

Many statistical methods have been developed for dose-finding studies, with a basic assumption that toxicity monotonically increases with respect to the dose. The standard 3 + 3 design is an algorithm-based procedure that typically defines the MTD as the highest dose with a toxicity probability less than 33% (Storer 1989). Although the 3 + 3 design is widely used in practice due to its simplicity, the estimates of the toxicity probabilities are not reliable (O'Quigley and Chevret 1991). As an alternative, the model-based continual reassessment method (CRM) proposed by O'Quigley, Pepe, and Fisher (1990) links the true toxicity probabilities and the prespecified toxicity probabilities with a single unknown parameter. During the trial conduct using the CRM, the unknown parameter is continuously updated as more data accumulate. Other related phase I trial designs include the Bayesian decision-theoretic approach by Whitehead and Brunier (1995); random walk rules by Durham, Flournoy, and Rosenberger (1997); dose escalation with overdose control by Babb, Rogatko, and Zacks (1998); and the biased-coin design with an isotonic regression estimator by Stylianou and Flournoy (2002).

Focusing on the CRM, Faries (1994) and Goodman, Zahurak, and Piantadosi (1995) developed practical improvements for the design, by enlarging the cohort size and limiting each dose escalation by one dose level. Møller (1995) extended the CRM using a preliminary up-and-down design in order to reach the neighborhood of the target dose. Piantadosi, Fisher, and Grossman (1998) used a simple dose–toxicity model to guide data interpolation. Heyd and Carlin (1999) would terminate the trial earlier if the width of the 95% posterior probability interval for the MTD became sufficiently narrow. Ishizuka and Ohashi (2001) proposed monitoring a posterior density function of toxicity in order to prevent patients from being treated at overly toxic doses. Leung and Wang (2002) applied decision theory to optimize the number of patients allocated to the MTD. Braun (2002) extended the CRM to model bivariate competing outcomes. Yuan, Chappell, and Bailey (2007) developed a quasi-likelihood approach to accommodating multiple toxicity grades. To improve the robustness of the CRM, Yin and Yuan (2009a) proposed using multiple sets of prespecified toxicity probabilities in the CRM model and taking a Bayesian model averaging (BMA) approach to estimate the true toxicity probabilities.

Dose finding based solely on toxicity, while ignoring efficacy, may not be the best strategy. There has been increasing research in dose-finding methods that jointly model toxicity and efficacy (Gooley et al. 1994; O'Quigley, Hughes, and Fenton 2001; among others). In particular, Thall and Cook (2004) proposed to partition the two-dimensional toxicity–efficacy probability domain by introducing equivalence contours. However, the trade-off contour was constructed with a polynomial model based on only three physician-specified equivalent points, which might be subjective. Yin, Li, and Ji (2006) developed a toxicity–efficacy odds-ratio contour as a trade-off for dose finding, which is more objective, intuitive, and easily interpretable. Furthermore, Yuan and Yin (2009) extended toxicity–efficacy joint modeling to time-to-event outcomes and constructed the trade-off based on survival curves.

All of the aforementioned methods were developed for single-agent dose-finding trials, and therefore cannot address drug-combination studies, a rapidly growing area of clinical research. Combining different agents can impart the advantages of inducing a synergistic treatment effect, targeting different disease pathways, and achieving a high-dose intensity with nonoverlapping toxicities. However, complex drug–drug interactive effects often lead to an unknown toxicity order (i.e., the usual monotonic toxicity order with respect to the dose is lost). Drug-combination studies can be formulated in a more general framework, that of a trial with several different drugs, each at a prespecified set of doses, or a study of a single agent at a set of doses, adding a change to different administration schedules. Along this direction, Korn and Simon (1993) introduced a tolerable dose diagram to provide guidance in targeting specific MTD combinations. Kramar, Lebecq, and Candalh (1999) proposed searching over a selected subset of drug combinations that still maintains the monotonic order. Kuzuya et al. (2001) proposed fixing one agent at each dose level and varying the other in a trial combining paclitaxel and carboplatin to treat ovarian cancer. Thall et al. (2003) proposed a six-parameter model to define the toxicity probability for the combination of gemcitabine and cyclophosphamide. Conaway, Dunbar, and Peddada (2004) examined the simple and partial orders for drug combinations based on the pool-adjacent-violators algorithm. Wang and Ivanova (2005) studied a logistic regression model with the standardized doses of the two drugs as covariates. Yuan and Yin (2008) developed a sequential CRM for drug-combination trials that uses the partial order of the two-dimensional dose-finding space. By introducing latent 2×2 contingency tables, Yin and Yuan (2009b) pooled indistinguishable toxicity probabilities together to construct a binomial likelihood for combinations of two agents. Yin and Yuan (2009c, 2010) proposed a copula-type regression to model the joint toxicity probability, which incorporates the prior information on the toxicity probabilities when each drug is administered alone.

Following a phase I drug-combination trial, there may be several MTDs identified, which are carried forward for Phase II testing. Phase II trials typically serve as a drug screening process in terms of efficacy or antidisease activities. Simultaneously examining several MTDs naturally leads to a multiarm study, in which adaptive randomization is often used to assign more patients to a more efficacious treatment arm (Yuan and Yin 2010).

To illustrate recent developments in Bayesian approaches for adaptive designs, in this chapter we discuss four innovative Bayesian adaptive designs: the BMA-CRM in phase I dose-finding trials (Yin and Yuan 2009a), jointly modeling toxicity and efficacy in phase I/II trials (Yin, Li, and Ji 2006), copula-type regression in phase I drug-combination trials (Yin and Yuan 2009c), and adaptive randomization in Phase I/II drug-combination trials.

3.2 Bayesian Model Averaging Continual Reassessment Method

3.2.1 Continual Reassessment Method

Let $(d_1, \ldots, d_J)$ denote a set of J prespecified doses for the drug under investigation, and let $(p_1, \ldots, p_J)$ be the corresponding prespecified toxicity probabilities, also known as the "skeleton," satisfying $p_1 < \ldots < p_J$. Let ϕ_T be the target toxicity rate. The CRM assumes a working dose–toxicity model,

$$\text{pr}(\text{toxicity at} \, d_j) = \pi_j(\alpha) = p_j^{\exp(\alpha)}, \quad j = 1, \ldots, J,$$

where α is an unknown parameter (O'Quigley and Shen 1996). Parabolic tangent or logistic structures can also be used to model the dose–toxicity curve (O'Quigley, Pepe, and Fisher 1990).

Let D denote the observed data: y_j out of n_j patients treated at dose level j have experienced the dose-limiting toxicity (DLT). Based on the binomial distribution, the likelihood function is

$$L(D \mid \alpha) \propto \prod_{j=1}^{J} \{p_j^{\exp(\alpha)}\}^{y_j} \{1 - p_j^{\exp(\alpha)}\}^{n_j - y_j}.$$

Using Bayes' theorem, the posterior means of the toxicity probabilities can be computed by

$$\hat{\pi}_j = \int p_j^{\exp(\alpha)} \frac{L(D \mid \alpha) f(\alpha)}{\int L(D \mid \alpha) f(\alpha) d\alpha} d\alpha,$$

where $f(\alpha)$ is a prior distribution for α, for example, $\alpha \sim N(0, \sigma^2)$. After updating the posterior estimates of the dose–toxicity probabilities, the dose recommended for the next cohort of patients is the one that has a toxicity probability closest to the target ϕ_T. That is, a new cohort of patients is assigned to dose level j^* with $j^* = \text{argmin}_{j \in (1, \ldots, J)} |\hat{\pi}_j - \phi_T|$. The trial continues until the exhaustion of the total sample size, and then the dose with a posterior toxicity probability closest to ϕ_T is selected as the MTD.

To improve the practical performance of the CRM, the modified version of the CRM (Goodman, Zahurak, and Piantadosi 1995; Møller 1995; Chevret 2006) requires that the cohort size is three; dose escalation is restricted to one level of change only; and if pr(toxicity at the lowest dose $> \phi_T$) > 0.9, the trial is terminated for safety.

3.2.2 Bayesian Model Averaging CRM

Although the practical modifications improve the operating characteristics of the CRM. There is an important unresolved issue: the set of prespecified toxicity probabilities (skeleton) in the CRM is arbitrary and subjective. Using different skeletons may lead to quite different design properties, and the performance of the CRM can be severely compromised if the elicited toxicity probabilities in the skeleton do not fit the assumed dose–toxicity model. Unfortunately, practitioners usually have no information to justify whether a specific skeleton is reasonable because the underlying true toxicity probabilities are unknown. To overcome the arbitrariness of the skeleton, Yin and Yuan (2009a) proposed the BMA-CRM by using multiple skeletons in the CRM combined with the BMA approach, which provides a better predictive performance than any single model (Raftery, Madigan, and Hoeting 1997; Hoeting et al. 1999).

Let $(M_1, \ldots, M_K)$ be the models corresponding to each set of the prespecified toxicity probabilities $\{(p_{11}, \ldots, p_{1J}), \ldots, (p_{k1}, \ldots, p_{kJ})\}$. Model M_k in the CRM is given by

$$\pi_{kj}(\alpha_k) = p_{kj}^{\exp(\alpha_k)}, \quad j = 1,\ldots,J,$$

which is based on the kth skeleton $(p_{k1}, \ldots, p_{kJ})$. Let $\mathrm{pr}(M_k)$ be the prior model probability, then the likelihood function under model M_k is

$$L(D \mid \alpha_k, M_k) \propto \prod_{j=1}^{J} \{p_{kj}^{\exp(\alpha_k)}\}^{y_j} \{1 - p_{kj}^{\exp(\alpha_k)}\}^{n_j - y_j}.$$

The posterior model probability for M_k is given by

$$\mathrm{pr}(M_k \mid D) = \frac{L(D \mid M_k)\mathrm{pr}(M_k)}{\sum_{i=1}^{K} L(D \mid M_i)\mathrm{pr}(M_i)},$$

where $L(D \mid M_k)$ is the marginal likelihood of model M_k,

$$L(D \mid M_k) = \int L(D \mid \alpha_k, M_k) f(\alpha_k \mid M_k) d\alpha_k,$$

and $f(\alpha_k \mid M_k)$ is the prior distribution of α_k under model M_k.

The BMA estimate for the toxicity probability at each dose level is

$$\bar{\pi}_j = \sum_{k=1}^{K} \hat{\pi}_{kj} \mathrm{pr}(M_k \mid D), \quad j = 1,\ldots,J,$$

where $\hat{\pi}_{kj}$ is the posterior mean of the toxicity probability at dose level j under model M_k,

$$\hat{\pi}_{kj} = \int p_{kj}^{\exp(\alpha_k)} \frac{L(D \mid \alpha_k, M_k) f(\alpha_k \mid M_k)}{\int L(D \mid \alpha_k, M_k) f(\alpha_k \mid M_k) d\alpha_k} d\alpha_k.$$

By assigning $\hat{\pi}_{kj}$ a weight of $\text{pr}(M_k \mid D)$, BMA automatically favors the best fitting model, and also provides a coherent mechanism to account for the model uncertainty associated with each skeleton.

3.2.3 Dose-Finding Algorithm

Patients in the first cohort are treated at the lowest dose d_1, or the physician-specified dose. The dose-finding algorithm of the BMA-CRM is described below.

1. Let j^{curr} denote the current dose level, and we find dose level j^* that has a toxicity probability closest to ϕ_T, $j^* = \text{argmin}_{j \in (1,\ldots,J)} |\bar{\pi}_j - \phi_T|$. If $j^{\text{curr}} > j^*$, we de-escalate the dose level to $j^{\text{curr}} - 1$; if $j^{\text{curr}} < j^*$, we escalate the dose level to $j^{\text{curr}} + 1$; otherwise, the dose stays at the same level as j^{curr} for the next cohort of patients.
2. Once the maximum sample size is reached, the dose that has the toxicity probability closest to ϕ_T is selected as the MTD.

In addition, we require an early termination of a trial for safety, if

$$\sum_{k=1}^{K} \text{pr}\{\pi_{k1}(\alpha_k) > \phi_T \mid M_k, D\}\text{pr}(M_k \mid D) > 90\%.$$

3.2.4 Simulation Study

We investigated the operating characteristics of the BMA-CRM through simulation studies. We considered eight doses and prepared four sets of initial guesses of the toxicity probabilities:

$$(p_1,\ldots,p_8) = \begin{cases} (0.02,0.06,0.08,0.12,0.20,0.30,0.40,0.50), & \text{skeleton1} \\ (0.01,0.05,0.09,0.14,0.18,0.22,0.26,0.30), & \text{skeleton2} \\ (0.10,0.20,0.30,0.40,0.50,0.60,0.70,0.80), & \text{skeleton3} \\ (0.20,0.30,0.40,0.50,0.60,0.65,0.70,0.75), & \text{skeleton4.} \end{cases}$$

We refer to the individual CRM using each of these four skeletons as CRM 1, CRM 2, CRM 3, and CRM 4. The target toxic probability was $\phi_T = 30\%$. We took a prior distribution of $\alpha \sim N(0,4)$ and assigned a prior model probability of 1/4 to each CRM model; that is, $\text{pr}(M_k) = 1/4$ for $k = 1,\ldots,4$. We took a cohort size of 3, and treated the first cohort of patients at the lowest dose level. The maximum sample size was 30. For each scenario, we carried out 10,000 simulated trials.

In Table 3.1, we summarize the simulation results for three different scenarios. In scenario 1, the seventh dose is the MTD; and the four individual CRMs selected the MTD with quite different probabilities: particularly, CRM 2 had the lowest MTD selection percentage of 30.8%, while incorrectly selected the eighth dose with the highest percentage of 56.9%; and the BMA-CRM had an MTD selection percentage of 51.5%. In scenario 2, for which the MTD is at the sixth dose level, the MTD selection percentage using the BMA-CRM was the second best among all of the five designs. The worst skeleton in Scenario 2 corresponds to CRM 2, which yielded an MTD selection percentage of less than 30%. In Scenario 3, which has the third dose as the MTD, CRM 1 behaved the worst with an MTD selection percentage of less than 50% compared to MTD selection percentages of more than 60% for the others.

TABLE 3.1 Simulation Study Comparing the CRM and BMA-CRM, With a Toxicity Target $\phi_T = 30\%$

Design	Recommendation Percentage at Dose Level 1	2	3	4	5	6	7	8	Average # Toxicity
Scenario 1	2	3	4	6	8	10	30	50	
CRM 1	0	0	0	0.1	1.4	16.0	**52.6**	29.9	4.7
# patients	3.2	3.0	3.0	3.1	3.6	4.7	5.7	3.6	
CRM 2	0	0	0	0.1	1.0	11.2	**30.8**	56.9	5.6
# patients	3.2	3.0	3.1	3.1	3.2	3.5	4.3	6.6	
CRM 3	0	0	0	0.8	4.6	22.1	**59.3**	13.1	3.9
# patients	3.2	3.0	3.2	3.5	4.1	5.2	6.4	1.4	
CRM 4	0	0	0	0.6	3.6	18.0	**44.8**	33.0	4.7
# patients	3.2	3.0	3.1	3.5	3.8	4.2	5.2	3.8	
BMA-CRM	0	0	0	0.2	1.5	16.2	**51.5**	30.6	4.7
# patients	3.2	3.0	3.1	3.2	3.5	4.4	6.3	3.2	
Scenario 2	2	6	8	12	20	30	40	50	
CRM 1	0	0	0	2.9	23.9	**43.6**	22.7	6.9	5.9
# patients	3.2	3.1	3.2	3.6	6.3	6.6	3.0	0.8	
CRM 2	0	0	0.3	4.3	17.1	28.4	25.5	24.4	6.5
# patients	3.2	3.1	3.4	3.8	4.6	4.8	3.8	3.2	
CRM 3	0	0	0.6	6.3	32.6	**40.8**	18.1	1.6	5.2
# patients	3.2	3.1	3.6	4.8	6.9	5.7	2.4	0.2	
CRM 4	0	0	0.4	7.5	27.8	**35.3**	20.7	8.2	5.5
# patients	3.2	3.1	3.6	4.9	6.4	4.8	2.9	1.0	
BMA-CRM	0	0	0.3	4.3	23.9	**41.6**	22.7	7.3	5.7
# patients	3.2	3.1	3.4	4.3	5.9	5.8	3.3	0.8	
Scenario 3	6	15	30	55	60	65	68	70	
CRM 1	0.9	27.8	**48.5**	21.0	1.5	0.2	0	0	9.1
# patients	4.3	7.4	9.7	6.5	1.9	0.2	0	0	
CRM 2	0.2	22.6	**60.8**	15.1	1.0	0.2	0	0	8.8
# patients	3.9	7.5	11.7	5.1	1.5	0.3	0	0	
CRM 3	0.3	19.6	**65.1**	14.4	0.6	0	0	0	8.4
# patients	4.1	7.2	13.0	5.0	0.6	0	0	0	
CRM 4	0.4	19.3	**65.6**	14.2	0.5	0	0	0	8.5
# patients	4.1	7.2	12.7	5.2	0.7	0.1	0	0	
BMA-CRM	0.3	20.6	**62.0**	16.1	0.9	0	0	0	8.6
# patients	4.1	7.2	12.2	5.6	0.8	0.1	0	0	

Source: Yin, G. and Yuan, Y., *Journal of the American Statistical Association*, 104, 954–68, 2009a.
Note: MTD is shown in boldface.

We further examined the relationship between the performance of each CRM and the corresponding posterior model probability using the BMA approach. We took 30 cohorts of size 3 and simulated 5000 trials. For each trial, we computed the posterior model probabilities for each CRM after every cohort was sequentially accrued. In Figure 3.1, we present the average of these posterior model probabilities versus the accumulating number of cohorts. Figure 3.1 shows that the posterior model probabilities of the four CRM models started separating after approximately 4–8 cohorts, and eventually stabilized in an order that correctly matches the performance of each CRM. These simulations demonstrated the robustness of the BMA-CRM.

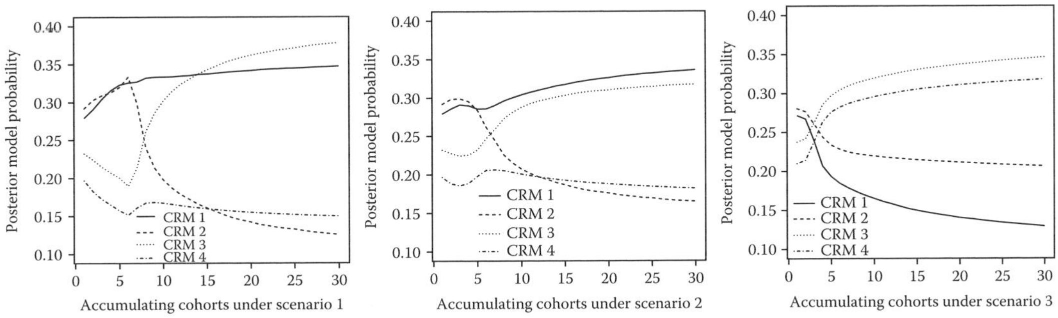

FIGURE 3.1 Posterior model probabilities of four individual CRMs vs. the accumulating number of cohorts under Scenarios 1, 2, and 3.

3.3 Jointly Modeling Toxicity and Efficacy in Phase I/II Design

3.3.1 Likelihood and Prior

In a typical phase I/II clinical trial, the interest is focused on finding the dose that optimizes the trade-off between toxicity and efficacy. Let p_j and r_j be the probabilities of toxicity and efficacy associated with dose level j. We assume a monotonically increasing order of toxicity probabilities with respect to the doses, but no such constraint for efficacy.

Let X_{ij} denote the binary toxicity outcome for subject i under dose level j, and let Y_{ij} denote the binary efficacy outcome of the same subject; that is, $X_{ij} = 1$ with probability p_j, or 0 with probability $1 - p_j$; and $Y_{ij} = 1$ with probability r_j, or 0 with probability $1 - r_j$. Following the global cross-ratio model (Dale 1986), at dose level j, we define $\pi_{xy}^{(j)} = \text{pr}(X_{ij} = x, Y_{ij} = y)$, and $\theta_j = \pi_{00}^{(j)}\pi_{11}^{(j)} / (\pi_{01}^{(j)}\pi_{10}^{(j)})$. The joint probabilities $\pi_{xy}^{(j)}$ can be obtained from the association parameter θ_j and the marginal probabilities p_j and r_j:

$$\pi_{11}^{(j)} = \begin{cases} \dfrac{a_j - \sqrt{a_j^2 + b_j}}{2(\theta_j - 1)} & \theta_j \neq 1 \\ p_j r_j & \theta_j = 1, \end{cases}$$

$$\pi_{10}^{(j)} = p_j - \pi_{11}^{(j)}, \quad \pi_{01}^{(j)} = r_j - \pi_{11}^{(j)}, \quad \pi_{00}^{(j)} = 1 - p_j - r_j + \pi_{11}^{(j)},$$

where $a_j = 1 + (p_j + r_j)(\theta_j - 1)$ and $b_j = -4\theta_j(\theta_j - 1)p_j r_j$. If n_j subjects are treated at dose d_j, then the likelihood function is

$$L(p_1,\ldots,p_J; r_1,\ldots,r_J; \theta_1,\ldots,\theta_J \mid D) \propto \prod_{j=1}^{J} \prod_{i=1}^{n_j} \prod_{x=0}^{1} \prod_{y=0}^{1} \{\pi_{xy}^{(j)}\}^{I(X_{ij}=x, Y_{ij}=y)}, \tag{3.1}$$

where $I(\bullet)$ is the indicator function.

We apply two different transformations for the p's and r's in the prior specification with or without incorporating the monotonic ordering constraint. To model toxicity, let

$$\xi_1 = \log\frac{p_1}{1-p_1}, \quad \xi_j = \log\left(\frac{p_j}{1-p_j} - \frac{p_{j-1}}{1-p_{j-1}}\right), \quad j = 2,\ldots,J,$$

and then

$$p_1 = \frac{e^{\xi_1}}{1+e^{\xi_1}}, \quad p_j = \frac{e^{\xi_1}+\cdots+e^{\xi_j}}{1+e^{\xi_1}+\cdots+e^{\xi_j}}.$$

Clearly, the p_j's satisfy the monotonic toxicity condition. For efficacy, we do not enforce the ordering constraint, and define

$$\zeta_1 = \log\frac{r_1}{1-r_1}, \quad \zeta_j = \log\left(\frac{r_j}{1-r_j}\right) - \log\left(\frac{r_{j-1}}{1-r_{j-1}}\right), \quad j = 2,\ldots,J,$$

and thus,

$$r_1 = \frac{e^{\zeta_1}}{1+e^{\zeta_1}}, \quad r_j = \frac{e^{\zeta_1+\cdots+\zeta_j}}{1+e^{\zeta_1+\cdots+\zeta_j}}.$$

For ease of computation, we take the prior distributions for the θ_j's to be independent from a log-normal distribution. Let $\boldsymbol{\xi} = (\xi_1,\ldots,\xi_J)^T$, and $\boldsymbol{\zeta}$ and $\boldsymbol{\theta}$ be defined similarly, then the joint posterior distribution is given by

$$f(\boldsymbol{\xi},\boldsymbol{\zeta},\boldsymbol{\theta} \mid D) \propto L(\boldsymbol{\xi},\boldsymbol{\zeta},\boldsymbol{\theta} \mid D) f(\boldsymbol{\xi},\boldsymbol{\zeta}) f(\theta_1)\ldots f(\theta_J),$$

where $L(\boldsymbol{\xi}, \boldsymbol{\zeta}, \boldsymbol{\theta}|D)$ is the likelihood after reparameterization, and $f(\boldsymbol{\xi}, \boldsymbol{\zeta})$ and $f(\theta_j)$ are the prior distributions. We typically assign noninformative priors to the model parameters, such that the likelihood dominates the posterior estimation and inference. To implement Gibbs sampling, we derive the full conditional distribution for each model parameter and obtain the posterior samples using the adaptive rejection Metropolis sampling algorithm (Gilks, Best, and Tan 1995).

3.3.2 Odds-Ratio Trade-Off

We define a set of admissible doses, $d_j \in \mathcal{A}$, if dose d_j satisfies

$$\text{pr}(p_j < \phi_T) > p^*, \quad \text{pr}(r_j > \phi_E) > r^*,$$

where ϕ_T and ϕ_E are prespecified upper toxicity and lower efficacy boundaries, and p^* and r^* are fixed probability cutoffs.

As shown in Figure 3.2, we expect the efficacy and toxicity probabilities (r_j, p_j) of the target dose to be closest to the lower-right corner (1, 0) in the two-dimensional domain. The horizontal and vertical lines crossing point (r_j, p_j) partition the probability space into four rectangles. The toxicity–efficacy odds ratio

$$\omega_j = \frac{p_j/(1-p_j)}{r_j/(1-r_j)} = \frac{p_j(1-r_j)}{r_j(1-p_j)},$$

is exactly the ratio of the areas between the lower-right and the upper-left rectangles. Clearly, a dose with a smaller value of ω_j is more desirable. Figure 3.2 also shows the equivalent odds-ratio contours, along which all of the points have the same toxicity–efficacy odds ratio.

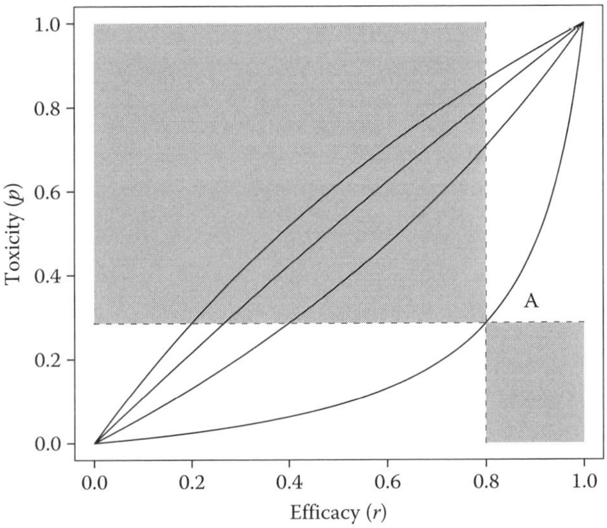

FIGURE 3.2 Toxicity–efficacy odds-ratio trade-off contours with point A (r_j, p_j) corresponding to dose level j.

We start by treating patients in the first cohort at the lowest dose level, with a restriction that untried doses cannot be skipped during dose escalation. The dose-finding algorithm is described as follows:

1. Let j^* be the highest tried dose level. If $\text{pr}(p_{j*} < \phi_T) > p^\dagger$ for some chosen cutoff probability of escalation, $p^\dagger \geq p^*$, we escalate to dose level $j^* + 1$.
2. Otherwise, the next cohort of patients are treated at the dose with the smallest odds ratio in $\mathcal{A}$. If $\mathcal{A}$ is an empty set, then the trial is terminated and no dose is selected.
3. Once the maximum sample size is reached, the dose with the minimum toxicity–efficacy odds ratio in $\mathcal{A}$ is recommended.

3.3.3 Simulation Studies

We conducted simulations to examine the operating characteristics of the Bayesian toxicity–efficacy odds-ratio design. We considered five doses (0.25, 0.5, 0.75, 1, 2); the maximum sample size for each trial was 60; and the cohort size was three. We took $\phi_T = \phi_E = 0.3$, $p^* = 0.25$, $r^* = 0.1$, and $p^\dagger = 0.5$, and for each configuration, we simulated 1000 trials. The bivariate binary outcomes were generated from the Dale model based on prespecified marginal probabilities of toxicity and efficacy with $\theta_j = 1$. After 1000 burn-ins, we recorded every fifth sample out of 5000 iterations to reduce the autocorrelation in the Markov chain.

For comparison, we examined an alternative criterion, which selects the dose with the largest $\pi_{01}^{(j)} = \text{pr}(T = 0, E = 1)$ to treat the next cohort of patients. Table 3.2 summarizes the simulation results under four scenarios using the ω_j and $\pi_{01}^{(j)}$ criteria, respectively. In Scenario 1, toxicity increases substantially with respect to the dose but efficacy does not change much. The two designs yielded similar dose selection percentages and treated most of the patients at dose level 1. In Scenario 2, efficacy increases dramatically but toxicity does not change much. Both designs selected the fifth dose with the highest percentages. In Scenario 3, the fifth dose is considered overly toxic, and the designs mainly selected the third and fourth doses. In Scenario 4, all of the five doses are excessively toxic and thus none of them should be selected.

By jointly modeling toxicity and efficacy in dose-finding trials, more information can be incorporated into the trial design. Furthermore, seamlessly transiting from Phase I to Phase II eliminates the gap between these two phases, and expedites the drug development process.

TABLE 3.2 Simulation Study with Different Probabilities of Toxicity and Efficacy (p_j, r_j) Under the Dale Model for Five Dose Levels

	Selection Percentage of Dose (# of Patients)					
	1	2	3	4	5	None
Scenario 1	(15, 55)	(25, 58)	(35, 60)	(45, 62)	(55, 65)	
ω_j	.1444	.2414	.3590	.5015	.6581	
	57.4 (30.1)	22.1 (13.5)	6.4 (6.0)	1.4 (2.6)	.1 (1.1)	12.6
$\pi_{01}^{(j)}$	.4675	.4350	.3900	.3410	.2925	
	53.7 (28.7)	23.4 (14.4)	8.2 (7.0)	2.4 (2.8)	.3 (1.0)	12.0
Scenario 2	(1, 5)	(2, 20)	(3, 35)	(4, 60)	(5, 80)	
ω_j	.1919	.0816	.0574	.0278	.0132	
	0 (3.1)	1.3 (4.2)	6.3 (6.6)	28.0 (16.0)	**61.5** (28.5)	2.9
$\pi_{01}^{(j)}$	.0495	.1960	.3395	.5760	.7600	
	0 (3.1)	.3 (3.3)	1.6 (4.4)	17.1 (12.5)	**79.1** (35.7)	1.9
Scenario 3	(1, 20)	(3, 40)	(4, 60)	(5, 70)	(35, 75)	
ω_j	.0404	.0464	.0278	.0226	.1795	
	4.8 (6.4)	15.2 (10.4)	35.1 (17.2)	**38.5** (18.2)	4.3 (6.6)	2.1
$\pi_{01}^{(j)}$	.1980	.3880	.5760	.6650	.4875	
	.5 (3.6)	5.6 (6.4)	30.0 (16.8)	**53.4** (23.3)	9.1 (9.2)	1.4
Scenario 4	(30, 5)	(40, 20)	(50, 35)	(60, 50)	(70, 60)	
ω_j	8.1429	2.6667	1.8571	1.5000	1.5556	
	0 (3.8)	.4 (2.6)	0 (1.4)	0 (.3)	0 (.1)	99.6
$\pi_{01}^{(j)}$	.0350	.1200	.1750	.2000	.1800	
	0 (4.0)	.8 (3.3)	.1 (1.6)	0 (.4)	0 (.1)	99.1

Source: Yin, G., Li, Y., and Ji, Y., *Biometrics*, 62, 777–84, 2006.

Note: In each scenario, the first row represents the true probabilities $100 \times (p_j, r_j)$; the second gives the true values of ω_j; the third exhibits the dose selection percentages and numbers of treated patients; and the last two rows correspond to the design using $\pi_{01}^{(j)}$.

3.4 Drug-Combination Trial

3.4.1 Copula-Type Regression

Before several drugs are combined, the toxicity profile of each individual drug needs to be thoroughly investigated. It is important to incorporate this rich prior information in drug-combination trials to improve the efficiency of the design. Considering a drug-combination trial with two agents, say A and B, let p_j be the prespecified toxicity probability corresponding to A_j, the jth dose of drug A, $p_1 < \ldots < p_J$; and q_k be that of B_k, the kth dose of drug B, $q_1 < \ldots < q_K$. Although toxicity monotonically increases with the dose when each drug is administered alone, the ordering of the toxicity probabilities of the combined drugs is less obvious. The maximum dose for each drug in the combination (i.e., A_J and B_K) is often the individual MTD that has already been determined in the single-agent trials. The remaining lower doses are some fractions of the MTD. Therefore, the upper bounds p_J and q_K are known, and typically given as less than 40%. This shrinks the specification range of the p_j's and q_k's immensely and thus reduces the variability and arbitrariness of these prespecified probabilities.

As in the CRM, we take p_j^{α} and q_k^{β} as the true toxicity probabilities for drug A and drug B, respectively, where $\alpha > 0$ and $\beta > 0$ are unknown parameters with prior means centered at one. A reasonable model to link the joint toxicity probability π_{jk} of (A_j, B_k) with p_j and q_k needs to satisfy the following conditions:

i. if $p_j^{\alpha}=0$ and $q_k^{\beta}=0$, then $\pi_{jk}=0$;
ii. if $p_j^{\alpha}=0$ then $\pi_{jk}=q_k^{\beta}$ and if $q_k^{\beta}=0$ then $\pi_{jk}=p_j^{\alpha}$;
iii. if either $p_j^{\alpha}=1$ or $q_k^{\beta}=1$, then $\pi_{jk}=1$.

We link π_{jk} with $(p_j^{\alpha}, q_k^{\beta})$ through a copula-type regression model (Nelsen 1999),

$$\pi_{jk}=1-\{(1-p_j^{\alpha})^{-\gamma}+(1-q_k^{\beta})^{-\gamma}-1\}^{-1/\gamma}, \tag{3.2}$$

where the association parameter $\gamma>0$ characterizes the drug–drug interactive effect. Note that $\lim_{p_j \to 1}(1-p_j^{\alpha})^{-\gamma}=\infty$, and thus $\pi_{jk}=1$ as p_j goes to 1. Moreover, if only one drug is tested, say $p_j>0$ and $q_k=0$, (3.2) reduces to the CRM, with $\pi_j=p_j^{\alpha}$. In Figure 3.3, we illustrate the joint toxicity probability surface based on (3.2) with $\alpha=\beta=2$ and $\gamma=1.5$ in the two-dimensional probability space. If the target toxicity probability is 40%, as shown by the horizontal plane, there is an intersection curve representing the MTD contour for the two drugs.

We can construct the likelihood function based on the binomial distribution with probabilities π_{jk}. If y_{jk} out of n_{jk} patients treated at dose levels (j, k) have experienced toxicity, the likelihood is given by

$$L(\alpha,\beta,\gamma \mid D) \propto \prod_{j=1}^{J}\prod_{k=1}^{K} \pi_{jk}^{y_{jk}}(1-\pi_{jk})^{n_{jk}-y_{jk}},$$

and correspondingly, the posterior distribution is

$$f(\alpha,\beta,\gamma \mid D) \propto L(\alpha,\beta,\gamma \mid D) f(\alpha) f(\beta) f(\gamma),$$

where $f(\alpha)$, $f(\beta)$, and $f(\gamma)$ are gamma prior distributions with mean one.

3.4.2 Dose-Finding Algorithm

Let ϕ_T be the target toxicity rate, and c_e and c_d be the fixed probability cutoffs for dose escalation and de-escalation, respectively. Patients are treated in cohorts of size 3. As demonstrated in Figure 3.4, dose escalation or de-escalation is restricted to only one dose level of change, and simultaneously escalating

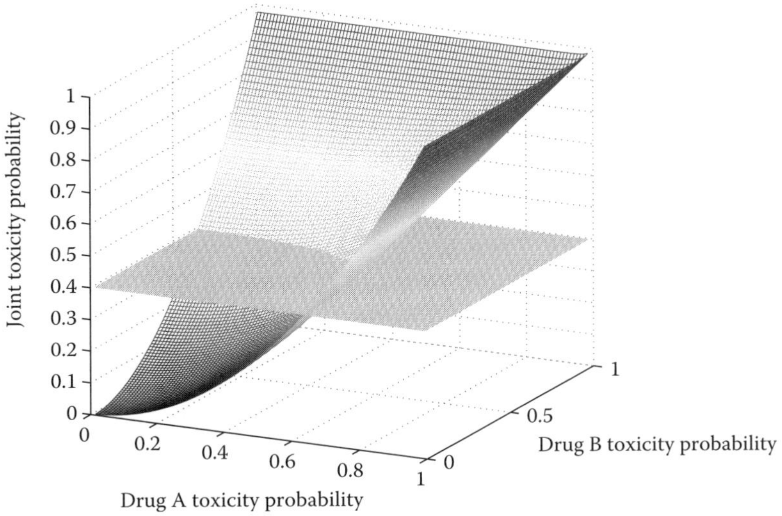

FIGURE 3.3 Diagram of a drug-combination trial.

or de-escalating both agents along the diagonal direction is not allowed. The dose-finding algorithm works as follows:

1. Patients in the first cohort are treated at the lowest dose combination (A_1, B_1).
2. At the current dose combination (A_j, B_k)
   i. If $\text{pr}(\pi_{jk} < \phi_T) > c_e$, the dose is escalated to an adjacent dose combination with the toxicity probability higher than the current and closest to ϕ_T. If the current dose combination is (A_J, B_K), the doses stay at the same levels.
   ii. If $\text{pr}(\pi_{jk} > \phi_T) > c_d$, the dose is de-escalated to an adjacent dose combination with the toxicity probability lower than the current and closest to ϕ_T. If the current dose combination is (A_1, B_1), the trial is terminated.
   iii. Otherwise, the next cohort of patients continues to be treated at the same dose combination.
3. Once the maximum sample size is reached, the dose combination with the toxicity probability closest to ϕ_T is selected as the MTD combination.

3.4.3 Simulation Study

We investigated the Bayesian copula-type dose-finding method through simulation studies under four scenarios, as listed in Table 3.3. Drug A had five dose levels and drug B had four. The target toxicity probability was $\phi_T = 40\%$, and the sample size was 60, with a cohort size of 3. We set $c_e = 0.8$ and $c_d = 0.45$, and took Gamma(2, 2) as the prior distribution for α and β, and Gamma(0.1, 0.1) for γ. We simulated 2000 trials under each scenario, and for each simulation, we recorded 2000 posterior samples after 100 burn-in iterations. Because the toxicity rates of the MTDs for Drug A and Drug B when

TABLE 3.3 Simulation for the Two-Drug Combinations With a Target Toxicity Probability of 40%

Dose Level	Drug A									
	1	2	3	4	5	1	2	3	4	5
Drug B										
			Scenario 1				Selection Probability			
4	0.54	0.67	0.75	0.81	0.86	0.9	0.1	0	0	0
3	0.48	0.59	0.68	0.75	0.81	10.2	1.7	0.1	0	0
2	**0.40**	0.45	0.59	0.67	0.74	**24.9**	11.6	1.7	0.1	0
1	0.24	**0.40**	0.47	0.56	0.64	3.1	**19.1**	6.2	0.3	0
			Scenario 2							
4	0.49	0.58	0.68	0.75	0.81	5.0	1.5	0	0	0
3	**0.40**	0.49	0.59	0.68	0.75	**17.6**	11.6	1.4	0.1	0
2	0.27	**0.40**	0.45	0.59	0.67	7.3	**19.2**	9.3	1.7	0.1
1	0.18	0.29	**0.40**	0.47	0.56	0.1	5.1	**11.2**	5.0	0.3
			Scenario 3							
4	0.31	**0.40**	0.50	0.61	0.75	3.8	**11.7**	8.5	1.3	0.1
3	0.23	0.34	**0.40**	0.53	0.67	0.7	5.9	**12.7**	8.0	1.2
2	0.16	0.25	0.34	**0.40**	0.52	0	0.7	3.5	**12.0**	10.3
1	0.09	0.16	0.18	0.22	**0.40**	0	0	0.3	3.5	**15.8**
			Scenario 4							
4	0.79	0.85	0.89	0.92	0.94	0	0	0	0	0
3	0.74	0.81	0.86	0.89	0.92	0	0	0	0	0
2	0.67	0.76	0.81	0.86	0.89	0	0	0	0	0
1	0.57	0.67	0.74	0.79	0.84	0.1	0	0	0	0

Source: Yin, G. and Yuan, Y., *Journal of the Royal Statistical Society C*, 58, 211–24, 2009c.

administered alone were 0.4 and 0.3, respectively, we specified the p_j's as (0.08, 0.16, 0.24, 0.32, 0.4) for Drug A; and the q_k's as (0.075, 0.15, 0.225, 0.3) for Drug B.

In the first three scenarios, there are two, three, and four MTDs, respectively. The Bayesian copula-type design selected the MTD combinations with quite high percentages. Scenario 4 examines the situation in which all of the drug combinations are overly toxic. The design successfully terminated 99.9% of the simulated trials early without any selection. The overall performance of the Bayesian copula-type design is satisfactory. The design allows for freedom of dose movement in the two-dimensional space. It continuously updates the posterior estimates of toxicity probabilities for all of the dose combinations based on the accumulated data and efficiently searches for the target across the entire drug-combination space.

3.5 Adaptive Randomization with Drug Combinations

3.5.1 Bayesian Adaptive Randomization

In a drug-combination trial, once Phase I dose finding is complete, due to the toxicity equivalence contour as shown in Figure 3.4, we may identify multiple, say K, dose combinations that are at a similar toxicity level. These K dose combinations satisfy the same safety requirements, and will be further investigated in a K-arm Phase II trial to evaluate their efficacy. Let $(r_1,\ldots,r_K)$ denote the response rates of these K admissible doses. If we observe that y_k out of n_k patients treated in arm k have responded, we can model efficacy using the following Bayesian hierarchical model,

$$y_k \sim \text{Binomial}(n_k, r_k), \quad r_k \sim \text{Beta}(\eta_1, \eta_2),$$

where we assign noninformative gamma prior distributions to η_1 and η_2.

In such a randomized multiarm trial, adaptive randomization provides a mechanism to mitigate the problem of randomly assigning patients to inferior treatments by skewing assignment probabilities toward more efficacious treatment arms. A common practice is to take the assignment probability proportional to the estimated response rate of each arm (i.e., $r_k/\Sigma_{k=1}^{K} r_k$), which, however, does not take into account the variability of the estimated response rates. An alternative is to compare the r_k's to a fixed value, say r_0, and take the assignment probability proportional to the posterior probability $\text{pr}(r_k > r_0|D)$. When two or more r_k's are much higher or lower than r_0, the corresponding posterior probabilities

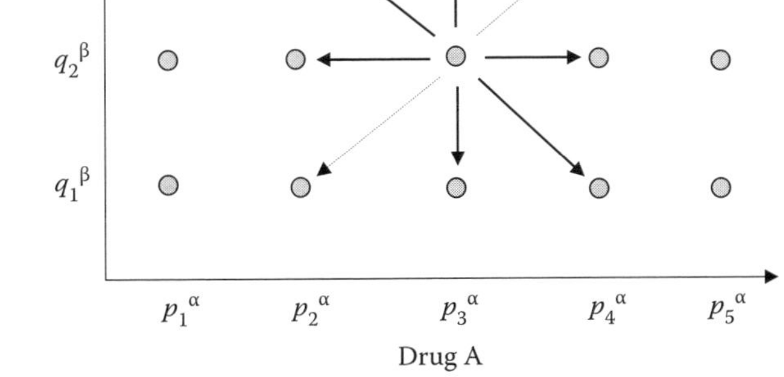

FIGURE 3.4 Joint toxicity probability surface and MTD contour for the two-drug combinations.

$\text{pr}(r_k > r_0|D)$ are either very close to 1 or 0, and thus the superior arm cannot be distinguished. A remedy is to use one arm as the reference, say the first treatment arm, and then randomize patients based on $R_k/\Sigma_{k=1}^{K} R_k$ with $R_k = \text{pr}(r_k > r_1|D)$ for $k > 1$, while setting $R_1 = 0.5$. Unfortunately, it cannot fully resolve the problem. In a two-arm trial, because $R_1 = 0.5$, arm 1 has an assignment probability of at least 1/3 (even if $R_2 = \text{pr}(r_2 > r_1|D) = 1$, i.e., treatment 2 is definitely superior to treatment 1), regardless of the efficacy of that treatment.

To overcome these difficulties, we propose a new Bayesian adaptive randomization scheme based on a moving reference instead of fixing the reference as a constant r_0 or r_1. Our method simultaneously accounts for the magnitude and uncertainty of the estimated r_k as follows:

1. Let $\bar{\mathcal{A}}$ and $\mathcal{A}$ denote the sets of treatment arms that have and have not been assigned randomization probabilities, respectively. We start with $\mathcal{A} = \{1,\ldots,K\}$ and $\bar{\mathcal{A}} = \{\cdot\}$ an empty set.
2. Take $\bar{r} = \Sigma_{k\in\mathcal{A}} r_k/\Sigma_{k\in\mathcal{A}} 1$ as the reference to determine $R_k = \text{pr}(r_k > \bar{r}|D)$, for $k \in \mathcal{A}$, and identify arm ℓ such that $R_\ell = \min_{k\in\mathcal{A}} R_k$.
3. Assign arm ℓ a randomization probability of π_ℓ, where

$$\pi_\ell = \frac{R_\ell}{\sum_{k\in\mathcal{A}} R_k}\left(1 - \sum_{k'\in\bar{\mathcal{A}}} \pi_{k'}\right),$$

   and then move arm ℓ from $\mathcal{A}$ to $\bar{\mathcal{A}}$.
4. Repeat Steps 2–3 until all of the arms are assigned randomization probabilities, $(\pi_1,\ldots,\pi_k)$.

As illustrated in Figure 3.5, once an arm is assigned a randomization probability, it will be removed from the admissible set $\mathcal{A}$. Thus the reference $\bar{r}$ is moving in the sense that, during the randomization

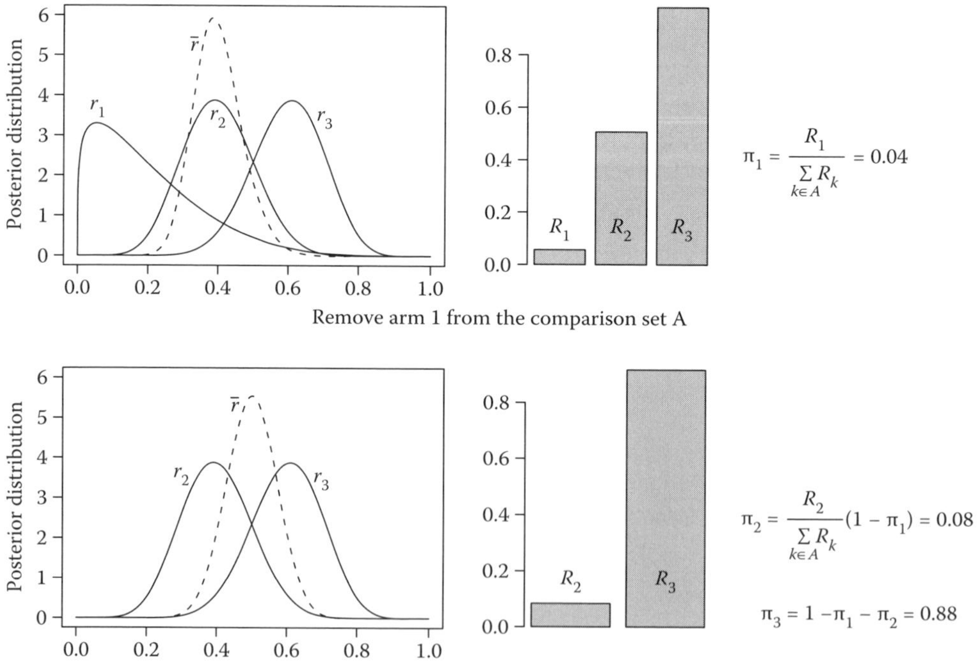

FIGURE 3.5 Illustration of the adaptive randomization for a three-arm trial. Based on the posterior distributions of r_1, r_2, r_3, and $\bar{r}$, we calculate $R_k = \text{pr}(r_k > \bar{r}|D)$ for $k = 1, 2, 3$; and assign the arm with the smallest value of R_k (i.e., arm 1) a randomization probability π_1. After spending π_1, we remove arm 1 from the comparison set $\mathcal{A}$ and distribute $1 - \pi_1$ to the remaining two arms in a similar manner.

process, it keeps changing based on the remaining arms in $\mathcal{A}$. By doing so, we obtain a zoomed-in comparison and achieve a high resolution to distinguish different treatments. We conducted a Phase II simulation study of randomizing a total of 100 patients to three treatment arms. We used a beta-binomial model to update the posterior estimates of the efficacy rates (r_1, r_2, r_3). We simulated 1000 trials under each of the three scenarios given in Table 3.4. The new Bayesian adaptive randomization with a moving reference efficiently allocated the majority of patients to the most efficacious arm, and often performed better than when using Arm 1 as the reference.

In Figure 3.6, we show the randomization probabilities averaged over 1000 simulations with respect to the accumulative number of patients. Using a moving reference, the Bayesian adaptive randomization has a substantially higher resolution to distinguish and separate treatment arms in terms of efficacy compared to using Arm 1 as the reference: for example, in Scenario 1, the curves are well

TABLE 3.4 Number of Patients Randomized to Each Treatment Arm Using the Adaptive Randomization With a Fixed vs. a Moving Reference

	Response Probability			Fixed Reference			Moving Reference		
Scenario	Arm 1	Arm 2	Arm 3	Arm 1	Arm 2	Arm 3	Arm 1	Arm 2	Arm 3
1	0.1	0.2	**0.3**	27.7	31.8	**40.6**	12.5	29.0	**58.5**
2	**0.3**	0.1	0.2	**61.1**	13.7	25.2	**58.4**	13.1	28.5
3	0.01	0.01	**0.5**	25.8	25.1	**49.1**	5.3	5.3	**89.4**

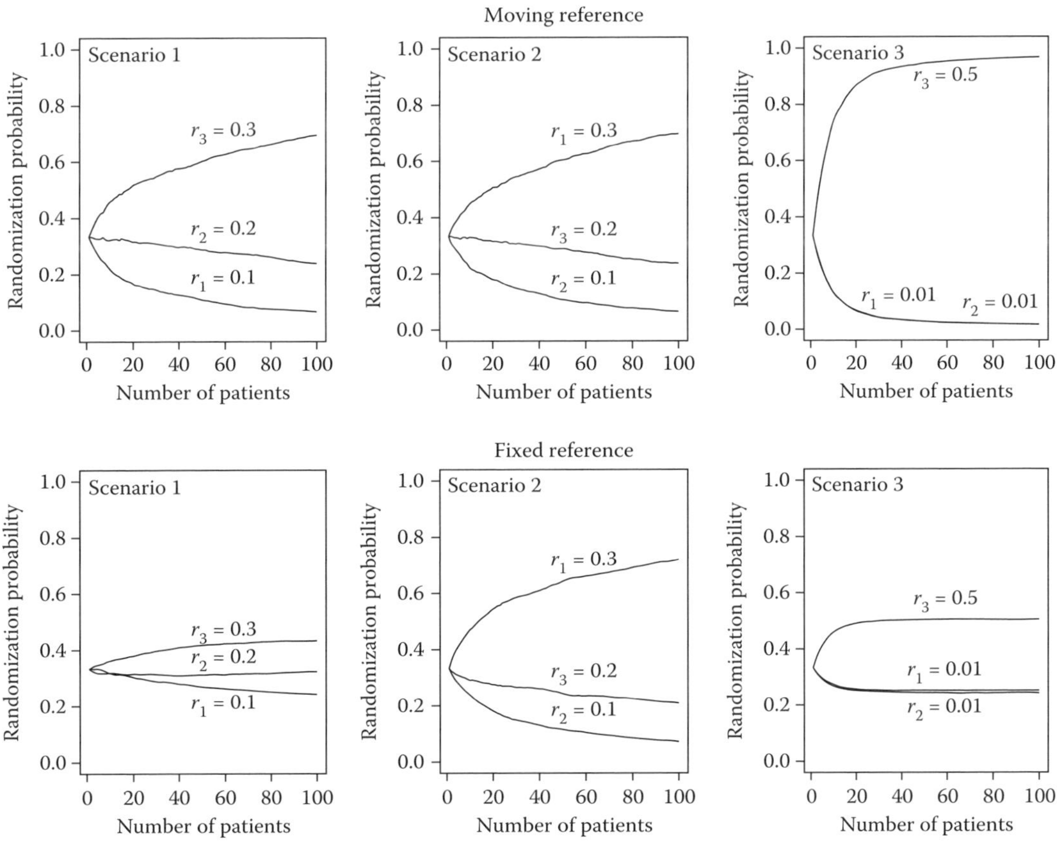

FIGURE 3.6 Randomization probabilities of the Bayesian adaptive randomization with a moving reference versus a fixed reference at Arm 1.

separated after 20 (using the moving reference) versus 40 patients (using Arm 1 as the reference) were randomized.

3.5.2 Phase I/II Design in Drug-Combination Trials

We seamlessly integrated the designs in Phase I and Phase II for combined therapies, as displayed in Figure 3.7. To examine the operating characteristics of the Phase I/II design, we simulated

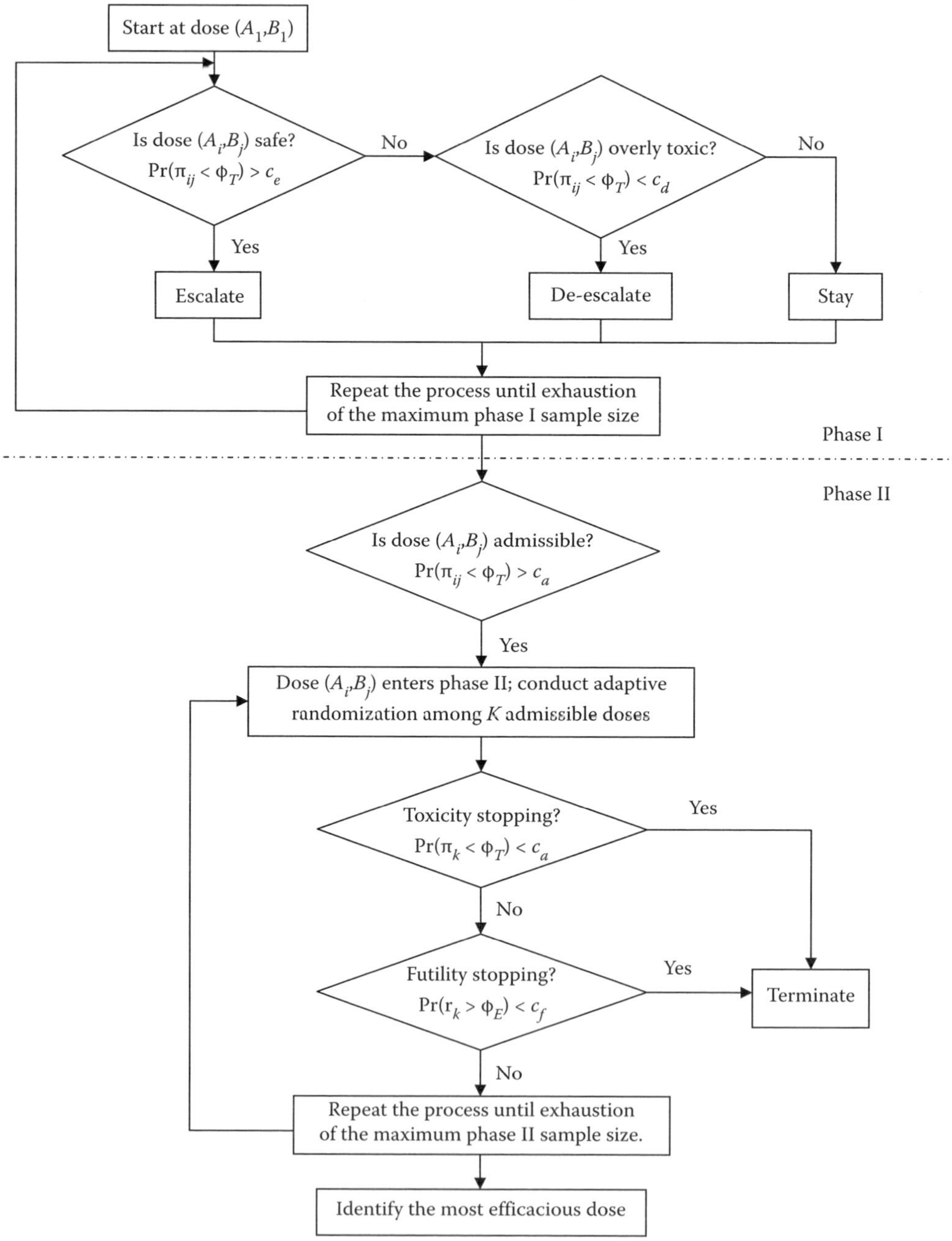

FIGURE 3.7 Diagram of the Phase I/II trial design for drug-combination trials.

TABLE 3.5 Selection Probability and Number of Patients Treated at Each Pair of Doses in the Phase I/II Drug-Combination Design

		Drug A											
	Drug	True Toxicity			True Efficacy			Simulation Results					
Scenario	B	1	2	3	1	2	3	Selection Percentage			Number of Patients		
1	2	0.1	0.15	0.45	0.20	0.40	0.60	1.0	25.2	18.3	8.8	17.0	15.3
	1	0.05	0.15	**0.20**	0.10	0.30	**0.50**	0.0	10.7	**42.8**	8.5	11.3	**18.0**
2	2	0.10	**0.20**	0.50	0.20	**0.40**	0.55	4.0	**44.5**	2.8	11.3	**21.2**	8.1
	1	0.05	0.15	0.40	0.10	0.30	0.50	0.30	24.0	19.2	9.7	15.8	11.4
3	2	0.10	0.15	**0.20**	0.20	0.30	**0.5**	1.7	7.0	**67.1**	8.3	10.9	**31.3**
	1	0.05	0.10	0.15	0.10	0.20	0.40	0	1.9	19.8	8.2	7.9	11.9
4	2	0.10	0.40	0.60	0.30	0.50	0.60	16.3	25.4	0.2	16.1	15.1	3.7
	1	0.05	**0.20**	0.50	0.20	**0.40**	0.55	3.9	**46.2**	3.1	14.2	**22.3**	5.7
5	2	0.10	**0.20**	0.50	0.20	**0.40**	0.50	4.2	**41.8**	9.3	10.6	**20.3**	10.7
	1	0.05	0.15	**0.20**	0.10	0.30	**0.40**	0.5	10.7	**29.8**	9.5	12.1	**15.0**
6	2	0.40	0.72	0.90	0.44	0.58	0.71	0.5	0	0	3.6	1.6	0.3
	1	**0.23**	0.40	0.59	**0.36**	0.49	0.62	**23.9**	3.7	0	**20.9**	6.0	0.8

1000 trials with three dose levels of Drug A and two dose levels of Drug B. The sample size was 80 patients: 20 for Phase I and 60 for Phase II. We specified the prior toxicity probabilities of Drug A as (0.05, 0.1, 0.2), and those for Drug B as (0.1, 0.2). The target toxicity upper limit $\phi_T = 0.33$, and the target efficacy lower limit $\phi_E = 0.2$. We used $c_e = 0.8$ and $c_d = 0.45$ to direct dose escalation and de-escalation, and $c_a = 0.45$ to define the set of admissible doses in Phase I. We applied the toxicity stopping rule of $\text{pr}(\pi_k < \phi_T) < c_a$ and the futility stopping rule of $\text{pr}(r_k > \phi_E) < c_f$ with $c_f = 0.1$ in Phase II. The decisions of dose assignment and adaptive randomization were made after observing the outcomes of every patient. For each simulated trial, we recorded 2000 posterior samples after 100 burn-in iterations.

Under six scenarios in Table 3.5, we report the selection probability and the number of patients treated at each dose combination. Overall, our method performed very well by yielding high selection probabilities of the target dose combinations, and assigning more patients to the more efficacious doses.

3.6 Conclusion

We have focused on Bayesian adaptive designs in Phase I and Phase I/II dose-finding trials. The BMA-CRM eliminates the arbitrariness in the specification of the skeleton by incorporating the uncertainties associated with each skeleton into the BMA procedure. It is robust, and straightforward to implement using the Gaussian quadrature approximation or the Markov chain Monte Carlo (MCMC).

Phase I/II trial designs simultaneously evaluate toxicity and efficacy to identify the most appropriate dose using the odds-ratio trade-off. The odds ratio has an objective interpretation of quantifying the relative degree of toxicity versus efficacy. The design efficiently uses all of the available data resources and seamlessly bridges the Phase I and II trials.

To accommodate the enormous need for designing clinical trials with drug combinations, a copula-type model can be used to link the joint toxicity probability with the toxicity probabilities of each drug. The Bayesian copula-type design can fully evaluate the joint toxicity profile of the combined drugs, as well as preserve their single-agent properties. It efficiently reorders the toxicity probabilities of the dose combinations based on the accrued data, so that each newly arrival cohort of patients will receive the most appropriate dose. In a typical drug-combination trial, the doses of each drug are often bounded by the corresponding single-agent MTDs for which the toxicity probabilities are known from previous studies. Therefore, the prespecified toxicity probabilities of each drug are much more accurate than the usual CRM for single-agent cases in the entire range of (0, 1).

Due to the toxicity equivalence contour in the two-dimensional dose-combination space, multiple MTD combinations with similar toxicity may be identified in Phase I. Thus, Phase II with adaptive randomization is natural and ethical in order to assign more patients to more efficacious doses. The Bayesian MCMC procedure can coherently update the posterior estimates for the model parameters as more patients enter the trial and more outcomes are observed. The Bayesian adaptive designs are flexible, able to incorporate prior knowledge, and achieve the goals of pulling information and borrowing strength from all the aspects of the trial.

References

Babb, J., Rogatko, A., and Zacks, S. (1998). Cancer phase I clinical trials: Efficient dose escalation with overdose control. *Statistics in Medicine,* 17:1103–20.

Braun, T. M. (2002). The bivariate continual reassessment method: Extending the CRM to phase I trials of two competing outcomes. *Controlled Clinical Trials,* 23:240–56.

Chevret, S. (2006). *Statistical Methods for Dose-Finding Experiments.* England: John Wiley and Sons Ltd.

Conaway, M. R., Dunbar, S., and Peddada, S. D. (2004). Designs for single- or multiple-agent phase I trials. *Biometrics,* 60:661–69.

Dale, J. R. (1986). Global cross-ratio models for bivariate, discrete, ordered responses. *Biometrics,* 42:909–17.

Durham, S. D., Flournoy, N., and Rosenberger, W. F. (1997). A random walk rule for Phase I clinical trials. *Biometrics,* 53:745–60.

Faries, D. (1994). Practical modification of the continual reassessment methods for Phase I cancer clinical trials. *Journal of Biophamaceutical Statistics,* 4:147–64.

Gilks, W. R., Best, N. G., and Tan, K. K. C. (1995). Adaptive rejection Metropolis sampling within Gibbs sampling. *Applied Statistics,* 44:455–72.

Goodman, S. N., Zahurak, M. L., and Piantadosi, S. (1995). Some practical improvements in the continual reassessment method for phase I studies. *Statistics in Medicine,* 14:1149–61.

Gooley, T. A., Martin, P. J., Fisher, L. D., and Pettinger, M. (1994). Simulation as a design tool for phase I/II clinical trials: An example from bone marrow transplantation. *Controlled Clinical Trial,* 15:450–62.

Heyd, J. M., and Carlin, P. B. (1999). Adaptive design improvements in the continual reassessment method for phase I studies. *Statistics in Medicine,* 18:1307–21.

Hoeting, J. A., Madigan, D., Raftery, A. E., and Volinsky, C. T. (1999). Bayesian model averaging: A tutorial. *Statistical Science,* 14:382–401.

Ishizuka, N., and Ohashi, Y. (2001). The continual reassessment method and its applications: A Bayesian methodology for phase I cancer clinical trials. *Statistics in Medicine,* 20:2661–81.

Korn, E. L., and Simon, R. (1993). Using the tolerable-dose diagram in the design of phase I combination chemotherapy trials. *Journal of Clinical Oncology,* 11:794–801.

Kramar, A., Lebecq, A., and Candalh, E. (1999). Continual reassessment methods in phase I trials of the combination of two drugs in oncology. *Statistics in Medicine,* 18:1849–64.

Kuzuya, K., Ishikawa, H., Nakanishi, T., Kikkawa, F., Nawa, A., Fujimura, H., Iwase, A., et al. (2001). Optimal doses of paclitaxel and carboplatin combination chemotherapy for ovarian cancer: A phase I modified continual reassessment method study. *International Journal of Clinical Oncology,* 6:271–78.

Leung, D. H.-Y., and Wang, Y.-G. (2002). An extension of the continual reassessment method using decision theory. *Statistics in Medicine,* 21:51–63.

Møller, S. (1995). An extension of the continual reassessment methods using a preliminary up-and-down design in a dose finding study in cancer patients, in order to investigate a greater range of doses. *Statistics in Medicine,* 14:911–22.

Nelsen, R. B. (1999). *An Introduction to Copulas*. New York: Springer-Verlag.

O'Quigley, J., and Chevret, S. (1991). Methods for dose finding studies in cancer clinical trials: A review and results of a Monte Carlo study. *Statistics in Medicine,* 10:1647–64.

O'Quigley, J., Hughes, M. D., and Fenton, T. (2001). Dose-finding designs for HIV studies. *Biometrics,* 57:1018–29.

O'Quigley, J., Pepe, M., and Fisher, L. (1990). Continual reassessment method: A practical design for phase 1 clinical trials in cancer. *Biometrics,* 46:33–48.

O'Quigley, J., and Shen, L. Z. (1996). Continual reassessment method: A likelihood approach. *Biometrics,* 52:673–84.

Piantadosi, S., Fisher, J., and Grossman, S. (1998). Practical implementation of a modified continual reassessment method for dose finding trials. *Cancer Chemotherapy and Pharmacology,* 41:429–36.

Raftery, A. E., Madigan, D., and Hoeting, J. A. (1997). Bayesian model averaging for linear regression models. *Journal of the American Statistical Association,* 92:179–91.

Storer, B. E. (1989). Design and analysis of phase I clinical trials. *Biometrics,* 45:925–37.

Stylianou, M., and Flournoy, N. (2002). Dose finding using the biased coin up-and-down design and isotonic regression. *Biometrics,* 58:171–77.

Thall, P. F., and Cook, J. (2004). Dose-finding based on toxicity-efficacy trade-offs. *Biometrics,* 60:684–93.

Thall, P. F., Millikan, R. E., Müller, P., and Lee, S.-J. (2003). Dose-finding with two agents in Phase I oncology trials. *Biometrics,* 59:487–96.

Wang, K., and Ivanova, A. (2005). Two-dimensional dose finding in discrete dose space. *Biometrics,* 61:217–22.

Whitehead, J., and Brunier, H. (1995). Bayesian decision procedures for dose determining experiments. *Statistics in Medicine,* 14:885–93.

Yin, G., Li, Y., and Ji, Y. (2006). Bayesian dose-finding in Phase I/II clinical trials using toxicity and efficacy odds ratios. *Biometrics,* 62:777–84.

Yin, G., and Yuan, Y. (2009a). Bayesian model averaging continual reassessment method in phase I clinical trials. *Journal of the American Statistical Association,* 104:954–68.

Yin, G., and Yuan, Y. (2009b). A latent contingency table approach to dose-finding for combinations of two agents. *Biometrics,* 65:866–75.

Yin, G., and Yuan, Y. (2009c). Bayesian dose-finding in oncology for drug combinations by copula regression. *Journal of the Royal Statistical Society C,* 58:211–24.

Yin, G., and Yuan, Y. (2010). Rejoinder to the correspondence of Gasparini, Bailey and Neuenschwander on "Bayesian dose finding in oncology for drug combinations by copula regression." *Journal of Royal Statistical Society C-Applied Statistics,* 59:544–46.

Yuan, Y., and Yin, G. (2008). Sequential continual reassessment method for two-dimensional dose finding. *Statistics in Medicine,* 27:5664–78.

Yuan, Y., and Yin, G. (2009). Bayesian dose finding by jointly modeling toxicity and efficacy as time-to-event outcomes. *Journal of Royal Statistical Society C,* 58:719–36.

Yuan, Y., and Yin, G. (2010). Bayesian Phase I/II drug-combination trial design in oncology. *Annals of Applied Statistics,* in revision.

Yuan, Z., Chappell, R., and Bailey, H. (2007). The continual reassessment method for multiple toxicity grades: A Bayesian quasi-likelihood approach. *Biometrics,* 63:173–79.

4

The Impact of Protocol Amendments in Adaptive Trial Designs

Shein-Chung Chow
Duke University School of Medicine

Annpey Pong
Merck Research Laboratories

4.1 Introduction

In one of their publications, the Pharmaceutical Research Manufacturer Association (PhRMA) Working Group on Adaptive Design defines an adaptive design as a clinical trial design that uses accumulating data to decide on how to modify aspects of the study as it continues, without undermining the validity and integrity of the trial (Gallo et al. 2006). PhRMA's definition emphasizes the feature by design adaptations rather than ad hoc adaptations. Based on adaptations applied, Chow, Chang, and Pong (2005) classified adaptive trials into different types of adaptive design including adaptive group sequential design (see e.g., Kelly, Stallard, and Todd 2005; Kelly et al. 2005), adaptive dose finding design (see, e.g., Bornkamp et al. 2007; Krams et al. 2007), and (two-stage) adaptive seamless design (see, e.g., Maca et al. 2006; Chow 2008). An adaptation is referred to as a modification or a change made to trial procedures and/or statistical methods before, during, and after the conduct of a clinical trial. By definition, adaptations that are commonly employed in clinical trials can be classified into the categories of prospective adaptation, concurrent adaptation, and retrospective adaptation. Prospective adaptations include, but are not limited to, stopping a trial early due to safety, futility, or efficacy at interim analysis, dropping the losers (or inferior treatment groups), sample size reestimation, and so on. Thus, prospective adaptations are usually referred to as *by design* adaptations described in the PhRMA white paper (Gallo et al. 2006). Concurrent (or ad hoc) adaptations include, but are not limited to, any modifications made to trial procedure such as inclusion/exclusion criteria, evaluability criteria, dose/regimen, and treatment duration, and so on. Retrospective adaptation is usually referred to as changes in the statistical analysis plan, which often occur prior to database lock or unblinding. In practice, prospective and ad hoc adaptations are implemented by study protocol and protocol amendments, respectively. Note that for significant (or major) adaptations (changes) in the statistical analysis plan, a protocol amendment is necessarily implemented. It also should be noted that by design adaptations are not flexible as an adaptive design means to be. On the other hand, ad hoc adaptations via protocol amendments reflects real clinical practice, which give clinical investigators a lot of flexibility for identifying best clinical benefits of the test treatment under investigation. Retrospective adaptations derive the most appropriate statistical methods for data analysis without undermining the validity and integrity of the trial. In this chapter, our emphasis will be placed on the impact of protocol amendments in clinical trials utilizing adaptive design methods.

In clinical trials, it is not uncommon to issue protocol amendments during the conduct of a clinical trial. The protocol amendments are necessary to describe what changes have been made and the rationales or justifications (both statistically and clinically) behind the changes to ensure the validity and integrity of the clinical trial. As a result of the changes or modifications, the original target patient population under study could have become a similar but different patient population. If the changes or modifications are made frequently during the conduct of the trial, the target patient population is in fact a moving target patient population. In practice, there is a risk that major (or significant) modifications made to the trial procedures and/or statistical procedures could lead to a totally different trial, which cannot address the scientific/medical questions that the clinical trial is intended to answer. In practice, it should be recognized that protocol amendments are not given gifts. Potential risks for introducing additional bias/variation as the result of modifications made should be carefully evaluated before the issue of a protocol amendment. It is important to identify, control, and hopefully eliminate/minimize the sources of bias/variation. Thus, it is of interest to measure the impact of changes or modifications that are made to the trial procedures and/or statistical methods after the protocol amendment.

In current practice, standard statistical methods are applied to the data collected from the actual patient population regardless of the frequency of changes (protocol amendments) that have been made during the conduct of the trial provided that the overall type I error is controlled at the prespecified level of significance. This, however, has raised a serious regulatory/statistical concern on whether the resultant statistical inference (e.g., independent estimates, confidence intervals, and p-values) drawn on the originally planned target patient population based on the clinical data from the actual patient population (as the result of the modifications made via protocol amendments) are accurate and reliable? After some modifications are made to the trial procedures and/or statistical methods, the target patient population may have become a similar but different patient population, but also the sample size may not achieve the desired power for detection of a clinically important effect size of the test treatment at the end of the study. In practice, we expect to lose power when the modifications have led to a shift in mean response and/or inflation of variability of the response of the primary study endpoint. As a result, the originally planned sample size may have to adjust. Thus, it is suggested that the relative efficiency at each protocol amendment be taken into consideration for derivation of an adjusted factor for sample size in order to achieve the desired power.

In this chapter, the concept of moving target patient population as the result of protocol amendments is introduced. Also the derivation of a sensitivity index for measuring the degree of population shift is included. The method with covariate adjustment proposed by Chow and Shao (2005) is discussed. Also included in this chapter are alternative approaches considering random covariate and Bayesian approach. Inference based on mixture distribution is described. Brief concluding remarks are given at last.

4.2 Moving Target Patient Population

For a given clinical trial in practice, it is not uncommon to have three to five protocol amendments after the initiation of the clinical trial. One of the major impacts of many protocol amendments is that the target patient population may have been shifted during the process, which may have resulted in a totally different target patient population at the end of the trial. A typical example is the case when significant adaptation (modification) is applied to inclusion/exclusion criteria of the study. Denoted by (μ, σ) the target patient population. After a given protocol amendment, the resultant (actual) patient population may have been shifted to (μ_1, σ_1), where $\mu_1 = \mu + \varepsilon$ is the population mean of the primary study endpoint and $\sigma_1 = C_\sigma$ $(C > 0)$ is the population standard deviation of the primary study endpoint. The shift in target patient population can be characterized by

$$E_1 = \left|\frac{\mu_1}{\sigma_1}\right| = \left|\frac{\mu+\varepsilon}{C\sigma}\right| = |\Delta| \left|\frac{\mu}{\sigma}\right| = |\Delta| E,$$

where

$$\Delta = \frac{1+\varepsilon/\mu}{C},$$

and E and E_1 are the effect size before and after population shift, respectively. Chow, Shao, and Hu (2002) and Chow and Chang (2006) refer to Δ as a sensitivity index measuring the change in effect size between the actual patient population and the original target patient population.

Denote by (μ_i, σ_i) the actual patient population after the ith modification of trial procedure, where $\mu_i = \mu + \varepsilon_i$ and $\sigma_i = C_i\sigma$, $i = 0,1, \ldots, K$. Note that $i = 0$ reduces to the original target patient population (μ, σ). That is, when $i = 0$, $\varepsilon_0 = 0$ and $C_0 = 1$. After K protocol amendments, the resultant actual patient population becomes (μ_K, σ_K), where $\mu_K = \mu + \sum_{i=1}^{K} \varepsilon_i$ and $\sigma_K = \prod_{i=1}^{K} C_i\sigma$. It should be noted that (ε_i, C_i), $i = 1, \ldots, K$ are in fact random variables. As a result, the resultant actual patient population following certain modifications to the trial procedures is a *moving* target patient population rather than a fixed target patient population.

As indicated in Chow and Chang (2006), the impact of protocol amendments on statistical inference due to shift in target patient population (moving target patient population) can be studied through a model that link the moving population means with some covariates (Chow and Shao 2005). However, in many cases, such covariates may not exist or they may exist but are not observed. In this case, it is suggested that inference on Δ be considered to measure the degree of shift in location and scale of patient population based on a mixture distribution by assuming the location or scale parameter is random (Chow, Chang, and Pong 2005). In what follows, statistical inference for the original target patient population for simple cases proposed by Chow and Shao (2005) is briefly described. Some recommendations for improvement are also outlined.

4.3 Statistical Inference with Covariate Adjustment

As indicated earlier, statistical methods of analyzing clinical data should be modified when there are protocol amendments during the trial, since any protocol deviations and/or violations may introduce bias to the conclusion drawn based on the analysis of data assuming without any changes made to the study protocol. For example, the target patient population of the clinical trial is typically defined through the patient inclusion/exclusion criteria. If the patient inclusion/exclusion criteria are modified during the trial, then the resulting data may not be from the target patient population in the original protocol and, thus, statistical methods of analysis have to be modified to reflect this change.

4.3.1 Approach with Fixed Covariate

Chow and Shao (2005) modeled the population deviations due to protocol amendments using some covariates and developed a valid statistical inference that is outlined in this section. For convenience sake, we denote the target patient population by $\mathcal{P}_0$. Parameters related to $\mathcal{P}_0$ are indexed by a subscript 0. For example, in a comparative clinical trial comparing a test treatment and a control, the effect size of the test treatment (or a given study endpoint) is $\mu_{0T} - \mu_{0C}$, where μ_{0T} and μ_{0C} are, respectively, the population means of the test treatment and the control for patients in $\mathcal{P}_0$.

Suppose that there are a total of K possible protocol amendments. Let $\mathcal{P}_k$ be the patient population after the kth protocol amendment, $k = 1, \ldots, K$. As indicated earlier, a protocol change may result in a patient population similar but slightly different from the original target patient population; that is, $\mathcal{P}_k$ may be different from $\mathcal{P}_0$, $k = 1, \ldots, K$. For example, when patient enrollment is too slow due to stringent patient inclusion/exclusion criteria, a typical approach is to relax the inclusion/exclusion criteria to increase the enrollment, which results in a patient population larger than the target patient population. Because of the possible population deviations due to protocol amendments, standard statistical methods may not be appropriate and may lead to invalid inference/conclusion regarding the target patient population.

Let μ_k be the mean of the study variable related to the patient population $\mathcal{P}_k$ after the kth protocol amendment, $k = 1, \ldots, K$. Note that the subscript T or C to indicate the test treatment and the control is omitted for simplicity in general discussion. Suppose that, for each k, clinical data are observed from n_k patients so that the sample mean $\bar{y}_k$ is an unbiased estimator of μ_k, $k = 0, 1, \ldots, K$. Ignoring the difference among $\mathcal{P}_k$'s results in an estimator $\bar{y} = \sum_k n_k \bar{y}_k / \sum_k n_k$, which is an unbiased estimator of a weighted average of μ_k's, not the original defined treatment effect μ_0.

In many clinical trials protocol changes are made by using one or a few covariates. Modifying patient inclusion/exclusion criteria, for example, may involve patient age or ethnic factors. Treatment duration, study dose/regimen, factors related to laboratory testing or diagnostic procedures are other examples of such covariates. Let $\mathbf{x}$ be a (possibly multivariate) covariate whose values are distinct for different protocol amendments. Throughout this article we assume that

$$\mu_k = \beta_0 + \beta' \mathbf{x}_k, \quad k = 0, 1, \ldots, K, \tag{4.1}$$

where β_0 is an unknown parameter, β is an unknown parameter vector whose dimension is the same as $\mathbf{x}$, β' denotes the transpose of β, and $\mathbf{x}_k$ is the value of $\mathbf{x}$ under the kth amendment (or the original protocol when $k = 0$). If values of $\mathbf{x}$ are different within a fixed population $\mathcal{P}_k$, then $\mathbf{x}_k$ is a characteristic of $\mathbf{x}$ such as the average of all values of $\mathbf{x}$ within $\mathcal{P}_k$.

Although $\mu_1, \ldots, \mu_K$ are different from μ_0, Model 4.1 relates them with the covariate $\mathbf{x}$. Statistical inference on μ_0 (or more generally, any function of $\mu_0, \mu_1, \ldots, \mu_K$) can be made based on Model 4.1 and data from $\mathcal{P}_k$, $k = 0,1, \ldots, K$.

4.3.1.1 Conditional Inference

We first consider inference conditional on a fixed set of $K \geq 1$ protocol amendments. Following the notation in the previous section, let $\bar{y}_k$ be the sample mean based on n_k clinical data from $\mathcal{P}_k$, which is an unbiased estimator of μ_k, $k = 0,1, \ldots, K$. Again, a subscript T or C should be added when we consider the test treatment or the control. Under Model 4.1, parameters β_0 and β can be unbiased and estimated by

$$\begin{pmatrix} \hat{\beta}_0 \\ \hat{\beta} \end{pmatrix} = (\mathbf{X}'\mathbf{W}\mathbf{X})^{-1}\mathbf{X}'\mathbf{W}\bar{\mathbf{y}}, \tag{4.2}$$

where $\bar{\mathbf{y}} = (\bar{y}_0, \bar{y}_1, \ldots, \bar{y}_K)'$, $\mathbf{X}$ is a matrix whose kth row is $(1, \mathbf{x}_k')$, $k = 0,1, \ldots, K$, and $\mathbf{W}$ is a diagonal matrix whose diagonal elements are $n_0, n_1, \ldots, n_K$. Here, we assume that the dimension of $\mathbf{x}$ is less or equal to K so that $(\mathbf{X}'\mathbf{W}\mathbf{X})^{-1}$ is well defined. To estimate μ_0, we may use the following unbiased estimator:

$$\hat{\mu}_0 = \hat{\beta}_0 + \hat{\beta}' \mathbf{x}_0.$$

For inference on μ_0, we need to derive the sampling distribution of $\hat{\mu}_0$. Assume first that, conditional on the given protocol amendments, data from each $\mathcal{P}_k$ are normally distributed with a common standard deviation σ. Since each $\bar{y}_k$ is distributed as $N(\mu_k, \sigma^2/n_k)$ and it is reasonable to assume that data from different $\mathcal{P}_k$'s are independent, $\hat{\mu}_0$ is distributed as $N(\mu_0, \sigma^2 c_0)$ with

$$c_0 = (1, \mathbf{x}_0)(\mathbf{X}'\mathbf{W}\mathbf{X})^{-1}(1, \mathbf{x}_0)'.$$

Let s_k^2 be the sample variance based on the data from $\mathcal{P}_k$, $k = 0,1, \ldots, K$. Then, $(n_k - 1)s_k^2/\sigma^2$ has the chi-square distribution with $n_k - 1$ degrees of freedom and, consequently, $(N - K)s^2/\sigma^2$ has the chi-square distribution with $N - K$ degrees of freedom, where

$$s^2 = \sum_k (n_k - 1)s_k^2/(N - K),$$

and $N = \Sigma_k n_k$. Confidence intervals for μ_0 and testing hypotheses related to μ_0 can be carried out using the t-statistic $t = (\hat{\mu}_0 - \mu_0)/\sqrt{c_0 s^2}$.

When $\mathcal{P}_k$'s have different standard deviations and/or data from $\mathcal{P}_k$ are not normally distributed, we have to use approximation by assuming that all n_k's are large. By the central limit theorem, when all n_k's are large, $\hat{\mu}_0$ is approximately normally distributed with mean μ_0 and variance

$$\tau^2 = (1, \mathbf{x}_0)(\mathbf{X}'\mathbf{W}\mathbf{X})^{-1}\mathbf{X}'\mathbf{W}\Sigma\mathbf{X}(\mathbf{X}'\mathbf{W}\mathbf{X})^{-1}(1, \mathbf{x}_0)', \tag{4.3}$$

where Σ is the diagonal matrix whose kth diagonal element is the population variance of $\mathcal{P}_k$, $k = 0,1, \ldots, K$. Large sample statistical inference can be made by using the z-statistic $z = (\hat{\mu}_0 - \mu_0)/\hat{\tau}$ (which is approximately distributed as the standard normal), where $\hat{\tau}$ is the same as τ with the kth diagonal element of Σ estimated by s_k^2, $k = 0, 1, \ldots, K$.

4.3.1.2 Unconditional Inference

In practice, protocol amendments are usually made in a random fashion; that is, the investigator of an on-going trial decides to make a protocol change with certain probability and, in some cases, changes are made based on the accrued data of the trial. Let C_K denote a particular set of K protocol amendments as described in the previous sections and let C be the collection of all possible sets of protocol amendments. For example, suppose that there are a total of M possible protocol amendments indexed by 1, …, M. Let C_k be a subset of $K \le M$ integers; that is,

$$C_K = \{i_1, \ldots, i_K\} \subset \{1, \ldots, M\}.$$

Then, C_K denotes the set of protocol amendments $i_1, \ldots, i_K$ and C is the collection of all subsets of {1, …, M}. In a particular problem, C_K is chosen based on a (random) decision rule ξ (often referred to as adaptation rule) and $P(C_K) = P(\xi = C_K)$, the probability that C_K is the realization of protocol amendments, is between 0 and 1 and $\sum_{C_K \in C} P(C_K) = 1$.

For a particular C_K, let z_{C_K} be the z-statistic defined in the previous section and let $\mathcal{L}(z_{C_K} \mid \xi = C_K)$ be the conditional distribution of z_ξ given $\xi = C_K$. Suppose that $\mathcal{L}(z_{C_K} \mid \xi = C_K)$ is approximately standard normal for almost every sequence of realization of ξ. We now show that $\mathcal{L}(z_\xi)$, the unconditional distribution of z_ξ, is also approximately standard normal. According to Theorem 1 in Liu, Proschan, and Pledger (2002),

$$\mathcal{L}(z_\xi) = E\left[\sum_{C_K \in C} \mathcal{L}(z_{C_K} \mid \xi = C_K) I_{\xi = C_K}\right], \tag{4.4}$$

where $I_\xi = C_K$ is the indicator function of the set $\{\xi = C_K\}$ and the expectation E is with respect to the randomness of ξ. For every fixed real number t, by the assumption,

$$P(z_{C_K} \le t \mid \xi = C_K) \to \Phi(t), \tag{4.5}$$

where Φ is the standard normal distribution function. Multiplying $I_\xi = C_K$ to both sides of Equation 4.5 leads to

$$P(z_{C_K} \le t \mid \xi = C_K) I_{\xi=C_K} \to \Phi(t) I_{\xi=C_K}. \tag{4.6}$$

Since the left-hand side of Equation 4.6 is bounded by 1, by the dominated convergence theorem,

$$\begin{aligned} E\left[P(z_{C_K} \le t \mid \xi = C_K) I_{\xi=C_K}\right] &\to E\left[\Phi(t) I_{\xi=C_K}\right] \\ &= \Phi(t) E\left[I_{\xi=C_K}\right] \\ &= \Phi(t) P(C_K). \end{aligned} \tag{4.7}$$

It follows from Equations 4.4 and 4.7 that

$$\begin{aligned} P(z_\xi \le t) &= \sum\nolimits_{C_K \in C} E\left[P(z_{C_K} \le t \mid \xi = C_K) I_{\xi=C_K}\right] \\ &\to \sum\nolimits_{C_K \in C} \Phi(t) P(C_K) \\ &= \Phi(t). \end{aligned}$$

Hence, a large sample inference can be made using the z-statistic z_ξ.

It should be noted that the finite distribution of z_ξ given by Equation 4.4 may be very complicated. Furthermore, Assumption 4.5; that is, $\mathcal{L}(z_{C_K} \mid \xi = C_K)$ is approximately standard normal for almost every sequence of realization of ξ, has to be verified in each application (via the construction of z_{C_K} and asymptotic theory such as the central limit theorem). Assumption 4.5 certainly holds when the adaptation rule ξ and z_{C_K} are independent for each $C_K \in \mathcal{C}$. For example, when protocol changes are modifying patient inclusion/exclusion criteria, the adaptation rule ξ is related to patient recruiting and, thus, is typically independent of the main study variable such as the drug efficacy. Another example is the adjustments of study dose/regimen because of safety considerations, which may be approximately independent with the drug efficacy. Some other examples can be found in Liu, Proschan, and Pledger (2002).

4.3.2 Alternative Approach with Random Covariate

As indicated earlier, Chow and Shao (2005) assumed x_{ik} is fixed and known so that α_i and β_i can be estimated through a regression between $\bar{y}_{ik}$ and $\bar{x}_{ik}$, where $\bar{y}_{ik}$ and $\bar{x}_{ik}$ are the sample mean of the study endpoint and the sample mean of the fixed known x-covariates, respectively, under treatment i after modification k, $i = 1, \ldots, I$, $k = 0,1, \ldots, K$. Once α_i and β_i are estimated, μ_{i0} can be estimated from $\mu_{i0} = \alpha_i + \beta_i' \bar{x}_{i0}$. In practice, however, x_{ik} is often an observed random covariate vector and Model 4.1 should be replaced by

$$\mu_{ik} = \alpha_i + \beta_i' \nu_{ik}, \quad k = 0,1,\ldots,K, i = 1,\ldots,I, \tag{4.8}$$

where v_{ik} is the population mean of the covariate under treatment i after modification k. Let y_{ikj} be the observed study endpoint from the jth patient under treatment i after amendment k and x_{ikj} be the associated observed covariate, $j = 1, \ldots, n_{ik}$, $k = 0,1, \ldots, K$, $i = 1, \ldots, I$. There is room for improvement by the following two directions.

First, under Model 4.8, we estimate μ_{ik} by $\bar{y}_{ik}$ (the sample mean of $y_{ik1},\ldots,y_{ikn_{ik}}$) and v_{ik} by $\bar{x}_{ik}$ (the sample mean of $x_{ik1},\ldots,x_{ikn_{ik}}$). Then, we estimate α_i and β_i by the weighted least squares estimates $\hat{\alpha}_i$ and $\hat{\beta}_i$ in a "regression" between $\bar{y}_{ik}$ and $\bar{x}_{ik}$ for each fixed i. The parameter μ_{i0} is estimated by $\hat{\mu}_{i0} = \hat{\alpha}_i + \hat{\beta}_i \bar{x}_{i0}$. Statistical inference (such as hypothesis testing and confidence intervals) can be made using $\hat{\mu}_{i0}$ and its exact or asymptotic distribution can be derived accordingly. Second, a more efficient statistical inference can be made if we replace Model 4.8 by the following stronger model:

$$E(y_{ikj} \mid x_{ikj}) = \alpha_i + \beta_i' x_{ikj}, \quad j = 1,\ldots,n_{ik}, k = 0,1,\ldots,K, I = 1,\ldots,I. \tag{4.9}$$

Under this model, we can first fit a regression between y_{ikj} and x_{ikj} for each fixed i to obtain least squares estimates $\hat{\alpha}_i$ and $\hat{\beta}_i$. Then, μ_{i0} is estimated by $\hat{\mu}_{i0} = \hat{\alpha}_i + \hat{\beta}_i' \bar{x}_{i0}$. Statistical inference can be made using $\hat{\mu}_{i0}$ and its exact or asymptotic distribution can be derived. Note that Model 4.9 is stronger than Model 4.8 so that we need to balance the gain in efficiency over bias due to the violation of Model 4.9.

As an alternative to Model 4.8, we may consider a random-deviation model. Suppose that there exist random variables δ_{ik}, $k = 1, \ldots, K$, $i = 1, \ldots, I$, such that

$$\mu_{ik} = \mu_{i0} + \delta_{ik}, \quad k = 1,\ldots,K, i = 1,\ldots,I. \tag{4.10}$$

This means that the population mean after the kth protocol amendment deviates from the mean of the target population by a random effect δ_{ik}. Of course, we may consider combining Models 4.1 and 4.10:

$$\mu_{ik} = \alpha_i + \beta_i' x_{ik} + \delta_{ik}, \quad k = 1,\ldots,K, i = 1,\ldots,I.$$

Under Model 4.10 and the assumptions that, conditional on δ_{ik}'s, y_{ikj}'s are independent with mean μ_{ik} in Model 4.10 and variance σ^2, where y_{ikj} is the study endpoint for the jth patient under treatment i after modification k. Then, the observed data follow a mixed effects model. Consequently, existing statistical procedures for mixed effects models can be applied to the estimation or inference. A further assumption can be imposed to Model 4.10:

$$y_{ikj} = \mu_{i0} + \lambda_k + \gamma_{ik} + \varepsilon_{ikj}, \quad i = 1,\ldots,I, k = 1,\ldots,K, \tag{4.11}$$

where λ_k's are independently distributed as $N(0,\sigma_\lambda^2)$, γ_{ik}'s are independently distributed as $N(0,\sigma_\gamma^2)$, which reflect the "interaction" between treatment and λ_k, ε_{ikj} are independently distributed as $N(0, \sigma^2)$, and λ_k's, γ_{ik}'s, and ε_{ikj}'s are independent. Note that μ_{i0}'s are the parameters of interest and the null hypothesis of interest is usually

$$\mu_{10} = \cdots = \mu_{I0} \quad \text{versus} \quad \mu_{i0}'s \text{ are not all equal.} \tag{4.12}$$

Testing Hypothesis 4.12 under Model 4.11 is straightforward if the data are balanced in the sense of $n_{ik} = n$ for all i and k. For an unbalanced case where n_{ik}'s are not the same, there is no simple commonly accepted testing procedure. Gallo and Khuri (1990) derived an exact test for Hypothesis 4.12 under the unbalanced mixed effects Model 4.11. Although other refinements were developed in Öfversten (1993), Christensen (1996), and Khuri, Mathew, and Sinha (1998), these existing tests do not have explicit forms; so their computation is complicated. Thus, an exact test for Hypothesis 4.12 can be developed, which has similar power to that in Gallo and Khuri (1990). Let $n = \min_{i=1,\ldots,I,k=0,1,\ldots,K}(n_{ik})$ and $(a_{ik1},\ldots,a_{ikn_{ik}})' = \Gamma_{n_{ik}}(1, t_{ij}^{1/2} J'_{n_{ik}-1})'$, $i=1,\ldots,I, k=0,1,\ldots,K$, where $t_{ik} = n^{-1} - n_{ik}^{-1} / n_{ik} - 1$ (when $n_{ik} = 1$, a_{ik1} is understood as 1), J_m is the m-vector of ones, and

$$\Gamma_m = \begin{pmatrix} \frac{1}{\sqrt{m}} & \frac{-1}{\sqrt{2}} & \frac{-1}{\sqrt{6}} & \cdots & \frac{-1}{\sqrt{m(m-1)}} \\ \frac{1}{\sqrt{m}} & \frac{1}{\sqrt{2}} & \frac{-1}{\sqrt{6}} & \cdots & \frac{-1}{\sqrt{m(m-1)}} \\ \frac{1}{\sqrt{m}} & 0 & \frac{2}{\sqrt{6}} & \cdots & \frac{-1}{\sqrt{m(m-1)}} \\ \vdots & \vdots & \vdots & \ddots & \vdots \\ \frac{1}{\sqrt{m}} & 0 & 0 & \cdots & \frac{m-1}{\sqrt{m(m-1)}} \end{pmatrix}.$$

Consider the transformation $r_{ik} = \bar{y}_{ik} + \sum_{j=1}^{n_{ik}} a_{ikj}(y_{ikj} - \bar{y}_{ik})$. Then, r_{ik}'s follow the mixed effects model

$$r_{ik} = \mu_i + \lambda_k + e_{ik}, \quad i=1,\ldots,I, k=0,1,\ldots,K, \tag{4.13}$$

where the λ_k's and the e_{ik}'s are independent, $\lambda_k \sim N(0,\sigma_\lambda^2)$, and $e_{ik} \sim N(0, \sigma_\gamma^2 + \sigma^2/n)$. Note that Model 4.13 is a mixed effects model with no interaction, no replicates, and homogenous error variance $\sigma_\gamma^2 + \sigma^2/d$. Under such a "balanced" and "additive" model, it is apparent that we can obtain an exact test for Hypothesis 4.12 based on the F-ratio [SSA/(I-1)]/[SSAB/(I-1)(K-1)], where

$$\text{SSA} = (K+1)\sum_{i=1}^{I}\left(\frac{1}{K+1}\sum_{k=0}^{K} r_{ik} - \frac{1}{I(K+1)}\sum_{i=1}^{I}\sum_{k=0}^{K} r_{ik}\right)^2$$

and

$$\text{SSAB} = \sum_{i=1}^{I}\sum_{k=0}^{K}\left(r_{ik} - \frac{1}{K+1}\sum_{k=0}^{K} r_{ik} - \frac{1}{I}\sum_{i=1}^{I} r_{ik} + \frac{1}{I(K+1)}\sum_{i=1}^{I}\sum_{k=0}^{K} r_{ik}\right)^2.$$

4.3.3 Bayesian Approach

Under Model 4.10, we may adopt a Bayesian approach. For simplicity, consider the case where $I = 2$ and $n_{ik} = n$ for all i and k. Let $\theta_k = \mu_{1k} - \mu_{2k} = \theta + \delta_k$, $k = 1, \ldots, K$, where $\theta = \mu_{10} - \mu_{20}$ and $\delta_k = \delta_{1k} - \delta_{2k}$. Let $d_k = \bar{y}_{1k} - \bar{y}_{2k}$, $k = 0, 1, \ldots, K$, where $\bar{y}_{ik}$ is the sample mean of the study endpoint under treatment i after modification k. Assume that δ_k's and d_k's are independent, $d_k \sim N(0, \sigma^2)$, and $\delta_k \sim N(0, \tau^2)$. The unknown parameters are θ, σ, and τ.

Suppose that the null hypothesis of interest is $\theta = 0$. Under the Bayesian frame work, we need priors for θ, σ^2, and τ^2. Once priors are chosen, we can calculate the posterior probability $P(\theta = 0|d)$, where $d = (d_0, d_1, \ldots, d_K)$. Suppose that the prior for $1/\sigma^2$ is $\Gamma(\alpha_1, \gamma_1)$ and the prior for $1/\tau^2$ is $\Gamma(\alpha_0, \gamma_0)$, where γ_0, γ_1, α_0, α_1 are known, the prior for θ has a point mass p at 0 and, for $\theta \neq 0$, the prior has a density $f(\theta)=1-p/\eta\sqrt{2\pi}\exp(-\theta^2/2\eta^2)$, $\theta \neq 0$, and p and η are assumed to be known. Then, $P(\theta = 0|d) = B/B + C$, where

$$B=\frac{p\left(\sqrt{\frac{n}{2\pi}}\right)^K}{\Gamma(\alpha_1)\gamma_1^{\alpha_1}\Gamma(\alpha_0)\gamma_0^{\alpha_0}}\int_0^\infty\int_0^\infty\frac{\left(\sigma^2\right)^{-1-1/2-\alpha_1}\left(\tau^2\right)^{-1-\alpha_0}}{(n\tau^2+\sigma^2)^{(K-1)/2}}$$

$$\times\exp\left(-\frac{1}{\sigma^2\gamma_1}-\frac{1}{\tau^2\gamma_0}-\frac{nd_0^2}{2\sigma^2}-\frac{n\sum_{k=1}^K d_k^2}{2(n\tau^2+\sigma^2)}\right)d\sigma^2 d\tau^2$$

and

$$C=\frac{(1-p)n^{K/2}}{\eta(2\pi)^K\Gamma(\alpha_1)\gamma_1^{\alpha_1}\Gamma(\alpha_0)\gamma_0^{\alpha_0}}\int_0^\infty\int_0^\infty\left(\sigma^2\right)^{-1-K/2-\alpha_1}\left(\tau^2\right)^{-1-(K-1)/2-\alpha_0}$$

$$\times\left(\frac{2\pi\sigma^2\tau^2}{n\tau^2+\sigma^2}\right)^{(K-1)/2}\sqrt{\frac{2\pi}{\left(\frac{n(K-1)}{n\tau^2+\sigma^2}+\frac{1}{\eta^2}+\frac{n}{\sigma^2}\right)}}\exp\left(-\frac{1}{\sigma^2\gamma_1}-\frac{1}{\tau^2\gamma_0}\right)$$

$$\times\exp\left(-\frac{1}{2}\left(\frac{n\sum_{k=1}^K d_k^2}{n\tau^2+\sigma^2}+\frac{nd_0^2}{\sigma^2}\right)+\frac{\left(\frac{n\sum_{k=1}^K d_k}{n\tau^2+\sigma^2}+\frac{nd_0}{\sigma^2}\right)^2}{2\left(\frac{n(K-1)}{n\tau^2+\sigma^2}+\frac{1}{\eta^2}+\frac{n}{\sigma^2}\right)}\right)d\sigma^2 d\tau^2.$$

For future methodology development based on statistical inference with covariate adjustment, it is of interest to consider (i) a more complex situations such as unequal sample sizes n_{ik} and/or unequal variances after protocol amendments, (ii) deriving approximations to the integrals involved in the posterior probabilities, (iii) studying robustness of the choices of prior parameters, and (iv) alternative forms of null hypotheses such as $-a \leq \theta \leq a$ with a given $a > 0$.

4.4 Inference Based on Mixture Distribution

The primary assumption of the above approaches is that there is a relationship between μ_{ik}'s and a covariate vector x. As indicated earlier, such covariates may not exist or may not be observable in practice. In this case, Chow, Chang, and Pong (2005) suggested assessing the sensitivity index and consequently deriving a unconditional inference for the original target patient population assuming that the shift parameter (i.e., ε) and/or the scale parameter (i.e., C) is random. It should be noted that effect of ε_i could be offset by C_i for a given modification i as well as by (ε_j C_j) for another modification j. As a result, estimates of the effects of (ε_i, C_i), $i = 1, \ldots, K$ are difficult, if not impossible, to obtain. In practice, it is desirable to limit the combined effects of (ε_i, C_i), $i = 0, \ldots, K$ to an acceptable range for a valid and unbiased assessment of treatment effect regarding the target patient population based on clinical data collected from the actual patient population.

The shift and scale parameters (i.e., ε and C) of the target population after a modification (or a protocol amendment) is made can be estimated by

$$\hat{\varepsilon}=\hat{\mu}_{Actual}-\hat{\mu},$$

and

$$\hat{C} = \hat{\sigma}_{Actual} / \hat{\sigma},$$

respectively, where $(\hat{\mu}, \hat{\sigma})$ and $(\hat{\mu}_{Actual}, \hat{\sigma}_{Actual})$ are some estimates of (μ, σ) and $(\mu_{Actual}, \sigma_{Actual})$, respectively. As a result, the sensitivity index can be estimated by

$$\hat{\Delta} = \frac{1 + \hat{\varepsilon} / \hat{\mu}}{\hat{C}}.$$

Estimates for μ and σ can be obtained based on data collected prior to any protocol amendments are issued. Assume that the response variable x is distributed as $N(\mu, \sigma^2)$. Let x_{ij}, $i = 1, \ldots, n_j$; $j = 0, \ldots, m$ be the response of the ith patient after the jth protocol amendment. As a result, the total number of patients is given by

$$n = \sum_{j=0}^{m} n_j.$$

Note that n_0 is the number of patients in the study prior to any protocol amendments. Based on x_{0i}, $i = 1, \ldots, n_0$, the maximum likelihood estimates (MLEs) of μ and σ^2 can be obtained as follows:

$$\hat{\mu} = \frac{1}{n_0} \sum_{i=1}^{n_0} x_{0i}, \tag{4.14}$$

$$\hat{\sigma}^2 = \frac{1}{n_0} \sum_{i=1}^{n_0} (x_{0i} - \hat{\mu})^2. \tag{4.15}$$

To obtain estimates for μ_{Actual} and σ_{Actual} for illustration purpose, in what follows, we will only consider the case where μ_{Actual} is random and σ_{Actual} is fixed.

4.4.1 The Case Where μ_{Actual} is Random and σ_{Actual} is Fixed

We note that the test statistic is dependent of sampling procedure (it is a combination of protocol amendment and randomization). The following theorem is useful. We will frequently use the well-known fact that linear combination of independent variables with normal distribution or asymptotic normal distribution follows a normal distribution. Specifically

---

Theorem 1

Suppose that $X|_{\mu} \sim N(\mu, \sigma^2)$ and $\mu \sim N(\mu_{\mu}, \sigma_{\mu}^2)$, *then:*

$$X \sim N(\mu_{\mu}, \sigma^2 + \sigma_{\mu}^2)$$

Proof

Consider the following characteristic function of a normal distribution $N(t; \mu, \sigma^2)$

$$\phi_0(w) = \frac{1}{\sqrt{2\pi\sigma^2}} \int_{-\infty}^{\infty} e^{iwt - \frac{1}{2\sigma^2}(t-\mu)^2} dt = e^{iw\mu - \frac{1}{2}\sigma^2 w^2}.$$

For distribution $X|_\mu \sim N(\mu, \sigma^2)$ *and* $\mu \sim N(\mu_\mu, \sigma_\mu^2)$, *the characteristic function after exchange the order of the two integrations is given by*

$$\phi(w) = \int_{-\infty}^{\infty} e^{iw\mu - \frac{1}{2}\sigma^2 w^2} N(\mu; \mu_\mu, \sigma_\mu^2) d\mu = \int_{-\infty}^{\infty} e^{iw\mu - \frac{\mu-\mu_\mu}{2\sigma_\mu^2} - \frac{1}{2}\sigma^2 w^2} d\mu.$$

Note that

$$\int_{-\infty}^{\infty} e^{iw\mu - \frac{(\mu-\mu_\mu)^2}{2\sigma_\mu^2}} d\mu = e^{iw\mu - \frac{1}{2}\sigma^2 w^2}$$

is the characteristic function of the normal distribution. It follows that

$$\phi(w) = e^{iw\mu - \frac{1}{2}(\sigma^2 + \sigma_\mu^2) w^2},$$

which is the characteristic function of $N(\mu_\mu, \sigma^2 + \sigma_\mu^2)$. *This completes the proof.* ▪

For convenience's sake, we set $\mu_{Actual} = \mu$ and $\sigma_{Actual} = \sigma$ for the derivation of estimates of ε and C Assume that x conditional on μ, i.e., $x|\mu = \mu_{Actual}$ follows a normal distribution $N(\mu, \sigma^2)$ That is,

$$x|_{\mu=\mu_{Actual}} \sim N(\mu, \sigma^2), \tag{4.16}$$

where μ is distributed as $N(\mu_\mu, \sigma_\mu^2)$ and σ, μ_μ, and σ_μ are some unknown constants. Thus, the unconditional distribution of x is a mixed normal distribution given below

$$\int N(x; \mu, \sigma^2) N(\mu; \mu_\mu, \sigma_\mu^2) d\mu = \frac{1}{\sqrt{2\pi\sigma^2}} \frac{1}{\sqrt{2\pi\sigma_\mu^2}} \int_{-\infty}^{\infty} e^{-\frac{(x-\mu)^2}{2\sigma^2} - \frac{(\mu-\mu_\mu)^2}{2\sigma_\mu^2}} d\mu, \tag{4.17}$$

where $x \in (-\infty, \infty)$ It can be verified that the above mixed normal distribution is a normal distribution with mean μ_μ and variance $\sigma^2 + \sigma_\mu^2$ (see proof given in the next section). In other words, x is distributed as $N(\mu_\mu, \sigma^2 + \sigma_\mu^2)$.

Note that when μ_{Actual} is random and σ_{Actual} is fixed, the shift from the target patient population to the actual population could be substantial especially for large μ_μ and σ_μ^2.

Maximum Likelihood Estimation Given a protocol mendment j and independent observations x_{ji}, $I = 1,2,\ldots,n_j$ the likelihood function is given by

$$l_j = \prod_{i=1}^{n_j} \left(\frac{1}{\sqrt{2\pi\sigma^2}} e^{-\frac{(x_{ij}-\mu_j)^2}{2\sigma^2}} \right) \frac{1}{\sqrt{2\pi\sigma_\mu^2}} e^{-\frac{(\mu_j-\mu_\mu)^2}{2\sigma_\mu^2}}, \tag{4.18}$$

where μ_j is the population mean after the jth protocol amendment. Thus, given m protocol amendments and observations x_{ji} $i = 1, \ldots, n_j$; $j = 0, \ldots, m$, the likelihood function can be written as

$$L = \prod_{j=0}^{m} l_j = \left(2\pi\sigma^2\right)^{-\frac{n}{2}} \prod_{j=0}^{m} \left[e^{-\sum_{i=1}^{n_j} \frac{(x_{ij}-\mu_j)^2}{2\sigma^2}} \frac{1}{\sqrt{2\pi\sigma_\mu^2}} e^{-\frac{(\mu_j-\mu_\mu)^2}{2\sigma_\mu^2}} \right]. \tag{4.19}$$

Hence, the log-likelihood function is given by

$$\begin{aligned} LL = &-\frac{n}{2}\ln\left(2\pi\sigma^2\right) - \frac{m+1}{2}\ln\left(2\pi\sigma_\mu^2\right) \\ &- \frac{1}{2\sigma^2}\sum_{j=0}^{m}\sum_{i=1}^{n_j}(x_{ij}-\mu_j)^2 - \frac{1}{2\sigma_\mu^2}\sum_{j=0}^{m}(\mu_j-\mu_\mu)^2. \end{aligned} \tag{4.20}$$

Based on Equation 4.20, the MLEs of μ_μ σ_μ^2 , and σ^2 can be obtained as follows:

$$\tilde{\mu}_\mu = \frac{1}{m+1}\sum_{j=0}^{m}\tilde{\mu}_j, \tag{4.21}$$

where

$$\tilde{\mu}_j = \frac{1}{n_j}\sum_{i=1}^{n_j} x_{ji}, \tag{4.22}$$

$$\tilde{\sigma}_\mu^2 = \frac{1}{m+1}\sum_{j=0}^{m}(\tilde{\mu}_j - \tilde{\mu}_\mu)^2, \tag{4.23}$$

and

$$\tilde{\sigma}^2 = \frac{1}{n}\sum_{j=0}^{m}\sum_{i=1}^{n_j}(x_{ji} - \tilde{\mu}_j)^2. \tag{4.24}$$

Note that $\partial LL / \partial \mu_j = 0$ leads to

$$\tilde{\sigma}_\mu^2 \sum_{i=1}^{n_j} x_{ji} + \tilde{\sigma}^2\tilde{\mu}_\mu - (n_j\tilde{\sigma}_\mu^2 + \tilde{\sigma}^2)\tilde{\mu}_j = 0.$$

In general, when $\tilde{\sigma}_\mu^2$ and $\tilde{\sigma}^2$ are compatible and n_j is reasonably large, $\tilde{\sigma}^2\tilde{\mu}_\mu$ is negligible as compared to $\tilde{\sigma}_\mu^2 \sum_{i=1}^{n_j} x_{ji}$ and $\tilde{\sigma}^2$ is negligible as compared to $n_j\tilde{\sigma}_\mu^2$. Thus, we have the Approximation 4.22, which greatly simplifies the calculation. Based on these MLEs, estimates of the shift parameter (i.e., ε) and the scale parameter (i.e., C) can be obtained as follows

$$\tilde{\varepsilon} = \tilde{\mu} - \hat{\mu},$$

$$\tilde{C} = \frac{\tilde{\sigma}}{\hat{\sigma}},$$

respectively. Consequently the sensitivity index can be estimated by simply replacing ε, μ, and C with their corresponding estimates $\tilde{\varepsilon}, \tilde{\mu}$, and $\tilde{C}$.

Random Protocol Deviations or Violations In the above derivation, we account for the sequence of protocol amendments assuming that the target patient population has been changed (or shifted) after each protocol amendment. Alternatively, if the cause of the shift in target patient population is not due to the sequence of protocol amendments but random protocol deviations or violations, we may obtain the following alternative (conditional) estimates.

Given m protocol deviations or violations and independent observations x_{ji} i 1, …, n_j; $j = 0, \ldots, m$, the likelihood function can be written as

$$L = \prod_{j=0}^{m} \prod_{i=1}^{n_j} l_{ji}$$

$$= \prod_{j=0}^{m} \left[\left(2\pi\sigma^2\right)^{-\frac{n_j}{2}} e^{-\sum_{i=1}^{n_j} \frac{(x_{ij}-\mu_j)^2}{2\sigma^2}} \left(2\pi\sigma_\mu^2\right)^{-\frac{n_j}{2}} e^{-\frac{n_j(\mu_j-\mu_\mu)^2}{2\sigma_\mu^2}} \right].$$

Thus, the log-likelihood function is given by

$$LL = -\frac{n}{2}\ln\left(2\pi\sigma^2\right) - \frac{n}{2}\ln\left(2\pi\sigma_\mu^2\right) - \frac{1}{2\sigma^2}\sum_{j=0}^{m}\sum_{i=1}^{n_j}(x_{ij}-\mu_j)^2 - \frac{1}{2\sigma_\mu^2}\sum_{j=0}^{m}\left[n_j(\mu_j-\mu_\mu)^2\right]. \tag{4.25}$$

As a result, the MLEs of μ_μ, σ_μ^2, and σ^2 are given by

$$\tilde{\mu}_\mu = \frac{1}{n}\sum_{j=0}^{m}\sum_{i=1}^{n_j} x_{ji} = \hat{\mu}, \tag{4.26}$$

$$\tilde{\sigma}_\mu^2 = \frac{1}{n}\sum_{j=0}^{m}\left[n_j(\tilde{\mu}_j - \tilde{\mu}_\mu)^2\right], \tag{4.27}$$

$$\tilde{\sigma}^2 = \frac{1}{n}\sum_{j=0}^{m}\sum_{i=1}^{n_j}(x_{ji} - \tilde{\mu}_j)^2, \tag{4.28}$$

where

$$\tilde{\mu}_j \approx \frac{1}{n_j}\sum_{i=1}^{n_j} x_{ji}.$$

Similarly, under random protocol violations, the estimates of μ_μ, σ_μ^2, and σ^2 can also be obtained based on the unconditional probability distribution described in Equation 4.17 as follows. Given m protocol amendments and observations x_{ji}, $i = 1, \ldots, n_j$; $j = 0,\ldots, m$, the likelihood function can be written as

$$L = \prod_{j=0}^{m}\prod_{i=1}^{n_j}\left(\frac{1}{\sqrt{2\pi(\sigma^2+\sigma_\mu^2)}}e^{-\frac{(x_{ji}-\mu_\mu)^2}{2(\sigma^2+\sigma_\mu^2)}}\right).$$

Hence, the log-likelihood function is given by

$$LL = -\frac{n}{2}\ln\left[2\pi(\sigma^2+\sigma_\mu^2)\right] + \sum_{j=0}^{m}\sum_{i=1}^{n_j}\frac{(x_{ji}-\mu_\mu)^2}{2(\sigma^2+\sigma_\mu^2)}. \quad (4.29)$$

Based on Equation 4.29, the MLEs of μ_μ, σ_μ^2, and σ^2 can be easily found. However, it should be noted that the MLE for μ_μ and $\sigma_*^2 = (\sigma^2 + \sigma_\mu^2)$ are unique but the MLE for σ^2 and σ_μ^2 are not unique. Thus, we have

$$\tilde{\mu} = \tilde{\mu}_\mu = \frac{1}{n}\sum_{j=0}^{m}\sum_{i=1}^{n_j} x_{ji},$$

$$\tilde{\sigma}^2 = \tilde{\sigma}_*^2 = \frac{1}{n}\sum_{j=0}^{m}\sum_{i=1}^{n_j}(x_{ji}-\tilde{\mu})^2.$$

In this case, the sensitivity index equal to 1. In other words, random protocol deviations or violations (or the sequence of protocol amendments) does not have an impact on statistical inference on the target patient population. However, it should be noted that the sequence of protocol amendments usually result in a moving target patient population in practice. As a result, the above estimates of μ_μ and σ_*^2 are often misused and misinterpreted.

4.4.2 Sample Size Adjustment

4.4.2.1 Test for Equality

To test whether there is a difference between the mean response of a test compound as compared to a placebo control or an active control agent, the following hypotheses are usually considered:

$$H_0: \varepsilon = \mu_1 - \mu_2 = 0 \text{ vs } H_a: \varepsilon \neq 0.$$

Under the null hypothesis, the test statistic is given by

$$z = \frac{\tilde{\mu}_1 - \tilde{\mu}_2}{\tilde{\sigma}_p}, \tag{4.30}$$

where $\tilde{\mu}_1$ and $\tilde{\mu}_2$ can be estimated from Equations 4.21 and 4.22 and σ_p^2 can be estimated using estimated variances from Equations 4.23 through 4.24. Under the null hypothesis, the test statistic follows a standard normal distribution for large sample. Thus, we reject the null hypothesis at the α level of significance if $z > z_{\alpha 2}$.

Under the alternative hypothesis that $\varepsilon \neq 0$, the power of the above test is given by

$$\Phi\left(\frac{\varepsilon}{\tilde{\sigma}_p} - z_{\alpha/2}\right) + \Phi\left(\frac{-\varepsilon}{\tilde{\sigma}_p} - z_{\alpha/2}\right) \approx \Phi\left(\frac{|\varepsilon|}{\tilde{\sigma}_p} - z_{\alpha/2}\right). \tag{4.31}$$

Since the true difference ε is an unknown, we can estimate the power by replacing ε in Equation 4.31 with the estimated value $\tilde{\varepsilon}$. As a result, the sample size needed to achieve the desired power of $1 - \beta$ can be obtained by solving the following equation

$$\frac{|\varepsilon|}{\tilde{\sigma}_e \sqrt{\frac{2}{n}}} - z_{\alpha/2} = z_{\beta}, \tag{4.32}$$

where n is the sample size per group, and

$$\tilde{\sigma}_e = \sqrt{\frac{n}{2} \tilde{\sigma}_p^2} = \sqrt{\frac{\tilde{\sigma}^2}{(m+1)^2} \sum_{j=0}^{m} \left(\frac{n}{n_j}\right) + \frac{n\tilde{\sigma}_\mu^2}{(m+1)}} \tag{4.33}$$

for homogeneous variance condition and balance design. This leads to the sample size formulation

$$n = \frac{4(z_{1-\alpha/2} + z_{1-\beta})^2 \tilde{\sigma}_e^2}{\varepsilon^2}, \tag{4.34}$$

where ε $\tilde{\sigma}^2$, $\tilde{\sigma}_\mu^2$, m, and $r_j = n_j / n$ are estimates at the planning stage of a given clinical trial. The sample size can be easily solved iteratively. Note that if $n_j = n / m + 1$, then

$$n = \frac{4(z_{1-\alpha/2} + z_{1-\beta})^2 \left(\tilde{\sigma}^2 + \frac{n\tilde{\sigma}_\mu^2}{m+1}\right)}{\varepsilon^2}.$$

Solving the above equation for n, we have

$$n = \frac{1}{R} \frac{4(z_{1-\alpha/2} + z_{1-\beta})^2 (\tilde{\sigma}^2 + \tilde{\sigma}_\mu^2)}{\varepsilon^2} = \frac{1}{R} n_{classic}, \tag{4.35}$$

where R is the relative efficiency given by

$$R=\frac{n_{classic}}{n}=\left(1+\frac{\tilde{\sigma}_{\mu}^{2}}{\tilde{\sigma}^{2}}\right)\left(1-\frac{4(z_{1-\alpha/2}+z_{1-\beta})^{2}}{\varepsilon^{2}}\frac{\tilde{\sigma}_{\mu}^{2}}{m+1}\right). \tag{4.36}$$

Table 4.1 provides various m and $\tilde{\sigma}_{\mu}^{2}$ with respect to R. As it can be seen from Table 4.1, an increase of m will result in a decrease of n. Consequently, a significant decrease of the desired power of the intended trial when no amendment $m = 0$ and $\tilde{\sigma}_{\mu}^{2}=0,\ R=1$.

4.4.2.2 Test for Noninferiority/Superiority

As indicated by Chow, Shao, and Wang (2003), the problem of testing noninferiority and (clinical) superiority can be unified by the following hypotheses:

$$H_0:\varepsilon=\mu_1-\mu_2\le\delta \text{ vs } H_a:\varepsilon>\delta,$$

where δ is the noninferiority or superiority margin. When $\delta > 0$, the rejection of the null hypothesis indicates the superiority of the test compound over the control. When $\delta < 0$, the rejection of the null hypothesis indicates the noninferiority of the test compound against the control. Under the null hypothesis, the test statistic

$$z=\frac{\tilde{\mu}_1-\tilde{\mu}_2-\delta}{\tilde{\sigma}_p} \tag{4.37}$$

follows a standard normal distribution for large sample. Thus, we reject the null hypothesis at the α level of significance if $z > z_{\alpha}$.

Under the alternative hypothesis $\varepsilon > 0$, the power of the above test is given by

$$\Phi\left(\frac{\varepsilon-\delta}{\tilde{\sigma}_e\sqrt{\frac{2}{n}}}-z_{\alpha/2}\right). \tag{4.38}$$

The sample size required for achieving the desired power of $1 - \beta$ can be obtained by solving the following equation

$$\frac{\varepsilon-\delta}{\tilde{\sigma}_e\sqrt{\frac{2}{n}}}-z_{\alpha/2}=z_{\beta}. \tag{4.39}$$

TABLE 4.1 Relative Efficiency

m	$\frac{\tilde{\sigma}_{\mu}^{2}}{\tilde{\sigma}^{2}}$	$\frac{\tilde{\sigma}_{\mu}^{2}}{\varepsilon^{2}}$	R
0	0.05	0.005	0.83
1	0.05	0.005	0.94
2	0.05	0.005	0.98
3	0.05	0.005	0.99
4	0.05	0.005	1.00

Note: $\alpha = 0.05$, $\beta = 0.1$.

This leads to

$$n = \frac{2(z_{1-\alpha} + z_{1-\beta})^2 \tilde{\sigma}_e^2}{(\varepsilon - \delta)^2}, \tag{4.40}$$

where $\tilde{\sigma}_e^2$ is given by Equation 4.33, and ε, $\tilde{\sigma}^2$, $\tilde{\sigma}_\mu^2$, m, and $r_j = n_j / n$ are estimates at the planning stage of a given clinical trial. The sample size can be easily solved iteratively. If $n_j = n / m + 1$, then the sample size can be explicitly written as

$$n = \frac{1}{R} \frac{(z_{1-\alpha} + z_{1-\beta})^2 \tilde{\sigma}^2}{(\varepsilon - \delta)^2}, \tag{4.41}$$

where R the relative efficiency given by

$$R = \frac{n}{n_{classic}} = \left(1 - \frac{(z_{1-\alpha} + z_{1-\beta})^2}{(\varepsilon - \delta)^2} \frac{\tilde{\sigma}_\mu^2}{m+1} \right). \tag{4.42}$$

It should be noted that α level for testing noninferiority or superiority should be 0.025 instead of 0.05 because when $\delta = 0$, the test statistic should be the same as that for testing equality. Otherwise, we may claim superiority with a small δ that is close to zero for observing an easy statistical significance. In practice, the choice of δ plays an important role for the success of the clinical trial. It is suggested that δ should be chosen in such a way that it is both statistically and clinically justifiable. Along this line, Chow and Shao (2006) provided some statistical justification for the choice of δ in a clinical trial.

4.4.2.3 Test for Equivalence

For testing equivalence, the following hypotheses are usually considered:

$$H_0 : |\varepsilon| = |\mu_1 - \mu_2| > \delta \text{ vs } H_a : |\varepsilon| \le \delta,$$

where δ is the equivalence limit. Thus, the null hypothesis is rejected and the test compound is concluded to be equivalent to the control if

$$\frac{\tilde{\mu}_1 - \tilde{\mu}_2 - \delta}{\tilde{\sigma}_p} \le -z_\alpha \text{ or } \frac{\tilde{\mu}_1 - \tilde{\mu}_2 - \delta}{\tilde{\sigma}_p^2} \ge z_\alpha. \tag{4.43}$$

It should be noted that the FDA recommends an equivalence limit of (80%, 125%) for bioequivalence based on geometric means using log-transformed data.

Under the alternative hypothesis that $|\varepsilon| \le \delta$, the power of the test is given by

$$\begin{aligned} &\Phi\left(\frac{\delta - \varepsilon}{\tilde{\sigma}_e \sqrt{\frac{2}{n}}} - z_\alpha \right) + \Phi\left(\frac{\delta + \varepsilon}{\tilde{\sigma}_e \sqrt{\frac{2}{n}}} - z_\alpha \right) - 1 \\ &\approx 2\Phi\left(\frac{\delta - |\varepsilon|}{\tilde{\sigma}_e \sqrt{\frac{2}{n}}} - z_\alpha \right) - 1. \end{aligned} \tag{4.44}$$

As a result, the sample size needed in order to achieve the desired power of $1 - \beta$ can be obtained by solving the following equation

$$\frac{\delta - |\varepsilon|}{\tilde{\sigma}_e \sqrt{\frac{2}{n}}} - z_\alpha = z_{\beta/2}. \tag{4.45}$$

This leads to

$$n = \frac{2(z_{1-\alpha} + z_{1-\beta/2})^2 \tilde{\sigma}_e^2}{(|\varepsilon| - \delta)^2}, \tag{4.46}$$

where $\tilde{\sigma}_e^2$ is given by Equation 4.33. If $n_j = n / m + 1$, then the sample size is given by

$$n = \frac{1}{R} \frac{(z_{1-\alpha} + z_{1-\beta/2})^2 \tilde{\sigma}^2}{(|\varepsilon| - \delta)^2}, \tag{4.47}$$

where R is the relative efficiency given by

$$R = \frac{n}{n_{classic}} = \left(1 - \frac{(z_{1-\alpha} + z_{1-\beta/2})^2}{(|\varepsilon| - \delta)^2} \frac{\tilde{\sigma}_\mu^2}{m+1}\right). \tag{4.48}$$

4.4.3 Remarks

In the previous section, we only consider the case where μ_{Actual} is random and σ_{Actual} is fixed. In practice, other cases such as (i) μ_{Actual} is fixed but σ_{Actual} is random, and (ii) both μ_{Actual} and σ_{Actual} are random and do exist. Following a similar idea as described in this section, estimates for μ_{Actual} and σ_{Actual} can be similarly obtained although closed forms of the MLEs may not exist. In this case, the method of EM algorithm may be applied. In addition, since n_j (sample size after the jth protocol amendment) and m (number of protocol amendments) could also be random variables, the following cases that (i) μ_{Actual} σ_{Actual} and n_j are all random, and (ii) μ_{Actual} σ_{Actual} n_j and m are all random may be of interest for obtaining unconditional inference for the original target patient population and/or the actual patient population.

4.5 Concluding Remarks

As pointed out by Chow and Chang (2006), the impact on statistical inference due to protocol amendments could be substantial especially when there are major modifications, which have resulted in a significant shift in mean response and/or inflation of the variability of response of the study parameters. It is suggested that a sensitivity analysis with respect to changes in study parameters be performed to provide a better understanding on the impact of changes (protocol amendments) in study parameters on statistical inference. Thus, regulatory's guidance on *what range of changes in study parameters are considered acceptable?* are necessary. As indicated earlier, adaptive design methods are very attractive to the clinical researchers and/or sponsors due to its flexibility especially in clinical trials of early clinical development. However, it should be noted that there is a high risk for a clinical trial using adaptive design methods failing in terms of its scientific validity and/or its limitation of providing useful information with a desired power especially when the sizes of the trials are relatively small and there are a number of protocol amendments. In addition, statistically it is a challenge to clinical researchers when there are missing values. Missing values could be due to the causes that relate to or are unrelated to the changes or modifications made in the protocol amendments. In this case, missing values must be handled carefully to provide an unbiased assessment and interpretation of the treatment effect.

For some types of protocol amendments, the method proposed by Chow and Shao (2005) gives valid statistical inference for characteristics (such as the population mean) of the original patient population. The key assumption in handling population deviation due to protocol amendments has to be verified in each application. Although a more complicated model (such as a nonlinear model in x) may be considered, Model 4.43 leads to simple derivations of sampling distributions of the statistics used in inference. The other difficult issue in handling protocol amendments (or, more generally, adaptive designs) is the fact that the decision rule for protocol amendments (or the adaptation rule) is often random and related to the main study variable through the accrued data of the on-going trial. Chow and Shao (2005) showed that if an approximate pivotal quantity conditional on each realization of the adaptation rule can be found, then it is also approximately pivotally unconditional and can be used for unconditional inference. Further research on the construction of approximate pivotal quantities conditional on the adaptation rule in various problems is needed.

For sample size calculation and adjustment in adaptive trial designs, it should be noted that sample size calculation based on data collected from pilot studies may not be as stable as expected. Lee, Wang, and Chow (2007) indicated that sample size calculation based on $s^2/\hat{\delta}^2$ is rather unstable. The asymptotic bias of $E(\hat{\theta} = s^2/\hat{\delta}^2)$ is given by

$$E(\hat{\theta}) - \theta = N^{-1}(3\theta^2 - \theta) = 3N^{-1}\theta^2\{1 + o(1)\}.$$

As an alternative, it is suggested that the median of $s^2/\hat{\delta}^2$; that is, $P[s^2/\hat{\delta}^2 \le \eta_{0.5}] = 0.5$ be considered. It can be shown that the asymptotic bias of the median of $s^2/\hat{\delta}^2$ is given by

$$\eta_{0.5} - \theta = -1.5N^{-1}\theta\{1 + o(1)\},$$

whose leading term is linear in θ. As it can be seen, the bias of the median approach can be substantially smaller than the mean approach for a small sample size and/or small effect size. However, in practice, we do not know the exact value of the median of $s^2/\hat{\delta}^2$. In this case, a bootstrap approach may be useful. In practice, when a shift in patient population has occurred, it is recommended the following sample size adjustment based on the shift in effect size be considered:

$$N_S = \min\left\{N_{\max}, \max\left(N_{\min}, \operatorname{sign}(E_0 E_S)\left|\frac{E_0}{E_S}\right|^a N_0\right)\right\},$$

where N_0 and N_s are the required original sample size before population shift and the adjusted sample size after population shift, respectively, $N_{\max}$ and $N_{\min}$ are the maximum and minimum sample sizes, a is a constant that is usually selected so that the sensitivity index Δ is within an acceptable range, and $\operatorname{sign}(x) = 1$ for $x > 0$; otherwise $\operatorname{sign}(x) = -1$.

References

Bornkamp, B., Bretz, F., Dmitrienko, A., Enas, G., Gaydos, B., Hsu, C. H., Konig, F., et al. (2007). Innovative approaches for designing and analyzing adaptive dose-ranging trials. *Journal of Biopharmaceutical Statistics*, 17:965–95.

Chow, S. C. (2008). On two-stage seamless adaptive design in clinical trials. *Journal of Formosan Medical Association*, 107(2):S51–S59.

Chow, S. C., and Chang, M. (2006). *Adaptive Design Methods in Clinical Trials*. New York: Chapman and Hall/CRC Press, Taylor and Francis.

Chow, S. C., Chang, M., and Pong, A. (2005). Statistical consideration of adaptive methods in clinical development. *Journal of Biopharmaceutical Statistics*, 15:575–91.

Chow, S. C., and Shao, J. (2005). Inference for clinical trials with some protocol amendments. *Journal of Biopharmaceutical Statistics*, 15:659–66.

Chow, S. C., and Shao, J. (2006). On margin and statistical test for noninferiority in active control trials. *Statistics in Medicine*, 25:1101–13.

Chow, S. C., Shao, J., and Hu, O. Y. P. (2002). Assessing sensitivity and similarity in bridging studies. *Journal of Biopharmaceutical Statistics*, 12:385–400.

Chow, S. C., Shao, J., and Wang, H. (2003). *Sample Size Calculation in Clinical Research*, 2nd ed. New York: Chapman and Hall/CRC Press, Taylor & Francis.

Christensen, R. (1996). Exact tests for variance components. *Biometrics*, 52:309–14.

Gallo, P., Chuang-Stein, C., Dragalin, V., Gaydos, B., Krams, M., and Pinheiro, J. (2006). Adaptive design in clinical drug development—An executive summary of the PhRMA Working Group (with discussions). *Journal of Biopharmaceutical Statistics*, 16 (3): 275–83.

Gallo, J., and Khuri, A. I. (1990). Exact tests for the random and fixed effects in an unbalanced mixed two-way cross-classification model. *Biometrics*, 46:1087–95.

Kelly, P. J., Sooriyarachchi, M. R., Stallard, N., and Todd, S. (2005). A practical comparison of group-sequential and adaptive designs. *Journal of Biopharmaceutical Statistics*, 15:719–38.

Kelly, P. J., Stallard, N., and Todd, S. (2005). An adaptive group sequential design for phase II/III clinical trials that select a single treatment from several. *Journal of Biopharmaceutical Statistics*, 15:641–58.

Khuri, A. I., Mathew, T., and Sinha, B. K. (1998). *Statistical Tests for Mixed Linear Models*. New York: John Wiley and Sons.

Krams, M., Burman, C. F., Dragalin, V., Gaydos, B., Grieve, A. P., Pinheiro, J., and Maurer, W. (2007). Adaptive designs in clinical drug development: Opportunities challenges, and scope reflections following PhRMA's November 2006 Workshop. *Journal of Biopharmaceutical Statistics*, 17:957–64.

Lee, Y., Wang, H., and Chow, S. C. (2010). A bootstrap-median approach for stable sample size determination based on information from a small pilot study. Submitted.

Liu, Q., Proschan, M. A., and Pledger, G. W. (2002). A unified theory of two-stage adaptive designs. *Journal of American Statistical Association*, 97:1034–041.

Maca, J., Bhattacharya, S., Dragalin, V., Gallo, P., and Krams, M. (2006). Adaptive seamless phase II/III designs—Background, operational aspects, and examples. *Drug Information Journal*, 40:463–74.

Öfversten, J. (1993). Exact tests for variance components in unbalanced mixed linear models. *Biometrics*, 49:45–57.

5

From Group Sequential to Adaptive Designs

Christopher Jennison
University of Bath

Bruce W. Turnbull
Cornell University

5.1 Introduction

In long-term experiments, it is natural to wish to examine the data as they accumulate instead of waiting until the conclusion. However it is clear that, with frequent looks at the data, there is an increased probability of seeing spurious results and making a premature and erroneous decision. To overcome this danger of overinterpretation of interim results, special statistical analysis methods are required. To address this need, the first classic books on sequential analysis were published by Wald (1947), motivated primarily by quality control applications, and by Armitage (1960) for medical trials. In this chapter, we shall be concerned with the latter application. The benefits of monitoring data in clinical trials are obvious:

Administrative. One can check on accrual, eligibility, and compliance, and generally ensure the trial is being carried out as per protocol.

Economic. Savings in time and money can result if the answers to the research questions become evident early—before the planned conclusion of the trial.

Ethical. In a trial comparing a new treatment with a control, it may be unethical to continue subjects on the control (or placebo) arm once it is clear that the new treatment is effective. Likewise if it becomes apparent that the treatment is ineffective, inferior, or unsafe, then the trial should not continue.

It is now standard practice for larger Phase III clinical trials to have a Data Monitoring Committee (DMC) to oversee the study and consider the option of early termination. Note that many of the same considerations apply to animal and epidemiologic studies as well.

It was soon recognized by researchers that fully sequential procedures, with continuous monitoring of the accumulating data, were often impractical and, besides that, much of the economic savings could be achieved by procedures that examined the data on a limited number of occasions throughout the trial—at 6 month intervals, for example, in a multiyear trial. The corresponding body of statistical analysis and design techniques has become known as *group sequential methodology* because the accumulated data are examined after observing each successive *group* of new observations. There is a large body of literature in the biostatistical and medical journals and there have been several comprehensive books published. These include Whitehead (1997), Jennison and Turnbull (2000), and Proschan, Lan, and Wittes (2006). Of related interest are books on the practical considerations for the operation of DMCs by Ellenberg, Fleming, and DeMets (2002) and Herson (2009) and a collection of case studies by DeMets, Furberg, and Friedman (2006).

In this chapter, we shall survey some of the major ideas of group sequential methodology. For more details, the readers should refer to the aforementioned books. In particular, we shall cite most often the book by Jennison and Turnbull (2000)—hereafter referred to as "JT," because clearly it is the most familiar to us! In the spirit of this current volume, we shall also show how much flexibility and adaptability are already afforded by "classical" group sequential procedures (GSPs). Then, we shall show how these methods can naturally be embodied in the more recently proposed adaptive procedures, and vice versa, and consider the relative merits of the two types of procedures. We conclude with some discussion and also provide a list of sources of computer software to implement the methods we describe.

5.2 The Canonical Joint Distribution of Test Statistics

The statistical properties of a GSP will depend on the joint distribution of the accumulating test statistics being monitored and the decision rules that have been specified in the protocol. We start with the joint distribution. For motivation, consider the simple "prototype" example of a balanced two-sample normal problem. Here we sequentially observe responses $X_{A1}, X_{A2}, \ldots$ from Treatment A and $X_{B1}, X_{B2}, \ldots$ from Treatment B. We assume that the $\{X_{Ai}\}$ and $\{X_{Bi}\}$ are independent and normally distributed with common variance σ^2 and unknown means μ_A and μ_B, respectively. Here $\theta = \mu_A - \mu_B$ is the parameter of primary interest.

At interim analysis (or "look" or "stage") k ($k = 1, 2, \ldots$), we have cumulatively observed the first n_k responses from each treatment arm with $n_1 < n_2 < \ldots$. Then the standardized test statistic based on all the responses so far is $Z_k = \sum_{i=1}^{n_k}(X_{Ai} - X_{Bi})/(\sigma\sqrt{2n_k})$. It is easy to verify that the joint distribution of $Z_1, \ldots, Z_K$ has the defining properties:

$$\begin{aligned} &\text{(i)} \quad (Z_1,\ldots,Z_K) \text{ is multivariate normal,} \\ &\text{(ii)} \quad E(Z_k) = \theta\sqrt{\mathcal{I}_k}, \quad k=1,\ldots,K, \text{ and} \\ &\text{(iii)} \quad Cov(Z_{k_1}, Z_{k_2}) = \sqrt{(\mathcal{I}_{k_1}/\mathcal{I}_{k_2})}, \quad 1 \le k_1 \le k_2 \le K, \end{aligned} \tag{5.1}$$

where $\mathcal{I}_k = n_k/(2\sigma^2)$ is termed the *information* or *information level* at stage k.

If a GSP with up to K analyses yields the sequence of statistics $Z_1, \ldots, Z_K$ for the parameter of interest θ, and their joint distribution satisfies Equation 5.1, we say that these statistics have the *canonical joint distribution* with information levels $\{\mathcal{I}_1, \ldots, \mathcal{I}_K\}$ for θ. In fact, this canonical joint distribution arises in a great many situations, not just the balanced two sample normal problem defined above; see Jennison and Turnbull (1997). The list includes unbalanced two-sample comparisons; comparison of normal responses adjusted for baseline covariates; longitudinal data; parallel and crossover designs, and so on. Calculation of the $\{Z_k\}$ defined above requires σ^2 to be known, but if the variance is unknown the theory applies approximately to the sequence of t-statistics. The same canonical joint distribution also holds approximately for binary and survival data. The specific details on how to construct the appropriate $\{Z_k\}$ and $\{\mathcal{I}_K\}$ sequences in each application are described in Chapter 3 of JT. Typically, Z_k is the Wald statistic for testing $\theta = 0$ and $\mathcal{I}_k$ is the reciprocal of the variance of the maximum likelihood (or other efficient) estimator of θ, each based on the accumulated data at stage k. The key conclusion is that statistical properties based on particular decision boundaries can be computed from Equation 5.1 and the results will be applicable to a very wide variety of situations, enabling a unified theory.

5.3 Hypothesis Testing Problems and Decision Boundaries with Equally Spaced Looks

A decision boundary provides critical values for Z_k at each stage k, which determine whether to stop or continue the trial. If the decision is to stop, the action to be taken is also specified. Various shapes for boundaries have been proposed and these shapes depend on the hypotheses about θ to be tested. Initially, we assume a maximum number of looks K is specified and these are to be taken at equal increments of information—that is, $\mathcal{I}_k = (k/K)\mathcal{I}_K$, for $k = 1, \ldots, K$. Later we shall relax this assumption, but it will still be convenient to use the equal information increment assumption initially for planning purposes.

5.3.1 Two-Sided Tests

For a two-sided test, the hypotheses are:

$$H_0 : \theta = 0 \quad \text{versus} \quad H_A : \theta \neq 0.$$

We set Type I and Type II error probability constraints:

$$\Pr_{\theta=0}\{\text{Reject } H_0\} = \alpha, \tag{5.2}$$

$$\Pr_{\theta=\pm\delta}\{\text{Reject } H_0\} = 1 - \beta. \tag{5.3}$$

Here α and β are specified (typical values might be $\alpha = 0.05$ and $\beta = 0.1$ or 0.2), and δ is a given effect size that it is important to detect. A fixed sample test ($K = 1$) that meets these requirements would reject H_0 when $|Z| \geq z_{\alpha/2}$ and requires information

$$\mathcal{I}_{f,2} = (z_{\alpha/2} + z_\beta)^2 / \delta^2, \tag{5.4}$$

where z_γ denotes the upper 100 γ percentage point of the standard normal distribution.

The decision boundary for a procedure with a maximum of K looks takes the form:

$$
\begin{array}{ll}
\multicolumn{2}{l}{\text{After group } k = 1, \ldots, K-1} \\
\quad \text{if } |Z_k| \geq c_k & \text{stop, reject } H_0 \\
\quad \text{otherwise} & \text{continue to group } k+1, \\
\multicolumn{2}{l}{\text{After group } K} \\
\quad \text{if } |Z_K| \geq c_K & \text{stop, reject } H_0 \\
\quad \text{otherwise} & \text{stop and report failure to reject } H_0, \text{ i.e., "accept" } H_0.
\end{array}
$$

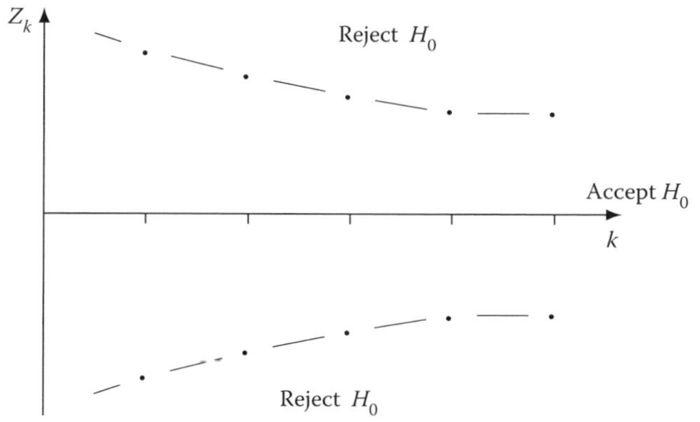

FIGURE 5.1 Two-sided decision boundary for $K = 5$.

A typical boundary for $K = 5$ is illustrated in Figure 5.1.

From Equation 5.1 we see that, in this case of equally spaced information increments, the joint distribution of $Z_1, \ldots, Z_K$ under H_0 does not depend on $\mathcal{I}_K$. Therefore the Type I error rate depends solely on the choice of $c_1, \ldots, c_K$. Once these are chosen to satisfy Equation 5.2, $\mathcal{I}_K$ can be chosen to satisfy Equation 5.3. However, there are still many ways to choose the $\{c_k\}$ to satisfy Equation 5.2. Wang and Tsiatis (1987) suggested a family of boundaries indexed by the parameter γ, in which $c_k = C(k/K)^\gamma$ for $k = 1, \ldots, K$. The value of C is determined by Equation 5.2 and depends on K, α, and the value of γ. Taking $\gamma = 0$ yields a Pocock (1977) boundary where c_k remains constant over k. We denote by $C_p(K, \alpha)$ the value of C for this test with K analyses and type I error probability α, then $c_k = C_p(K, \alpha)$ for each $k = 1, \ldots, K$. The case $\gamma = -1/2$ yields an O'Brien and Fleming (1979) boundary. For this case, we denote the value of C in the Wang and Tsiatis formula by $C_B(K, \alpha)$ and the boundary is $c_k = C_B(K, \alpha)\sqrt{(K/k)}$ for $k = 1, \ldots, K$. These values of c_k decrease with k—similar to those depicted in Figure 5.1. Tables of the constants $C_p(K, \alpha)$ and $C_B(K, \alpha)$ can be found in Pocock (1977), O'Brien and Fleming (1979) and in JT, Chapter 2. The tables in JT also give values of the so-called inflation factor, denoted by R. Then the value of $\mathcal{I}_k$ needed to satisfy Equation 5.3 can be found from the formula $\mathcal{I}_k = R\mathcal{I}_{f,2}$, where $\mathcal{I}_{f,2}$ is given by Equation 5.4. We reproduce Tables 2.1 through 2.4 of JT, Chapter 2 here for ease of reference as Tables 5.1 through 5.4. The constants $C_p(K, \alpha)$ and $C_B(K, \alpha)$ are given in Tables 5.1 and 5.2 and inflation factors $R_p(K, \alpha)$ and $R_B(K, \alpha)$ in Tables 5.3 and 5.4. We discuss the construction of the entries in these tables of constants in Section 5.4.

As an example, suppose we specify an O'Brien and Fleming GSP with a maximum of $K = 5$ analyses and $\alpha = 0.05$. From Table 2.3 of JT, we see that for $\gamma = -1/2$ the constant $C = 2.04$ and the boundary values are $c_1 = 4.56$, $c_2 = 3.23$, $c_3 = 2.63$, $c_4 = 2.28$, and $c_5 = 2.04$. These values can be compared with the fixed sample critical value of $z_{0.025} = 1.96$. The wider boundary values are to compensate for the fact that the test statistic is being examined multiple times (here five). Suppose we additionally ask for power $1 - \beta = 0.9$ at effect size $\pm\delta$. From Table 2.4 of JT, the inflation factor is $R = 1.026$, which means that the maximum information needed will be 2.6% more than the fixed sample test would require. For the prototype two-sample normal problem described at the beginning of Section 5.2, the fixed sample information $\mathcal{I}_{f,2} = (z_{\alpha/2} + z_\beta)^2/\delta^2$ corresponds to a sample size $n_f = 2\sigma^2\mathcal{I}_{f,2}$ per treatment arm. Of course, with the group sequential stopping rule there is a good possibility of stopping earlier than stage K. For example, if $\mu_A - \mu_B = \delta$ the expected information and number of observations at termination are only 76% of their values for the fixed sample test. For $\mu_A - \mu_B = 1.5\delta$ this proportion is 56%; see JT, Table 2.5. The modest increase in maximum information ($R > 1$) is a small price to pay for the advantages of possible early stopping.

Note that this decision boundary does not permit early stopping to accept H_0 (i.e., for *futility*). It is possible to have an "inner wedge" boundary that does allow such a feature, but we shall not discuss this further here. For complete details see JT, Chapter 5.

TABLE 5.1 Constants $C_P(K, \alpha)$ for Pocock Two-Sided Tests With K Groups of Observations and Type I Error Probability α

	$C_P(K, \alpha)$		
K	$\alpha = 0.01$	$\alpha = 0.05$	$\alpha = 0.10$
1	2.576	1.960	1.645
2	2.772	2.178	1.875
3	2.873	2.289	1.992
4	2.939	2.361	2.067
5	2.986	2.413	2.122
6	3.023	2.453	2.164
7	3.053	2.485	2.197
8	3.078	2.512	2.225
9	3.099	2.535	2.249
10	3.117	2.555	2.270
11	3.133	2.572	2.288
12	3.147	2.588	2.304
15	3.182	2.626	2.344
20	3.225	2.672	2.392

Source: From Jennison, C. and Turnbull, B. W., *Group Sequential Methods with Applications to Clinical Trials*. Boca Raton, FL: Chapman & Hall/CRC, 2000. With permission.

TABLE 5.2 Constants $C_B(K, \alpha)$ for O'Brien & Fleming Two-Sided Tests with K Groups of Observations and Type I Error Probability α

	$C_B(K, \alpha)$		
K	$\alpha = 0.01$	$\alpha = 0.05$	$\alpha = 0.10$
1	2.576	1.960	1.645
2	2.580	1.977	1.678
3	2.595	2.004	1.710
4	2.609	2.024	1.733
5	2.621	2.040	1.751
6	2.631	2.053	1.765
7	2.640	2.063	1.776
8	2.648	2.072	1.786
9	2.654	2.080	1.794
10	2.660	2.087	1.801
11	2.665	2.092	1.807
12	2.670	2.098	1.813
15	2.681	2.110	1.826
20	2.695	2.126	1.842

Source: From Jennison, C. and Turnbull, B. W., *Group Sequential Methods with Applications to Clinical Trials*. Boca Raton, FL: Chapman & Hall/CRC, 2000. With permission.

TABLE 5.3 Constants $R_P(K, \alpha, \beta)$ to Determine Group Sizes for Pocock Two-Sided Tests with K Groups of Observations, Type I Error Probability α and Power $1 - \beta$

	$R_P(K, \alpha, \beta)$					
	$1 - \beta = 0.8$			$1 - \beta = 0.9$		
K	$\alpha = 0.01$	$\alpha = 0.05$	$\alpha = 0.10$	$\alpha = 0.01$	$\alpha = 0.05$	$\alpha = 0.10$
1	1.000	1.000	1.000	1.000	1.000	1.000
2	1.092	1.110	1.121	1.084	1.100	1.110
3	1.137	1.166	1.184	1.125	1.151	1.166
4	1.166	1.202	1.224	1.152	1.183	1.202
5	1.187	1.229	1.254	1.170	1.207	1.228
6	1.203	1.249	1.277	1.185	1.225	1.249
7	1.216	1.265	1.296	1.197	1.239	1.266
8	1.226	1.279	1.311	1.206	1.252	1.280
9	1.236	1.291	1.325	1.215	1.262	1.292
10	1.243	1.301	1.337	1.222	1.271	1.302
11	1.250	1.310	1.348	1.228	1.279	1.312
12	1.257	1.318	1.357	1.234	1.287	1.320
15	1.272	1.338	1.381	1.248	1.305	1.341
20	1.291	1.363	1.411	1.264	1.327	1.367

Source: From Jennison, C. and Turnbull, B. W., *Group Sequential Methods with Applications to Clinical Trials.* Boca Raton, FL: Chapman & Hall/CRC, 2000. With permission.

TABLE 5.4 Constants $R_B(K, \alpha, \beta)$ to Determine Group Sizes for O'Brien & Fleming Two-Sided Tests with K Groups of Observations, Type I Error Probability α and Power $1 - \beta$

	$R_P(K, \alpha, \beta)$					
	$1 - \beta = 0.8$			$1 - \beta = 0.9$		
K	$\alpha = 0.01$	$\alpha = 0.05$	$\alpha = 0.10$	$\alpha = 0.01$	$\alpha = 0.05$	$\alpha = 0.10$
1	1.000	1.000	1.000	1.000	1.000	1.000
2	1.001	1.008	1.016	1.001	1.007	1.014
3	1.007	1.017	1.027	1.006	1.016	1.025
4	1.011	1.024	1.035	1.010	1.022	1.032
5	1.015	1.028	1.040	1.014	1.026	1.037
6	1.017	1.032	1.044	1.016	1.030	1.041
7	1.019	1.035	1.047	1.018	1.032	1.044
8	1.021	1.037	1.049	1.020	1.034	1.046
9	1.022	1.038	1.051	1.021	1.036	1.048
10	1.024	1.040	1.053	1.022	1.037	1.049
11	1.025	1.041	1.054	1.023	1.039	1.051
12	1.026	1.042	1.055	1.024	1.040	1.052
15	1.028	1.045	1.058	1.026	1.042	1.054
20	1.030	1.047	1.061	1.029	1.045	1.057

Source: From Jennison, C. and Turnbull, B. W., *Group Sequential Methods with Applications to Clinical Trials.* Boca Raton, FL: Chapman & Hall/CRC, 2000. With permission.

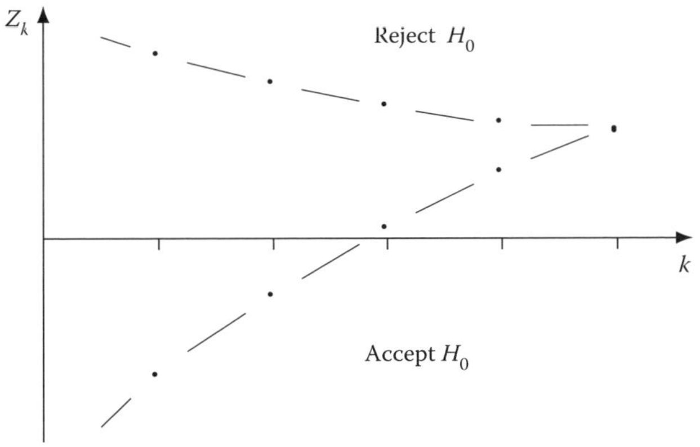

FIGURE 5.2 Decision boundary for a one-sided test with $K = 5$.

5.3.2 One-Sided Tests

Here we test

$$H_0:\theta=0 \quad \text{versus} \quad H_A:\theta>0. \tag{5.5}$$

We set Type I and Type II error probability constraints:

$$\Pr_{\theta=0}\{\text{Reject } H_0\}=\alpha, \tag{5.6}$$

$$\Pr_{\theta=\delta}\{\text{Reject } H_0\}=1-\beta. \tag{5.7}$$

Typical values might be $\alpha = 0.025$ and $\beta = 0.1$ or 0.2. A fixed sample test ($K = 1$) that meets these requirements would reject H_0 when $Z \geq z_\alpha$ and requires information

$$I_{f,1}=(z_\alpha+z_\beta)^2/\delta^2. \tag{5.8}$$

The decision boundary for a procedure with a maximum of K looks takes the form:

$$\begin{array}{ll} \text{After group } k=1,\ldots,K-1 & \\ \quad \text{if } |Z_k|\geq b_k & \text{stop, reject } H_0 \\ \quad \text{if } |Z_k|\leq a_k & \text{stop, accept } H_0 \\ \quad \text{otherwise} & \text{continue to group } k+1, \\ \text{After group } K & \\ \quad \text{if } Z_K\geq b_K & \text{stop, reject } H_0 \\ \quad \text{if } Z_K< a_K & \text{stop, accept } H_0, \end{array} \tag{5.9}$$

where $a_K = b_K$ to ensure termination at analysis K; see Figure 5.2. Typically, tests are designed with analyses at equally spaced information levels (or "group sizes") so $\Delta_1 = \ldots = \Delta_K$ where $\Delta_k = \mathcal{I}_k - \mathcal{I}_{k-1}$, $k = 2, \ldots, K$, and $\Delta_1 = \mathcal{I}_1$. Then, for given K, the maximum information $\mathcal{I}_K$ and boundary values (a_k, b_k), $k = 1, \ldots, K$, can be chosen to satisfy Equations 5.6 and 5.7. Several suggestions for choice of boundary values are described in JT, Chapter 4 and results presented there show savings in expected sample size are achieved under $\theta = 0$ and $\theta = \delta$, and also at intermediate values of θ. We shall discuss this one-sided testing problem in more detail later when we look at the case of unequal and unpredictable increments of information between looks.

5.3.3 One-Sided Tests with a Nonbinding Lower Boundary

The upper boundary in Figure 5.2 is often called the efficacy boundary and the lower one the futility boundary. Sometimes the futility boundary is considered just a guideline; that is, somewhat arbitrary and *nonbinding*, so that investigators may decide to continue a study even though the futility boundary has been crossed with $Z_k < a_k$. In order to protect the Type I error in this case, the left-hand side of Equation 5.6 must be computed assuming $a_1 = \; = a_{K-1} = -\infty$ (i.e., with no lower boundary). This leads to a higher efficacy boundary and a small decrease in power, but the Type I error probability will be maintained whatever futility boundary is actually used—a feature that is often important. If the efficacy boundary is constructed this way, it is still useful to have a futility boundary in mind as a guide to stopping for negative results, but applying this futility boundary can only decrease the Type I error and so Equation 5.6 is always assured.

5.3.4 Other Boundaries

Various other shapes of boundaries could be considered. For example, in a one-sided or two-sided test it may be desirable to stop early only for futility and not for efficacy. Alternatively, the goal might be to demonstrate equivalence or noninferiority. We shall not consider these more specialized situations further here but direct the reader to the references cited in Section 5.1.

5.4 Computations for Group Sequential Tests: Armitage's Iterated Integrals

This section covers some technical computational details and may be omitted at a first reading. We discuss how the Type I error, power, expected information (or sample size), and other statistical properties of GSPs like the one-sided and two-sided tests discussed in Section 5.3 can be computed. Our calculations are relevant for any of the models for accumulating data for which the canonical representation Equation 5.1 applies.

Let $\mathcal{C}_1, \ldots, \mathcal{C}_K$ be subsets of the real line $\Re = (-\infty, \infty)$ representing the continuation regions of a group sequential test. That is, if stage k has been reached, then the procedure stops if $Z_k \notin \mathcal{C}_k$, but otherwise it continues to stage $k + 1$. The sets $\mathcal{C}_k$ need not be intervals, but we must have $\mathcal{C}_K = \varnothing$, the empty set, to ensure termination by stage K. The stopping region at stage k is $\mathcal{C}_k^c$, the complement of $\mathcal{C}_k$, and this may be further partitioned into several sets, indicating the appropriate action to be taken upon stopping. If the only action upon stopping is to choose between accepting and rejecting a null hypothesis H_0, then we have two sets, $\mathcal{A}_k$ and $\mathcal{B}_k$ say, where we stop to accept H_0 at stage k if $Z_k \in \mathcal{A}_k$, and stop to reject H_0 at stage k if $Z_k \in \mathcal{B}_k$. In this case $\mathcal{A}_k \cup \mathcal{B}_k \cup \mathcal{C}_k = (-\infty, \infty)$ is a partition of the real line.

As an example, the two-sided procedures of Section 5.3, are of the above form with

$$\begin{aligned} &\mathcal{A}_k = \varnothing, && \mathcal{B}_k = (-\infty, -c_k) \cup (c_k, \infty), && \mathcal{C}_k = (-c_k, c_k), && \text{for } k = 1, \ldots, K-1, \\ &\mathcal{A}_K = (-c_K, c_K), && \mathcal{B}_K = (-\infty, -c_K) \cup (c_K, \infty), && \mathcal{C}_K = \varnothing. \end{aligned}$$

Similarly, the one-sided procedures of Section 5.3 are of this form but with

$$\mathcal{A}_k = (-\infty, a_k), \qquad \mathcal{B}_k = (b_k, \infty), \qquad \mathcal{C}_k = (a_k, b_k), \qquad k = 1, \ldots, K,$$

where $a_K = b_K$ so $C_K = \emptyset$. Decision boundaries of the other procedures we have mentioned (inner wedge designs, equivalence tests, etc.) can also be described in this way.

We define the stopping time T by

$$T = \min\{k: Z_k \notin C_k\}. \tag{5.10}$$

Note that $1 \leq T \leq K$ since $C_K = \emptyset$. We assume $Z_1, \ldots, Z_K$ have the canonical joint distribution given in Equation 5.1 and define

$$G_k(z;\theta) = \Pr_\theta\{Z_k \leq z, T \geq k\}$$

and

$$g_k(z;\theta) = \frac{\partial}{\partial z} G_k(z;\theta) \tag{5.11}$$

for $k = 1, \ldots, K$, $-\infty < z < \infty$ and $-\infty < \theta < \infty$.

From the subdensity $g_k(z;\theta)$ given by Equation 5.11, we can obtain all the quantities we need. For example, the distribution of the stopping stage is

$$\Pr_\theta\{T = k\} = \int_{C_k^c} g_k(z;\theta)dz, \quad k = 1,\ldots,K.$$

Similarly, the probability that the procedure stops and takes the action associated with the sets $\{\mathcal{A}_k\}$, say, is

$$\Pr_\theta\{\cup_{k=1}^K \mathcal{A}_k\} = \sum_{k=1}^K \int_{\mathcal{A}_k} g_k(z;\theta)dz.$$

This last expression allows us to compute the size and power of our tests.

The quantities $\{g_k(z;\theta)\}$ involve complicated multinormal integrals, the numerical computation of which would appear to be quite difficult, especially for larger values of K, say $K > 5$. However, the computation is facilitated by noting the Markov structure of the sequence $Z_1, Z_2, \ldots$. The recursive formulae of Armitage, McPherson, and Rowe (1969) can be used to calculate each $g_k(z;\theta)$ in turn. These formulae are:

$$g_1(z;\theta) = \varphi(z - \theta\sqrt{\mathcal{I}_1}), \tag{5.12}$$

and for $k = 2, \ldots, K$,

$$g_k(z;\theta) = \int_{C_{k-1}} g_{k-1}(u;\theta)\frac{\sqrt{\mathcal{I}_k}}{\sqrt{\Delta_k}}\varphi\left(\frac{z\sqrt{\mathcal{I}_k} - u\sqrt{\mathcal{I}_{k-1}} - \Delta_k\theta}{\sqrt{\Delta_k}}\right)du, \tag{5.13}$$

where $\varphi(z) = (2\pi)^{-1/2}\exp(-z^2/2)$ denotes the standard normal density.

These equations follow directly from the joint distribution of $\{Z_1, \ldots, Z_K\}$ given by Equation 5.1. The first Equation 5.12 is immediate and Equation 5.13 follows by noting that Equation 5.1 implies the sequence of score statistics $Z_k\sqrt{\mathcal{I}_k}$, $k = 1, \ldots, K$, is Markov with independent normal increments. Thus

$$Z_k\sqrt{\mathcal{I}_k} - Z_{k-1}\sqrt{\mathcal{I}_{k-1}} \sim N(\theta\Delta_k, \Delta_k)$$

and is independent of $Z_1, \ldots, Z_{k-1}$. As before, $\Delta_k = \mathcal{I}_k - \mathcal{I}_{k-1}$ denotes the increment in information between analyses $k - 1$ and k and for notational completeness we define $Z_0 = \mathcal{I}_0 = 0$.

It follows that only a succession of $K - 1$ univariate integrations is needed to evaluate the subdensities $g_k(z; \theta)$ and related probabilities and not a rather complicated K-fold multivariate integral. More details on these computations are given in JT, Chapter 19.

In fact, the computations can be simplified even more by realizing that we only need to carry out the recursive integrations for one value of θ, say $\theta = 0$. Emerson and Fleming (1990) note the following "handy formula" that is useful in converting a subdensity g_k evaluated under one value of θ for computations at another:

$$g_k(z;\theta) = g_k(z;0)\exp(\theta z\sqrt{\mathcal{I}_k} - \theta^2\mathcal{I}_k/2), \quad k = 1,\ldots,K. \tag{5.14}$$

This result clearly holds for $k = 1$. If we assume the result holds for $k - 1$, use of Equation 5.13 and some algebraic manipulation shows it holds for k and then Equation 5.14 follows by induction. This is an example of a likelihood ratio identity; see Siegmund (1985, Propositions 2.24 and 3.2).

The computational methods described in this section are used by the various commercial and free software packages that are widely available to aid implementation of group sequential designs and monitoring of accumulating data. More information on available computer software is provided in Section 5.9.

5.5 Error Spending Procedures for Unequal, Unpredictable Increments of Information

While monitoring the trial, the increments of information at successive analyses may not be equal. For example, if the meetings of the DMC are planned for certain calendar times, variations in subject accrual will imply unequal and unpredictable increments in information. In our normal prototype example of Section 5.2, the information level $\mathcal{I}_k$ at stage k depends on the value of σ^2, which may be unknown and, while the information levels at analysis k can be estimated using the current estimate of σ^2 in the formula $\mathcal{I}_k = n_k/(2\sigma^2)$, this value will not be known in advance. Similarly, if we are collecting binary data and comparing proportions based on a normal approximation to the binomial, the variance will be unknown (JT, Section 3.6) and variance estimates from the accumulating data must be used. In a two-armed trial, when the difference between two treatments is adjusted for baseline covariates, the information at each stage depends on the baseline data that are only observed as subjects enter the study. For survival data endpoints, information is approximately proportional to the total number of events that have occurred so, again, increments are likely to be unequal and unpredictable.

Lan and DeMets (1983) presented two-sided tests that "spend" Type I error as a function of observed information. These methods start with the definition of a (Type I) error spending function $f(\mathcal{I})$. A typical function is depicted in Figure 5.3. It can be any nondecreasing function with $f(0) = 0$ and $f(\mathcal{I}) = \alpha$ for $\mathcal{I} \geq \mathcal{I}_{max}$. The choice of $\mathcal{I}_{max}$ is discussed below.

The critical value c_k for the stopping boundary at analysis k is chosen to give cumulative Type I error probability $f(\mathcal{I}_k)$ at stage k. The null hypothesis H_0 is accepted if $\mathcal{I}_{max}$ is reached without earlier rejection of H_0. The critical values $\{c_k\}$ are computed iteratively. At the first analysis, the information $\mathcal{I}_1$ is observed and c_1 is obtained by solving the equation: $\Pr_{\theta=0}\{|Z_1| \geq c_1\} = f(\mathcal{I}_1)$. The test stops and rejects H_0 if $|Z_1| > c_1$ and continues otherwise. Now suppose we are at stage $k \geq 2$ and we have observed $\mathcal{I}_1, \ldots, \mathcal{I}_k$. Having already obtained critical values $c_1, \ldots, c_{k-1}$ at the previous analyses, we compute the current critical value c_k by solving for it in the equation:

$$\Pr_{\theta=0}\{|Z_1| < c_1, \ldots, |Z_{k-1}| < c_{k-1}, |Z_k| \geq c_k\} = f(\mathcal{I}_k) - f(\mathcal{I}_{k-1}).$$

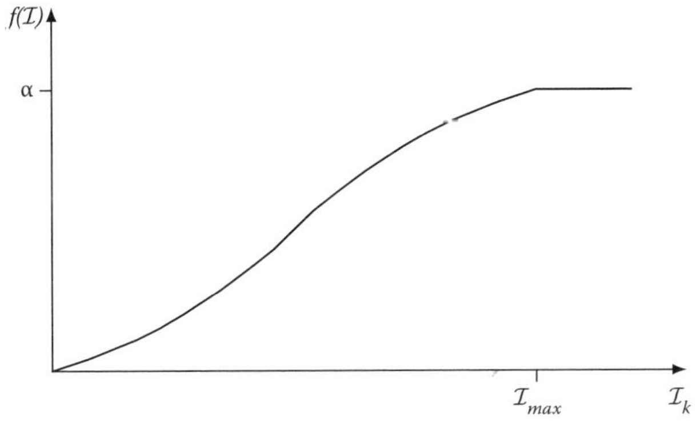

FIGURE 5.3 A typical error spending function.

This equation can be solved numerically using the computational formulae of Section 5.4. Note that computation of c_k does *not* depend on future information levels, $\mathcal{I}_{k+1}, \mathcal{I}_{k+2}, \ldots$. In a "maximum information design" the study continues until a boundary is crossed or an analysis reached with $\mathcal{I}_k \geq \mathcal{I}_{max}$. The maximum number of analyses K does not have to be prespecified in advance but if a particular maximum K is so specified, the study terminates at analysis K with $f(\mathcal{I}_K)$ defined to be α even if $\mathcal{I}_K < \mathcal{I}_{max}$. The value of $\mathcal{I}_{max}$ should be chosen to meet the desired power requirement under a typical or anticipated sequence of information levels. A usual choice is the equally spaced one; that is, $\mathcal{I}_k = (k/K)\mathcal{I}_{max}$ for $k = 1, \ldots, K$ with a prespecified K. Chapter 7 of JT presents the family of error spending functions $f(\mathcal{I}) = \min\{\alpha, \alpha(\mathcal{I}/\mathcal{I}_{max})^{\rho}\}$, $\mathcal{I} \geq 0$, referred to as the "ρ-family," where the index ρ can take positive values. If ρ is large then less of the error is spent early and the decision boundary at $\pm c_k$ is wider there; conversely, early boundaries are narrower when ρ is smaller. For equally spaced looks, the choice of $\rho = 1$ approximates a Pocock (1977) boundary, while $\rho = 3$ approximates an O'Brien and Fleming (1979) boundary.

The error spending construction ensures the Type I error probability is equal to α for any observed sequence of information levels $\{\mathcal{I}_k\}$. This property relies on the fact that the sequence $\{Z_k\}$ follows the canonical joint distribution of Equation 5.1, given the observed $\{\mathcal{I}_k\}$. It is therefore essential that the values of $Z_1, \ldots, Z_{k-1}$ do not affect the next information level $\mathcal{I}_k$ and this precludes, for example, deciding to conduct the next analysis sooner when the current test statistic is close to a boundary. Examples of how such practices can inflate the Type I error probability are given in JT, Section 7.4. We shall discuss *adaptive* methods that do allow such response-dependent choice of group sizes in Sections 5.4 and 5.8, but note for now that these procedures have to be defined in special ways in order to protect Type I error in the presence of such adaptation.

We can construct a one-sided error spending test analogously. We define two nondecreasing functions $f(\mathcal{I})$ and $g(\mathcal{I})$ with $f(0) = g(0) = 0$, $f(\mathcal{I}_{max}) = \alpha$ and $g(\mathcal{I}_{max}) = \beta$, specifying how the Type I and II error probabilities are spent as a function of the accruing information. In a similar manner to the two-sided case, we successively construct pairs of critical values (a_k, b_k) so that

$$\Pr_{\theta=0}\{\text{Reject } H_0 \text{ by analysis } k\} = f(\mathcal{I}_k) \quad \text{and} \quad \Pr_{\theta=\delta}\{\text{Accept } H_0 \text{ by analysis } k\} = g(\mathcal{I}_k).$$

The value of $\mathcal{I}_{max}$ should be chosen so that the boundaries converge at the final analysis under a typical sequence of information levels, for example, $\mathcal{I}_k = (k/K)\mathcal{I}_{max}$, $k = 1, \ldots, K$, for an anticipated value K. If we reach $\mathcal{I}_K > \mathcal{I}_{max}$ (over-running) then solving for a_K and b_K is liable to yield $a_K > b_K$. In this case, keeping b_K as calculated and reducing a_K to b_K guarantees the Type I error rate at α and gains extra power. If the final analysis K is reached with $\mathcal{I}_K$ still less than $\mathcal{I}_{max}$ (under-running), again keeping b_K as calculated preserves the Type I error rate at α. However, this time we must increase a_K to b_K and the attained power will be slightly below $1 - \beta$.

Finally we note that, for a fixed sequence of information levels there is a one-to-one correspondence between the procedures of Sections 5.3.1 and 5.3.2 defined directly in terms of boundaries for Z-values and the procedures discussed here, which are defined by error spending functions.

5.6 *P*-Values and Confidence Intervals

So far we have concentrated on the design and monitoring of a group sequential study in a hypothesis testing framework. However, once we have ended the study, we are usually interested in more than just a decision to accept or reject the null hypothesis. In this section, we shall consider the construction of P-values (which measure the evidence against the null hypothesis) and of confidence intervals (which give a range of effect sizes θ "consistent" with observed data). Both are to be computed once the procedure has terminated. We shall also, in Section 5.6.3, describe repeated confidence intervals (RCIs) and repeated P-values that may be used at any interim analysis. The methods described here apply to the one-sided and two-sided procedures of Sections 5.3.1 and 5.3.2 that use parametric boundaries, as well as the error spending tests of Section 5.5.

5.6.1 *P*-Values on Termination

We use the notation of Section 5.4. Let Ω be the sample space defined by the group sequential design; that is, the set of all pairs (k, z) where $z \notin C_k$ so the test can terminate with $(T, Z_T) = (k, z)$. We denote the observed value of (T, Z_T) by (k^*, z^*). The P-value is the minimum significance level under which a test defined on the sample space Ω can reject H_0 on seeing the observed outcome (k^*, z^*), smaller P-values indicating stronger evidence against H_0. For a continuous response distribution, the P-value should be uniformly distributed under H_0; that is, $\Pr\{P\text{-value} \le p\} = p$ for all $0 \le p \le 1$.

The P-value for testing H_0 on observing (k^*, z^*) can also be stated as

$$\Pr_{\theta=0}\{\text{Observe}\,(k,z)\,\text{as extreme or more extreme than}\,(k^*,z^*)\},$$

where "extreme" refers to the ordering of Ω implicit in the construction of tests of H_0 at different significance levels. However, there is no single natural ordering of the points in Ω and several different orderings have been proposed (see JT, Section 8.4). Suppose a GSP has continuation regions (a_k, b_k), $k = 1, \ldots,$ $K - 1$, then in the "stagewise" ordering of Ω we say (k', z') is higher than (k, z), denoted $(k', z') \succ (k, z)$, if any one of the following three conditions holds:

$$(i) k' = k \text{ and } z' \ge z, \quad (ii) k' < k \text{ and } z' \ge b_{k'}, \quad (iii) k' > k \text{ and } z \le a_k.$$

When the GSP is a one-sided test, it is natural to consider a one-sided P-value for testing H_0: $\theta = 0$ versus $\theta > 0$,

$$\Pr_{\theta=0}\{(T,Z_T) \succ (k^*,z^*)\},$$

so higher outcomes in the ordering give greater evidence against H_0.

If the GSP is a two-sided test of H_0: $\theta = 0$ versus $\theta \ne 0$ with continuation regions $(-c_k, c_k)$, we start with the same overall ordering (with $-c_k$ and c_k in place of a_k and b_k in the above definition) but now consider outcomes in both tails of the ordering when defining a two-sided P-value. Consider an O'Brien and Fleming two-sided procedure with $K = 5$ stages, $\alpha = 0.05$, and equal increments in information. As stated in Section 5.3.1, the critical values are $c_1 = 4.56$, $c_2 = 3.23$, $c_3 = 2.63$, $c_4 = 2.28$, and $c_5 = 2.04$. The stagewise ordering for this GSP is depicted in Figure 5.4.

Suppose we observe the values shown by stars in Figure 5.4, $Z_1 = 3.2$, $Z_2 = 2.9$, and $Z_3 = 4.2$, so the boundary is crossed for the first time at the third analysis and the study stops to reject H_0 with $T = 3$ and $Z_T = 4.2$. The two-sided P-value is given by

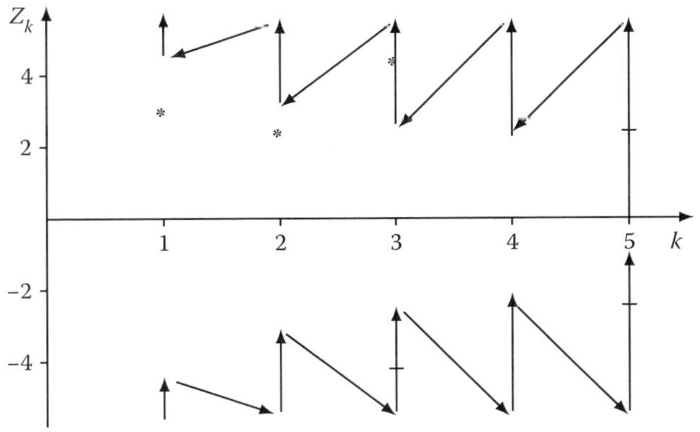

FIGURE 5.4 Stagewise ordering for an O'Brien and Fleming design with five analyses and $\alpha = 0.05$.

$$\Pr_{\theta=0}\{|Z_1| \geq 4.56 \text{ or } |Z_2| \geq 3.23 \text{ or } |Z_3| \geq 4.2\},$$

which can be calculated to be 0.0013, using the methods of Section 5.4.

Other orderings are possible, but the stagewise ordering has the following desirable properties:

i. If the group sequential test has two-sided Type I error probability α, the P-value is less than or equal to α precisely when the test stops with rejection of H_0.
ii. The P-value on observing (k^*, z^*) does not depend on values of $\mathcal{I}_k$ and c_k for $k > k^*$, which means the P-value can still be computed in an error spending test where information levels at future analyses are unknown.

5.6.2 A Confidence Interval on Termination

We can use a similar reasoning to construct a confidence interval (CI) for θ upon termination. Suppose the test terminates at analysis k^* with $Z_{k^*} = z^*$. A 100(1−α)% confidence interval for θ contains precisely those values θ for which the observed outcome (k^*, z^*) is in the "middle (1−α)" of the probability distribution of outcomes under θ.

This can be seen to be the interval (θ_1, θ_2) where

$$\Pr_{\theta=\theta_1}\{(T, Z_T) \succ (k^*, z^*)\} = \alpha/2$$

and

$$\Pr_{\theta=\theta_2}\{T, Z_T) \prec (k^*, z^*)\} = \alpha/2.$$

This follows from the relation between a 100(1−α)% confidence interval for θ and the family of level α two-sided tests of hypotheses $H\colon \theta = \tilde{\theta}$.

Consider our previous example where an O'Brien and Fleming two-sided procedure with $K = 5$ stages and $\alpha = 0.05$ ended at stage $T = 3$ with $Z_3 = 4.2$ and suppose the observed information levels are $\mathcal{I}_1 = 20$, $\mathcal{I}_2 = 40$, and $\mathcal{I}_3 = 60$. In this case, the computation using Armitage's iterated integrals (Section 5.4) yields a 95% CI of (0.20, 0.75) for θ. In contrast, the "naive" fixed sample CI would be (0.29, 0.79) but it is not appropriate to use this interval: failure to take account of the sequential stopping rule means that the coverage probability of this form of interval is *not* 1−α.

Note that there is a consistency of hypothesis testing and the CI on termination. Suppose a group sequential study is run to test H_0: $\theta = 0$ versus $\theta \neq 0$ with Type I error probability α. Then, a 1−α confidence interval on termination should contain $\theta = 0$ if and only if H_0 is accepted. This happens automatically if outcomes for which we reject H_0 are at the top and bottom ends of the sample space ordering—and any sensible ordering does this.

5.6.3 Repeated Confidence Intervals and Repeated *P*-Values

Repeated confidence intervals (RCIs) for a parameter θ are defined as a sequence of intervals I_k, $k = 1, \ldots, K$, for which a simultaneous coverage probability is maintained at some level, 1–α say. The defining property of a (1–α)-level sequence of RCIs for θ is

$$\Pr_{\theta}\{\theta \in I_k \text{ for all } k = 1,\ldots,K\} = 1-\alpha \text{ for all } \theta. \tag{5.15}$$

The interval I_k provides a statistical summary of the information about the parameter θ at the kth analysis, automatically adjusted to compensate for repeated looks at the accumulating data. As such, it can be presented to a data monitoring committee (DMC) to be considered with all other relevant information when discussing early termination of a study. The construction and use of RCIs is described in JT, Chapter 9.

If τ is *any* random stopping time taking values in $\{1, \ldots, K\}$, the guarantee of simultaneous coverage stated in Equation 5.15 implies that the probability I_τ contains θ must be at least 1–α; that is,

$$\Pr_{\theta}\{\theta \in I_\tau\} \geq 1-\alpha \text{ for all } \theta. \tag{5.16}$$

This property shows that an RCI can be used to summarize information about θ on termination and the confidence level 1–α will be maintained, regardless of how the decision to stop the study was reached. In contrast, the methods of Section 5.6.2 for constructing confidence intervals on termination rely on a particular stopping rule being specified at the outset and strictly enforced.

When a study is monitored using RCIs, the intervals computed at interim analyses might also be reported at scientific meetings. The basic property stated in Equation 5.15 ensures that these interim results will not be "overinterpreted." Here, overinterpretation refers to the fact that, when the selection bias or optional sampling bias of reported results is ignored, data may seem more significant than warranted, and this can lead to adverse effects on accrual and drop-out rates, and to pressure to unblind or terminate a study prematurely.

Repeated *P*-values are defined analogously to RCIs. At the kth analysis, a two-sided repeated *P*-value for H_0: $\theta = \theta_0$ is defined as $P_k = \max\{\alpha: \theta_0 \in I_k(\alpha)\}$, where $I_k(\alpha)$ is the current $(1 - \alpha)$-level RCI. In other words, P_k is that value of α for which the kth $(1 - \alpha)$-level RCI contains the null value, θ_0, as one of its endpoints. The construction ensures that, for any $p \in (0, 1)$, the overall probability under H_0 of ever seeing a repeated *P*-value less than or equal to p is no more than p and this probability is exactly p if all repeated *P*-values are always observed. Thus, the repeated *P*-value can be reported with the usual interpretation, yet with protection against the multiple-looks effect.

The RCIs and *P*-values defined in this section should not be confused with the CIs and *P*-values discussed in Sections 5.6.1 and 5.6.2, which are valid only at termination of a sequential test conducted according to a strictly enforced stopping rule. Monitoring a study using RCIs and repeated *P*-values allows flexibility in making decisions about stopping a trial at an interim analysis. These methodologies can, therefore, be seen as precursors to more recent adaptive methods, also motivated by the desire for greater flexibility in monitoring clinical trials.

5.7 Optimal Group Sequential Procedures

5.7.1 Optimizing Within Classes of Group Sequential Procedures

We have described a variety of group sequential designs for one-sided and two-sided tests with early stopping to reject or accept the null hypothesis. Some tests have been defined through parametric descriptions of their boundaries, others through error spending functions. Since a key aim of interim monitoring is to terminate a study as soon as is reasonably possible, particularly under certain values of the treatment difference, it is of interest to find tests with optimal early stopping properties. These designs may be applied directly or used as benchmarks to assess the efficiency of designs that are attractive for other reasons. In our later discussion of flexible "adaptive" group sequential designs, we shall see the importance of assessing efficiency in order to quantify a possible trade-off between flexibility and efficiency.

In formulating a group sequential design, we first specify the hypotheses of the testing problem and the Type I error rate α and power $1 - \beta$ at $\theta = \delta$. Let $\mathcal{I}_f$ denote the information needed by the fixed sample test; that is, $\mathcal{I}_{f,2}$ as given by Equation 5.4 for a two-sided test with error probabilities α and β, or $\mathcal{I}_{f,1}$ as given by Equation 5.8 for a one-sided test with the error probability constraints of Equations 5.6 and 5.7. We specify the maximum number K of possible analyses and the maximum information that may be required $\mathcal{I}_{max} = R\mathcal{I}_f$, where R is the inflation factor. As special cases, K or R could be set to ∞ if we do not wish to place an upper bound on them. With these constraints, we look within the specified family of GSPs for the one that minimizes the average information on termination $E(\mathcal{I}_T)$ either at one θ value or averaged over several θ values.

To find the optimum procedure for a given sequence of information levels $\{\mathcal{I}_k\}$, we must search for boundary values $\{c_k\}$ for a two-sided test or $\{(a_k, b_k)\}$ for a one-sided test that minimize the average expected sample size criterion subject to the error probability constraints. This involves searching in a high dimensional space. Rather than search this space directly, we create a related sequential Bayes decision problem with a prior on θ, sampling costs, and costs for a wrong decision. The solution for such a problem can be found by a backward induction (dynamic programming) technique. Then, a two-dimensional search over cost parameters leads to a Bayes problem whose solution is the optimal GSP with error rates equal to the values α and β being sought. This is essentially a Lagrangian method for solving a constrained optimization problem; see Eales and Jennison (1992, 1995) and Barber and Jennison (2002) for more details.

5.7.2 Optimizing with Equally Spaced Information Levels

Let us consider one-sided tests with $\alpha = 0.025$, power $1 - \beta = 0.9$, $\mathcal{I}_{max} = R\mathcal{I}_{f,1}$, and K analyses at equally spaced information levels $\mathcal{I}_k = (k/K)\mathcal{I}_{max}$. For our optimality criterion, here we shall take $\int f(\theta)E_\theta(\mathcal{I}_T)d\theta$, where $f(\theta)$ is the density of a $N(\delta, \delta^2/4)$ distribution and $\mathcal{I}_T$ denotes the information level on termination. This average expected information is centered on θ values around $\theta = \delta$ but puts significant weight over the range 0–2δ, encompassing both the null hypothesis and effect sizes well in excess of the value δ at which power is set. This is a suitable criterion when δ is a minimal clinically significant effect size and investigators are hoping the true effect is larger than this.

Table 5.5 shows the minimum expected value of $\int f(\theta)E_\theta(\mathcal{I}_T)d\theta$ for various combinations of K and R. These values are stated as percentages of the required fixed sample information $\mathcal{I}_{f,1}$ and as such are

TABLE 5.5 Minimum Values of $\int f(\theta)E_\theta(\mathcal{I}_T)d\theta$ Expressed as a Percentage of $\mathcal{I}_{f,1}$

	R						
K	1.01	1.05	1.1	1.15	1.2	1.3	Minimum over *R*
2	79.3	74.7	73.8	74.1	74.8	77.1	73.8 at *R* = 1.1
3	74.8	69.0	67.0	66.3	66.1	66.6	66.1 at *R* = 1.2
4	72.5	66.5	64.2	63.2	62.7	62.5	62.5 at *R* = 1.3
5	71.1	65.1	62.7	61.5	60.9	60.5	60.5 at *R* = 1.3
10	68.2	62.1	59.5	58.2	57.5	56.7	56.4 at *R* = 1.5
20	66.8	60.6	58.0	56.6	55.8	54.8	54.2 at *R* = 1.6

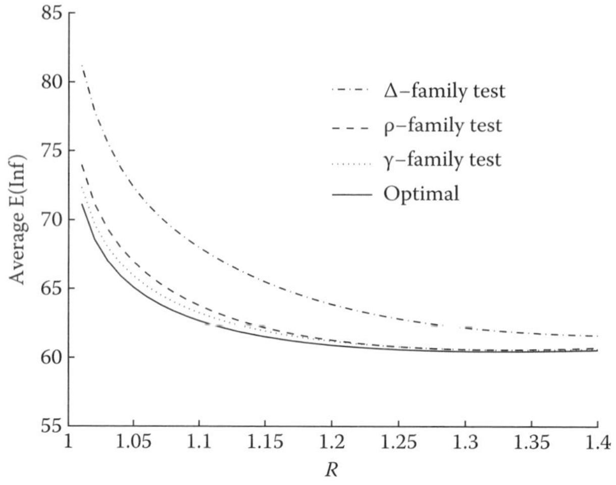

FIGURE 5.5 $\int f(\theta)E_\theta(\mathcal{I}_T)d\theta$ as a percentage of $\mathcal{I}_{f,1}$ plotted against the inflation factor R for four families of tests with $K = 5$ equally spaced looks, $\alpha = 0.025$, and $\beta = 0.1$.

invariant to the value of the effect size δ. For fixed R, it can be seen that the average $E(\mathcal{I}_T)$ decreases as K increases, but with diminishing returns. For fixed K, the average $E(\mathcal{I}_T)$ decreases as R increases up to a point, R^* say. For values of $R > R^*$, the larger increments in information (group sizes) implicit in the definition $\mathcal{I}_k = (k/K)R\mathcal{I}_{f,1}$, are suboptimal. It is evident that including just a single interim analysis ($K = 2$) can significantly reduce $E(\mathcal{I}_T)$. If the resources are available to conduct more frequent analyses, we would recommend taking $K = 4$ or 5 and $R = 1.1$ or 1.2 to obtain most of the possible reductions in expected sample size offered by group sequential testing.

We can use our optimal tests to assess parametric families of group sequential tests that have been proposed for this one-sided testing problem. The assessment is done by comparing the criterion $\int f(\theta)E_\theta(\mathcal{I}_T)d\theta$ for each test against that for the corresponding optimal procedure. We consider three families of tests:

A. In Section 5.5 we introduced the ρ family of error spending tests with Type I and II error spending functions $f(x) = \min\{\alpha, \alpha(x/\mathcal{I}_{max})^\rho\}$ and $g(x) = \min\{\beta, \beta(x/\mathcal{I}_{max})^\rho\}$, respectively. For given $\mathcal{I}_{max}$, the requirement that the upper and lower decision boundaries of a one-sided test meet at $\mathcal{I}_{max}$ determines the value of ρ and vice versa. Since $\mathcal{I}_{max} = R\mathcal{I}_{f,1}$ the inflation factor R is also determined by ρ.
B. Hwang, Shih, and DeCani (1990) proposed another family of error spending tests in which cumulative error spent is proportional to $(1-e^{-\gamma\mathcal{I}_k/\mathcal{I}_{max}})/(1-e^{-\gamma})$ instead of $(\mathcal{I}_k/\mathcal{I}_{max})^\rho$ in the ρ family defined in (A). In this case, the parameter γ determines the inflation factor R and vice versa.
C. Pampallona and Tsiatis (1994) proposed a parametric family for monitoring successive values of Z_k. This family is indexed by a parameter Δ and the boundaries for Z_k involve $\mathcal{I}_k^{\Delta-1/2}$. The parameter Δ determines the inflation factor R and vice versa.

Figure 5.5 shows values of $\int f(\theta)E_\theta(\mathcal{I}_T)d\theta$ plotted against R for these three families of tests for the case of $K = 5$ equally sized groups, $\alpha = 0.05$, and $1 - \beta = 0.9$. The fourth and lowest curve is the minimum possible average $E_\theta(\mathcal{I}_T)$ for each value of R, obtained by our optimal tests.

It can be seen that both error spending families are highly efficient but the Pampallona and Tsiatis (1994) tests are noticeably suboptimal.

5.7.3 Optimizing Over Information Levels

We can extend the computations of the previous section to permit the optimal choice of cumulative information levels $\mathcal{I}_1, \ldots, \mathcal{I}_K$ with $\mathcal{I}_K \leq R\mathcal{I}_f$, as well as optimizing over the decision boundary values

$\{(a_k, b_k)\}$. In particular, allowing the initial information level $\mathcal{I}_1$ to be small may be advantageous if it is important to stop very early when there is a large treatment benefit—the "home run" treatment. We still use dynamic programming to optimize for a given sequence $\mathcal{I}_1, \ldots, \mathcal{I}_K$, but add a further search over these information levels by, say, the Nelder and Mead (1965) algorithm applied to a suitable transform of $\mathcal{I}_1, \ldots, \mathcal{I}_K$.

Allowing a free choice of the sequence of information levels enlarges the class of GSPs being considered, resulting in more efficient designs. We shall see in the next section that there are tangible benefits from this approach, particularly for $K = 2$.

Although we consider arbitrary sequences $\mathcal{I}_1, \ldots, \mathcal{I}_K$, these information levels and the boundary values (a_k, b_k), $k = 1, \ldots, K$, are still set at the start of the study and cannot be updated as observations accrue. Relaxing this requirement leads to a further enlargement of the candidate procedures, which we discuss in the next section.

5.7.4 Procedures with Data Dependent Increments in Information

The option of scheduling each future analysis in a response-dependent manner has some intuitive appeal. For example, it would seem reasonable to choose smaller group sizes when the current test statistic lies close to a stopping boundary and larger group sizes when well away from a boundary. Schmitz (1993) refers to such designs as "sequentially planned decision procedures." Here, at each analysis $k = 1, \ldots, K - 1$, the next cumulative information level $\mathcal{I}_{k+1}$ and critical values (a_{k+1}, b_{k+1}) are chosen based on the currently available data. The whole procedure can be designed to optimize an efficiency criterion subject to the upper limit $\mathcal{I}_K \le R\mathcal{I}_f$. There is an uncountable number of decision variables to be optimized as one defines $\mathcal{I}_{k+1}(z_k)$, $a_{k+1}(z_k)$, and $b_{k+1}(z_k)$ for each value of $\mathcal{I}_k$ and every z_k in the continuation region $C_k = (a_k, b_k)$. However, by means of discretization of the $\mathcal{I}_k$ scale, the dynamic programming optimization computation, though still formidable, can be carried out. Note that, while the Schmitz designs are adaptive in the sense that future information levels are allowed to depend on current data, these designs are not "flexible". The way in which future information levels are chosen, based on past and current information levels and Z-values, is specified at the start of the study—unlike the flexible, adaptive procedures we shall discuss in Section 5.8.

The question arises as to how much extra efficiency can be obtained by allowing unequal but prespecified information levels (Section 5.7.3) or, further, allowing these information levels to be data dependent (Schmitz, 1993). Jennison and Turnbull (2006a) compare families of one-sided tests of H_0: $\theta = 0$ versus H_1: $\theta > 0$ with $\alpha = 0.025$ and power $1 - \beta = 0.9$ at $\theta = \delta$. They use the same efficiency criterion $\int f(\theta)E_\theta(\mathcal{I}_T)\,d\theta$ we have considered previously, subject to the constraint on maximum information $\mathcal{I}_K \le R\mathcal{I}_f$. We can define three nested classes of GSPs:

1. GSPs with equally spaced information levels,
2. GSPs permitting unequally spaced but fixed information levels,
3. GSPs permitting data dependent increments in information according to a prespecified rule.

Table 5.6, which reports cases in Table 1 of Jennison and Turnbull (2006a) with $R = 1.2$, shows the optimal values of the efficiency criterion for these three classes of GSPs as a percentage of the fixed sample information for values of $K = 1$–6, 8, and 10. We see that the advantage of varying group sizes *adaptively* is small, but it is present. On the other hand, such a procedure is much more complex than its nonadaptive counterparts.

Although we have focused on a single efficiency criterion $\int f(\theta)E_\theta(\mathcal{I}_T)d\theta$, the same methods can be applied to optimize with respect to other criteria, such as $E_\theta(\mathcal{I}_T)$ at a single value of θ or averaged over several values of θ. Results for other criteria presented in Eales and Jennison (1992, 1995) and Barber and Jennison (2002) show qualitatively similar features to those we have reported here. Optimality criterion can also be defined to reflect both the cost of sampling and the economic utility of a decision and the time at which it occurs; see Liu, Anderson, and Pledger (2004).

TABLE 5.6 Optimized $\int f(\theta)E_\theta(\mathcal{I}_T)d\theta$ as a Percentage of $\mathcal{I}_{f,1}$ for Tests with Inflation Factor $R = 1.2$

K	1. Optimal GSP with K Equal Group Sizes	2. Optimal GSP with K Optimized Group Sizes	3. Optimal Adaptive Design of Schmitz
1	100.0	100.0	100.0
2	74.8	73.2	72.5
3	66.1	65.6	64.8
4	62.7	62.4	61.2
5	60.9	60.5	59.2
6	59.8	59.4	58.0
8	58.3	58.0	56.6
10	57.5	57.2	55.9

5.8 Tests Permitting Flexible, Data Dependent Increments in Information

5.8.1 Flexible Redesign Protecting the Type I Error Probability

In the Schmitz (1993) GSPs of Section 5.7.4, the future information increments (group sizes) and critical values are permitted to depend on current and past values of the test statistic Z_k, assuming of course that the stopping boundary had not been crossed. These procedures are not flexible in that the rules for making the choices are prespecified functions of currently available Z_k values. With this knowledge, it is possible *ab initio* to compute a procedure's statistical properties, such as Type I and II error probabilities and expected information at termination. However, what can be done if an unexpected event happens in mid-course and we wish to make some ad hoc change in the future information increment levels? This is often referred to as flexible *sample size reestimation* or *sample size modification.*

Consider the application of a classical group sequential one-sided design. The trial is under way and, based on data observed at analysis j, it is desired to increase future information levels. If we were to do this and continue to use the original values (a_k, b_k) for $k > j$ in the stopping rule of Equation 5.9, the Type I error rate would no longer be guaranteed at α. If arbitrary changes in sample size are allowed, the Type I error rate is typically inflated; see Cui, Hung, and Wang (1999, Table A1) and Proschan and Hunsberger (1995). However, as an exception, note that if it is *preplanned* that increases in sample size are only permitted when the interim treatment estimate is sufficiently high (conditional power greater than 0.5), this implies that the actual overall Type I error rate may be reduced; see Chen, DeMets, and Lan (2004).

Suppose, however, that we do go ahead with this adaptation and the cumulative information levels are now $\tilde{\mathcal{I}}^{(1)},\ldots,\tilde{\mathcal{I}}^{(K)}$; here, $\tilde{\mathcal{I}}^{(k)} = \mathcal{I}_k$ for $k \le j$ but the $\tilde{\mathcal{I}}^{(k)}$ differ from the originally planned $\mathcal{I}_k$ for $k > j$. Let $\tilde{Z}^{(k)}$ be the usual Z-statistic *formed from data in stage k alone* and $\tilde{\Delta}_k = \tilde{\mathcal{I}}^{(k)} - \tilde{\mathcal{I}}^{(k-1)}$. Again, the $\tilde{\Delta}_k$ are as originally planned for $k \le j$ but they depart from this plan for $k > j$. We *can* still maintain the Type I error probability using the original boundary if we use the statistics $\tilde{Z}^{(k)}$ in the appropriate way. Note that, even though the information increment $\tilde{\Delta}^{(k)}$ is an ingredient of the statistic $\tilde{Z}^{(k)}$ and, for $k > j$, this can depend on knowledge of the previously observed $\tilde{Z}^{(1)},\ldots,\tilde{Z}^{(k-1)}$, each $\tilde{Z}^{(k)}$ has a standard normal $N(0, 1)$ distribution under $\theta = 0$ conditionally on the previous responses and $\tilde{\Delta}^{(k)}$. It follows that this distribution holds unconditionally under H_0, so we may treat $\tilde{Z}^{(1)}$, $\tilde{Z}^{(2)}$, ... as independent $N(0, 1)$ variables. The standard distribution of the $\{\tilde{Z}^{(k)}\}$ under H_0 means we can use the original boundary values in Equation 5.9 and maintain the specified Type I error rate α, provided we monitor the statistics

$$\tilde{Z}_k = (w_1\tilde{Z}^{(1)} + \cdots + w_k\tilde{Z}^{(k)})/(w_1^2 + \cdots + w_k^2)^{1/2}, \quad k = 1,\ldots,K, \tag{5.17}$$

where the weights $w_k = \sqrt{\Delta_k}$ are the square roots of the *originally planned* information increments. With this definition, the $\tilde{Z}_k$ follow the canonical joint distribution of Equation 5.1 under H_0 that was originally anticipated; see Lehmacher and Wassmer (1999) or Cui, Hung, and Wang (1999). Under the alternative $\theta > 0$, the $\tilde{Z}^{(k)}$ are not independent after adaptation and if information levels are increased, then so are the means of the Z-statistics, which leads to the desired increase in power.

Use of a procedure based on Equation 5.17 is an example of a *combination test.* In particular Equation 5.17 is a *weighted inverse normal combination* statistic (Mosteller and Bush, 1954). Other combination test statistics can be used in place of Equation 5.17, such as the inverse χ^2 statistic proposed by Bauer and Köhne (1994). However, use of Equation 5.17 has two advantages: (i) we do not need to recalculate the stopping boundaries $\{(a_k, b_k)\}$, and (ii) if no adaptation occurs, we have $\tilde{Z}_k = Z_k$, $k = 1, 2, \ldots$, and the procedure proceeds as originally planned.

5.8.2 Efficiency of Flexible Adaptive Procedures

We have seen in Section 5.8.1, by using Equation 5.17, how the investigator has the freedom to modify a study in light of accruing data and still maintain the Type I error rate. But what is the cost, if any, of this flexibility? To examine this question, we need to consider specific strategies for adaptive design. Jennison and Turnbull (2006a) discuss the example of a GSP with $K = 5$ analyses testing H_0: $\theta \le 0$ against $\theta > 0$ with Type I error probability $\alpha = 0.025$ and power $1 - \beta = 0.9$ at $\theta = \delta$. A fixed sample size test for this problem requires information $\mathcal{I}_f = \mathcal{I}_{f,1}$, as given by Equation 5.8. Suppose the study is designed as a one-sided test from the ρ-family of error-spending tests, as described in Section 5.5, and we choose index $\rho = 3$. The boundary values $a_1, \ldots, a_5$ and $b_1, \ldots, b_5$ are chosen to satisfy

$$\Pr_\theta\{Z_1 > b_1 \text{ or } \ldots \text{ or } Z_1 \in (a_1,b_1),\ldots,Z_{k-1} \in (a_{k-1},b_{k-1}), Z_k > b_k\} = (\mathcal{I}_k / \mathcal{I}_{max})^3 \alpha,$$

$$\Pr_\theta\{Z_1 < a_1 \text{ or } \ldots \text{ or } Z_1 \in (a_1,b_1),\ldots,Z_{k-1} \in (a_{k-1},b_{k-1}), Z_k < a_k\} = (\mathcal{I}_k / \mathcal{I}_{max})^3 \beta$$

for $k = 1, \ldots, 5$. At the design stage, equally spaced information levels $\mathcal{I}_k = (k/5)\mathcal{I}_{max}$ are assumed and calculations show that a maximum information $\mathcal{I}_{max} = 1.049\mathcal{I}_f$ is needed for the boundaries to meet up with $a_5 = b_5$. The boundaries are similar in shape to those in Figure 5.2.

Suppose external information becomes available at the second analysis, leading the investigators to seek conditional power of 0.9 at $\theta = \delta/2$ rather than $\theta = \delta$. Since this decision is independent of data observed in the study, one might argue that modification could be made without prejudicing the Type I error rate. However, it would be difficult to prove that the data revealed at interim analyses had played no part in the decision to redesign. Following the general strategy described in Cui, Hung, and Wang (1999), it is decided to change the information increments in the third, fourth, and fifth stages to $\tilde{\Delta}_k = \gamma\Delta_k$ for $k = 3$, 4, and 5. The factor γ depends on the data available at Stage 2 and is chosen so that the conditional power under $\theta = \delta/2$, given the observed value of Z_2, is equal to $1 - \beta = 0.9$. However, γ is truncated to lie in the range 1–6, so that sample size is never reduced and the maximum total information is increased by at most a factor of 4. Figure 5.6 shows that the power curve of the adaptive test lies well above that of the original group sequential design. The power 0.78 attained at $\theta = 0.5\delta$ falls short of the target of 0.9 because of the impossibility of increasing conditional power when the test has already terminated to accept H_0 and the truncation of γ for values of Z_2 just above a_2.

It is of interest to assess the cost of the delay in learning the ultimate objective of the study. Our comparison is with a ρ-family error-spending test with $\rho = 0.75$, power 0.9 at 0.59δ and the first four analyses at fractions 0.1, 0.2, 0.45, and 0.7 of the final information level $\mathcal{I}_5 = \mathcal{I}_{max} = 3.78\mathcal{I}_f$. This choice ensures that the power of the nonadaptive test is everywhere as high as that of the adaptive test, as seen in Figure 5.6, and the expected information curves of the two tests are of a similar form. Figure 5.7 shows the expected information on termination as a function of θ/δ for these two tests; the vertical axis is in

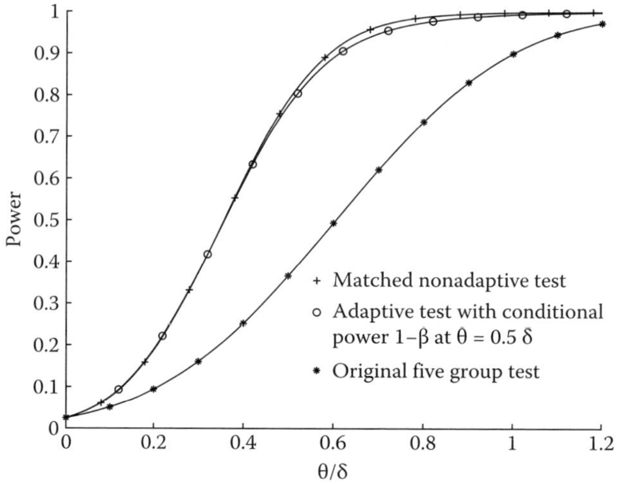

FIGURE 5.6 Power curves of the original test, the adaptive design with sample size revised at look 2 to attain conditional power 0.9 at $\theta = 0.5\ \delta$, and the matched nonadaptive test. (From Jennison, C. and Turnbull, B. W., *Biometrika*, 93, 1–21, 2006a. With permission.)

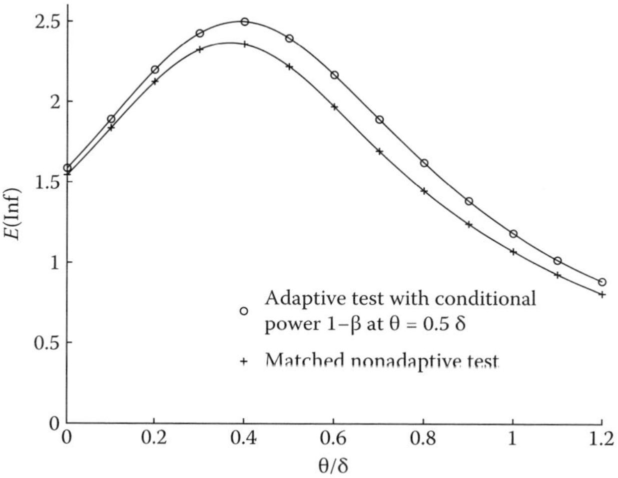

FIGURE 5.7 Expected information functions $E_\theta(\mathcal{I}_T)$ of the adaptive design and matched nonadaptive design, expressed in units of $\mathcal{I}_f$. (From Jennison, C. and Turnbull, B. W., *Biometrika*, 93, 1–21, 2006a. With permission.)

units of $\mathcal{I}_f$. Together, Figures 5.6 and 5.7 demonstrate that the nonadaptive test dominates the adaptive test in terms of both power and expected information over the range of θ values. Also, the nonadaptive test's maximum information level of $3.78\mathcal{I}_f$ is 10% lower than the adaptive test's $4.20\mathcal{I}_f$.

It is useful to have a single summary of relative efficiency when two tests differ in both power and expected information. If test A with Type I error rate α at $\theta = 0$ has power function $1 - b_A(\theta)$ and expected information $E_{A,\theta}(\mathcal{I})$ under a particular $\theta > 0$, Jennison and Turnbull (2006a) define its efficiency index at θ to be

$$EI_A(\theta) = \frac{(z_\alpha + z_{b_A(\theta)})^2}{\theta^2} \frac{1}{E_{A,\theta}(\mathcal{I})},$$

the ratio of the information needed to achieve power $1 - b_A(\theta)$ in a fixed sample test to $E_{A,0}(\mathcal{I})$. In comparing tests A and B, we take the ratio of their efficiency indices to obtain the efficiency ratio

$$ER_{A,B}(\theta) = \frac{EI_A(\theta)}{EI_B(\theta)} \times 100 = \frac{E_{B,\theta}(\mathcal{I})}{E_{A,\theta}(\mathcal{I})} \frac{(z_\alpha + z_{b_A(\theta)})^2}{(z_\alpha + z_{b_B(\theta)})^2} \times 100.$$

This can be regarded as a ratio of expected information adjusted for the difference in attained power. The plot of the efficiency ratio in Figure 5.8 shows the adaptive design is considerably less efficient than the simple group sequential test, especially for $\theta > \delta/2$, and this quantifies the cost of delay in learning the study's objective.

Another motivation for sample size modification is the desire to increase sample size on seeing low interim estimates of the treatment effect. Investigators may suppose the true treatment effect is perhaps smaller than they had hoped and aim to increase, belatedly, the power of their study. Or they may hope that adding more data will make amends for an unlucky start. We have studied such adaptations in response to low interim estimates of the treatment effect and found inefficiencies similar to, or worse than, those in the preceding example. The second example in Jennison and Turnbull (2006a) concerns such adaptation using the Cui, Hung, and Wang (1999) procedure. We have found comparable inefficiencies when sample size is modified to achieve a given conditional power using the methods of Bauer and Köhne (1994), Proschan and Hunsberger (1995), Shen and Fisher (1999), and Li et al. (2002). When adaptation is limited to smaller increases in sample size, the increase in power is smaller but efficiency loss is still present.

We saw in Section 5.7.4 that the preplanned adaptive designs of Schmitz (1993) can be slightly more efficient than conventional group sequential tests. One must, therefore, wonder why the adaptive tests that we have studied should be less efficient than competing group sequential tests, sometimes by as much as 30 or 40%. We can cite three contributory factors:

1. *Use of nonsufficient statistics.* In Jennison and Turnbull (2006a), it is proved that all admissible designs (adaptive or nonadaptive) are Bayes procedures. Hence, their decision rules and sample size rules must be functions of sufficient statistics. Adaptive procedures using combination test statistics (Equation 5.17) with their unequal weighting of observations are not based on sufficient statistics. Thus, they cannot be optimal designs for any criteria. Since the potential benefits of adaptivity are slight, any departure from optimality can leave room for an efficient nonadaptive design, with the

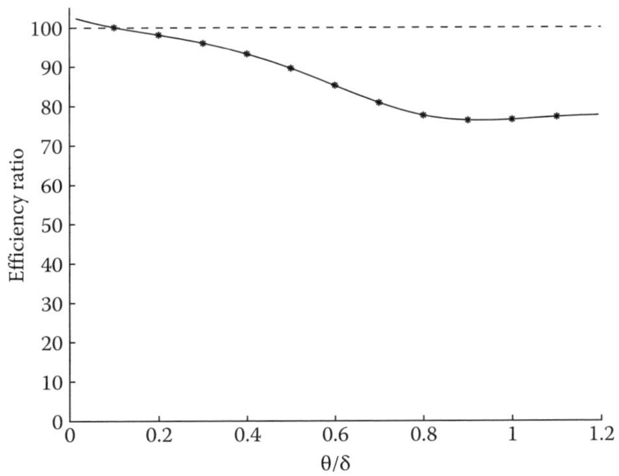

FIGURE 5.8 Efficiency ratio between the adaptive design and matched nonadaptive design. (From Jennison, C. and Turnbull, B. W., *Biometrika*, 93, 1–21, 2006a. With permission.)

same number of analyses, to do better. Note that this is a stronger conclusion than that of Tsiatis and Mehta (2003) who allow the comparator nonadaptive design to have additional analyses.

2. *Suboptimal sample size modification rule.* Rules based on conditional power differ qualitatively from those arising in the optimal adaptive designs of Section 5.7.4. Conditional power rules invest a lot of resource in unpromising situations with a low interim estimate of the treatment effect. The optimal rule shows greater symmetry, taking higher sample sizes when the current test statistic is in the middle of the continuation region, away from both boundaries. The qualitative differences between these two types of procedure are illustrated by the typical shapes of sample size functions shown in Figures 5.9 and 5.10.
3. *Over-reliance on a highly variable interim estimator of* θ. The sample size modification rules of many adaptive designs involve the current interim estimator of effect size, often as an assumed value in a conditional power calculation. Since this estimator is highly variable, use of this estimate leads to random variation in sample size, which is in itself inefficient; see Jennison and Turnbull (2003) for further discussion of this point in the context of a two-stage design.

Our conclusion in this section is that group sequential tests provide an efficient and versatile mechanism for conducting clinical trials, but it can be useful to have adaptive methods to turn to when a

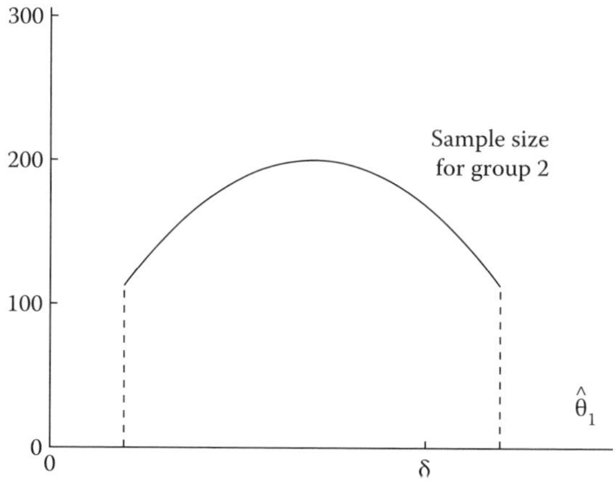

FIGURE 5.9 Typical shape of sample size function for an optimal adaptive test.

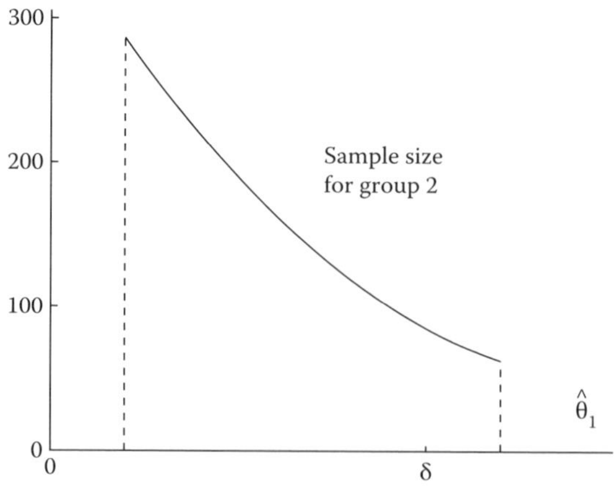

FIGURE 5.10 Typical shape of sample size function for a conditional power adaptive design.

study's sample size is found to be too small. Our first example depicts a situation where a change in objective could not have been anticipated at the outset and an adaptive solution is the only option. While good practice at the design stage should ensure that a study has adequate power, it is reassuring to know there are procedures available to rescue an under-powered study while still protecting the Type I error rate. What we do not recommend is the use of such adaptive strategies as a substitute for proper planning. Investigators may have different views on the likely treatment effect, but it is still possible to construct a group sequential design that will deliver the desired overall power with low expected sample size under the effect sizes of most interest; for further discussion of how to balance these objectives, see Schäfer and Müller (2004) and Jennison and Turnbull (2006b).

5.9 Discussion

In Sections 5.2 to 5.6 we described the classical framework in which group sequential tests are set, presented an overview of GSPs defined by parametric boundaries or error spending functions, and discussed inference on termination of a GSP. These classical GSPs are well studied; optimal tests have been derived for a variety of criteria and error spending functions identified that give tests with close to optimal performance.

The GSPs adapt to observed data in the most fundamental way by terminating the study when a decision boundary is crossed. Error spending designs have the flexibility to accommodate unpredictable information sequences. In cases where information depends on nuisance parameters that affect the variance of the outcome variable, Mehta and Tsiatis (2001) propose "information monitoring" designs in which updated estimates of nuisance parameters are incorporated in error spending tests. Overall, classical group sequential methodology is versatile and can handle a number of the problems that more recent adaptive methods have been constructed to solve.

A question that poses problems for both group sequential and adaptive methods is how to deal with delayed responses that arrive after termination of a study. Stopping rules are usually defined on the assumption that no more responses will be observed after the decision to terminate, but it is not uncommon for such data to accrue, particularly when there is a significant delay between treatment and the time the primary response is measured. Group sequential methods that can handle such delayed data and methods for creating designs that do this efficiently are described by Hampson (2009).

We discussed in Sections 5.7.4 and 5.8 how data dependent modification of group sizes can be viewed as a feature of both classical GSPs and adaptive designs. It is our view that the benefits of such modifications are small compared to the complexity of these designs. There is also a danger that interpretability may be compromised; indeed, Burman and Sonesson (2006) give an example where adaptive redesign leads to a complete loss of credibility.

A key role that remains for flexible adaptive methods is to help investigators respond to unexpected external events. As several authors have pointed out, it is good practice to design a study as efficiently as possible given initial assumptions, so the benefits of this design are obtained in the usual circumstances where no mid-course change is required. However, if the unexpected occurs, adaptations can be made following the methods described in Section 5.8 or, more generally, by maintaining the conditional Type I error probability, as suggested by Denne (2001) and Müller and Schäfer (2001). Finally, the use of flexible adaptive methods to rescue an under-powered study should not be overlooked: while it is easy to be critical of a poor initial choice of sample size, it would be naive to think that such problems will cease to arise.

It should be clear from our exposition that group sequential and adaptive methods involve significant computation. Fortunately, there is a growing number of computer software packages available for implementing these methods to design and monitor clinical trials. Self-contained programs include EAST (http://www.cytel.com/Products/East/), ADDPLAN (http://www.addplan.com/), PEST (http://www.maths.lancs.ac.uk/department/research/statistics/mps/pest), NCSS/PASS (http://www.ncss.com/passsequence.html), and ExpDesign Studio (Chang 2008).

Several useful macros written for SAS are detailed in Dmitrienko et al. (2005, Chapter 4). The add-on module S+SeqTrial (http://www.spotfire.tibco.com/products/splus-seqtrial.aspx) is available for use with S-PLUS.

A number of Web sites offer software that can be freely downloaded. The gsDesign package (http://cran.r-project.org/) is one of several packages for use with *R*. The Web site http://www.biostat.wisc.edu/landemets/ contains FORTRAN programs for error spending procedures. Our own FORTRAN programs, related to the book JT, are available at http://people.bath.ac.uk/mascj/book/programs/general. For a review of the capabilities of all these software packages, we refer the reader to the article by Wassmer and Vandemeulebroecke (2006).

Our comments on adaptive design in this chapter relate to sample size modification as this is the key area of overlap with GSPs. Adaptive methods do, of course, have a wide range of further applications—as the other chapters in this book demonstrate.

References

Armitage, P. (1960). *Sequential Medical Trials,* 1st ed. Springfield: Thomas.

Armitage, P., McPherson, C. K., and Rowe, B. C. (1969). Repeated significance tests on accumulating data. *Journal of the Royal Statistical Society, A,* 132:235–44.

Barber, S., and Jennison, C. (2002). Optimal asymmetric one-sided group sequential tests. *Biometrika,* 89:49–60.

Bauer, P., and Köhne, K. (1994). Evaluation of experiments with adaptive interim analyses. *Biometrics,* 50:1029–41.

Burman, C.-F., and Sonesson, C. (2006). Are flexible designs sound? *Biometrics,* 62:664–69.

Chang, M. (2008). *Classical and Adaptive Clinical Trial Designs Using ExpDesign Studio.* New York: Wiley.

Chen, J. Y. H., DeMets, D. L., and Lan, K. K. G. (2004). Increasing the sample size when the unblinded interim result is promising. *Statistics in Medicine,* 23: 1023–38.

Cui, L., Hung, H. M. J., and Wang, S.-J. (1999). Modification of sample size in group sequential clinical trials. *Biometrics,* 55:853–57.

DeMets, D. L., Furberg, C. D., and Friedman, L. M., eds. (2006). *Data Monitoring in Clinical Trials.* New York: Springer.

Denne, J. S. (2001). Sample size recalculation using conditional power. *Statistics in Medicine,* 20:2645–60.

Dmitrienko, A., Molenberghs, G., Chuang-Stein, C., and Offen, W. (2005). *Analysis of Clinical Trials Using SAS: A Practical Guide.* Cary: SAS Institute Press.

Eales, J. D., and Jennison, C. (1992). An improved method for deriving optimal one-sided group sequential tests. *Biometrika,*79:13–24.

Eales, J. D., and Jennison, C. (1995). Optimal two-sided group sequential tests. *Sequential Analysis,* 14:273–86.

Ellenberg, S. S., Fleming, T. R., and DeMets, D. L. (2002). *Data Monitoring Committees in Clinical Trials: A Practical Perspective.* West Sussex: Wiley.

Emerson, S. S., and Fleming, T. R. (1990). Parameter estimation following group sequential hypothesis testing. *Biometrika,* 77:875–92.

Hampson, L. V. (2009). *Group Sequential Tests for Delayed Responses.* PhD thesis, University of Bath.

Herson, J. (2009). *Data and Safety Monitoring Committees in Clinical Trials.* Boca Raton, FL: Chapman & Hall/CRC.

Hwang, I. K., Shih, W. J., and DeCani, J. S. (1990). Group sequential designs using a family of type I error probability spending functions. *Statistics in Medicine,* 9:1439–45.

Jennison, C., and Turnbull, B. W. (1997). Group sequential analysis incorporating covariate information. *Journal of the American Statistical Association,* 92:1330–41.

Jennison, C., and Turnbull, B. W. (2000). *Group Sequential Methods with Applications to Clinical Trials.* Boca Raton, FL: Chapman & Hall/CRC.

Jennison, C., and Turnbull, B. W. (2003). Mid-course sample size modification in clinical trials based on the observed treatment effect. *Statistics in Medicine,* 22:971–93.

Jennison, C., and Turnbull, B. W. (2006a). Adaptive and nonadaptive group sequential tests. *Biometrika,* 93:1–21.

Jennison, C., and Turnbull, B. W. (2006b). Efficient group sequential designs when there are several effect sizes under consideration. *Statistics in Medicine,* 35:917–32.

Lan, K. K. G., and DeMets, D. L. (1983). Discrete sequential boundaries for clinical trials. *Biometrika,* 70:659–63.

Lehmacher, W., and Wassmer, G. (1999). Adaptive sample size calculation in group sequential trials. *Biometrics,* 55:1286–90.

Li, G., Shih, W. J., Xie, T., and Lu, J. (2002). A sample size adjustment procedure for clinical trials based on conditional power. *Biostatistics,* 3:277–87.

Liu, Q., Anderson, K. M., and Pledger, G. W. (2004). Benefit-risk evaluation of multi-stage adaptive designs. *Sequential Analysis,* 23:317–31.

Mehta, C. R., and Tsiatis, A. A. (2001). Flexible sample size considerations using information-based interim monitoring. *Drug Information Journal,* 35:1095–1112.

Mosteller, F., and Bush, R. R. (1954). Selected quantitative techniques. In *Handbook of Social Psychology,* Vol. 1, ed. G. Lindsey, 289–334. Cambridge: Addison-Wesley.

Müller, H.-H., and Schäfer, H. (2001). Adaptive group sequential designs for clinical trials: Combining the advantages of adaptive and of classical group sequential procedures. *Biometrics,* 57:886–91.

Nelder, J. A., and Mead, R. (1965). A simplex method for function minimization. *Computer Journal,* 7:308–13.

O'Brien, P. C., and Fleming, T. R. (1979). A multiple testing procedure for clinical trials. *Biometrics,* 35:549–56.

Pampallona, S., and Tsiatis, A. A. (1994). Group sequential designs for one-sided and two-sided hypothesis testing with provision for early stopping in favor of the null hypothesis. *Journal of Statistical Planning and Inference,* 42:19–35.

Pocock, S. J. (1977). Group sequential methods in the design and analysis of clinical trials. *Biometrika,* 64:191–99.

Proschan, M. A., and Hunsberger, S. A. (1995). Designed extension of studies based on conditional power. *Biometrics,* 51:1315–24.

Proschan, M. A., Lan, K. K. G., and Wittes, J. T. (2006). *Statistical Monitoring of Clinical Trials.* New York: Springer.

Schäfer, H., and Müller, H.-H. (2004). Construction of group sequential designs in clinical trials on the basis of detectable treatment differences. *Statistics in Medicine,* 23:1413–24.

Schmitz, N. (1993). *Optimal Sequentially Planned Decision Procedures.* Lecture Notes in Statistics, 79. New York: Springer-Verlag.

Shen, Y., and Fisher, L. (1999). Statistical inference for self-designing clinical trials with a one-sided hypothesis. *Biometrics,* 55:190–97.

Siegmund, D. (1985). *Sequential Analysis.* New York: Springer-Verlag.

Tsiatis, A. A., and Mehta, C. (2003). On the inefficiency of the adaptive design for monitoring clinical trials. *Biometrika,* 90:367–78.

Wald, A. (1947). *Sequential Analysis.* New York: Wiley.

Wang, S. K., and Tsiatis, A. A. (1987). Approximately optimal one-parameter boundaries for group sequential trials. *Biometrics,* 43:193–200.

Wassmer, G., and Vandemeulebroecke, M. (2006). A brief review on software developments for group sequential and adaptive designs. *Biometrical Journal,* 48:732–37.

Whitehead, J. (1997). *The Design and Analysis of Sequential Clinical Trials,* 2nd ed. Chichester: Wiley.

6

Determining Sample Size for Classical Designs

Simon Kirby
and Christy
Chuang-Stein
Pfizer, Inc.

6.1 Introduction

In clinical trials, we collect data to answer important scientific questions on the effect of interventions in humans. It is essential that before conducting a trial we ask how much information is necessary to answer the questions at hand. Since the amount of information is highly related to the number of subjects included in the trial, determining the number of subjects to include in a trial is an important part of trial planning.

It is not surprising then that determining sample size was among the first tasks when statisticians started to support clinical trials. As a result, determining sample size has been the subject of research interest for many statisticians over the past 50 years and numerous publications have been devoted to this subject (e.g., Lachin 1981; Donner 1984; Noether 1987; Dupont and Plummer 1990; Shuster 1990; Lee and Zelen 2000; Senchaudhuri et al. 2004; O'Brien and Castelloe 2007; Chow, Shao, and Wang 2008; Machin et al. 2008). Much of the research efforts led to closed-form (albeit often approximate) expressions for the needed sample size.

When designing a trial, one needs to take into consideration how the data will be analyzed. Efficiency in the analysis should generally translate into a reduction in the sample size. Our experience suggests that this has not always been the case. In many situations, a conservative approach is adopted in the hope that the extra subjects will provide some protection against unanticipated complications. In some cases, however, even a seemingly conservative approach might not be enough because of the very conservative approach used to handle missing data. Equally important, there are situations when the estimation of sample size is based on the ideal situation with complete balance between treatment groups with no missing data. The latter often leads to underpowered studies.

Earlier work on sample size focused on instances when closed-form expressions could be derived. Because study designs and analytical methods have become increasingly more complicated, there is an increasing trend to use simulation to evaluate the operating characteristics of a design and the associated decision rule. This trend has intensified during the past 10 years with a greater adoption of adaptive designs. The need to use simulation to assess the performance of an adaptive design has even spilled over to the more traditional designs where adaptations are not a design feature.

In addition to scientific considerations, sample size has budgetary and ethical implications. An institutional review board (IRB), before approving a proposed trial, needs to know the extent of human exposure planned for the trial. If the trial is not capable of answering the scientific question it sets out to answer, it may not be ethical to conduct the trial in the first place. If the trial is enrolling more subjects than existing safety experience could comfortably support, the study will need a more extensive monitoring plan to ensure patient safety. In either case, the number of subjects planned for the study will be a critical factor in deciding whether the proposed study plan is scientifically defensible.

The decision on sample size is typically based on many assumptions. The validity of these assumptions could often be verified using interim data. As a result, sample size determined at the design stage could be adjusted if necessary. This subject is covered in other chapters of this book.

In this chapter, we will focus on sample sizes for classical designs that are not adaptive in nature. In Section 6.2, we will first look at the sample size needed to support hypothesis testing. In this context, we will examine Normal endpoints, binary endpoints, ordinal endpoints, and survival endpoints. In Section 6.3, we discuss sample size determination under some nonstandard approaches that have been developed recently. In Section 6.4, we highlight a few additional issues to consider when determining the sample size. We finish this chapter with some further comments in Section 6.5.

6.2 The Hypothesis Testing Approach

In this section, we will look at sample size to support hypothesis testing. In this case, a sample size is chosen to control the probability of rejecting the null hypothesis H_0 when it is true (Type I error rate, α) and to ensure a certain probability of accepting the alternative hypothesis H_1 when the treatment effect is of a prespecified magnitude δ covered by the alternative hypothesis (Power, $1 - \beta$). The quantity β is called the Type II error rate. For convenience, we will use α to denote Type I error rate generically whether the test is one-sided or two-sided. It should be understood that if we choose to conduct a one-sided test for simplicity when the situation calls for a two-sided test, the Type I error rate for the one-sided test should be half of that set for the two-sided test.

Setting the power equal to $(1 - \beta)$ when the effect size is δ means that there is a probability of $(1 - \beta)$ rejecting H_0 when the treatment effect is equal to δ. It is important to realize that this does not mean that the observed treatment effect will be greater than δ with probability $(1 - \beta)$. In practice, the treatment effect of interest is usually taken to be either a minimum clinically important difference (MCID) or a treatment effect thought likely to be true. According to ICH E9, an MCID is defined as "the minimal effect which has clinical relevance in the management of patients."

There are an enormous number of scenarios that could be considered. We are selective in our coverage picking either situations that are more commonly encountered or that can be easily studied to obtain insights into a general approach. While we cover different types of endpoints in this section, we focus more on endpoints that follow a Normal distribution. In addition, we focus primarily on estimators that are either the treatment effects themselves or some monotonic functions of the treatment effects.

6.2.1 Sample Size to Show Superiority of a Treatment

The majority of confirmatory trials are undertaken to show that an investigative intervention is superior to a placebo or a control treatment. In this subsection we will consider how to determine the sample size to demonstrate superiority.

Dupont and Plummer (1990) propose a general approach for superiority testing when the estimator of the treatment effect or a monotonic function of the effect follows a Normal or approximately Normal distribution. We will adopt their general approach in setting up the framework for sample size determination.

Let the parameter θ be a measure of the true treatment effect. We are interested in testing the null hypothesis of $H_0 : \theta \leq \theta_0$ against the one-sided alternative $H_1 : \theta > \theta_0$ at the nominal significance level α. Denote the function of θ that we are interested in by $f(\theta)$. Assume our test is to have a 100(1 – β)% power to reject H_0 when $\theta = \theta_A > \theta_0$. According to Dupont and Plummer, the required total sample size n_{tot} needs to satisfy the following relationship

$$f(\theta_0)+Z_\alpha\frac{\sigma(\theta_0)}{\sqrt{n_{tot}}}=f(\theta_A)-Z_\beta\frac{\sigma(\theta_A)}{\sqrt{n_{tot}}}. \tag{6.1}$$

In Equation 6.1, $\sigma(\theta)/\sqrt{n_{tot}}$ is the standard error of the estimator for $f(\theta)$ and Z_α and Z_β are the upper 100α% and 100β% percentiles of the standard Normal distribution. Equation 6.1 represents the amount of overlap of the distributions of the estimator when $\theta = \theta_0$ and $\theta = \theta_A$ that gives the desired Type I and Type II error rates. This is illustrated in Figure 6.1 when the estimator follows a Normal distribution and $f(\theta) = \theta$. Equation 6.1 can be used with suitable substitutions for a variety of data types and situations as we will illustrate throughout this chapter.

6.2.1.1 Normally Distributed Data

6.2.1.1.1 Two Parallel Groups Design

We first consider the simple situation when subjects are allocated randomly in equal proportion to two treatments and we wish to compare the mean responses to the two treatments. Denote the mean responses to the experimental treatment and control by μ_E and μ_C, respectively. Assume that the treatment effect of the experimental treatment over the control is measured by the difference $\mu_E - \mu_C$. Without loss of generality, we assume that a positive difference suggests that the experimental treatment is more efficacious. An estimate for $\mu_E - \mu_C$ is the observed difference $\bar{y}_E - \bar{y}_C$ where $\bar{y}$ is the sample mean response for a respective treatment group. For known common variance σ^2, the difference in sample means $\bar{y}_E - \bar{y}_C$ has a Normal distribution with standard error of $\sqrt{2\sigma^2/n}$ where n is the common sample size for each group.

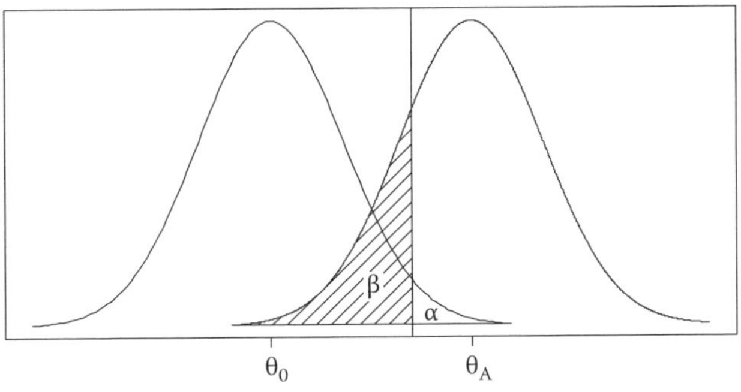

FIGURE 6.1 Distributions of the test statistic under the null hypothesis ($\theta = \theta_0$) and the alternative hypothesis ($\theta = \theta_A$) under the assumption that the test statistic has a Normal distribution.

For simplicity, assume that the null hypothesis is $H_0 : \mu_E - \mu_C \leq 0$ and the alternative hypothesis is $H_1 : \mu_E - \mu_C > 0$. We want the study to have a power of $(1 - \beta)$ to reject H_0 when the treatment effect is δ at the one-sided $100\alpha\%$ level. The sample size requirement in Expression 6.1 (with $n = n_{tot}/2$) becomes

$$Z_\alpha\sqrt{\frac{2\sigma^2}{n}} = \delta - Z_\beta\sqrt{\frac{2\sigma^2}{n}}. \tag{6.2}$$

Solving Equation 6.2 for n, we obtain the following well-known formula for the sample size for each group

$$n = \frac{2\sigma^2(Z_\alpha + Z_\beta)^2}{\delta^2}. \tag{6.3}$$

For unequal randomization with $r = n_E / n_C$, Equation 6.2 becomes

$$Z_\alpha\sqrt{\frac{(1+r)^2\sigma^2}{rn_{tot}}} = \delta - Z_\beta\sqrt{\frac{(1+r)^2\sigma^2}{rn_{tot}}}. \tag{6.4}$$

Solving Equation 6.4 for n_{tot} leads to

$$n_{tot} = \frac{(r+1)^2\sigma^2(Z_\alpha + Z_\beta)^2}{r\delta^2}. \tag{6.5}$$

From Equation 6.5, we can obtain the sample sizes for the two groups as $n_E = (r/(r + 1))n_{tot}$ and $n_C = (1/(r + 1))n_{tot}$.

When σ^2 is unknown the standard error of the difference in sample means can be estimated by

$$\sqrt{\frac{s^2}{n_E} + \frac{s^2}{n_C}},$$

where s^2 is the usual unbiased estimate of the common within-group variance. Under the null hypothesis, the difference in sample means divided by the standard error of the difference above has a t-distribution with $(n_{tot} - 2)$ degrees of freedom. It has a noncentral t-distribution when the true treatment difference is equal to δ. In this case, Equation 6.4 can be used with the standard Normal distribution replaced by the appropriate values of the t-distribution.

$$t_{(\alpha,n_{tot}-2)}\sqrt{\frac{(1+r)^2\sigma^2}{rn_{tot}}} = \delta - t_{(\beta,n_{tot}-2)}\sqrt{\frac{(1+r)^2\sigma^2}{rn_{tot}}}.$$

In the above equation $t_{(\gamma,n_{tot}-2)}$ is the upper 100γth percentile of a t-distribution with $(n_{tot} - 2)$ degrees of freedom. In this case, n_{tot} is given by

$$n_{tot} = \frac{(r+1)^2\sigma^2(t_{(\alpha,n_{tot}-2)} + t_{(\beta,n_{tot}-2)})^2}{r\delta^2}. \tag{6.6}$$

Because n_{tot} appears on both sides, some iteration is required to find the value of n_{tot} to satisfy the relationship in Equation 6.6. Equation 6.5 can be used as a starting point for this iteration. When the two treatment groups are expected to have different variances σ_E^2 and σ_C^2, Satterthwaite (1946) proposed to replace the equal-variance expression in Equation 6.6 by the following approximation

$$n_{tot} = \frac{[(1+r)\sigma_E^2 + r(r+1)\sigma_C^2](t_{(\alpha,df^*)} + t_{(\beta,df^*)})^2}{r\delta^2}, \tag{6.7}$$

where df^* is given by

$$df^* = \frac{\left(\dfrac{\sigma_E^2}{n_E} + \dfrac{\sigma_C^2}{n_C}\right)^2}{\left(\dfrac{\left(\dfrac{\sigma_E^2}{n_E}\right)^2}{n_E - 1}\right) + \left(\dfrac{\left(\dfrac{\sigma_C^2}{n_C}\right)^2}{n_C - 1}\right)}.$$

Again, iteration will be necessary to solve for n_{tot} in Equation 6.7. A starting point is to substitute in values for the standard Normal distribution in place of the t-distribution values.

6.2.1.1.2 2 × 2 Crossover Design

Consider a 2 × 2 crossover design where each sequence (e.g., AB and BA) is to be randomly assigned to n patients, resulting in a total of $n_{tot} = 2n$ subjects in the trial. Assume that the data will be analyzed using an analysis of variance model that contains additive terms for subject, period, and treatment. The sample size requirement in Equation 6.1 for a difference between treatment means of $\delta > 0$ with a known within subject variance σ_{ws}^2 states that

$$Z_\alpha \sqrt{\frac{2\sigma_{ws}^2}{n_{tot}}} = \delta - Z_\beta \sqrt{\frac{2\sigma_{ws}^2}{n_{tot}}}.$$

Hence the required total number of subjects is

$$n_{tot} = \frac{2\sigma_{ws}^2 (Z_\alpha + Z_\beta)^2}{\delta^2}. \tag{6.8}$$

For unknown variance Equation 6.8 becomes

$$n_{tot} = \frac{2\sigma_{ws}^2 (t_{\alpha,res} + t_{\beta,res})^2}{\delta^2}. \tag{6.9}$$

In Equation 6.9, *res* denotes the residual degrees of freedom from the analysis of variance. Some iteration is necessary to obtain the total number of subjects n_{tot}.

6.2.1.1.3 One-Way Analysis of Variance

For a one-way analysis of variance model with g (>2) treatments, if a single hypothesis is to be tested, it is usually about a linear contrast of the treatment means $\Sigma_{i=1}^g c_i\mu_i$ where $\Sigma_{i=1}^g c_i = 0$. We denote the value of this contrast when the treatment means are in the space covered by the alternative hypothesis by $\delta = \Sigma_{i=1}^g c_i \mu_{Ai}$. The alternative space in this case consists of all g-plets that are not all equal.

In this case the requirement represented by Equation 6.1 with equal treatment allocation and appropriate t-distribution substitution, becomes

$$t_{(\alpha,n_{tot}-g)}\sqrt{\frac{\sigma^2}{n}\sum_{i=1}^{g}c_i^2} = \delta - t_{(\beta,n_{tot}-g)}\sqrt{\frac{\sigma^2}{n}\sum_{i=1}^{g}c_i^2}.$$

The required sample size per group is

$$n = \frac{\sigma^2 \sum_{i=1}^{g} c_i^2 (t_{(\alpha,n_{tot}-g)} + t_{(\beta,n_{tot}-g)})^2}{\delta^2}. \tag{6.10}$$

A starting point for iteration is Equation 6.3 with $2\sigma^2$ replaced by $\sigma^2\Sigma_{i=1}^{g}c_i^2$.

6.2.1.1.4 Model-Based Design: E_{max} Models

An increasingly popular model for describing the relationship between dose and response in a dose-ranging study is the E_{max} model (Kirby, Brain, and Jones 2010) described in Equation 6.11.

$$Y = E_0 + \frac{E_{max} \times Dose^{\lambda}}{ED50^{\lambda} + Dose^{\lambda}} + \varepsilon. \tag{6.11}$$

In Equation 6.11, Y is the response while parameters E_0, E_{max}, $ED50$, and λ represent respectively, the placebo response, the maximum response attributable to the treatment, the dose that gives half of the treatment-induced response, and the shape of the dose–response curve. The error term, ε is usually assumed to be Normally and independently distributed with a constant variance. Setting $\lambda = 1$ gives the simpler 3-parameter E_{max} model.

Several questions are often of interest when employing the E_{max} model. For example, one can ask whether there is evidence of a dose–response relationship, whether the difference in response between a dose and placebo is likely to exceed a threshold of interest, and what dose gives a certain response above the placebo. For the first question, one can use an F test that looks at the additional sum of squares explained by the E_{max} model beyond that explained by the model, which predicts a constant response at all doses.

The test of whether the difference in response between a dose and the placebo exceeds a value of interest could be based on

$$\frac{\hat{E}_{max} \times Dose_i^{\hat{\lambda}}}{\hat{ED50}^{\hat{\lambda}} + Dose_i^{\hat{\lambda}}}. \tag{6.12}$$

In Equation 6.12, all estimates are maximum likelihood estimates. To find the asymptotic variance for the estimated difference in Equation 6.12, we could use the delta method (Morgan 2000). We could construct a statistic based on Equation 6.12 and its approximate asymptotic variance.

One could estimate the dose that will give a certain response Δ above that of a placebo. The estimated dose, given in Equation 6.13, could be obtained by solving the estimated E_{max} model. The delta method can again be used to obtain an approximate variance for the estimated dose. If the primary objective of fitting an E_{max} model is to identify a dose with a desirable property, the analysis will focus on estimation instead of hypothesis testing.

$$\hat{E}D_{\Delta} = \frac{\hat{E}D50}{\left(\dfrac{\hat{E}_{\max}}{\Delta} - 1\right)^{1/\lambda}}. \tag{6.13}$$

In the first two cases, power calculations are best done by simulation. Simulation is also the best approach to quantify the width of the confidence interval for the dose of interest in the third case. One can vary the sample size in the simulation to identify the smallest sample size that will meet the desirable properties under different assumptions on the parameters in the E_{max} model. We want to remind our readers that the E_{max} model (particular the 4-parameter one) may not fit a particular set of data in the sense that the fitting process might not converge. As a result, substitute models (Kirby, Brain, and Jones 2010) often need to be specified as a step-down option both in the protocol as well as when setting up the simulation program.

6.2.1.1.5 Model-Based Design: A Repeated Measures Model

Let Y_{ij} denote the response of the jth repeated measurement on the ith subject. We assume that the following repeated measures model is adequate to describe Y_{ij} under a two-treatment parallel group design:

$$Y_{ij} = \beta_0 + \beta_1 x_i + \varepsilon_{ij}, \quad j = 1,\ldots,k \quad i = 1,\ldots,2n. \tag{6.14}$$

In Equation 6.14, x_i is an indicator variable for treatment assignment (equal allocation). We assume that the errors have a known constant variance and that the correlation between any two measurements on the same individual is constant and equal to ρ. In addition, we assume that our interest is the time-averaged difference in response between two treatment groups. The variance of this time-averaged response for a subject is $\sigma^2[1 + (k - 1)\rho] / k$.

According to Equation 6.1, the sample size required to detect a difference of $\delta > 0$ needs to satisfy

$$Z_{\alpha}\sqrt{\frac{2\sigma^2[1+(k-1)\rho]}{kn}} = \delta - Z_{\beta}\sqrt{\frac{2\sigma^2[1+(k-1)\rho]}{kn}}.$$

The above equation leads to the following requirement for the necessary sample size in each group:

$$n = \frac{2\sigma^2[1+(k-1)\rho](Z_{\alpha}+Z_{\beta})^2}{k\delta^2}. \tag{6.15}$$

Equation 6.15 can be modified to reflect a different correlation matrix R between repeated measurements. This can be done by replacing $[1 + (k - 1)\rho] / k$ by $(\mathbf{1}'R^{-1}\mathbf{1})^{-1}$ where $\mathbf{1}$ is a k by 1 vector of ones and R^{-1} is the inverse matrix of R (Diggle et al. 2002).

6.2.1.2 Binary Data

6.2.1.2.1 Two Parallel Groups Design

An approximation for the required sample size under an r:1 randomization ratio (n_E/n_C) to detect a difference δ (> 0) in the response rates between two treatment groups could be obtained by noting that the sample size requirement (Equation 6.1) in this case becomes

$$Z_{\alpha}\sqrt{\frac{(1+r)^2\,pq}{rn_{tot}}} = \delta - Z_{\beta}\sqrt{\frac{(1+r)p_E q_E}{rn_{tot}} + \frac{(1+r)\,r\,p_C q_C}{rn_{tot}}}.$$

In the above expression, p_E and p_C represent the response rate in the experimental and the control group under the alternative hypothesis and $p_E - p_C = \delta$. p is the response rate among all subjects from the two groups combined, $q = 1 - p$, $q_C = 1 - p_C$, and $q_E = 1 - p_E$. Solving for n_{tot} in the above gives

$$n_{tot} = \frac{\left(Z_\alpha \sqrt{\frac{(1+r)^2 pq}{r}} + Z_\beta \sqrt{\frac{(1+r)}{r}(p_E q_E + r p_C q_C)} \right)^2}{\delta^2}. \tag{6.16}$$

6.2.1.2.2 *Chi-Square Test for Two Parallel Groups Design*

The sample size requirement for a chi-square test without continuity correction is

$$Z_\alpha \sqrt{\frac{(1+r)^2 pq}{r n_{tot}}} = \delta - Z_\beta \sqrt{\frac{(1+r)^2 pq}{r n_{tot}}},$$

where p, q, and δ were defined in the previous subsection. The above leads to the following expression for n_{tot}:

$$n_{tot} = \frac{(r+1)^2 (Z_\alpha + Z_\beta)^2 pq}{r\delta^2}. \tag{6.17}$$

6.2.1.2.3 *Fisher's Exact Test for Two Parallel Groups Design*

Under the null hypothesis that the response rates in the two groups are the same and conditional on the total number of responses (T) observed, the number of responses for the experimental treatment group follows a hypergeometric distribution

$$P(Y_E = i | T, n_E, n_C) = \frac{\binom{n_E}{i}\binom{n_C}{T-i}}{\binom{n_E + n_C}{T}}. \tag{6.18}$$

The exact p-value is defined as

$$\sum_{i=T_E}^{T} \frac{\binom{n_E}{i}\binom{n_C}{T-i}}{\binom{n_E + n_C}{T}}. \tag{6.19}$$

In Equation 6.19, T_E represents the observed responses in the experimental group.

In this case, sample size determination will be conducted through simulation or enumeration. For a prespecified configuration (p_E, p_C) under the alternative hypothesis and fixed n_E and n_C the power of Fisher's exact test can be obtained by summing the probabilities of all the outcomes such that the exact p-value is less than α.

6.2.1.2.4 Model-Based Design: Linear Trend Test for Proportions

When there are multiple doses in a study and the primary interest is to ascertain a dose–response relationship based on a binary endpoint, a common analytical approach is to conduct a trend test. Following Nam (1987), we assume there are k groups representing a placebo and (k-1) doses. Denote the binomial outcome among the n_i subjects at dose level x_i by Y_i (i = 0, …, k-1) and $x_0 = 0$ represents the placebo group. Thus, Y_i has a binomial distribution $B(n_i, p_i)$. We assume that $\{p_i\}$ follows a linear trend on the logistic scale; that is,

$$p_i = \frac{\exp(\gamma + \lambda x_i)}{1 + \exp(\gamma + \lambda x_i)}.$$

Defining

$$Y = \sum_i y_i, U = \sum_i y_i x_i, n_{tot} = \sum_i n_i, \bar{p} = \frac{Y}{N}, \bar{q} = 1 - \bar{p}, \text{and } \bar{x} = \sum_i \frac{n_i x_i}{n_{tot}},$$

it can be shown that Y and U are jointly sufficient for the parameters γ and λ. The conditional mean of U given Y, under the null hypothesis (all $\{p_i\}$ are the same), is

$$\bar{p}\left(\sum_i n_i x_i\right).$$

$$U' = U - \bar{p}\left(\sum_i n_i x_i\right) = \sum_i y_i (x_i - \bar{x})$$

has an approximate Normal distribution under the null hypothesis with a variance equal to

$$pq\left[\sum_i n_i (x_i - \bar{x})^2\right] \text{where } p = \sum n_i p_i / n_{tot} \text{ and } q = 1 - p.$$

The variance of U' under the alternative hypothesis is equal to

$$\sum_i n_i p_i q_i (x_i - \bar{x})^2.$$

For $\delta = \Sigma_i n_i p_i (x_i - \bar{x}), > 0$ under the alternative hypothesis assuming a positive trend between the response rate and the dose, the sample size requirement (Equation 6.1) becomes:

$$Z_\alpha \sqrt{pq \sum_i n_i (x_i - \bar{x})^2} = \sum_i n_i p_i (x_i - \bar{x}) - Z_\beta \sqrt{\sum_i n_i p_i q_i (x_i - \bar{x})^2}.$$

Letting

$$r_i = \frac{n_i}{n_0} \text{ and } A = \sum_i r_i p_i (x_i - \bar{x})$$

the sample size for the control group can be written as

$$n_0 = \frac{\left(Z_\alpha \sqrt{pq\sum_i r_i(x_i-\bar{x})^2} + Z_\beta \sqrt{\sum_i r_i p_i q_i (x_i-\bar{x})^2}\right)^2}{A^2}. \tag{6.20}$$

From n_0, one can find the necessary sample size n_i. The above is also the sample size for the Cochran-Armitage test without continuity correction.

6.2.1.2.5 Model-Based Design: Logistic Regression

In the simplest case with two treatment groups and a binary outcome, one could analyze the data by fitting the following logistic regression model

$$\log\left(\frac{p_i}{1-p_i}\right) = \alpha + \beta x_i,$$

where $x_i = 1$ for the experimental treatment and 0 for the control. In the above logistic regression model, β represents the additional effect associated with the experimental treatment. The parameter β can be written as

$$\log\left[\frac{p_E(1-p_C)}{(1-p_E)p_C}\right],$$

which is the logarithmic odds ratio of responding on the experimental treatment relative to the control treatment. This log odds ratio can be estimated by

$$\log\left[\frac{\hat{p}_E(1-\hat{p}_C)}{(1-\hat{p}_E)\hat{p}_C}\right],$$

where $\hat{p}_E$ and $\hat{p}_C$ are the observed rates for the two groups, respectively. This estimate has an asymptotic Normal distribution with mean equal to the true log odds ratio and an asymptotic standard deviation of

$$\sqrt{\frac{1}{n_E p_E(1-p_E)} + \frac{1}{n_c p_C(1-p_C)}}.$$

In this case, the sample size requirement for $\delta = \log[p_E(1-p_C)/(1-p_E)p_C]$ in Equation 6.1 becomes

$$Z_\alpha \sqrt{\frac{1}{n_E p_E(1-p_E)} + \frac{1}{n_C p_C(1-p_C)}} = \delta - Z_\beta \sqrt{\frac{1}{n_E p_E(1-p_E)} + \frac{1}{n_C p_C(1-p_C)}}.$$

Let $r = n_E/n_C$, the resulting sample size for the control is given in Equation 6.21. From n_C, one can obtain the sample size for the experimental group:

$$n_C = \frac{(Z_\alpha + Z_\beta)^2}{\delta^2}\left[\frac{1}{rp_E(1-p_E)} + \frac{1}{p_C(1-p_C)}\right]. \tag{6.21}$$

Additional discussion on sample size determination when logistic regression analysis is used can be found in Agresti (2002).

6.2.1.2.6 Model-Based Design: A Repeated Measures Model

Suppose a binary response is repeatedly measured and Y_{ij} denotes the jth response of the ith subject. Assume $\Pr(Y_{ij} = 1) = p_E$ for the experimental treatment and $\Pr(Y_{ij} = 1) = p_C$ for the control treatment.

We will assume that we are interested in the average response rate over time. Under the assumption of a constant correlation (ρ) between any two measurements on the same subject, the variance of the difference in time averaged proportions (equal allocation) under the null hypothesis is

$$\frac{2pq[1+(k-1)\rho]}{kn},$$

where p is the probability of response for all subjects combined and $q = 1 - p$. Under the alternative hypothesis, the variance is

$$\frac{(p_E q_E + p_C q_C)[1+(k-1)\rho]}{kn}.$$

Thus sample size requirement (Equation 6.1) for $\delta = p_E - p_C > 0$ becomes

$$n = \frac{[1+(k-1)\rho]\left[Z_\alpha\sqrt{2pq} + Z_\beta\sqrt{(p_E q_E + p_C q_C)}\right]^2}{k\delta^2}. \tag{6.22}$$

If we allow for a general correlation matrix R as in the case of a continuous endpoint, we can replace $[1 + (k - 1)\rho] / k$ by $(\mathbf{1}'R^{-1}\mathbf{1})^{-1}$ in the above expression. This is similar to the repeated measures case with a continuous endpoint.

6.2.1.3 Ordinal Data

When the number of ordinal categories is at least five and the sample size is reasonable, ordinal data are often analyzed as if they are continuous using scores assigned to the ordinal categories (Chuang-Stein and Agresti 1997). When this is the case, the methods discussed earlier for Normally distributed data can be considered for use.

6.2.1.3.1 Mann–Whitney Test for Two Parallel Groups

For two samples Y_{Ei} $(i = 1,\ldots,n_E)$ and Y_{Cj} $(j = 1,\ldots n_C)$, the Mann–Whitney statistic is based on the number of times that $Y_{Ei} > Y_{Cj}$ for all possible pairs of (Y_{Ei}, Y_{Cj}); that is, $\#(Y_E > Y_C$; Noether 1987). The expectation of $\#(Y_E > Y_C)$ under the null hypothesis is $n_E n_C / 2$. It is $n_E n_C p''$ under the alternative hypothesis where $p'' = P(Y_E > Y_C)$. Noether also shows that the standard error of $\#(Y_E > Y_C)$ under the null hypothesis is

$$\sqrt{\frac{n_E n_C (n_{tot}+1)}{12}},$$

and states that this could be used as an approximation to the standard error under the alternative hypothesis. With this approximation, the requirement (Equation 6.1) for $\delta = n_E n_C p'' > n_E n_C / 2$ becomes

$$\frac{n_E n_C}{2} + Z_\alpha\sqrt{\frac{n_E n_C (n_{tot}+1)}{12}} = \delta - Z_\beta\sqrt{\frac{n_E n_C (n_{tot}+1)}{12}}.$$

Using $n_E = cn_{tot}$ (so $n_C = (1 - c)n_{tot}$), the required sample size can be written as being approximately equal to

$$n_{tot} = \frac{(Z_\alpha + Z_\beta)^2}{12c(1-c)\left(p'' - \frac{1}{2}\right)^2}. \tag{6.23}$$

6.2.1.3.2 Model-Based Design: Proportional Odds Model

The proportional odds model (McCullagh 1980) is a model frequently used to describe ordinal data. We will assume that the response categories are arranged from the most desired one (the lowest category) to the least desired one (the highest category). When treatment is the only covariate, the proportional odds model for two treatments is

$$\log\left(\frac{Q_{ij}}{1-Q_{ij}}\right) = \alpha_j + \beta x_i \quad \text{i=1,2} \quad \text{j=1,...,k-1.}$$

In the above expression, Q_{ij} is the cumulative probability that a response in the *i*th treatment group is in category *j* or a lower (better) category, α_j is a parameter for the *j*th category, β represents the additional effect associated with the experimental treatment group, and x_i is an indicator variable taking the value 1 for the experimental treatment and 0 for the control. The name proportional odds model comes from the fact that the odds ratio below is the same regardless of $j = 1,\ldots, k-1$. The logarithm of this constant odds ratio is equal to the parameter β.

$$\log\left[\frac{Q_{1j}(1-Q_{2j})}{Q_{2j}(1-Q_{1j})}\right] = \beta.$$

Denote the maximum likelihood estimate for β by $\hat{\beta}$. Whitehead (1993) provides the following approximation to the large sample variance of $\hat{\beta}$:

$$V(\hat{\beta}) - \frac{1}{\frac{n_E n_C n_{tot}}{3(n_{tot}+1)^2}\left[1 - \sum_{j=1}^{k}\left(\frac{n_j}{n_{tot}}\right)^3\right]}.$$

Assuming a randomization ratio r between n_E and n_C, and $n_{tot} / (n_{tot} + 1) \approx 1$, sample size requirement (Equation 6.1) for $\delta = \log[Q_{Ej}(1 - Q_{Cj})/Q_{Cj}(1 - Q_{Ej})]$ becomes:

$$Z_\alpha \sqrt{\frac{1}{\frac{rn_{tot}}{3(r+1)^2}\left[1 - \sum_{j=1}^{k} \bar{p}_j^3\right]}} = \delta - Z_\beta \sqrt{\frac{1}{\frac{rn_{tot}}{3(r+1)^2}\left[1 - \sum_{j=1}^{k} \bar{p}_j^3\right]}},$$

where $\bar{p}_j$ is the average proportion responding in the *j*th category in the combined group under the alternative hypothesis. Solving for n_{tot} gives

$$n_{tot} = \frac{3(r+1)^2(Z_\alpha + Z_\beta)^2}{r\delta^2\left(1 - \sum_{j=1}^{k} \bar{p}_j^3\right)}. \tag{6.24}$$

6.2.1.4 Survival Data

6.2.1.4.1 Log-Rank Test

We will consider two treatment groups. Assume that the event of interest occurs at time t_j ($t_1 < t_2 < \ldots < t_r$) in the combined groups. The log-rank test comparing the two groups is based on

$$U = \sum_{j=1}^{r} (d_{Ej} - e_{Ej}),$$

where d_{Ej} is the observed number of subjects with the event in the experimental treatment group at time t_j and e_{Ej} is the corresponding expected number under the null hypothesis that the log hazard ratio between the two treatments

$$\phi(t) = \log(\psi(t)) = \log\left(\frac{h_E(t)}{h_C(t)}\right)$$

is zero at all time points. According to Sellke and Siegmund (1983), the distribution of U is approximately Normal with mean ϕV and variance V

$$V = \sum_{j=1}^{r} \frac{n_{Ej}\, n_{Cj}\, d_j(n_j - d_j)}{n_j^2(n_j - 1)}$$

for small values of ϕ.

In the above, n_j denotes the total number of subjects at risk for the event at time t_j and d_j ($= d_{Ej} + d_{Cj}$) is the number of events at t_j combined over the two groups. The log rank test is the most powerful nonparametric test to detect proportional hazards alternatives (Hopkin 2009). The latter includes the special case when the time-to-event distribution is exponential for both groups. The sample size requirement (Equation 6.1) for $\delta = \phi_A < 0$ becomes

$$-Z_\alpha \sqrt{V} = \delta\, V + Z_\beta \sqrt{V}.$$

When the number of events is few relative to the number at risk for the event, V can be approximated by (Collett 2003):

$$V = \sum_{j=1}^{r} \frac{n_{Ej}\, n_{Cj}\, d_j}{n_j^2}.$$

Further, if ϕ_A is small and an equal randomization ratio is employed, then V can be further simplified to $V = \sum_{j=1}^{r} d_j / 4$.

Using this simplification and rewriting the sample size requirement in terms of the total number of events d, we have

$$d = \frac{4(Z_\alpha + Z_\beta)^2}{\delta^2}. \quad (6.25)$$

When there are tied survival times, the use of the log rank test corresponds to the use of the score test for the discrete proportional hazards model. Please see Collett (2003) for more details. Assuming exponential time-to-event distributions, finding the number of subjects needed to produce the number of events in Equation 6.25 requires additional assumptions such as recruitment rate, recruitment period, and the length of follow-up.

6.2.2 Sample Size for Studies to Show Noninferiority

A different objective to that of proving superiority is to prove that an experimental treatment is at least within a certain treatment effect range of the active control in a randomized trial. To do this, the range or a noninferiority margin, $\delta_{non-\inf}$ (>0), needs to be defined. The noninferiority margin needs to be prespecified in the protocol. The choice of the margin should be based on a combination of statistical reasoning and clinical judgment, taking into consideration the particular disease area (ICH 1998; EMEA 2005). The margin should be set in such a way that if the margin requirement is met by the experimental treatment in a trial, the experimental treatment would have beaten a placebo if a placebo could have been included in the trial. In addition, by meeting the margin requirement, the experimental treatment is not substantially inferior to the control. For this chapter, we will assume that a margin has been carefully chosen for the noninferiority study being planned.

Assume again that higher values are indicative of a more desirable result and that θ represents the difference between the new treatment and the control (new treatment – control). With the definition of the noninferiority margin, the null hypothesis can be expressed as $H_0 : \theta \leq -\delta_{non-\inf}$ against the one-sided alternative $H_1 : \theta > -\delta_{non-\inf}$.

For θ set to $-\delta_{non-\inf}$ under the null hypothesis and set to 0 under the alternative hypothesis, Expression 6.1 becomes

$$-\delta_{non-\inf} + Z_\alpha \frac{\sigma(\theta=-\delta_{non-\inf})}{\sqrt{n_{tot}}} = -Z_\beta \frac{\sigma(\theta=0)}{\sqrt{n_{tot}}}.$$

For example, when the data are Normally distributed with a known and common variance in a parallel group design with equal randomization allocation, the sample size requirement becomes

$$-\delta_{non\ \inf} + Z_\alpha \sqrt{\frac{2\sigma^2}{n}} = -Z_\beta \sqrt{\frac{2\sigma^2}{n}}.$$

The above expression gives the required sample size per group as

$$n = \frac{2\sigma^2 (Z_\alpha + Z_\beta)^2}{\delta^2_{non-\inf}}. \tag{6.26}$$

We want to point out that if the null hypothesis H_0 is to be tested at a significance level of $\alpha/2$, we will need to replace Z_α in Equation 6.26 by $Z_{\alpha/2}$. The latter is usually what is required of confirmatory noninferiority trials even though we are only interested in a one-sided alternative hypothesis.

6.2.3 Sample Size for Studies to Show Equivalence

Occasionally the objective of a study is to show that two treatments are equivalent. This is often the case in bioequivalence studies (Patterson and Jones 2006). In general, the significance level for a bioequivalence study is set at a level higher than that for testing clinical equivalence.

In a similar manner to the case of noninferiority, the equivalence decision starts with the choice of an equivalence margin δ_{equiv} (>0). Assume that the probability to claim equivalence when the absolute difference between the two groups is δ_{equiv} is to be capped at α. One approach is to construct a symmetric 100(1–2α)% confidence interval for θ and conclude equivalence if the entire confidence interval falls within the interval $(-\delta_{equiv}, \delta_{equiv})$. An alternative approach that is operationally the same as the symmetric confidence interval approach is to conduct two sets of one-sided tests, each at a significance level of α. The two sets of tests are $H_{01}: \theta \leq -\delta_{equiv}$ versus $H_{11}: \theta > -\delta_{equiv}$ and $H_{02}: \theta \geq \delta_{equiv}$ versus $H_{12}: \theta < \delta_{equiv}$. Equivalence will be concluded if both H_{01} and H_{02} are rejected at the α level. Chow and Shao (2002) discussed differences between the testing and the confidence interval approach if other 100(1–2α)% confidence intervals are constructed.

Using the condition in Equation 6.1 with θ set to $-\delta_{equiv}$ under H_{01} and θ set to 0 under H_{11}, the sample size requirement for the first set of null and alternative hypotheses needs to satisfy

$$-\delta_{equiv} + Z_\alpha \frac{\sigma(\theta = -\delta_{equiv})}{\sqrt{n_{tot}}} = -Z_\beta \frac{\sigma(\theta = 0)}{\sqrt{n_{tot}}}.$$

This gives the expression for sample size to be

$$n_{tot} = \frac{\left(Z_\alpha \sigma(\theta = -\delta_{equiv}) + Z_\beta \sigma(\theta = 0)\right)^2}{\delta_{equiv}^2}. \tag{6.27}$$

The same sample size expression is obtained by considering the second set of hypotheses with θ set to δ_{equiv} under H_{02} and to 0 under H_{12}.

For comparing the means of two groups under a parallel group design with equal randomization allocation where data are Normally distributed with a known common variance, the sample size requirement can be expressed as

$$-\delta_{equiv} + Z_\alpha \sqrt{\frac{2\sigma^2}{n}} = -Z_\beta \sqrt{\frac{2\sigma^2}{n}},$$

leading to the required sample size per treatment group as

$$n = \frac{2\sigma^2 (Z_\alpha + Z_\beta)^2}{\delta_{equiv}^2}. \tag{6.28}$$

6.2.4 Information-Based Approach to Sample Sizing

Rather than considering the number of subjects required, a recent approach considers the amount of information required about the parameter of interest to ensure a prespecified power at an allowed Type I error rate. This is the case with the time-to-event endpoints considered earlier where the requirement is expressed in terms of the number of events to be observed. Information-based planning can be particularly useful for a group sequential design when the number of subjects required may depend on assumptions about nuisance parameters such as the variance for a continuous endpoint and the response rate of the control group for a binary endpoint (Mehta and Tsiatis 2001). We will use a simple example to illustrate the idea behind information-based sample size planning.

Suppose we are interested in comparing the means of two treatment groups for a parallel group design with n subjects per group and the variance for the two groups is assumed to be known and common between the groups. The information about the difference in the sample means is defined as

$n / (2\sigma^2)$, which is the inverse of the variance of the difference in sample means. Using Equation 6.3, we can demonstrate that

$$\frac{n}{2\sigma^2} = \frac{(Z_\alpha + Z_\beta)^2}{\delta^2}.$$

The advantage of the expression on the right-hand side of the above equation is that it does not contain the nuisance parameter σ^2 so it does not depend on a correct assumption about the value of this parameter. For a group sequential design, we can design the trial so that the trial achieves a prespecified maximum level of information if the trial reaches the target enrollment. This can be done by assessing the amount of information obtained at each interim analysis and comparing it with the maximum information required. The information available at each interim analysis can be estimated as the inverse of the variance of the estimator for the parameter of interest at the interim point.

Assume that the distribution of the test statistic under a fixed design is $Z \sim N(\theta\sqrt{I_{fixed}}, 1)$. The maximum information I_{max} under the group sequential version of the fixed design is related to I_{fixed} by $I_{max} = RI_{fixed}$ where R depends on the number of analyses (interim and final), α, β and the chosen function to describe the group sequential boundary (Jennison and Turnbull 2000). Some values for R are given in the book by Jennison and Turnbull. Values for other situations can be calculated using the general algorithm described by Jennison and Turnbull.

6.3 Other Approaches to Sample Sizing

6.3.1 Estimation

For many trials in the early phase of a product development program, the primary objective is to estimate the treatment effect or a dose–response relationship. For such trials, precision of the estimator is typically the basis for determining the necessary sample size. A common approach in this case is to put a bound on the expected distance between the point estimate and the upper (or lower) limit of a $100(1 - \alpha)\%$ confidence interval for the parameter of interest. For a symmetric confidence interval, such distance is simply one-half of the width of the confidence interval.

For an estimator of $f(\theta)$ that has a Normal or approximate Normal distribution with standard error of $\sigma(\theta)/\sqrt{n_{tot}}$, the requirement on the expected width of a symmetric confidence interval translates to

$$Z_{\alpha/2}\frac{\sigma(\theta)}{\sqrt{n_{tot}}} = \frac{w}{2},$$

where w is the width of the confidence interval. Solving for n_{tot} gives

$$n_{tot} = \frac{4Z_{\alpha/2}{}^2\sigma^2(\theta)}{w^2}. \tag{6.29}$$

For example, consider the case of two treatment groups in a parallel group design with n subjects per group. Assume the data follows a Normal distribution and the variance common to the two groups is known. The condition on the width of the confidence interval leads to

$$Z_{\alpha/2}\sqrt{\frac{2\sigma^2}{n}} = \frac{w}{2}, \tag{6.30}$$

which translates to the following requirement on n per group:

$$n = \frac{8Z_{\alpha/2}{}^2\sigma^2}{w^2}. \tag{6.31}$$

If the variance is common but unknown and the sample size is expected to be on the low side, a t-distribution might be a better choice than the Normal distribution in Equation 6.31. In this case, the sample size n needs to satisfy

$$t_{2(n-1),\alpha/2}\sqrt{\frac{2\sigma^2}{n}} = \frac{w}{2}.$$

The coverage probability obtained as described above will not be the nominal level 100(1 – α)%. This is because σ^2 needs to be estimated. For the coverage probability to be equal to 100(1 – γ)%, Kupper and Hafner (1989) show that we need to have

$$\Pr\left(s\sqrt{\frac{2}{n}}t_{2(n-1),\alpha/2} \le \frac{w}{2}\right) \ge 1-\gamma.$$

The above can be written as

$$\Pr\left(\frac{2(n-1)s^2}{\sigma^2} \le \frac{2n(n-1)(w/2)^2}{2\sigma^2 F_{1,2(n-1),\alpha}}\right) \ge 1-\gamma,$$

where $F_{1,2(n-1),\alpha}$ is the upper 100αth percentile of an F-distribution with (1,2(n-1)) df. As a result, n has to be at least large enough to satisfy the requirement in Equation 6.32.

$$\frac{2n(n-1)}{n_z} \ge \frac{\chi^2_{2(n-1),\gamma}F_{1,2(n-1),\alpha}}{\chi^2_{1,\alpha}}. \tag{6.32}$$

In Equation 6.32, $\chi^2_{q,\varsigma}$ is the upper 100ςth percentile of a χ^2-distribution with q df and n_z is the sample size in Equation 6.31.

Another situation where the objective is estimation rather than testing is the use of algorithm-based designs to estimate the maximum tolerated dose (MTD) in Phase I oncology trials. There are many variants of algorithm-based designs in this context. The simplest one is the 3 + 3 design that does not allow dose de-escalation. This design can be described as follows:

> Groups of 3 patients are entered at a dose level i. If no patient has a dose-limiting toxicity then the dose is escalated to the next dose i + 1. If at least two patients have dose-limiting toxicities then the previous dose i–1 will be considered the MTD. If only one patient has a dose-limiting toxicity, then three more patients will be treated at dose level i. If at most one of the six patients treated at dose i has a dose-limiting toxicity then the dose is escalated. If at least two out of six patients have a dose-limiting toxicity then the previous dose is considered the MTD. If dose escalation is still indicated at the last dose level then the MTD is at or above the last dose. If the trial stops at the first dose then the MTD is below the first dose. In either of these two cases the MTD is considered to not have been determined from the trial.

It is not possible to know in advance the exact number of patients needed in the design. Given the probability of toxicity at each dose level it is possible to derive an expression for the expected number of patients in the trial. The derivation of the expression is somewhat lengthy so we refer the readers to Lin and Shih (2001) for details.

6.3.2 Sample Sizing for Dual Criteria

Concerns about concluding a statistically significant but not clinically meaningful difference have led some authors to consider other possible success criteria (Kieser and Hauschke 2005; Chuang-Stein et al. 2010). One approach is to set dual success criteria requiring the difference to be statistically significant and a treatment effect estimate that is greater than some threshold.

Consider the case of comparing the means of two treatment groups with n per group under a parallel group design. Assume that the data are Normally distributed with a known common variance. Suppose the threshold for clinical relevance is chosen to be the MCID. When the true difference in treatment means is δ ($\delta > \text{MCID}$), n needs to satisfy the inequality in Equation 6.33 for the study to have a greater than $(1 - \gamma)$ chance to observe a difference in means at least as large as the MCID:

$$n \geq \frac{2\sigma^2 Z_\gamma^2}{(\delta - \text{MCID})^2}. \tag{6.33}$$

The right-hand side of the inequality in Equation 6.33 can be very large if δ is not much greater than the MCID. The ratio of sample size required to have an observed difference in means greater than the MCID and the usual sample size given by Expression 6.3 is

$$\frac{Z_\gamma^2}{(Z_{\alpha/2} + Z_\beta)^2} \frac{\delta^2}{(\delta - \text{MCID})^2}.$$

Setting $(1 - \beta) = (1 - \gamma) = 0.9$ and $\alpha = 0.05$, it can be shown that the requirement to observe a difference in means greater than the MCID will be more demanding than the requirement of statistical significance if $\delta < 1.65$*MCID. In other words, the true treatment difference needs to be quite a bit bigger than the MCID for the requirement on the observed difference to be less demanding than that of a statistical significance. This means that for the dual success criteria to be met with a reasonable sample size, the true treatment effect needs to be reasonably large.

Another possibility is to size a study to test the null hypothesis of $H_0 : \theta \leq \text{MCID}$ against the alternative hypothesis of $H_1 : \theta > \text{MCID}$. Again, consider the simple case of comparing the means of two treatment groups with equal sample size where the data follow a Normal distribution with known constant variance. The sample size requirement can be written as

$$\text{MCID} + Z_\alpha \sqrt{\frac{2\sigma^2}{n}} = \delta - Z_\beta \sqrt{\frac{2\sigma^2}{n}},$$

leading to

$$n = \frac{2\sigma^2 (Z_\alpha + Z_\beta)^2}{(\delta - \text{MCID})^2}. \tag{6.34}$$

The ratio of this expression to Equation 6.3 is $\delta^2 / (\delta - \text{MCID})^2$. The ratio is quite large when δ is close to (but greater than) the MCID. For example, if MCID = 0.3 and $\delta = 0.4$, the ratio is 16. The ratio decreases as δ increases. When $\delta = 2^*\text{MCID}$, the ratio is 4. Since the sample size for the expression in Equation 6.3 (based on a perceived treatment effect that is two times the MCID) is relatively small, the sample size required according to Equation 6.34 might not be prohibitively large. However, the implied requirement of a treatment effect of two times the MCID is unlikely to be met very often in practice!

6.3.3 Prespecifying Desirable Posterior False-Positive and False-Negative Probabilities

Lee and Zelen (2000) propose an approach aimed to achieve prespecified posterior false-positive and false-negative error probabilities conditional on the outcome of a trial. They consider the null and alternative hypotheses given by $H_0 : \theta = 0$ and $H_1 : \theta \neq 0$ and argue that for a trial to be considered ethical it is necessary that there is no prior reason to favor one treatment over another. Therefore, they assign equal prior probability $\pi / 2$ to $\theta > 0$ and $\theta < 0$, leaving a prior probability $(1 - \pi)$ to the null hypothesis H_0.

Let C be a binary outcome that reflects the outcome of the trial with " + " denoting success (i.e., rejecting H_0) and "–" denoting failure (i.e., failing to reject H_0) and T be a binary outcome denoting the true state of nature with " + " denoting $\theta \neq 0$ (H_1) and "–" denoting $\theta = 0$ (H_0). We have $\alpha = \Pr(C = + | T = -)$ and $\beta = \Pr(C = - | T = +)$.

The posterior false-negative and false-positive error probabilities can be defined as $\alpha^* = \Pr(T = + | C = -)$ and $\beta^* = \Pr(T = - | C = +)$. Using Bayes rule, we could obtain the posterior probabilities for making the correct decisions as follows:

$$P_1 = 1 - \alpha^* = \Pr(T = - | C = -) = \frac{(1-\alpha)(1-\pi)}{(1-\alpha)(1-\pi) + \beta\pi},$$

and

$$P_2 = 1 - \beta^* = \Pr(T = + | C = +) = \frac{(1-\beta)\pi}{(1-\beta)\pi + \alpha(1-\pi)}.$$

Consequently, α and β can be written in terms of P_1, P_2, and π as

$$\alpha = \frac{(1-P_2)(\pi + P_1 - 1)}{(1-\pi)(P_1 + P_2 - 1)},$$

and

$$\beta = \frac{(1-P_1)(P_2 - \pi)}{\pi(P_1 + P_2 - 1)}.$$

These relationships require that $P_1 > 1 - \pi$ and $P_2 > \pi$ to avoid the possibility that α and β are negative. These two conditions ensure that the posterior probabilities are larger than the respective prior probabilities and that the hypothesis testing is informative.

Lee and Zelen propose a trialist to specify P_1, P_2, and π that satisfy $P_1 > 1 - \pi$ and $P_2 > \pi$. From these three values, a trialist could derive α and β and proceed with the conventional sample size formulae using the obtained α and β. For example, if $\pi = 0.2$, $P_1 = 0.9$, and $P_2 = 0.60$, then α and β will be 0.1 and 0.4, respectively.

6.3.4 Assurance for Confirmatory Trials

In a similar manner to the approach of Lee and Zelen (2000), the assurance approach to determining the sample size makes use of a prior distribution for the treatment effect. The prior distribution is not used to calculate posterior error probabilities, but to calculate the probability of success for the final analysis based on a frequentist analysis at a conventional significance level α. Such an approach is likely to be of particular interest for Phase III trials, because it gives an assessment on the probability of reaching a successful trial outcome.

To illustrate the approach we consider again the situation of comparing the means of two treatment groups of equal sample size (n per group) and the data are Normally distributed with a known common variance. We assume that our prior knowledge about the treatment effect can be summarized by a Normal distribution with mean μ_0 and variance ν. We can combine this assumption with the sampling distribution for the difference in sample means to obtain the unconditional distribution for the difference in the sample means as below:

$$\int P(\bar{Y}_E - \bar{Y}_C | \delta) f(\delta) d\delta.$$

Let $\tau^2 = \sigma^2(2 / n)$. We can show that the unconditional distribution for $\bar{Y}_E - \bar{Y}_C$ is Normal with mean μ_0 and variance $\tau^2 + \nu$. The null hypothesis of $H_0 : \mu_E - \mu_C \leq 0$ is rejected in favor of the alternative hypothesis $H_1 : \mu_E - \mu_C > 0$ at a significance level α if the observed means in the two group satisfy $\bar{Y}_E - \bar{Y}_C > Z_\alpha \tau$. The probability of this happening is equal to

$$1 - \Phi\left(\frac{Z_\alpha \tau - \mu_0}{\sqrt{\tau^2 + \nu}}\right) = \Phi\left(\frac{-Z_\alpha \tau + \mu_0}{\sqrt{\tau^2 + \nu}}\right).$$

The above probability is termed assurance by O'Hagan, Stevens, and Campbell (2005).

If $-Z_\alpha \tau + \mu_0 > 0$, the assurance will be less than the usual power to detect a difference of μ_0. The latter is $\Phi[(-Z_\alpha \tau + \mu_0)/\tau]$. The motivation for considering assurance instead of power is that by the time a sponsor is planning a confirmatory trial, there should be reasonably good information about the treatment effect. Using this prior information in the above approach gives an assessment of the probability of achieving statistical significance given the relevant prior information. By comparison the traditional approach to sample sizing based on the concept of statistical power gives the probability of a statistically significant result conditional on the treatment effect being assumed to take a fixed value.

We would like to point out that there are situations when one cannot increase the assurance to a desirable level by simply increasing the sample size. In the example above, the maximum achievable assurance probability is $\Phi(\mu_0 / \sqrt{\nu})$, which is determined by the amount of prior information we have about the treatment effect. This limit reflects what is achievable given the prior information. Thus, if the assurance for a confirmatory trial is much lower than the usual power based on the traditional sample size consideration, one needs to pause and evaluate seriously the adequacy of prior information before initiating a confirmatory trial.

We would like to point out that success can be defined more broadly. For example, a successful outcome may be defined by a statistically significant difference plus a clinically meaningful point estimate for the treatment effect. Whatever the definition may be, one can apply the concept of assurance by averaging the probability of a successful outcome over the prior distribution for the treatment effect. Interested readers are referred to Carroll (2009) and Chuang-Stein et al. 2010.

6.4 Other Topics

6.4.1 Missing Data

A simple way to compensate for missing data is to increase the sample size from n_{tot} to

$$n_{tot}^{*} = \frac{n_{tot}}{1 - p_{miss}}, \tag{6.35}$$

where p_{miss} is the proportion of subjects with missing data.

The inflation noted in Expression 6.35 acts as if patients who dropped out early from the trial contribute no information to the analysis. While this practice creates a conservative sample size in most situations, some analytical approaches to handling missing data could require a different adjustment. For example, if missingness occurs completely at random and the primary analysis adopts the baseline carried forward procedure, then the mean treatment effect measured by change from baseline will be $(1 - p_{miss})\delta$, if δ is the true treatment effect. To detect an effect of the size $(1 - p_{miss})\delta$, we will need to increase the sample size to $n_{tot}(1 - p_{miss})^{-2}$ and not just $n_{tot}(1 - p_{miss})^{-1}$. For example, if $p_{miss} = 0.3$, the sample size will need to be at least twice as large as the originally estimated sample size n_{tot}. This represents a substantial increase and illustrates how procedures to handle missing data could substantially affect sample size decisions.

6.4.2 Multiple Comparisons

In many trials, there is interest in conducting several inferential tests and drawing definitive inferences from all these tests. The need to control the study-wise Type I error rate on such occasions has led to many proposals for multiple comparison procedures (Hochberg and Tamhane 1987). When determining the sample size for such a trial, it is important to take into consideration how the multiplicity adjustment will be carried out in the analysis. One approach that has been frequently used to determine sample size in the presence of multiple comparisons is to apply the Bonferroni procedure and use a conservative significance level for each individual test. The rationale is that because of the conservative nature of Bonferroni adjustment, the sample size obtained under this approach will generally lead to a higher power when a more efficient multiple comparison procedure is used.

Alternatively, one could use simulation to determine the necessary sample size. The greatest advantage of simulation is that it offers flexibility and can incorporate other considerations in sample size decisions. The latter includes methods to handle missing data and examine the impact of different missing patterns. For some trials, dropout occurs early due to intolerance to the study medications. In other trials, dropout could occur uniformly throughout the study duration. If a mixed model for repeated measures is used in the primary analysis, different missing patterns might have different impact on the analytical results. These different considerations could be included in extensive scenario planning at the design stage.

Another important consideration in sample size planning when multiple comparisons are involved is the definition of power. Many trialists employ a hierarchical testing strategy under, which tests are successively conducted until a nonsignificant conclusion is reached. While this sequential testing preserves the Type I error rate, it has an impact on the power for tests that are several steps beyond the initial one. Thus, if a specific comparison is of prime importance despite its location in the sequence of tests, it is important that we assess the chance of reaching this particular comparison. Simulation can help us with this assessment.

6.4.3 Reducing Sample Size Due to Efficiency Gain in an Adjusted Analysis

The inclusion of predictive covariates in either a linear model or a logistic model will increase the efficiency of testing for a treatment effect (Robinson and Jewell 1991). Let us first consider the linear model case where gender (denoted by Z) is predictive of a continuous outcome Y. The model in Equation 6.36 contains only the treatment assignment X ($x_i = 1$ if the ith subject receives the new treatment and $= 0$ otherwise). The model in Equation 6.37 contains a term representing gender (0 or 1) in addition to the treatment assignment. The variance of the two models are denoted by $\sigma^2_{Y.X}$ and $\sigma^2_{Y.XZ}$, respectively:

$$E(Y_i \mid x_i) = a^* + b_1^* x_i, \tag{6.36}$$

$$E(Y_i \mid x_i, z_i) = a + b_1 x_i + b_2 z_i. \tag{6.37}$$

We will assume that the response follows a Normal distribution and denote the maximum likelihood estimates for b_1^* and b_1 by $\hat{b}_1^*$ and $\hat{b}_1$, respectively. The asymptotic relative precision of $\hat{b}_1$ to $\hat{b}_1^*$ is

$$ARP(\hat{b}_1 \text{ to } \hat{b}_1^*) = \frac{\text{var}(\hat{b}_1^*)}{\text{var}(\hat{b}_1)} = \frac{1-\rho^2_{XZ}}{1-\rho^2_{YZ.X}}. \tag{6.38}$$

In Equation 6.38, ρ_{XZ} is the correlation between X and Z and $\rho_{YZ.X}$ is the partial correlation between Y and Z given X. In a randomized trial where a single randomization ratio is used, $\rho_{XZ} = 0$. As a result, $ARP(\hat{b}_1 \text{ to } \hat{b}_1^*) > 1$ unless $\rho_{YZ.X} = 0$. The latter condition fails when gender is predictive of response regardless of the treatment group. Therefore, the inclusion of a predictive covariate in a linear model will increase the precision of the estimate for the treatment effect.

For large trials, randomization generally creates reasonable balance between treatment groups. The point estimate for the treatment effect under the model in Equation 6.36 will be reasonably close to that under model Equation 6.37, so bias is usually not an issue. The major advantage of including predictive covariates is the gain in efficiency from a more precise treatment effect estimate.

The situation with a logistic model is more complicated. Imagine replacing the left-hand side of Equations 6.36 and 6.37 by $\log(p_i/(1-p_i))$ where $p_i = \Pr(Y_i = 1)$ and $1 - p_i = \Pr(Y_i = 0)$. The complication in this case comes from nonlinear models and the fact that models in Equations 6.36 and 6.37 estimate different parameters (Freedman 2008). The model in Equation 6.36 deals with population-based inference while the model in Equation 6.37 deals with inference conditional on the covariate (gender). As such, comparing the estimates for b_1^* and b_1 directly is not particularly meaningful. However, since both estimates have been used to test for a treatment effect, we will include some comments on their relative performance here.

Robinson and Jewell (1991) show that in the case of a logistic model, $\text{var}(\hat{b}_1) \geq \text{var}(\hat{b}_1^*)$. Also, the point estimate $\hat{b}_1$ tends to be larger than $\hat{b}_1^*$ in absolute value. However, the asymptotic relative efficiency of $\hat{b}_1$ to $\hat{b}_1^*$, measured in terms of statistical power to test for a treatment effect is ≥ 1. It is equal to 1 if and only if gender (in our example) is independent of (Y,X).

So, when the analysis is adjusted for predictive covariates, there is usually some gain in efficiency for testing the treatment effect. When planning the sample size for a trial, one should consider how such efficiency gain might be translated to a smaller sample size. This will not be an issue if the variance used in the planning is the residual error variance from a fitted model in a previous trial. On other hand, if the variance used in the planning is the within-group sample variance from the previous trial, then one could possibly use a sample size smaller than that based on the within-group sample variance. Although it is possible that a trialist might ultimately decide not to take advantage of this efficiency gain at the planning stage in order to provide some protection against uncertainties, this decision should be an informed articulation with full awareness of the implications.

6.5 Summary

In this chapter, we focus on sample size planning for classical designs where sample size is determined at the beginning of the trial. We cover different types of endpoints under both the modeling and non-modeling approaches. Despite this, our coverage is limited. There are many other scenarios that have been omitted from this chapter. For example, one could apply isotonic regression analysis when looking at a dose–response relationship.

We include closed-form formulae to handle simpler situations. Many of them are a convenient first-step in providing an approximate sample size for more complex situations. Traditionally sample sizing has focused heavily on hypothesis testing. We have shown how sample size could be determined for a model-based approach. Due to the heavy use of simulation and computing-intensive methodology, a trialist is no longer limited to closed-form formulae. Simulation can better handle more complicated situations. It allows us to address more real-world situations and better align sample size planning with the analytical strategy chosen for the trial.

A lot of attention is being devoted to making better decisions during the learn phase of a "learn-and-confirm" drug development paradigm (Sheiner 1997). The learn phase consists of proof of concept and dose-ranging studies. The primary objective of a proof-of-concept trial is often to make a correct decision, which means a go-decision if the investigative product is promising and a no-go decision if the investigative product is inactive. Without a strong prior belief on the effect of the new treatment, the probability of an erroneous go-decision and that of an erroneous no-go decision could be similarly important to a pharmaceutical sponsor. As a result, the metric for judging the quality of the decision could be a combination of these two probabilities. For a dose-ranging study, the primary objectives are often to ascertain a positive dose–response relationship and to identify the "right" dose to move into the confirmatory phase if the data support this decision. While we discuss sample size based on fitting a dose–response model in this chapter, we have not explicitly addressed the sample size required for sound dose selection. Because decisions in the learn phase are generally more fluid and unique to each situation, it is hard to provide explicit sample size formulation. Instead, a general framework for making decisions and evaluating the operating characteristics of the design (including sample size) may be the best recommendation to a trialist (Kowalski et al. 2007, Chuang-Stein et al. 2010).

Another trend in sample size planning is the awareness that our uncertainty in the treatment effect should be incorporated into the planning. The concept of statistical power should be combined with our knowledge on the treatment effect. This is especially true in the development of a pharmaceutical product where the ultimate goal is a valuable medicine and our knowledge about the product candidate accumulates over time. The chance of reaching that goal needs to be constantly evaluated and reevaluated to the extent that it becomes an integral part of the stage-gate decisions.

Increasingly, internal decisions by a pharmaceutical sponsor have taken on a Bayesian flavor and a critical question is the chance that the new product possesses certain properties deemed necessary for it to be commercially viable. As such, sample size, which is a strong surrogate for the cost of a clinical trial, needs to be planned with this new objective in mind.

Another realization is that despite the best planning, surprises can occur. It might turn out that the information we have accumulated so far based on a more homogeneous population does not appropriately reflect the treatment outcome in a more heterogeneous population. In many situations, it is critical to have the opportunity to recalibrate design parameters such as sample size and in some cases, the target population, as a trial progresses. It is conjectured that by recalibrating our design specifications, we will enable better decisions that could lead to a higher Phase III success rate (Chuang-Stein 2004). The latter is the topic of other chapters in this book.

References

Agresti, A. (2002). *Categorical Data Analysis*, 2nd ed. New Jersey: Wiley.

Caroll, J. K. (2009). Back to basics: Explaining sample size in outcome trials, are statisticians doing a thorough job? *Pharmaceutical Statistics*, DOI:10.1002/pst.362.

Chow, S. C., and Shao, J. (2002). A note on statistical methods for assessing therapeutic equivalence. *Controlled Clinical Trials*, 23: 515–20.

Chow, S. C., Shao, J., and Wang, H. (2008). *Sample Size Calculations in Clinical Research*, 2nd ed. Boca Raton, FL: Chapman and Hall.

Chuang-Stein, C. (2004). Seize the opportunities. *Pharmaceutical Statistics*, 3 (3): 157–59.

Chuang-Stein, C., and Agresti, A. (1997). Tutorial in biostatistics: A review of tests for detecting a monotone dose-response relationship with ordinal response data. *Statistics in Medicine*, 16: 2599–2618.

Chuang-Stein, C., Kirby, S., Hirsch, I., and Atkinson, G. (2010). A Quantitative Approach for Making Go/No Go Decisions in Drug Development (accepted for publication in *Drug Information Journal*).

Chuang-Stein, C., Kirby, S., Hirsch, I., and Atkinson, G. (2010). The role of the minimum clinically important difference and its impact on designing a trial. (submitted for publication).

Collett, D. (2003). *Modelling Survival Data in Medical Research,* 2nd ed. Boca Raton, FL: Chapman and Hall.

Diggle, P. J., Heagerty, P., Liang, K., and Zeger, S. L. (2002). *Analysis of Longitudinal Data,* 2nd ed. Oxford: Oxford University Press.

Donner, A. (1984). Approaches to sample size estimation in the design of clinical trials—A review. *Statistics in Medicine*, 3: 199–214.

Dupont, W. D., and Plummer, W. D., Jr. (1990). Power and sample size calculations. *Controlled Clinical Trials,* 11: 116–28.

EMEA. (2005). *Guideline on the Choice of the Non-Inferiority Margin 2005*. Available at http://www.emea.europa.eu/htms/human/humanguidelines/efficacy.htm

Freedman, D. A. (2008). Randomization does not justify logistic regression. *Statistical Science*, 23 (2): 237–49.

Hochberg, Y., and Tamhane, A. (1987). *Multiple Comparison Procedures*. New Jersey: John Wiley & Sons.

Hopkin, A. (2009). Log-rank test. *Wiley Encyclopedia of Clinical Trials*, New Jersey: Wiley.

ICH. (1998). *ICH-E9 Statistical Principles for Clinical Trials 1998*. Available at http://www.ich.org/LOB/media/MEDIA485.pdf

Jennison, C. J., and Turnbull, B. W. (2000). *Group Sequential Methods with Applications to Clinical Trials*. Boca Raton, FL: Chapman and Hall.

Kieser, M., and Hauschke, D. (2005). Assessment of clinical relevance by considering point estimates and associated confidence intervals. *Pharmaceutical Statistics*, 4: 101–7.

Kirby, S., Brain, P., and Jones, B. (2010). Fitting Emax models to clinical trial dose-response data (accepted for publication in *Pharmaceutical Statistics*).

Kowalski, K. G., Ewy, W., Hutmacher, M. W., Miller, R., and Krishnaswami, S. (2007). Model-based drug development—A new paradigm for efficient drug development. *Biopharmaceutical Report*, 15 (2): 2–22.

Kupper, L. L., and Hafner, K. B. (1989). How appropriate are popular sample size formulas? *The American Statistician*, 43 (2): 101–5.

Lachin, J. M. (1981). Introduction to sample size determination and power analysis for clinical trials. *Controlled Clinical Trials*, 2: 93–113.

Lee, S. J., and Zelen, M. (2000). Clinical trials and sample size considerations: Another perspective. *Statistical Science*, 15 (2): 95–110.

Lin, Y., and Shih, W. J. (2001). Statistical properties of the traditional algorithm-based designs for phase I cancer clinical trials. *Biostatistics*, 2: 203–15.

Machin, D., Campbell, M. J., Tan, S.-B., and Tan, S.-H. (2008). *Sample Size Tables for Clinical Studies*, 3rd ed. Chichester: Wiley-Blackwell.

Mehta C., and Tsiatis, A. A. (2001). Flexible sample size considerations using information-based interim monitoring. *Drug Information Journal*, 35: 1095–1112.

Morgan, B. J. T. (2000). *Applied Stochastic Modelling*. London: Arnold.

McCullagh, P. (1980). Regression models for ordinal data. *Journal of the Royal Statistical Society, Series B*, 42: 109–42.

Nam, J. (1987). A simple approximation for calculating sample sizes for detecting linear trend in proportions. *Biometrics*, 43: 701–5.

Noether, G. E. (1987). Sample size determination for some common nonparametric tests. *JASA*, 82 (398): 645–47.

O'Brien, R. G., and Castelloe, J. (2007). Sample-size analysis for traditional hypothesis testing: Concepts and Issues. Chapter 10 in *Pharmaceutical Statistics Using SAS: A Practical Guide*, eds. A. Dmitrienko, C. Chuang-Stein, and R. D'Agostino. Cary, NC: SAS Press.

O'Hagan, A., Stevens, J. W., and Campbell, M. J. (2005). Assurance in clinical trial design. *Pharmaceutical Statistics*, 4: 187–201.

Patterson, S., and Jones, B. (2006). *Bioequivalence and Statistics in Clinical Pharmacology*. Boca Raton, FL: Chapman and Hall.

Robinson, L. D., and Jewell, N. P. (1991). Some surprising results about covariate adjustment in logistic regression models. *International Statistical Review*, 58 (2): 227–40.

Satterthwaite, F. E. (1946). An approximate distribution of estimates of variance components. *Biometrics Bulletin*, 2: 110–14.

Sellke, T., and Siegmund, D. (1983). Sequential analysis of the proportional hazards model. *Biometrika*, 70: 315–26.

Senchaudhuri, P., Suru, V., Kannappan, A., Pradhan, V., Patel, A., Chandran, V. P., Deshmukh, A., Lande, B., Sampgaonkar, J., Mehta, C. and Patel, N. (2004). *StatXact PROCs for SAS Users: Statistical Software for Exact Nonparametric Inference*. Version 6. Cytel Software.

Sheiner, L. B. (1997). Learning versus confirming in clinical drug development. *Clinical Pharmacology & Therapeutics*, 61 (3): 275–91.

Shuster, J. J. (1990). *Handbook of Sample Size Guidelines for Clinical Trials*. Boca Raton, FL: CRC Press.

Whitehead, J. (1993). Sample size calculations for ordered categorical data. *Statistics in Medicine*, 12: 2257–71.

7

Sample Size Reestimation Design with Applications in Clinical Trials

Lu Cui
Eisai Inc.

Xiaoru Wu
Columbia University

7.1 Flexible Sample Size Design

In clinical trials, the traditional approach to demonstrate that a new drug is superior to a placebo uses a fixed sample size design. The number of subjects needed are calculated prior to the start of the study based on a targeted treatment difference δ_0 as well as the estimated variation of the response variable. As an example, consider a two arm clinical trial comparing a new test drug with a placebo. Assume that the outcomes of the primary efficacy measurement X for the placebo and Y for the new treatment follow the normal distributions with means μ_0 and μ_1, respectively, and a common variance $0.5\sigma^2$. The corresponding one-sided hypothesis then is

$$H_0:\delta=0 \quad vs. \quad H_1:\delta>0, \tag{7.1}$$

where $\delta=\mu_1-\mu_0$ is the treatment difference. Assuming that σ is known, for usual fixed sample size design, the number of subjects per treatment group needed to detect the treatment difference δ based on Z-test with the power $1-\beta$ at the significance level α is calculated as

$$N_{(1-\beta)}(\delta)=\frac{(z_\alpha+z_\beta)^2}{\delta^2}. \tag{7.2}$$

Here z is the upper percentile of the standard normal distribution. Write the Z statistic as

$$Z=\frac{\sum_{i=1}^{N} Z_i}{\sqrt{N}\sigma},$$

where $Z_i=Y_i-X_i$ and $N=N_{(1-\beta)}(\delta)$. For simplicity we further assume $\sigma=1$. In practice σ can often be estimated using historical data at the time of study design, or using blinded data during the trial (Gould 1992; Gould and Shi 1992; Shi 1993).

Since the true treatment difference is unknown, to calculate the sample size, δ in Equation 7.2 is replaced by a targeted treatment difference δ_0. The determination of δ_0 can be based on various considerations such as clinical, marketing, resource, or other considerations. However, it essentially needs to be in line with the true δ. Otherwise the calculated sample size can be off the target, leading to an under- or over-powered study depending on how δ_0 differs from δ. For fixed sample size design, choice of δ_0 is critically important, and once the sample size is calculated it can no longer be altered.

Accurately projecting the true treatment difference to determine the sample size is challenging. Because of lack of prior data, an accurate projection of δ can be difficult to obtain. This is particularly true when the study is for a drug in a new class or in a patient population that is somehow different from those in the earlier studies. For example, if a Phase III study is to enroll patients globally, the estimate of the treatment difference δ based on the data from small Phase II studies conducted in the United States will potentially be inaccurate. For a mega Phase III study requiring tens of thousands of subjects to detect a small treatment difference, the conflict between need and lack of good prior information at the design stage becomes more prominent. On one hand, a slight miss of the targeted δ may have significant impact on the projection of the total sample size and hence the power of the trial. On the other hand, limited resource and a tight timeline may prohibit conducting extensive Phase II studies to generate sufficient information for later design use.

To further illustrate the difficulty in sample size calculation, a concrete example is given in Liu, Zhu, and Cui (2008) involving two well-known randomized studies of Tamoxifen in preventing breast cancer in patients at high risk. One study, Breast Cancer Prevention Trial (BCPT) with a total $n = 13{,}388$ subjects shows a reduction in relative risk of breast cancer incidence of 49% as Tamoxifen versus the control. A similar study, Italian National Trial (INT), with $n = 5408$ shows only a risk reduction of 24% associated with the Tamoxifen use. The different outcomes from two similar studies surely puzzle later trial designers who may wonder what would be the right effect size to use in projecting the sample size. Unfortunately, in reality, a situation like this happens from time to time. Despite efforts made, the uncertainty associated with projecting δ is constantly presented and the reliability of the calculated sample size from time to time becomes questionable. To address this issue, flexible sample size design is proposed as an alternative approach to fixed sample size calculation.

Flexible sample size design implements the idea of internal data piloting to allow adjustment of final sample size based on interim data of a study (Wittes and Brittain 1990). This is different from traditional fixed sample size design in which the final sample size remains the same as the initial projection. Flexible sample size design has the advantage of utilizing internal trial data that is more relevant than external data, and can be more abundant than historical data from small early Phase II studies. Further, such internal data can be readily available when the trial has scheduled unblinded interim data monitoring. As compared to the fixed sample size method, there is a better chance for flexible sample size design to hit the target.

The objective of the flexible sample size design is to achieve a robust statistical power of the trial through interim sample size adjustment. Consider the hypothesis testing problem (Equation 7.1). If the true δ is known, the sample size N of the trial is calculated at δ according to Equation 7.2. Therefore N can be viewed as an ideal or reference sample size at which the trial will achieve the wanted power of $1 - \beta$. Now assume that the treatment difference δ at the design stage of the trial is known only up to a range, say $[\delta_L, \delta_U]$, where $0 < \delta_L < \delta_U$. The flexible sample size design starts with an initial estimate of the needed sample size, say, N_{int} per treatment group. The sample size then can be adjusted based on the accumulated interim data in an unblinded fashion. More precisely, the objective of a flexible sample size design is to achieve the power of $1 - \beta$ for any value of the true $\delta \in [\delta_L, \delta_U]$ with the final sample size N_{fin} per group close to the ideal one or N as if the final sample size was calculated when δ is known.

Traditional fixed sample size method is to calculate the total sample size as one number. Flexible sample size design, in general, is a strategy. As it will be seen below, it involves not only the calculation of the initial sample size but also the policy of sample size reestimation and change as well as the adjustment of test statistic or rejection critical value. For flexible sample size design the impact of a less accurate initial guess work on δ is reduced as compared to a fixed sample size method. The distinction between the two sample size methods leads to some essential differences with respect to their objective, performance, and implementation.

7.2 Sample Size Reestimation

Different approaches to flexible sample size designs have been proposed. Among them the traditional group sequential design (Jennison and Turnbull 2003; Tsiatis and Mehta 2003) and the sample size reestimation method are most often used. In the following, the discussion will focus on sample size reestimation method. The group sequential method, however, will be frequently mentioned for comparison purpose.

In a sample size reestimation design, the trial starts with an initial sample size N_{int} obtained based on historical data, or established based on a minimally acceptable size of the treatment difference from business, clinical, resource, regulatory, or other valid considerations. In an interim analysis, the treatment effect is assessed based on unblinded data, and the needed final sample size is recalculated as N_{fin}. Generally, N_{fin} is a random outcome depending on the observed treatment difference in the interim analysis.

For sample size reestimation method, with the interim unblinding, the type I error rate can be inflated if the statistical test at the end does not account for the interim unblinding and the random nature of N_{fin} (Cui, Hung, and Wang 1997; Cui, Hung, and Wang 1999; Shun et al. 2001). Therefore, the adjustment of test statistic or rejection rules is generally required in order to keep the type I error rate under control. To illustrate, let's consider a simple reestimation method proposed by Cui, Hung, and Wang (1997, 1999). We denote the method as the CHW method for easy reference though it is sometimes also called the weighted Z-test in literature.

Consider the hypothesis testing problem (Equation 7.1). Suppose that the targeted power is 1− β at statistical significance level α. To test the drug efficacy, it starts with a usual group sequential test with a total of K analyses including $K - 1$ interim analyses. For the purpose, an α-spending function is chosen and the corresponding critical values C_k, $k = 1, \ldots, K$, are determined. The test statistic, denoted by S, can be written as

$$S_k = \frac{1}{\sqrt{N_k}} \sum_{i=1}^{N_k} Z_i, k=1,\ldots,K, \tag{7.3}$$

where S_k is the value of S and N_k is the sample size per treatment group at the kth interim analysis, respectively. The null hypothesis H_0 is rejected if $S_k > C_k$, and otherwise the trial proceeds to the next analysis. At the Kth look, reject H_0 if $S_K > C_K$ or leave the trial inconclusive.

This group sequential test allows stopping the trial early for unexpected drug efficacy, but it does not allow increasing sample size. Therefore it is a flexible sample size design with fixed maximum information. The initial sample size N_{int} of this group sequential test is calculated and $N_{fin} \leq N_{int} = N_{max}$, where N_{max} is the maximum sample size of the trial.

To further improve sample size flexibility, it is decided to use a sample size reestimation strategy. This reestimation design, constructed on the top of the group sequential test, is initially the same as S. The final sample size, however, is reassessed later at the lth interim analysis. Assume that the reestimated total sample size is $N_{fin} = M$ per treatment group. Let $b = (M - N_l)/(N_{int} - N_l)$, where $b > 1$ if the reestimation leads to a sample size increase, or $b < 1$ if the sample size decreases. The new schedule for the interim analysis after the lth interim analysis then is at $M_{l+j} = b(N_{l+j} - N_l) + N_l$, $j = 1, \ldots K - l$, where $M_K = M$. If there is no sample size change after the lth analysis or $b = 1$ and $M_{l+j} = N_{l+j}$, the remaining analyses will be performed at the originally scheduled times.

The test statistic U of the reestimation design before and after the lth analysis is defined as $U_k = S_k$, $k = 1, \ldots, l$ and

$$U_{l+j} = S_l\sqrt{\frac{N_l}{N_{l+j}}} + \frac{\sum_{i=N_l+1}^{M_{l+j}} Z_i}{\sqrt{M_{l+j} - N_l}}\sqrt{\frac{N_{l+j} - N_l}{N_{l+j}}}, \tag{7.4}$$

$j = 1, \ldots, K - l$, respectively. Similar to group sequential test, the rejection of the null hypothesis is made if $U_k > C_k$ for some k, $k = 1, \ldots, K$. Otherwise, the trial is inconclusive.

Once the test statistic U is given, the final sample size needed under the reestimation design can be obtained using computer simulation. The final sample size is determined through the simulation as the one that delivers the wanted overall power. Analytically the final sample size $N_{\text{fin}} = M$ may be obtained using conditional power approach. Let $\hat{\delta}$ be the estimate of δ from the lth interim analysis. When $K = 2$, $l = 1$ and the sample size change is to target whatever to make the conditional power at the final analysis equal to $1 - \beta$ or

$$P(U_K > C_K \mid S_l, \hat{\delta}) = 1 - \beta,$$

the final sample size per treatment group as reestimated is

$$M = \left(\frac{\sqrt{\frac{N_K}{N_K - N_l}}\left(C_k - S_l\sqrt{\frac{N_l}{N_K}}\right) - z_\beta}{\hat{\delta}}\right)^2 + N_l. \tag{7.5}$$

For arbitrary K and l, the above calculated M still provides a good sample size guideline though may not be precise since not all remaining interim analyses after the sample size reestimation are taken into account in the calculation. Sample size change may subject to other requirements also. For example, the policy may allow both increase and decrease of sample size if the reestimated sample size is different from the initial sample size by a certain percentage. The policy may only allow a sample size increase if the goal is to avoid any potentially insufficient statistical power. Criterion or policy on how the sample size should be changed can further complicate the calculation of the final sample size. While in general a close form expression of the final sample size needed is difficult to obtain, M calculated above is often used as an approximation to the final sample size. Some commercial computational packages now are available to assist planning sample size reestimation design.

The CHW test has the following properties. First, it has type I error rate exactly at the significance level α regardless how the data driven sample size reestimation and change are made. Secondly, if sample size reestimation does not lead to sample size change, test statistic U reduces to the original group sequential test S. Therefore, S is a special case of U. Thirdly, it is easy to compute U after sample size reestimation as a simple weighted sum of the two usual group sequential test statistics before and after the sample size reestimation. The flexibility and the computational simplicity make the CHW method attractive from a practical point of view.

The potentially changeable initial sample size of the CHW method no longer has the usual meaning of the final sample size but serves as a reference scale only. An on-target initial sample size would require no further sample size modification. If the initial sample size is off the target, however, with the reestimated final sample size, the test statistic is adjusted by down-weighting or up-weighting the contribution from later enrolled subjects, depending on whether or not the initial sample size is under- or over-estimated, respectively. To illustrate this, consider a trial with two analyses including one interim analysis. The sample size reestimation is performed with 50% of the initially planned total sample size N_{int} per treatment group. The final test statistic U_2 after the mid-course sample size change then is

$$U_2 = S_1\sqrt{0.5} + \frac{\sum_{i=N_1+1}^{M} z_i}{\sqrt{M-N_1}}\sqrt{0.5},$$

where N_1 and $N_{\text{fin}} = M$ are the interim analysis and the modified final sample sizes, respectively. When an insufficient sample size is optimistically projected initially so that a later sample size increase is required, the weight 0.5 in the second term of U_2 down weighs the contribution from the more than a half of the total number of subjects enrolled after the interim analysis. Similarly, if a larger than needed initial sample size is conservatively used leading to the later decrease of the total sample size, the test statistic U_2 will up weigh the contribution from less than a half of the total number of subjects enrolled after the interim analysis. This intuitively makes sense, and should introduce no bias under the usual assumption on the homogeneity of the subjects enrolled over time.

When the outcome does not follow normal distribution, a large sample method can be used. The large sample version of the CHW method can be given in terms of Brownian motion process (Cui, Hung, and Wang 1999). This should cover various large sample tests including the usual rate test by normal approximation and log rank test.

Similar reestimation methods are proposed by various authors, including what is often called variance spending method (Fisher 1998; Shen and Fisher 1999) or the FS method, and inverted normal method by Lehmacher and Wassmer (1999) or the LW method. These methods share some conceptual similarities with the CHW method using reweighted test statistics but are applicable under slightly different conditions or expressed somehow in different forms.

For the same hypothesis testing problem with $K - 1$ interim analyses, Müller and Schäfer (2001, 2004) proposed a conditional error probability based reestimation method. Their method, allowing a flexible maximum sample size, is also referred to as an adaptive group sequential design to distinguish it from the traditional group sequential design. The MS method allows change of total sample size, timing of interim analysis as well as interim critical values as long as such change preserves the conditional type I error rate. Assume that a group sequential test is planned originally at times N_k, $k = 1, \ldots, K$ with critical values C_k, $k = 1, \ldots, K$, and that sample size reestimation is to be performed at the lth interim analysis. The MS method allows changing the timing of the interim analysis after the sample size reestimation to N'_k, and the critical values to C'_k, $k = 1, \ldots, K$. The type I error rate can be preserved if the conditional type I error probability based on the new test plan after the lth interim analysis or the conditional probability to reject the null hypothesis given the outcome at the lth interim analysis is the same as that based on the original test plan. As compared to the CHW method, the MS method is more general in the sense of allowing not only sample size reestimation but also other types of interim trial adaptations. However, it is computationally more intensive due to the need for determining C'_k to satisfy the conditional probability constrain. More reestimation methods along controlling conditional error probability can be found in Proschan and Hunsberger (1995), Chi and Liu (1999), Liu and Chi (2001), and Liu, Proschan, and Pledger (2002) under a two-stage design framework with a possibility to extend the trial from the first to the second stage. The concept of combining different stages or phases of clinical trials are explored utilizing meta-analysis technique (Bauer and Köhne 1994; Bauer and Röhmel 1995). An extension of this combination approach to multiple stages is proposed by Hartung and Knapp (HK method, 2003), which allows multiple extensions of a trial with flexible sample size increment determined by the available interim data.

Recent work by Gao, Ware, and Mehta (2008) studies the relationship among CHW, MS, and the method suggested by Proschan and Hunsberger. The authors show that under a simple configuration these methods are equivalent. By altering the critical values after the interim sample size reestimation, MS method achieves the same effect and level of type I error control as those from reweighing of the CHW method.

Discussion about parameter estimation under sample size reestimation can be found in Cheng and Shen (2002), Lawrence and Hung (2003), and Mehta et al. (2007). Applications of flexible sample size design to the problem of switching testing hypotheses between superiority and noninferiority can be found for example in Wang et al. (2001), Shi, Quan, and Li (2004), and Lai, Shih, and Zhu (2006). More reading on sample size reestimation method and its variation, and more generally on flexible sample size design can be found in Jennison and Turnbull (2006), Lan and Trost (1997), Denne and Jennison (2000), Chen, DeMets, and Lan (2004), Lai and Shih (2004), Lan et al. (2005), Hung et al. (2005), Chuang-Stein et al. (2006), Shi (2006), Bartroff and Lai (2008), and Bauer (2008).

7.3 Measure of Adaptive Performance

Setting the goal of flexible sample size design to achieve a robust power and an efficient sample size for all values of $\delta \in [\delta_L, \delta_U]$, Liu et al. define the optimal flexible sample size design as the one minimizing an average performance score (*APS*). In their definition, the true sample size under fixed sample size design, $N_{1-\beta}(\delta)$, as calculated in Equation 7.2 is used as the benchmark since this would be the best sample size one could calculate to achieve the desired power if the true δ was known. The final sample size N_{fin} can be compared with $N = N_{1-\beta}(\delta)$ and the difference between the two is reflected in the sample size ratio

$$SR(N_{\text{fin}} \mid \delta,\beta) = \frac{N_{\text{fin}}}{N_{1-\beta}(\delta)}, \tag{7.6}$$

or the sample size difference

$$SD(N_{\text{fin}} \mid \delta,\beta) = N_{\text{fin}} - N_{1-\beta}(\delta). \tag{7.7}$$

Either $SR = SR(N_{\text{fin}}|\delta, \beta)$ or $SD = SD(N_{\text{fin}}|\delta, \beta)$ can be used to measure the deviation of the final sample size from the ideal or reference sample size $N_{1-\beta}(\delta)$ at δ. For example, if *SR* is larger than 1, the trial is regarded oversized. This leads to the definition of an relative oversize score

$$ROS(\delta \mid f_1,\beta) = 100\% \times \frac{E[SR-1]_+}{f_1 - 1}.$$

In the above equation, $[x]+$ equals to x if $x > 0$ and equals to 0 otherwise, $f_1 > 1$ is a penalty factor. The sample size is viewed as excessive only when the final sample size N_{fin} exceeds $N_{1-\beta}(\delta)$ significantly or $E[SR-1]+ > f_1 - 1$. Similarly, if *SR* is smaller than 1, the trial is underpowered or undersized. This leads to the definition of the relative undersize function as

$$RUS(\delta \mid f_2,\beta) = 100\% \times \frac{E[1-SR]_+}{1-f_2},$$

where $0 \le f_2 < 1$. The relative undersize function can be defined alternatively in the power scale rather than the sample size scale as the relative underpower function

$$RUP(\delta \mid f_3,\beta) = 100\% \times \frac{[N_{1-\beta} - N_{\text{pow}}]_+}{N_{1-\beta} - N_{(1-f_3)\times(1-\beta)}},$$

where $0 \le f_3 < 1$ and N_{pow} is the fixed sample size calculated using Equation 7.2 by plugging in the power of the flexible sample trial evaluated at the true δ (Liu, Zhu, and Cui 2008).

The total penalty at each δ due to both oversize and underpower can be given as

$$R(\delta \mid f_1, f_3, \beta) = ROS(\delta \mid f_1, \beta) + RUP(\delta \mid f_3, \beta).$$

The APS then can be defined as a weighted average of the total penalty $R(\delta|f_1, f_3, \beta)$ or

$$APS(f_1, f_3, \beta) = \int_{\delta_L}^{\delta_U} R(\delta \mid f_1, f_3, \beta) w(\delta) d\delta, \tag{7.8}$$

where $w(\delta) \ge 0$ is a weight function. The choice of $w(\delta)$ can be a constant over $[\delta_L, \delta_U]$ if there is no information about which value of δ is more likely. Otherwise, for example, the choice can be a density of a truncated normal distribution if one believes that the values of δ is likely centered at a particular point of the interval. In the definitions of penalty function $R(\delta|f_1, f_3, \beta)$ and the average performance score *APS*, f_3 can be replaced by f_2 if undersize function *RUS* is used.

The definition of *APS* allows the summarization of the adaptive performance by a single value. Since *APS* penalizes both oversizing and undersizing the trial, a small value of *APS* implies a smaller deviation from both targeted power and reference sample size. Therefore, minimizing *APS* is desirable. This leads to Liu's definition.

Definition 1 An optimal flexible sample size design is one achieving the minimum *APS* in a set of flexible sample size designs.

Definition 1 targets sample size and power simultaneously. This is different from the traditional fixed sample size design under which the optimality focuses on statistical power only. Definition 1 also applies to fixed sample design, and *APS* can measure the performance of fixed sample size design when the value of δ falls somewhere in $[\delta_L, \delta_U]$.

As a single value representation of the adaptive performance of flexible sample size design, *APS* makes potentially complicated comparison among different flexible designs with respect to power, final sample size, and performance at different δ simple and in an integrated way. Although it can be difficult to prove the existence of an optimal design by Definition 1 in general, practically it would not be an issue since the comparison typically is within a finite set of candidate designs. Values of *APS* can be calculated for individual designs, and the optimal design with the smallest *APS* value can be determined. Illustrations in the use of *APS* will be given later in the discussion of performance assessment.

Average performance scores can be defined differently, for example, through the choice of parameters f_1, f_2, f_3 as well as the weight function $w(\delta)$. It may also be defined based on the sample size difference *SD* instead of the sample size ratio SR. This leads to the following definition of APS^*.

$$APS^* = \int_{\delta_L}^{\delta_U} \mid E(N_{\text{fin}}) - N_{(1-\beta)}(\delta) \mid w(\delta) d\delta, \tag{7.9}$$

where $w(\delta)$ is a weight function. Following the optimality definition of Liu et al. (2008), the optimal sample size design based on APS^* is the one with the minimum value of APS^*. This optimally chosen design is expected to behave similar to the fixed sample size design with the sample size $N_{(1-\beta)}(\delta)$ at all $\delta \in [\delta_L, \delta_U]$.

In general the computation of average performance score relies on numerical method except for simple cases. For example, it can be shown that the optimal fixed sample size design minimizing APS^* is the one with the sample size $N = N_{\text{int}} = N_{\text{fin}}$ calculated to target the center of the interval $[\delta_L, \delta_U]$ or

$\delta_0 = (\delta_L + \delta_U)/2$ when $w(\delta)$ is a uniform weight function. Without loss of generality, suppose $w(\delta) = 1$. The APS^* can be expressed as

$$APS^* = \int_{\delta_L}^{\delta_U} (z_\alpha + z_\beta)^2 \left| \frac{1}{\delta_0^2} - \frac{1}{\delta^2} \right| d\delta. \tag{7.10}$$

The value of APS^* decreases in δ_0 if δ_0 is smaller than δ_L, or increases if larger than δ_U. Otherwise,

$$APS^* = C \times \left[-\frac{4}{\delta_0} + \frac{\delta_L + \delta_U}{\delta_0^2} + \frac{1}{\delta_L} + \frac{1}{\delta_U} \right], \tag{7.11}$$

where $C = (z_\alpha + z_\beta)^2$. Further, letting the derivative of APS^* with respect to δ_0 be zero, one can show that the APS^* is minimized at $\delta_0 = (\delta_L + \delta_U)/2$. Therefore, when one only has the knowledge of the range of δ, the best fixed sample size strategy (avoiding oversizing or undersizing the trial) is to target the midpoint of the range, which agrees with intuition.

Other optimality definitions of flexible sample size design include the one proposed by Tsiatis and Mehta (2003) for group sequential designs. They consider a set of group sequential designs and suggest taking the advantage of the group sequential test and allowing early termination of the trial to gain sample size flexibility. In this sense, the group sequential design can be viewed as a special kind of flexible sample size design. The optimality by the definition of Tsiatis and Mehta (2003) can be described as follows.

Definition 2 Among all K-look group sequential designs with a given α-spending function, the optimal one has the largest power at δ in all interim and final analyses.

Using a similar approach to Neyman-Pearson Lemma and assuming a simple alternative, Tsiatis and Mehta (2003) show that the optimal group sequential design satisfying Definition 2 is the group sequential likelihood ratio test. Definition 2 is different from Definition 1 in several aspects. First, it only deals with group sequential design, not directly applying to other flexible sample size design. Secondly, it focuses on the power performance of a statistical test at the true δ but not all values of δ in $[\delta_L, \delta_U]$. Thirdly, it does not have a benchmark for or impose constraints on the final sample size. Definition 2 is a direct extension of the traditional concept of optimal test for fixed sample design to group sequential design. This trait is reflected in the limited adaptivity of the optimal design selected under Definition 2. Simulations in Tsiatis and Mehta (2003) show that an optimally chosen group sequential likelihood ratio test under Definition 2, like a fixed sample test, can have unstable power for different δ. The power can vary from about 90% for $\delta = 0.36$, 70% for $\delta = 0.22$ and to less than 20% as the treatment difference diminishes to $\delta = 0.08$. Optimally chosen group sequential likelihood ration test based on Definition 2 does not necessarily maintain a robust power over a range of δ.

The third definition of the optimality of flexible sample size design is proposed in Jennison and Turnbull (2006) for a two-way testing problem of Hypothesis 7.1 with the possibility of accepting or rejecting the null hypothesis. In the context of hypothesis testing only allowing rejection of the null, the definition can be stated as below.

Definition 3 An optimal sample size design in a set of sample size designs with power $1 - \beta$ at δ_L is the one minimizing the average of the mean final sample sizes at $\delta = \delta_L$ and $\delta = \delta_U$:

$$ASN = \frac{E_{\delta_L}(N_{\text{fin}}) + E_{\delta_U}(N_{\text{fin}})}{2}.$$

This definition targets a robust power of at least $1 - \beta$ over the range of δ and in the meantime minimizes the average of the most optimistic and pessimistic mean sample sizes. Definition 3 improves Definition 2 by taking final sample size into consideration. It is more in line with the objective of flexible sample size design. Definition 1 is more general as compared to Definition 3. Simulation study shows that under Definition 3, reestimation design often outperforms group sequential design in terms of achieving a smaller *ASN* (Jennison and Turnbull 2006). More performance comparison of reestimation design and others will be given in the next section.

7.4 Performance Comparison

When new flexible sample size designs are rapidly developed, how to compare the performance of different designs becomes a confusing issue. The question is particularly on the adaptive performance of sample size reestimation method versus the traditional group sequential method. Some early results (Jennison and Turnbull 2003; Tsiatis and Mehta 2003) raised concerns on the potential lack of efficiency of reestimation design as compared to group sequential design. More recent results, however, (Jennison and Turnbull 2006; Liu, Zhu, and Cui 2008) point to the opposite direction; namely, reestimation design in general seems to have a better adaptive performance. The latter assessment is more in line with intuitions knowing the ultimate flexibility of the reestimation design.

Possible reasons for a better adaptive performance of the reestimation design as compared to the group sequential design can be seen in several ways. For a group sequential test, once the initial total sample size is determined, there are limited ways to alter it and this sample size cannot be increased. Although the total sample size can be decreased via early termination of the study for efficacy based on interim analysis, there are only a few choices of alternative sample sizes. For example, if a group sequential design has a total sample size of 200 subjects per treatment group and has only two analyses including one interim analysis performed at 50% of the total sample size, this group sequential design has only two possible choices of the final sample size; namely, either 100 subjects or 200 subjects per treatment group. For a reestimation design with 200 subjects per treatment group as the initial sample size, the new sample size can be projected at the time of interim analysis when the first 100 subjects per treatment group are accrued. This new sample size in general can be any number larger than 100 as projected through sample size reestimation. No upsizing and limited downsizing of the trial and possible difficulty to stop the trial early due to a stringent stopping boundary used may significantly affect and limit the adaptive performance of a group sequential design. On the contrary, allowing continuous variation of the final sample size upward or downward gives reestimation design full flexibility to address the need for sample size change, potentially leading to a better adaptive performance. As mentioned in Jennison and Turnbull (2006), many reestimation designs as illustrated with the CHW and MS methods are generalization of group sequential method with a built-in interim analysis structure. When there is no sample size change, such reestimation designs reduce to group sequential design. Therefore the set of reestimation designs contain group sequential designs as a subset. From an optimization point of view, the optimal adaptive performance should be achieved in the larger set of reestimation designs than that within the set of group sequential design. Simulations as described later will show that this is the case.

The comparison of the adaptive performance of flexible sample size designs is closely related to the design objective, comparison criterion, and designs to be compared. When any of these factors are not clearly set up, confusions on the performance of flexible sample size designs arise. Incorrect conclusion can follow from either unfair comparisons or improperly extending the conclusion to the situation which the comparison does not really cover. An often seen mistake of this kind is to draw a conclusion on the adaptive performance of one class of flexible designs versus another via the comparison of only a few designs from each class. To compare the adaptive performance of different classes of flexible sample size designs, one needs a criterion for the comparison and needs to identify the best design in each class.

Liu et al. (2008) have studied the adaptive performance of sample size reestimation design in terms of *APS*, robustness of power over a prespecified range of δ and the average final sample size. They find that the best reestimation design in general outperforms the group sequential design. They consider the range of δ to be [0.1, 0.5] and a set of candidate designs, consisting of group sequential tests and reestimation designs (CHW and HK designs). Their group sequential tests have initial or the maximum sample sizes $N_{int} = 40, 80, \ldots, 1000$, four equally spaced analyses, and α-spending functions of O'Brien-Fleming or Pocock boundaries. Their reestimation designs include CHW designs with the same initial sample sizes, number of analyses, and α-spending functions with the maximum sample size caped at 1000. In addition, HK design is also considered. Stimulations suggest that the best group sequential methods with O'Brien-Fleming or Pocock α-spending functions are the ones with the initials sample size $N_{int} = 160$ or $N_{int} - 280$, respectively. The best CHW methods with O'Brien-Fleming or Pocock α-spending functions are the ones with the initials sample size $N_{int} = 160$ or $N_{int} = 240$, respectively. The following table summarizes the *APS* values of the best design in each of the five sample size design classes (Liu, Zhu, and Cui 2008).

Method	N_{int}	*APS*
GS/OB	160	75.4
GS/PO	280	55.5
RE/OB	160	50.3
RE/PO	240	37.2
HK		46.7

From the table, it can be seen that group sequential design with Pocock α-spending function outperforms group sequential design with the O'Brien-Fleming α-spending function. This intuitively makes sense since the latter makes early termination of the study more difficult so that the trial becomes less flexible. It is interesting to note that even with the O'Brien-Fleming α-spending function, CHW design still outperforms the group sequential design with Pocock α-spending function in terms of a smaller *APS* value. The HK method performs fairly well because of its constant monitoring and updating the final sample size as needed. The best overall performer is the CHW design with Pocock α-spending function and the initial sample size $N_{int} = 240$. It achieves the smallest *APS* as 37.2 in all candidate designs.

Figure 7.1 shows the power curves of the identified best performing design overall (CHW design with Pocock α-spending function and $N_{int} = 240$), the best group sequential design (group sequential likelihood ratio test with Pocock α-spending function and $N_{int} = 280$), and the fixed sample size design targeting the treatment difference at the center of the range of δ. The corresponding average sample size curves are provided in Figure 7.2 with an additional reference sample size curve for easy comparison. It is noticed that the best overall design indeed has a robust power over $[\delta_L, \delta_U]$. It achieves 90% of power or larger for $\delta \in [0.14, 0.5]$, which covers about 90% of the targeted range from 0.1 to 0.5. For about 98% of the targeted range of δ, it achieves 80% of power or larger. Significant drop in power of this CHW test occurs only when δ is very close to 0.1. The average final sample size of this CHW test varies within 20% of the reference sample size for most of the time. The average final sample size is about 35% below the reference sample size at the left end of the range and about 50% over at the right end of the range. At either extreme, the deviation of the average sample size from the reference sample size remains moderate. The performance of the best overall design is satisfactory and the design objective can be regarded as achieved.

Studying the performance of flexible sample size design under the two-way decision setting to allow either rejecting or accepting the null, Jennison and Turnbull show again that the reestimation design outperforms group sequential design under their original Definition 3 (Jennison and Turnbull 2006). The authors consider Müller and Schäfer's design, which allows arbitrary $K - 1$ interim analyses and

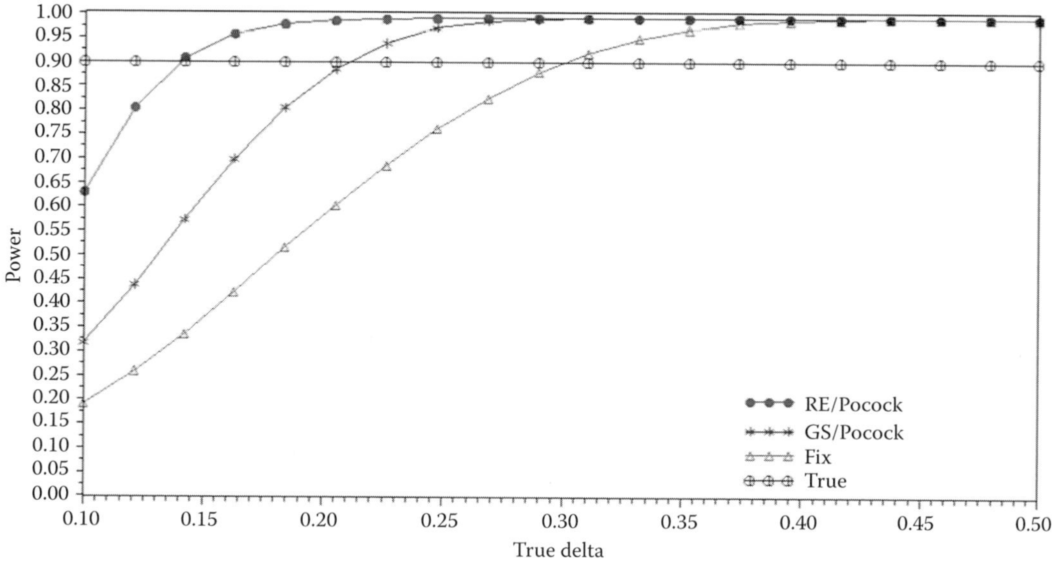

FIGURE 7.1 Power comparison of flexible sample size design.

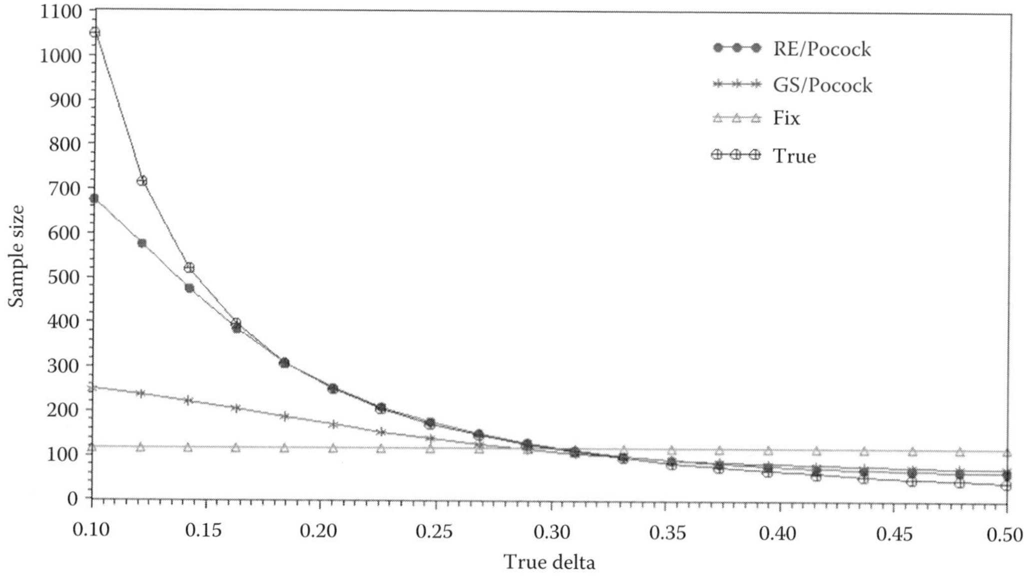

FIGURE 7.2 Average sample size of flexible sample size design.

has full freedom to choose next sample size increment and stopping critical values for rejecting or accepting the null hypothesis based on the current data. This reestimation design is compared with three types of group sequential designs with predetermined equal or unequal sample size increments, and a specific or arbitrary-error spending function. Their simulations show that the reestimation design outperforms three group sequential designs and always delivers the smallest average sample size.

Performance comparison of reestimation test and group sequential likelihood ratio test under Definition 2 is made indirectly in Tsiatis and Mehta (2003) through introduction of a group sequential test to approximate the reestimation test. Since the group sequential likelihood ratio test is the most efficient test among all group sequential designs, a better performance of the group sequential likelihood ratio test versus reestimation design might be inferred out if the group sequential approximation is valid or well represents the behavior of the reestimation method. The issue with this comparison is that such an approximation can be rough if it has only a few interim analyses. Further the comparison focuses only on the power performance of the tests at a single point δ. The conclusion of a better efficiency associated with group sequential likelihood ratio test may not be readily extended to all δ in $[\delta_L, \delta_U]$. As mentioned before, the simulations show an unstable power associated with the optimally chosen, under Definition 2, group sequential likelihood ratio test when the value of the true treatment difference δ drifts away from the targeted one. Our additional simulations also suggest that for an optimally chosen reestimation design under Definition 1, it would be difficult to construct an approximation group sequential likelihood ratio test as suggested in Tsiatis and Mehta (2003) with a reasonable number of interim analyses to outperform this reestimation design.

7.5 Implementation

For a fixed sample size design, the issue simply is to calculate the needed sample size based on projected treatment effect. Sample size reestimation design, as a sample size strategy, involves not only calculating the initial sample size as the first step but also an array of further operations with respect to reestimating sample size, adjusting test statistic to keep type I error rate under control, assessing and searching for better designs, and validating performance for a chosen design. Only after all the above are properly done, a sample size reestimation design becomes ready to go live or to be implemented in a clinical trial.

The work of sample size reestimation design begins with setting up the design objective. More precisely, it starts from the determination of the range of the unknown δ or $[\delta_L, \delta_U]$. This range typically is obtained as a confidence interval of δ based on available historical data at the time of design. A narrower or wider confidence interval can be used depending the confidence level of the designer's choice. As compared to the fixed sample size design requiring an on-target projection of the size of treatment difference, a less stringent requirement of the range of δ as the target in the reestimation design makes the task of sample size determination easier, though it by no means encourages a careless job. The obtained range of δ can be further refined by taking other factors into considerations. The requirement for a minimum δ allowed from marketing, resource, and clinical point of views can be considered. For example, based on a marketing strategy, a minimum value of δ allowed can be set up to make it in line with the effect sizes of competing drugs. For a sponsor with limited resources and a tight development timeline, a minimum δ can also be chosen to prevent overspending and to shorten the trial period. If there is a regulatory requirement on a minimum number of subjects in order for the trial to collect sufficient amount of safety information of the study drug, this requirement needs to be considered when setting up the upper limit of the range of δ. To be on the safe side, one may prefer a more robust range of δ and therefore choose a conservative initial estimate of the treatment difference to start. Generally, when all relevant factors are considered, a balanced solution and the final range $[\delta_L, \delta_U]$ can be obtained.

Once the range of δ is determined, one needs to choose candidate flexible designs among which the best design later will be determined. The candidate designs generally can be any designs as long as they have controlled type I error rate and allow change of the final sample size based on the interim data. For example, traditional group sequential design can be considered for its easy implementation and wide acceptance by regulatory agencies. For better flexibility and computational simplicity, one may choose the CHW method. For the maximum flexibility, Müller and Schäfer's method can also be added.

The pool of candidate designs generally include several sets of different types of designs such as group sequential designs and sample size reestimation designs with various configurations. A set of group sequential design may have a number of group sequential likelihood ratio tests with different initial sample sizes, α-spending functions, and different numbers and timings of interim analyses. The same thing can happen for a set of reestimation designs. Although there may be a large number of different designs in the pool of candidate design, their adaptive performance can be easily evaluated based on the average performance score, *APS*, as illustrated before.

For a reestimation design, when and how to perform interim sample size reestimation directly affects its efficiency. Obviously, reestimation design becomes useful only when there are more data at the time of reestimating the sample size than the data available at the design stage. In general, the sample size reestimation should not be performed too early before sufficient interim data accumulated or too late leaving little room for further improvement. Limited simulation has showed that a better time to perform sample size reestimation is at about 40–50% information time. Once the reestimated sample size is obtained, sample size change may be done according to a predetermined sample size change policy. For example, the sample size adjustment may only be performed if the calculated conditional power is smaller than the targeted one by certain percentage and if so only sample size increase is allowed. The sample size change policy may also limit the number of interim analyses for sample size reestimation and adjustment. Since too many interim analyses in general are not recommended due to concerns on trial integrity, a cap of maximum three or four interim analyses seems reasonable. Varying sample size change policy gives different candidate designs for performance evaluation.

Once the range of the unknown δ, the candidate design pool, and sample size reestimation and change policy are set up, it is ready to evaluate the performance of candidate designs based on certain criteria like *APS*. The evaluation usually is done through simulations. For each design, random trial outcomes are generated, the sample size is reestimated, and the final sample size is recorded. Repeating this process allows calculating the average final sample size and thus the performance score *APS*. After the average performance score is obtained for each candidate design, the one with the smallest average performance score can be chosen as the best design within each class or type of designs. The best overall design is the one with the minimum average performance score among all candidate designs. Besides the average performance score, other considerations may also help to make the decision. The implementation simplicity and regulatory acceptance are often used as additional criteria. When there are a number of designs with the smallest or near smallest *APS*, one needs to make further selection based on more detailed performance information. As a tool for performance assessment, the total penalty function $R(\delta | f_1, f_3, \beta)$ can be plotted against $\delta \in [\delta_L, \delta_U]$ to see where the penalty emphasizes (Liu, Zhu, and Cui 2008). It is possible for two designs to achieve similar *APS* values but one penalizes more on undersize and the other penalizes more on oversize. The preference then can be given to a particular one to best meet the trial requirements.

The final step in choosing a flexible design is design validation. The purpose of this validation is to demonstrate that an optimally chosen design meets the expectation and the design objectives. The power curve of the chosen design is provided to confirm a robust power over the range of δ. The average final sample size over the range can also be displayed. This final validation is necessary since the best sample size design is often chosen based on an optimality criterion that may not be intuitive or clearly shows its advantages in terms of power and final sample size. After the validation and confirmation, the chosen design can be implemented.

Regarding operational aspects, the way to handle unblinded interim analysis in a reestimation design is quite similar to that in the usual interim analysis requiring data unblinding. To ensure the integrity of the trial after interim unblinding, an independent data review body or data monitoring committee (DMC) can be used. The DMC and its independent statistician may perform unblinded interim analysis and sample size reestimation and adjustment according to a chosen method. The plan for sample size reestimation can be described in the protocol and interim analysis plan regarding the range of δ, the candidate designs to be considered and the performance assessment criteria. The technical details on the sample size change policy can be passed to the independent DMC statistician by the sponsor statistician but remains confidential to others in the project team. Without disclosure of the details of the analysis and the observed interim treatment outcome, the DMC can make a sample change recommendation with a proposed new sample size. This sample size reestimation can be easily combined with a required interim analysis for the usual drug safety and efficacy monitoring purposes. The use of DMC and independent statistician for sample size reestimation expands the traditional role of DMC, and can effectively help to minimize potential biases introduced from the interim unblinding. Even though, there may still be concerns on potential negative impact from the interim unblinding from regulatory perspectives, knowing a sponsor may be able to figure out the treatment effect size from a backward calculation based on the recommended new sample size. Generally, as long as the details on how the new sample size is calculated are kept confidential within statisticians, the likelihood for such a backward calculation of the treatment difference is low. The ultimate improvement of clinical trial quality justifies the use of sample size reestimation method and makes it a viable design option.

Sample size reestimation design as a kind of flexible sample size design improves clinical trial by providing more robust statistical power and efficient final sample size against potential misspecification of the targeted treatment difference. As compared to fixed sample size design, reestimation design is more complicated, requiring more careful thinking, planning, and execution. However, the extra work is worth the return of a better designed trial with a higher chance to succeed. Further, the use of sample size reestimation design expands the traditional role of statisticians in clinical trials and makes their work more challenging and interesting.

References

Bartroff, J., and Lai, T. L. (2008). Efficient adaptive designs with mid-course sample size adjustment in clinical trials. *Statistics in Medicine,* 27: 1593–1611.

Bauer, P. (2008). Adaptive designs: Looking for a needle in the haystack—A new challenge in medical research. *Statistics in Medicine,* 27: 1565–80.

Bauer, P., and Köhne, K. (1994). Evaluation of experiments with adaptive interim analyses. *Biometrics,* 50: 1029–41.

Bauer, P., and Röhmel, J. (1995). An adaptive method for establishing a dose relationship. *Statistics in Medicine,* 14: 1595–1607.

Chuang-Stein, C., Anderson, K., Gallo, P., and Collins, S. (2006). Sample size re-estimation: A review and recommendations. *Drug Information Journal,* 40: 475–84.

Chen, Y. H. J., DeMets, D., and Lan, K. K. G. (2004). Increasing the sample size when the unblinded interim result is promising. *Statistics in Medicine,* 23: 1023–38.

Cheng, Y., and Shen, Y. (2002). Estimation of a parameter and its exact confidence interval following sequential sample size re-estimation trials. *Biometrics,* 60: 910–18.

Chi, G. Y. H., and Liu, Q. (1999). The attractiveness of the concept of a prospectively designed two-stage clinical trial. *Journal of Biopharmaceutical Statistics,* 9: 537–47.

Cui, L., Hung, H. M., and Wang, S. J. (1997). Impact of changing sample size in a group sequential clinical trial. *ASA Proceedings of Biopharmaceutical Section,* 52–57.

Cui L., Hung, H. M., and Wang, S. J. (1999). Modification of sample size in group sequential clinical trials. *Biometrics,* 55: 853–57.

Denne, J. S., and Jennison, C. (2000). A group sequential *t*-test with updating of sample size. *Biometrika,* 87: 125–34.

Fisher, L. (1998). Self-designing clinical trials. *Statistics in Medicine,* 17: 1551–62.

Gao, P., Ware, J., and Mehta, C. (2008). Sample size re-estimation for adaptive sequential design in clinical trials. *Journal of Biopharmaceutical Statistics,* 18: 1184–96.

Gould, A. L. (1992). Interim analyses for monitoring clinical trials that do not materially affect the type I error rate. *Statistics in Medicine,* 11: 55–66.

Gould, A. L., and Shi W. J. (1992). Sample size re-estimation without unblinding for normally distributed outcomes with unknown variance. *Communications in Statistics—Theory and Methods,* 21: 2833–53.

Hartung, J., and Knapp, G. (2003). A new class of completely self-designing clinical trials. *Biometrical Journal,* 45: 3–19.

Hung, H. M., Cui, L., Wang, S. J., and Lawrence, J. (2005). Adaptive statistical analysis following sample size modification based on interim review of effect size. *Journal of Biopharmaceutical Statistics,* 15: 693–706.

Jennison, C., and Turnbull W. (2003). Mid-course sample size modification in clinical trials based on the observed treatment effect. *Statistics in Medicine,* 22: 971–93.

Jennison, C., and Turnbull, B. (2006). Efficient group sequential designs when there are several effect sizes under consideration. *Statistics in Medicine,* 25: 917–32.

Lai, T. L., and Shih, M. C. (2004). Power, sample size and adaptation considerations in the design of group sequential clinical trials. *Biometrika,* 91: 507–28.

Lai, T. L., Shih, M. C., and Zhu, G. (2006). Modified Haybittle-Peto group sequential designs for testing superiority and non-inferiority hypotheses in clinical trials. *Statistics in Medicine,* 25: 1149–67.

Lan, K. K., Soo, Y., Siu, C., and Wang, M. (2005). The use of weighted *Z*-tests in medical research. *Journal of Biopharmaceutical Statistics,* 15: 625–39.

Lan, K. K., and Trost, D. C. (1997). Estimation of parameters and sample size re-estimation. *Proceedings of American Statistical Association, Biopharmaceutical Section,* 48–51.

Lawrence, J., and Hung, H. M. (2003). Estimation and confidence intervals after adjusting the maximum information. *Biometrical Journal,* 45: 143–52.

Lehmacher, W., and Wassmer, G. (1999). Adaptive sample size calculations in group sequential trials. *Biometrics,* 55: 1286–90.

Liu, G. F., Zhu, G. R., and Cui, L. (2008). Evaluating the adaptive performance of flexible sample size designs with treatment difference in an interval. *Statistics in Medicine,* 27: 584–96.

Liu, Q., and Chi, G. Y. H. (2001). On sample size and inference for two-stage adaptive designs. *Biometrics,* 57: 172–77.

Liu, Q., Proschan, M. A., and Pledger, G. W. (2002). A unified theory of two-stage adaptive designs. *Journal of the American Statistical Association,* 97: 1034–41.

Mehta, C., Bauer, P., Posch, M., and Werner, B. (2007). Repeated confidence intervals for adaptive group sequential trials. *Statistics in Medicine,* 26: 5422–33.

Müller, H. H., and Schäfer, H. (2001). Adaptive group sequential designs for clinical trials: Combining the advantages of adaptive and of classical group sequential procedures. *Biometrics,* 57: 886–91.

Müller, H. H., and Schäfer, H. (2004). A general statistical principle for changing a design any time during the course of a clinical trial. *Statistics in Medicine,* 23: 2497–2508.

Proschan, M. A., and Hunsberger, S. A. (1995). Designed extension of studies based on conditional power. *Biometrics,* 51: 1315–24.

Shen, Y., and Fisher, L. (1999). Statistical inference for self-designing clinical trials with a one-sided hypothesis. *Biometrics,* 55: 190–97.

Shi, W. J. (1993). Sample size re-estimation for triple blind clinical trials. *Drug Information Journal,* 27: 761–64.

Shi, W. J. (2006). Group sequential, sample size re-estimation and two-stage adaptive designs in clinical trials: A comparison. *Statistics in Medicine,* 25: 933–41.

Shi, W. J., Quan, H., and Li, G. (2004). Two-stage adaptive strategy for superiority and non-inferiority hypotheses in active controlled clinical trials. *Statistics in Medicine,* 23: 2781–98.

Shun, Z., Yuan, W., Brady, W. E., and Hsu, H. (2001). Type I error in sample size re-estimation based on observed treatment difference (with commentary). *Statistics in Medicine,* 20: 497–513.

Tsiatis, A. A., and Mehta, C. (2003). On the inefficiency of the adaptive design for monitoring clinical trials. *Biometrika,* 90: 367–78.

Wang, S. J., Hung, H. M. J., Tsong, Y., and Cui, L. (2001). Group sequential test strategies for superiority and non-inferiority hypotheses in active controlled clinical trials. *Statistics in Medicine,* 20: 1903–12.

Wittes, J., and Brittain, E. (1990). The role of internal pilot studies in increasing the efficiency of clinical trials. *Statistics in Medicine,* 9: 65–72.

8

Adaptive Interim Analyses in Clinical Trials

Gernot Wassmer
University of Cologne

8.1 Introduction

Interim analyses in group sequential trials allow making conclusions on efficacy and safety before the planned end of the trial is reached. The practical use of group sequential designs, however, is limited since they do not allow for data-driven sample size reassessments or other design changes. The distinctive feature of classical methods in group sequential analyses is that they require a *data independent* choice of the group sample sizes and that external factors only may influence the change or modification of the design. On the other hand, redesigning a study *based on the results of an interim analysis* looks attractive. It is desirable to adjust or reassess, for example, sample size calculations that are merely based on facts that are available prior to the study.

In recent years, several methods were proposed that allow a flexible design through the use of adaptive interim analyses while maintaining the (overall) type I error rate. A strategy that copes well with the demands of practice is based on combining the p-values obtained from the separate stages by using a specific combination test. This strategy was initially proposed by Bauer (1989) and Bauer and Köhne (1994) where the focus was on two-stage designs and Fisher's combination test. Multistage designs were proposed as well that generalize the conventional groups sequential designs (e.g., Cui, Hung, and Wang 1999; Lehmacher and Wassmer 1999) and therefore are a powerful supplement to them. These designs allow for performing design changes during the course of a trial in a data-driven way. They even offer very general types of adaptation, such as selection of treatment arms, selection of endpoints, subgroup selection of patients (so-called enrichment designs), and even a data-driven modification of hypotheses when performing interim analyses.

A specific feature of these types of adaptations is that they need not to be prespecified during the planning stage. Specifically, the rule how the adaptations are performed is not fixed and hence the types of adaptations have some ad hoc character. Nevertheless, this does not introduce arbitrariness in these designs. The opposite is true: The increased flexibility must be handled extremely carefully, otherwise the integrity of the study is jeopardized. In other words, these designs cannot replace careful study designing, but they offer the possibility to perform confirmatory statistical analyses where in an interim analysis essential trial characteristics might be changed in a data-driven way.

A very important practical application of adaptive designs is the data-driven selection of treatment arms in multiarmed designs that can be combined with sample size reassessment strategies. This is usually applied in so-called adaptive seamless designs and might be considered as one of the most promising data-dependent adaptation strategies. Here an additional multiplicity issue due to multiple treatment comparisons arises. The closed testing principle according to Marcus, Peritz, and Gabriel (1976) offers a straightforward way to be applied in adaptive two- or multistage designs.

This article describes the statistical methodology that enables such types of confirmatory analyses. We start with the brief description of the general principle of conducting a confirmatory trial by the use of the combination testing principle. In this section we also consider the general principle of redesigning a trial by use of the conditional rejection probability (CRP) principle due to Müller and Schäfer (2001, 2004). A more thorough discussion and review of the basic concepts can be found in Vandemeulebroecke (2008) and references therein. In the next section we describe the most important applications of confirmatory adaptive designs that are sample size reassessment, treatment arm selection, patient enrichment strategies, and combinations of them. Particularly, we describe the application of the closed testing principle in adaptive interim analysis that enables a correct statistical analysis when changing, dropping, or adding hypotheses in a data-driven way (Hommel 2001).

8.2 Confirmatory Adaptive Designs

The motivation for confirmatory adaptive test designs is to define a statistical test that controls the Type I error rate even if data-driven modifications of the design were performed at the interim stage. The following description focuses on two-stage designs. Several authors (e.g., Proschan, Follmann, and Waclawiw 1992) have shown that this might result in a substantial increase of the originally assumed level of significance α. Originally, two concepts (Bauer and Köhne 1994; Proschan and Hunsberger 1995) were independently introduced that overcome this issue. They are closely related and essentially equivalent (see Chapter 11). Particularly, both can be defined in terms of one-sided p-values p_1 and p_2 from the separate stages of the trial and (Posch and Bauer 1999; Wassmer 1999). The only condition is that the distribution of the p-values is, under H_0, stochastically not smaller than the uniform. The procedures can therefore be applied in very different situations. The first procedure (Bauer and Köhne 1994) combines the p-values p_1 and p_2 through the use of an appropriate combination function $C(p_1, p_2)$. The second (Proschan and Hunsberger 1995) is based upon the specification of a conditional Type I error rate function $\alpha(p_1)$. The principle essentially states that at the final stage of the trial the hypothesis can be rejected if either $C(p_1, p_2)$ fulfills the condition for rejecting H_0 (that is defined by the combination test), or the p-value from the second-stage data, p_2, is smaller than or equal to $\alpha(p_1)$.

The Type I error rate of the procedure is not inflated, irrespective of how the adaptation in the interim analysis was carried out. This is even true if in the interim analysis the hypothesis to be tested was changed. At the end of the trial, if the combination test yields a significant result, the intersection $H_0^1 \cap H_0^2$ of the two hypotheses, H_0^1 and H_0^2, of the first and the second stage of the trial, respectively, are tested. A simple argument extends this to the hypothesis of interest at the final stage, H_0^2: H_0^2 can be rejected if the combination test and the test for H_0^2 itself is rejected at level α. This is the application of the closed testing procedure (CTP) due to Marcus, Peritz, and Gabriel (1976). Depending on the hypothesis H_0^2 was prespecified or not, one can use the combination test of the second-stage data alone for performing this test (see Section 8.3.2 for more details). The decisive advantage of the adaptive procedure is given by the fact that all information available after performing the first stage of the study may be used for planning and hence modifying the second stage. Possible modifications include changing the sample size, the test statistic, the number of treatment arms, the target population, the endpoint, or the selection of endpoints in a set of endpoints to be tested, and so on.

It is straightforward to extend these designs to designs with more than one interim analysis. Particularly, the use of the inverse normal combination function enables the formulation of adaptive designs within the (classical) group sequential testing approaches. For adaptive designs, this was proposed by Lehmacher and Wassmer (1999). To describe this approach, let

$$C(p_1,\ldots,p_k)=\frac{1}{\sqrt{k}}\sum_{i=1}^{k}\Phi^{-1}(1-p_i) \tag{8.1}$$

at each stage k of the procedure, $k = 1, \ldots, K$, where $\Phi^{-1}(\cdot)$ denotes the inverse of the standard normal cumulative distribution function (cdf). The procedure consists of specifying appropriate decision regions for Equation 8.1. Since, under H_0, the $\Phi^{-1}(1 - p_k)$'s are independent and standard normally distributed if the distribution of the p-values is equal to the uniform, the decision regions can be found within the class for classical group sequential test designs. The designs of Pocock (1977), O'Brien and Fleming (1979), designs due to Wang and Tsiatis (1987), or even more general designs (e.g., designs that incorporate the stopping for futility option, or error spending function designs due to Lan and DeMets 1983) may be used. See Jennison and Turnbull (2000) for a comprehensive review of group sequential designs. One can also specify designs where rejection of H_0 is intended only in the last stage of the trial. These approaches maintains α exactly for any, possibly data driven choice of sample sizes even though the type of the modifications needs not be prespecified at the start of the trial.

More generally, one might also consider the weighted inverse normal test statistic

$$C(p_1,\ldots,p_k)=\frac{1}{\sqrt{\sum_{i=1}^{k}w_i^2}}\sum_{i=1}^{k}w_i\cdot\Phi^{-1}(1-p_i), \tag{8.2}$$

where $\sum_{k=1}^{K}w_k^2=1$. Using Equation 8.2 one might apply test designs that are based on independent, normally distributed increments with possibly unequal stage sample sizes. The weights are chosen according to the planned information times (Lehmacher and Wassmer 1999). The crucial point is that these weight are fixed and may not be changed during the course of the trial. The resulting test procedure is equivalent to the method proposed by Cui, Hung, and Wang (1999) who used the error spending approach by maintaining the originally planned information rates for calculating the test statistic. They did not adopt the idea of p-value combination but of down-weighting the test statistic if a sample size increase was performed.

An even more general approach is given by the CRP principle due to Müller and Schäfer (2001, 2004). The idea of this approach is to consider, at some interim stage k of the trial, the conditional Type I error rate $\alpha(\boldsymbol{x}_k)$ that is defined as the conditional probability, under H_0, of rejecting H_0 in one of the subsequent stages, given the data observed up to this stage, $\boldsymbol{x}_k$. The remainder of the trial can be performed as a test at level $\alpha(\boldsymbol{x}_k)$ where the design of this test is arbitrary. That is, in an interim analysis one can choose a one-stage or a multistage design with appropriately chosen decision regions, new weights for combining the test statistic, or even a change in the hypotheses tested in further analyses. Particularly, this involves a free choice of the number of stages considered in a group sequential test design.

The CRP principle essentially coincides with the recursive application of combination tests as proposed by Brannath, Posch, and Bauer (2002) when testing means with normally distributed data, the variance is assumed to be known, and the inverse normal combination test was chosen as the adaptive test. For example, if a two-stage design was considered, the conditional error rate is simply the condition for the p-value for the second stage, p_2, to reject H_0. Generally, the calculation of the conditional Type I error rate is based on the original test statistic, for example, on the t-test statistic or the test statistic of the Dunnett, F, or some other test. In the t-test situation (i.e., if the variance is not assumed to be known), the calculation of the conditional Type I error rate may become complicated (Posch et al. 2004; Timmesfeld, Schäfer, and Müller 2007). An interesting application is for multiarmed designs as proposed by König et al. (2008). This application also depends on quite restrictive assumptions though (see Section 8.3.2). For most other testing situations, the (exact) implementation of the CRP approach is not yet feasible. Nevertheless, it can be replaced by the calculation of the conditional Type I error rate when using the inverse normal combination testing principle. The latter, by the way, even yields an exact level α testing procedure if an exact way for calculating the p-values for the separate stages is available.

8.3 Most Relevant Types of Adaptations

8.3.1 Adaptive Sample Size Recalculation

Historically, changing the sample size in an on-going trial based on the results observed so far was the first major issue for developing adaptive confirmatory designs. In a clinical trial with a continuous primary endpoint, sample size calculation is essentially (not exclusively) based on assumptions on the treatment effect and on the variability (variance) of the outcome measure. Conceptually, the treatment effect is the clinically relevant treatment effect; that is, the effect that is worth detecting with specified power, usually 80% or 90%. Practically, if a larger treatment effect is anticipated (clinicians are typically optimistic in this regard), this expected treatment effect is usually used for the sample size calculation, or the discussion ends with taking a value midway the expected and the clinically relevant effect. For the variance typically an estimate from other studies is available, and this estimate is used in the sample size calculation hoping that the estimate comes near to the true variability. Thus, if the treatment effect and variability estimates are correct, the probability to achieve a significant result is indeed equal to the specified power. If, on the other hand, the treatment effect is over- or underestimated, and/or the variance is under- or overestimated the power is smaller or larger than desired. In all these cases it seems reasonable to use the data observed so far in order to obtain information on the correctness of the estimates.

Using information about the variability is conceptually different from using information about the treatment effect (Proschan 2009). First, the latter requires a look at the data in a completely unblinded way, which is not true for the former. Further, if the sample size calculation was based on the minimum clinically relevant treatment effect, a sample size increase should not be taken into consideration, and a design that incorporates early stopping for efficacy (which is the classical group sequential test design) is exactly designed for the purpose of dealing with larger effect sizes (Jennison and Turnbull 2003). Hence, treatment effect estimates are often used in an immutable, data independent sense. All that is not true for the variability. If the sample size reestimation is performed only on the basis of the variance it was shown that one can analyze the data as if such reestimation was not performed. It can be shown that the Type I error rate is only slightly increased, and this increase can be considered as practically irrelevant. Thus, no specific statistical methodology is needed, and sample size reestimation can be done in the context of an internal pilot study design and even be performed in a blinded way. For a review if these methods see Friede and Kieser (2006) and Proschan (2009).

Things are different if the sample size is reestimated from the treatment effect. It was shown by Proschan and Hunsberger (1995) that, in a two-stage design, the actual Type I error rate can be more than doubled if sample size reestimation based on the interim results was performed. Hence, specific methodology is needed. The combination testing principle is one method. If the inverse normal combination test is used, the following property is useful and attractive: If no sample size reestimation was performed during the trial, the design that is based on the inverse normal method and the design that uses the (classical) group sequential approach coincides. This property exactly holds for normally distributed observations with a known variance. It is approximately true if the variance is unknown or the process of data accumulation is only asymptotically a process with independent and normally distributed increments. Note that it is theoretically true for all designs if the CRP principle is applied, but the CRP principle is not feasible in many cases.

Conditional power arguments can be used to argue for a sample size change for the subsequent stage(s) of the trial. If in a two-stage parallel group design the unweighted inverse normal method is used, the conditional power is given by

$$CP_{\vartheta}(z_1)=P_{\vartheta}\left(\frac{Z_1+Z_2}{\sqrt{2}}\geq u_2|z_1\right)=P_{\vartheta}\left(Z_2\geq\sqrt{2}u_2-z_1\right)=1-\Phi\left(\sqrt{2}\,u_2-z_1-\vartheta\sqrt{\frac{n_2}{2}}\right), \quad (8.3)$$

where ϑ is the unknown treatment effect, $z_i = \Phi^{-1}(1 - p_i)$, $i = 1, 2$, is the test statistic of the ith stage of the trial, and u_2 is the critical value for the second stage of the trial. The crucial point is the choice of ϑ.

A first choice for ϑ is the observed effect size estimate. This yields very large sample sizes if the effect size estimate is small. Another choice is the originally assumed effect size. This might be regarded as the more conservative approach and might be unreasonable if the observed effect size estimate is considerably larger than originally assumed effect size. An alternative is to consider the conditional power curve together with the likelihood function of the parameter of interest at given sample size. If this is considered together, it gives good insight about the chance for a success by the end of the trial. An example is shown in Figure 8.1 for a two-stage parallel group O'Brien and Fleming design with $u_1 = 2.797$, $u_2 = 1.977$, $n_1 = 20$ for each arm in the first stage and observed effect size 0.474 (which yields $z_1 = 1.5$). The variance is assumed to be known and equal to 1. The conditional power is calculated under the assumption of leaving the sample size unchanged (i.e., $n_2 = 20$).

This curve shows that under the observed effect size (0.474) the power is roughly 55%, but in areas where the likelihood function is considerably high, the power is increasing to about 90%. From this point of view, a sample size change is not reasonable at all, and this could be a good advice. Note that a conditional power requirement of 80% and setting $\vartheta = 0.474$ would require doubling the originally planned sample size.

When the trial starts, $CP_{\vartheta}(Z_1)$ from Equation 8.3 is a random variable with a distribution that depends on ϑ. Bauer and König (2006) investigated this distribution and showed that sample size calculations based on conditional power need to be handled very carefully. An interim treatment effect estimate and the corresponding conditional power calculation might mislead you to an erroneous increase or decrease of the sample size. Nevertheless, the best available information at a given point in time can be utilized for the sample size adjustment, and the risk of a false-negative study outcome can be reduced

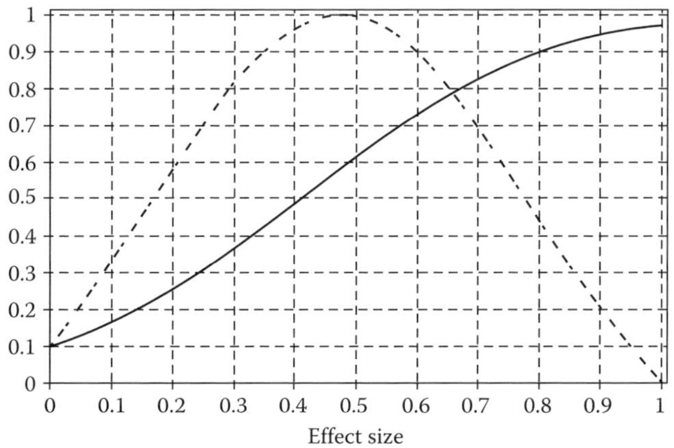

FIGURE 8.1 Conditional power (solid line) and Likelihood (dashed line).

considerably. When performed carefully, redesigning the sample size in an interim analysis on the basis of the results observed so far considerably improves the power of the trial. This was shown for continuous outcomes as well as for testing rates, and the hazard ratio in survival designs (Wassmer, Eisebitt, and Coburger 2001; Wassmer 2003, 2006). Note that these designs may become inefficient for substantial changes in sample size (Jennison and Turnbull 2003). This problem does not occur for small to moderate changes, which represents the practically relevant situation such that in general a careful reassessment of the necessary sample size and a potential change of it turns out to be a recommendable strategy in the progress of an adaptively planned confirmatory clinical trial.

8.3.2 Confirmatory Adaptive Designs in Multiarmed Trials

Monitoring pairwise comparisons in multiarmed clinical trial designs was adapted by Follmann, Proschan, and Geller (1994) and Proschan, Follmann, and Geller (1994). They derived critical values for the overall test statistic through simulation and showed that, in the all-pairs comparison setting, the procedure preserves the familywise error rate (FWER) in a strong sense if a treatment arm is dropped at some stage k of the trial if it was shown to be inferior. Hellmich (2001) showed that otherwise (e.g., if a superior treatment arm is dropped due to severe side effects) the FWER indeed is no more preserved. An alternative approach, where the number of treatment arm selections needs to be specified, was proposed by Stallard and Todd (2003; see also, Kelly, Stallard, and Todd 2005; Friede and Stallard 2008; Stallard and Friede 2008). A fully flexible approach is derived from the combination testing (or the CRP) principle together with the CTP. This approach will be reviewed in the following. Before we start, we emphasize that these designs enable valid statistical analysis if treatment selection procedures or other design adaptations were performed in interim analyses. They do not refer to the treatment selection or dose-finding procedures themselves. A discussion of these methods is provided in the Chapter 11 of this book. In other words, we discuss methods that are primarily conceived for Phase III, whereas proper dose finding (Phase II) is discussed in Chapter 11.

For simplicity, we consider the many-to-one comparison setting, where G experimental treatment groups are tested against a control group. Without loss of generality, we consider testing means μ_g of normally distributed variables (i.e., we are considering G elementary hypotheses):

$$H_0^g : \mu_0 = \mu_g, g = 1,\ldots,G.$$

The global hypothesis is

$$H_0 = \bigcap_{g=1}^{G} H_0^g : \mu_0 = \cdots = \mu_G.$$

When performing the closed test we also will consider intersection hypotheses that are, for example,

$$H_0^{23} = H_0^2 \cap H_0^3 : \mu_0 = \mu_2 = \mu_3,$$

and all elementary hypotheses H_0^g.

For the CTP we first derive the corresponding closed system of hypotheses consisting of all possible intersection hypotheses $H_0^{\mathcal{I}} = \bigcap_{i \in \mathcal{I}} H_0^i, \mathcal{I} \subseteq \{1,\ldots,G\}$. Then, for each of the hypotheses in the closed system of hypotheses we find a suitable local level-α test. In the simplest case, this is the Bonferroni test, but other tests (e.g., the Dunnett test) can also be used. Having observed the data, we reject $H_0^{\mathcal{I}}$ at FWER α, if all hypotheses $H_0^{\mathcal{J}}$ with $H_0^{\mathcal{J}} \subseteq H_0^{\mathcal{I}}$ are rejected, each at (local) level α.

An elementary hypothesis H_0^g is rejected if H_0^g itself and all hypotheses containing H_0^g are rejected, each at level α. In the many-to-one comparison setting, for $G = 3$ the closed system of hypotheses is illustrated in Figure 8.2 indicating how rejection of an elementary hypothesis is reached: Only if the global hypothesis can be rejected, hypotheses consisting of two elementary hypothesis are tested, only if an intersection hypothesis is rejected, subsequent elementary hypotheses are tested.

How to apply the closed testing principle within adaptive designs was proposed by several authors, for example, Bauer and Kieser (1999), Kieser, Bauer, and Lehmacher (1999), Hellmich (2001), Hommel (2001), or Posch et al. (2005). An excellent tutorial is provided by Bretz et al. (2009). The problem is essentially stated as follows: If one or more treatment arms were dropped in an interim analysis and hence the set of initial hypotheses was reduced, usually no data are available from the excluded treatment group(s). In this case, we define tests for intersection hypotheses for partly excluded treatment arms as tests for hypotheses for nonexcluded treatment arms. For example, if one treatment arm, s, is selected out of G treatment arms, all tests for intersection hypotheses containing H_0^s are formally defined as tests for H_0^s. This is a valid test procedure since $H_0^{\mathcal{J}} \subseteq H_0^s$ for all $s \in \mathcal{J}$ or equivalently: if H_0^s is rejected, $H_0^{\mathcal{J}}$ with $s \in \mathcal{J}$ is rejected in particular, under control of the FWER.

Generally, denoting $\mathcal{E} \subset \{1, \ldots, G\}$ the index set of all excluded H_0^g, a test for $H_0^{\mathcal{J}}$ with $\mathcal{J} \cap \mathcal{E} \neq \emptyset$ is performed as a test for $H_0^{\mathcal{J}\setminus\mathcal{E}}$. For example, when using Bonferroni tests, the adjusted p-value for the hypothesis $H_0^{\mathcal{J}}$ at stage k of the group sequential test procedure is given by

$$p_{\mathcal{J},k}^{\mathrm{BON}} = \min\{|\mathcal{J}\setminus\mathcal{E}| \min_{g\in\mathcal{J}\setminus\mathcal{E}}\{p_g\},1\}$$

Applying this testing procedure, at the first interim analysis, it is possible to stop the trial while showing significance of one (or more) treatment arms. This might be possible if the CTP already shows significance for these treatment arms. In an interim analysis, it is also possible to stop the trial due to futility arguments. This is usually based on conditional power calculations. However, it is expected that the first stage is specifically used to select a treatment arm to be considered in the subsequent stages of the trial and/or to reassess the sample size for the subsequent stages.

Let

$$C(p,q) = \frac{w_1\Phi^{-1}(1-p)+w_2\Phi^{-1}(1-q)}{\sqrt{w_1^2+w_2^2}}$$

denote the inverse normal test statistic with some prefixed weights w_1, w_2 (cf., Equation 8.2), p and q denoting the first and second stage p-values for elementary or intersection tests. At the second stage, the hypotheses belonging to the selected treatment arm s is rejected if

$$\min_{\mathcal{J}\ni s} C(p_{\mathcal{J}}, q_{\mathcal{J}\setminus\mathcal{E}}) \geq u_2, \tag{8.4}$$

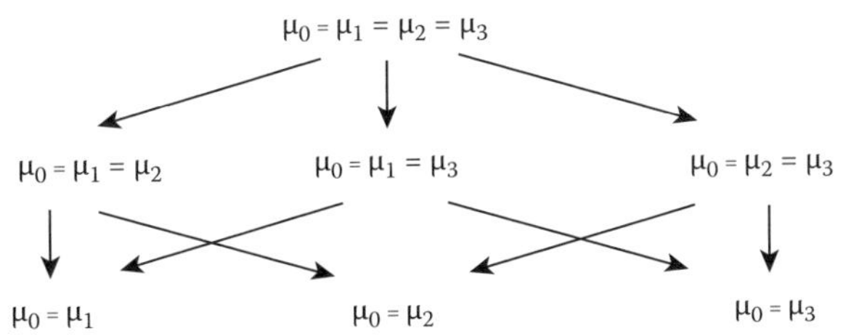

FIGURE 8.2 Closed system of hypotheses ($G = 3$).

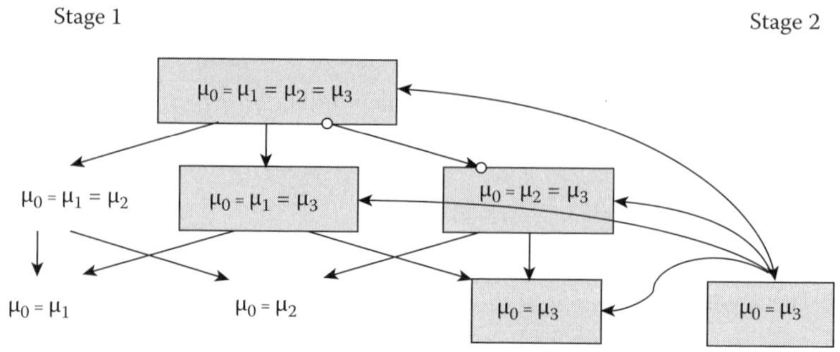

FIGURE 8.3 Two-stage closed testing procedure.

where u_2 denoted the critical value for the second stage of the group sequential test procedure.

If one treatment is selected, Equation 8.4 reduces to

$$\min_{\mathcal{J} \ni s} C(p_{\mathcal{J}}, q_k) \geq u_2 . \tag{8.5}$$

For $G = 3$ and $s = 3$, the latter case is illustrated in Figure 8.3, the curved arrows indicating what combination of tests have to be carried out and showing Equation 8.5 in order to show significance of the selected treatment arm.

This principle can easily be extended to multiple stages and/or to other combination functions (e.g., Fisher's combination test) and to the CRP approach.

8.3.2.1 Adaptive Dunnett Test

König et al. (2008) proposed a procedure that is based on the conditional Type I error rate of the single-stage Dunnett test. They showed that this procedure uniformly improves the Dunnett test if treatment arms were selected in an interim stage. The test coincides with the classical Dunnett test if no treatment arm selections (or other adaptations) were performed. Application within the CTP is straightforward. The procedure is different than the inverse normal method, when a Dunnett test is used for testing intersection hypotheses, and is generally more powerful. It can be shown that, however, the gain in power is only slight.

The proposed test is a two-stage procedure where in the interim analysis the conditional Type I error rate for the Dunnett test is calculated. Assume that the variance σ^2 is known and treatment means $\bar{x}_0, \ldots, \bar{x}_G$ from the first stage data with sample sizes $n_0, \ldots, n_G$ are calculated. Assume that the information rate $t_1 = n/N$ that relates the first stage sample size to the preplanned overall sample size N is planned (i.e., at first step we assume the ratios n_g/n_0 are constant over the two stages). The conditional Type I error rate is then given by

$$\alpha_G = \alpha_G(z_1^{(1)}, \ldots, z_G^{(1)}) = 1 - \int_{-\infty}^{\infty} \prod_{g \in \mathcal{G}} \Phi\left(\frac{c_G(\alpha) - \sqrt{t_1}\, z_g^{(1)} + \sqrt{1-t_1}\, \lambda_g x}{\sqrt{(1-t_1)(1-\lambda_g^2)}} \right) \varphi(x)\, dx , \tag{8.6}$$

where

$$\lambda_g = \sqrt{\frac{n_g}{n_0 + n_g}},$$

$$z_g^{(1)} = \frac{\bar{x}_g - \bar{x}_0}{\sigma\left(\sqrt{1/n_g + 1/n_0}\right)}, \; g = 1, \ldots, G, \text{and}$$

$c_G(\alpha)$ is the critical value for performing Dunnett's test at level α with G active treatments. Equation 8.6 can be computed numerically. At the interim stage, treatment selection and/or sample size recalculation (e.g., based on conditional power) can be performed. If the second stage test is a test at level α_G, the procedure preserves the overall level.

Assume a set $\mathcal{S} \subset \{1, \ldots, G\}$ of treatment arms were selected for the second stage. König et al. (2008) proposed two tests for the global test for $H_0 \cap H_0^S$ at the final stage. The first is to perform a conditional second stage Dunnett test at level α_G, the second is based on a corresponding unconditional test.

When the conditional second stage Dunnett test is selected, the p-value at the final analysis is given by

$$1-\int_{-\infty}^{\infty}\prod_{g\in\mathcal{S}}\Phi\left(\frac{\max_{g\in\mathcal{S}} z_g-\sqrt{t_1}\,z_g^{(1)}+\sqrt{1-t_1}\,\lambda_g x}{\sqrt{(1-t_1)(1-\lambda_g^2)}}\right)\varphi(x)dx, \quad (8.7)$$

where z_g is the observed overall test statistic for treatment arm g at the final stage. Equation 8.7 is similar to Equation 8.6, with $c_G(\alpha)$ replaced by the observed maximum statistic $\max_{g\in\mathcal{S}} z_g$, and the integration performed over selected treatment arms.

If the unconditional test is used, the p-value is calculated from the second stage data alone and given by

$$1-\int_{-\infty}^{\infty}\prod_{g\in\mathcal{S}}\Phi\left(\frac{\max_{g\in\mathcal{S}} z_g^{(2)}+\lambda_g x}{\sqrt{1-\lambda_g^2}}\right)\varphi(x)dx, \quad (8.8)$$

where $z_g^{(2)}$ is the observed test statistic for treatment arm g from the second stage data. Application of the tests based on Equations 8.6 through 8.8 within the CTP yields a multiple testing procedure for the considered closed system of hypotheses.

The test based on Equation 8.7 coincides with the classical Dunnett test if no treatment arms were selected. If sample size recalculations were performed the test based on Equation 8.7 assumes the λ_g, $g = 1, \ldots, G$, to be constant over the stages, otherwise the test based on Equation 8.8 should be used (where λ_g can be recalculated from the second stage data). Both tests require the variance to be known and therefore the sample sizes to be quite large in order to obtain valid approximate results. With the implemented Dunnett test, no formal stopping rules are foreseen; that is, the interim analysis is performed solely to perform a data dependent treatment arm selection and/or a sample size recalculation.

8.3.3 Patient Enrichment Designs

When reporting clinical trial results it is usually the case that results from a subgroup of patients also reported. It is well known that these results can only be interpreted in an exploratory sense. If one wants to confirm, for example, efficacy of a new treatment compared to a control in a subgroup of patients, an additional study has to be performed where the hypothesis concerning the subgroup of patients is specified in advance. It might also be the case that interim data suggest a population shift and it is desired to perform the remainder of the trial with the newly defined (sub)population. Within the frequentist framework, this can only be performed in an exploratory sense, and the final decision must be based on an additional trial. Or the subgroup is prespecified and a multiplicity issue arises that can be solved, for example, by performing a closed test procedure (cf., Brannath et al. 2009).

Adaptive designs, on the other hand, allow for identifying subgroups in interim analysis in a data-driven way. Wang, Hung, and O'Neill (2009) have shown how this can be done in the context of a so-called adaptive patient enrichment design. They define an adaptive enrichment design as a design that prospectively defines the investigation of the treatment effect in the originally planned (unselected) patient population and the prespecified patients subsets. Adaptive tests were defined as p-value combination tests or weighted Z-tests, which are equivalent to the inverse normal method. Through simulations they showed that the enrichment design outperforms the classical fixed design with a prespecified multiple testing procedure.

By use of the closed testing principle this procedure is described very easily because formally the same situation arises as for the multiarmed testing situation. The treatment arms stand for the prespecified subgroups of patients and the global hypothesis H_0 refers to the treatment effect in the entire (unselected) study population. Furthermore, treatment arm selection is formally identical to subgroup selection and hence the same procedure as described for the adaptive treatment selection applies. Specifically, for a two-stage design, if H_0^S refers to the hypothesis of no treatment effect in the selected subgroup, H_0^S can be rejected in the final stage if

1. The combination test that combines the p-values for H_0 and H_0^S for the first and the second stage data, respectively, and
2. The combination test that combines the p-values for H_0^S for the first and the second stage data, respectively,

can be rejected. Since typically the first stage p-value for H_0^S is smaller than the first-stage p-value for H_0 (otherwise subgroup selection is not meaningful in most cases), the first condition suffices to show efficacy for the subgroup of patients. In general, however, both conditions must be fulfilled.

Obviously, this procedure can be extended to the multistage case including sample size reassessment procedures at the interim analyses. It also applies to nested subsets of patients as described in Wang, Hung, and O'Neill (2009). In the context considered here, adaptive designs can select subgroups in an unprespecified way and allow for concluding efficacy at the final end of the trial. This is due to the fact that it is possible to include completely new hypotheses to the prespecified set of hypotheses (Hommel 2001). In this case, however, the test for the newly defined hypothesis is based on data only from the second stage. The practical applicability of this approach is questionable because the condition for the second stage p-value is the same as the condition for the p-value of a completely new study. Furthermore, since the combination test that combines the p-values for H_0 and H_0^S for the first- and the second-stage data, respectively, must be significant, too, in practically relevant cases there is no gain in power when performing such a design. Nevertheless, it shows that flexibility can also be applied with regard to an unforeseen selection of patient characteristics and hence these designs allow for dealing with the unexpected in a very general way.

8.4 Concluding Remarks

We described how to perform data-driven changes of the study design in the on-going trial under control of the Type I error. We focused on the three most relevant adaptations, namely sample size reassessment, treatment arm selection strategies, and patient enrichment designs. The procedures can be used in confirmatory trials. The considered type of confirmatory adaptive designs was introduced by Bauer (1989) and found enormous interest in the last two decades. Note that the term adaptive design was already used before this seminal paper (and actually is used) in a number of different meanings, but the possibility to learn from experience (a Bayesian principle) was the new and interesting issue that was introduced by these designs. It was the provocation that the rigid rules in the frequentist approach can be weakened and the way was open for great flexibility in performing clinical trials.

Unfortunately, this was also misunderstood at some places. It was thought that studies did not need to be adequately planned anymore and it was sufficient to perform one or more interim analyses in place of performing planning efforts. As a consequence, regulators were confronted with senseless statistical designs containing relevant deficiencies for conducting the trials. The EMA reflection paper (2007) was the response to this for some cases misapplied ways of conducting adaptive designs. The EMA paper highlights some major conceptual problems and discusses potential applications of adaptive designs from a regulators point of view. The draft guidance on "Adaptive Design Clinical Trials for Drugs and Biologics" of the U.S. Food and Drug Administration (FDA, 2010) is the second official statement from regulators dealing with their position on adaptive clinical trial designs.

There are two major issues that need to be clarified. First, in the discussion of adaptive designs the conduct of interim analysis per se can be criticized. For example, it is certainly true that performing interim analysis can jeopardize the integrity of the study, especially when interim analyses were performed in an unblinded way. Nevertheless, this is not a problem of adaptive design but of performing interim analyses in general. Hence, one must carefully distinguish between problems that are inherited from group sequential designs and problems that are specifically referring to adaptive designs. The conduct of interim analysis is usually performed within independent data monitoring committees (IDMCs). The role of IDMCs, however, goes beyond the scope of this article.

The second major issue relevant for the discussion is the need for a careful distinction between methodological possibilities and clinical applications to be recommended when performing adaptive confirmatory designs. Indeed, it is not recommended to exhaust the existing flexibility of adaptive designs. This is even more important as there is not very much experience available in conducting these designs. At the moment, we are on the way to finding reasonable adaptive strategies, the ones that were described in this paper appear to be most promising.

Acknowledgments

The author thank Marc Vandemeulebroecke and the referee for helpful comments on an earlier draft of the manuscript.

References

Bauer, P. (1989). Multistage testing with adaptive designs. *Biom. und Inform. in Med. und Biol.* 20: 130–48.

Bauer, P., and Kieser, M. (1999). Combining different phases in the development of medical treatments within a single trial. *Statistics in Medicine,* 18: 1833–48.

Bauer, P., and Köhne, K. (1994). Evaluation of experiments with adaptive interim analyses. *Biometrics,* 50: 1029–41.

Bauer, P., and König, F. (2006). The reassessment of trial perspectives from interim data—A critical view. *Statistics in Medicine,* 25: 23–36.

Brannath, W., Posch, M., and Bauer, P. (2002). Recursive combination tests. *Journal of the American Statistical Association,* 97: 236–44.

Brannath, W., Zuber, E., Branson, M., Bretz, F., Gallo, P., Posch, M., and Racine-Poon, A. (2009). Confirmatory adaptive designs with Bayesian decision tools for a targeted therapy on oncology. *Statistics in Medicine,* 28: 1445–63.

Bretz, F., König, F., Brannath, W., Glimm, E., and Posch, M. (2009). Tutorial in biostatistics: Adaptive designs for confirmatory clinical trials. *Statistics in Medicine,* 28: 1181–1217.

Cui, L., Hung, H. M. J., and Wang, S.-J. (1999). Modification of sample size in group sequential clinical trials. *Biometrics,* 55: 853–57.

EMA. (2007). Reflection paper on methodological issues in confirmatory clinical trials with an adaptive design. *European Medicines Agencies,* CHMP/EWP/2459/02.

FDA. (2010). Adaptive design clinical trials for drugs and biologics. *U.S. Food and Drug Administration, draft guidance.* Available at http://www.fda.gov/downloads/Drugs/GuidanceCompliance Regulatory Information/Guidances/UCM201790.pdf

Follmann, D. A., Proschan, M. A., and Geller, N. L. (1994). Monitoring pairwise comparisons in multi-armed clinical trials. *Biometrics,* 50: 325–36.

Friede, T., and Kieser, M. (2006). Sample size recalculation in internal pilot designs: A review. *Biometrical Journal,* 48: 1–19.

Friede, T., and Stallard, N. (2008). A comparison of methods for adaptive treatment selection. *Biometrical Journal,* 50: 767–81.

Hellmich, M. (2001). Monitoring clinical trials with multiple arms. *Biometrics,* 57: 892–98.

Hommel, G. (2001). Adaptive modifications of hypotheses after an interim analysis. *Biometrical Journal,* 43: 581–89.

Jennison, C., and Turnbull, B. W. (2000). *Group Sequential Methods with Applications to Clinical Trials.* Boca Raton: Chapman & Hall/CRC.

Jennison, C., and Turnbull, B. W. (2003). Mid-course sample size modification in clinical trial. *Statistics in Medicine,* 22: 971–93.

Kelly, P. J., Stallard, N., and Todd, S. (2005). An adaptive group sequential design for phase II/III clinical trials that select a single treatment from several. *Journal of Biopharmaceutical Statistics,* 15: 641–58.

Kieser, M., Bauer, P., and Lehmacher, W. (1999). Inference on multiple endpoints in clinical trials with adaptive interim analyses. *Biometrical Journal,* 41: 261–77.

König, F., Brannath, W., Bretz, F., and Posch, M. (2008). Adaptive dunnett tests for treatment selection. *Statistics in Medicine,* 27: 1612–25.

Lan, K. K. G., and DeMets, D. L. (1983). Discrete sequential boundaries for clinical trials. *Biometrika,* 70: 659–63.

Lehmacher, W., and Wassmer, G. (1999). Adaptive sample size calculations in group sequential trials. *Biometrics,* 55: 1286–90.

Marcus, R., Peritz, E., and Gabriel, K. R. (1976). On closed testing procedures with special reference to ordered analysis of variance. *Biometrika,* 63: 655–60.

Müller, H.-H., and Schäfer, H. (2001). Adaptive group sequential designs for clinical trials: Combining the advantages of adaptive and of classical group sequential approaches. *Biometrics,* 57: 886–91.

Müller, H. H., and Schäfer, H. (2004). A general statistical principle for changing a design any time during the course of a trial. *Statistics in Medicine,* 23: 2497–2508.

O'Brien, P. C., and Fleming, T. R. (1979). A multiple testing procedure for clinical trials. *Biometrics,* 35: 549–56.

Pocock, S. J. (1977). Group sequential methods in the design and analysis of clinical trials. *Biometrika,* 64: 191–99.

Posch, M., and Bauer, P. (1999). Adaptive two stage designs and the conditional error function. *Biometrical Journal,* 41: 689–96.

Posch, M., Koenig, F., Branson, M., Brannath, W., Dunger-Baldauf, C., and Bauer, P. (2005). Testing and estimating in flexible group sequential designs with adaptive treatment selection. *Statistics in Medicine,* 2443: 3697–3714.

Posch, M., Timmesfeld, N., König, F., and Müller, H.-H. (2004). Conditional rejection probabilities of Student's *t*-test and design adaptation. *Biometrical Journal,* 46: 389–403.

Proschan, M. A. (2009). Sample size re-estimation in clinical trials. *Biometrical Journal,* 51: 348–57.

Proschan, M. A., Follmann, D. A., and Geller, N. L. (1994). Monitoring multi-armed trials. *Statistics in Medicine,* 13: 1441–52.

Proschan, M. A., Follmann, D. A., and Waclawiw, M. A. (1992). Effects on assumption violations on type I error rate in group sequential monitoring. *Biometrics,* 48: 1131–43.

Proschan, M. A., and Hunsberger, S. A. (1995). Designed extension of studies based on conditional power. *Biometrics,* 51: 1315–24.

Stallard, N., and Friede, T. (2008). A group-sequential design for clinical trials with treatment selection. *Statistics in Medicine,* 27: 6209–27.

Stallard, N., and Todd, S. (2003). Sequential designs for phase III clinical trials incorporating treatment selection. *Statistics in Medicine,* 22: 689–703.

Timmesfeld, N., Schäfer, H., and Müller, H.-H. (2007). Increasing the sample size during clinical trials with t-distributed test statistics without inflating the type I error rate. *Statistics in Medicine,* 26: 2449–64.

Vandemeulebroecke, M. (2008). Group sequential and adaptive designs—A review of basic concepts and points of discussion. *Biometrical Journal,* 50: 541–57.

Wang, S.-J., Hung, H. M. J., and O'Neill, R. T. (2009). Adaptive patient enrichment designs in therapeutic trials. *Biometrical Journal,* 51: 358–74.

Wang, S. K., and Tsiatis, A. A. (1987). Approximately optimal one-parameter boundaries for group sequential trials. *Biometrics,* 43: 193–99.

Wassmer, G. (1999). *Statistical Test Procedures for Group Sequential and Adaptive Designs in Clinical Trials. Theoretical Concepts and Solutions in SAS.* (In german). Professorial dissertation. Cologne, Germany.

Wassmer, G. (2003). Data-driven analysis strategies for proportion studies in adaptive group sequential test designs. *Journal of Biopharmaceutical Statistics,* 13: 585–603.

Wassmer, G. (2006). Planning and analyzing adaptive group sequential survival trials. *Biometrical Journal,* 48.

Wassmer, G., Eisebitt, R., and Coburger, S. (2001). Flexible interim analyses in clinical trials using multi-stage adaptive test designs. *Drug Information Journal,* 35: 1131–46.

9

Classical Dose-Finding Trial

Naitee Ting
Boehringer-Ingelheim Pharmaceuticals, Inc.

9.1 Background and Clinical Development Plan

Classical drug development programs usually are referred to those for the treatment of chronic diseases. In most of the programs, Phase I clinical trials recruit healthy normal volunteers to study pharmacokinetics (PK), pharmacodynamics (PD), and the maximally tolerated dose (MTD) for the drug candidate. Patients with the target disease under study are recruited in Phase II. Therefore, under these development programs, drug efficacy cannot be studied at Phase I, and the first efficacy trial is designed in Phase II. One important step in early clinical development of a new drug is to draft a clinical development plan (CDP). Various clinical studies are designed and carried out according to this plan, and such a CDP is updated over time based on newly available information. Understanding of dose–response relationship should be one of the central components in CDP. Since dose finding is mainly addressed in Phase II, this chapter focuses on clinical trials to be designed during the Phase II clinical development.

The importance of dose-finding in clinical development is also noted by the regulatory agencies. This is reflected from the ICH-E4 (1994) guidance: "Assessment of dose–response should be an integral component of drug development with studies designed to assess dose–response an inherent part of establishing the safety and effectiveness of the drug. If development of dose–response information is built into the development process it can usually be accomplished with no loss of time and minimal extra effort compared to development plans that ignore dose–response."

In drug development, concerns for drugs to treat life-threatening disease such as cancer, can be very different from those for other drugs. In the early stage of developing a cancer drug, patients are recruited to trials under open-label treatment with the test drug and some effective background cancer therapy. Under this circumstance, doses of the test drug may be adjusted during the treatment period. Information obtained from these studies will then be used to help suggest dose regimen for future studies. Various study designs to handle these situations are available in statistical/oncology literatures. In some cases, drugs for life-threatening diseases are approved for the target patient population before large-scale Phase III studies are completed because of public need. When this is the case, additional clinical studies may be sponsored by National Institute of Health (NIH) or National Cancer Institute (NCI) in the United States. Many of the NIH/NCI studies are still designed for dose-finding or dose-adjustment purposes.

In the classical development programs for drugs to treat chronic diseases, considerations and plans regarding dose-finding should be in place starting from the nonclinical development stage. Across all Phases of clinical development, information to help with dose selection is needed. The key stage for finding the appropriate range of doses should be around Phase II. But critical information to help designing Phase II studies are obtained from nonclinical and Phase I studies. In certain situations—as the drug candidate belongs to a well-established drug class—where information from other drugs of the same class is available, clinical scientists need to make best use of the available information to help design Phase II studies. Hence one of the primary objectives in the earlier part of CDP should be to deliver useful data in order to help design dose ranging and dose selection studies in Phase II. Based on information collected from Phase I clinical studies, a number of Phase II studies should be planned and carried out: proof of concept (PoC), dose ranging, and dose finding studies. Some of these studies are carried out to measure the clinical endpoints; some others are to measure biomarkers. Choice of appropriate endpoints for each study should be considered in the CDP. Criteria to determine success should be also clarified in the CDP.

After the multiple dose PK is established for a drug candidate from Phase I studies, there is often an estimated MTD. In the CDP, considerations should be made to determine whether studies can be conducted simultaneously or sequentially. In other words, for a trial designed to study PK, this trial can also provide safety information to help estimate MTD. Meanwhile, another study can be designed to learn the food effect. In these development programs, we should try to maximize the amount of information that can be collected in each study and minimize the time to achieve these objectives. On the other hand, a PoC study or a dose ranging study cannot be designed without the MTD information. Hence these studies should be conducted after MTD information can be obtained from earlier studies. Therefore, the CDP needs to lay out the sequence of studies to be designed and executed over time, and estimation of the starting time of a new study should be based on critical information available to help design that study. Sometimes PoC and dose ranging studies are combined. All of these strategies need to be discussed while the CDP is being drafted.

In this chapter, Section 9.2 covers some dose-finding considerations in developing drugs for oncology. Section 9.3 discusses some challenges in designing classical dose-finding studies during Phase II. Section 9.4 attempts to simplify the objectives of these trials. Section 9.5 is about PK and PD. Section 9.6 introduces clinical simulations. Section 9.7 covers the concept of confirmation and exploration in clinical trial designs. Section 9.8 considers selection of Type I and II error rates. Section 9.9 covers analysis of dose-finding trials using the MCP-Mod method. Section 9.10 discusses range of doses. Section 9.11 introduces types of design other than the parallel group design. Section 9.12 presents an example, and Section 9.13 provides a summary.

9.2 Dose-Finding in Oncology

As indicated in Section 9.1, concerns in developing cancer drugs can be different from those in developing drugs to treat chronic diseases. In this section, an introduction of designing early Phase oncology clinical trials is provided by Ivanova (2006).

Phase I trials in oncology are conducted to obtain information on dose-toxicity relationship. Preclinical studies in animals define a dose with approximately 10% mortality (the murine LD10). One-tenth or two-tenths of the murine equivalent of LD10, expressed in milligrams per meters squared, is usually used as a starting dose in a Phase I trial. It is standard to choose a set of doses according to the modified Fibonacci sequence in which higher escalation steps have decreasing relative increments (100%, 65%, 50%, 40%, and 30% thereafter). Toxicity in oncology trials is graded using the National Cancer Institute Common Terminology Criteria for Adverse Events version 3.0 (available online from the Cancer Therapy Evaluation Program Web site http://ctep.cancer.gov). Toxicity is measured on a scale from 0 to 5. The dose limiting toxicity (DLT) is usually defined as treatment related nonhematological toxicity of grade 3 or higher, or treatment related hematological toxicity of grade 4 or higher. The toxicity outcome is typically binary (DLT/no DLT). The underlying assumption is that the probability of toxicity is a nondecreasing function of dose. The MTD is statistically defined as the dose at which the probability of toxicity is equal to the maximally tolerated level, Γ. Alternatively, the MTD can be defined as the dose just below the lowest dose level with unacceptable toxicity rate Γ_U, $\Gamma < \Gamma_U$ (Rosenberger and Haines 2002). For example, the MTD can be defined as the dose level just below the lowest dose level where two or more out of six patients had toxicity. In the first definition, the MTD can be uniquely determined for any monotone dose-toxicity relationship; in the second, the MTD depends on the set of doses chosen for the study. In Phase I oncology studies, Γ ranges from 0.1 to 0.35. In oncology, unlike many other areas of medicine, dose-finding trials do not treat healthy volunteers, but rather patients who are ill and for whom other treatments did not work. An important ethical issue to consider in designing such trials (Ratain et al. 1993) is the need to minimize the number of patients treated at toxic doses. Therefore, patients in oncology dose-finding trials are assigned sequentially starting with the lowest dose.

Von Békésy (1947) and Dixon and Mood (1954) described an up-and-down design where the dose level increases following a nontoxic response and decreases if toxicity is observed. This procedure clusters the treatment distribution around the dose for which the probability of toxicity is equal to $\Gamma = 0.5$. To target any quantile Γ, Derman (1957) modified the decision rule of the design using a biased coin. Durham and Flournoy (1994, 1995) considered two biased coin designs in the spirit of Derman. Wetherill (1963) and Tsutakawa (1967a, 1967b) proposed to assign patients in groups rather than one at a time. Group up-and-down designs can target a wide range of toxicity rates Γ. Storer (1989) and Korn et al. (1994) used decision rules of group designs to suggest several designs for dose-finding. Among the designs studied in Storer (1989) and Korn et al. (1994) were versions of the traditional or 3 + 3 design widely used in oncology.

Biased coin designs, group up-and-down designs, the traditional or 3 + 3 design and its extension A + B designs (Lin and Shih 2001) are often referred to as nonparametric designs. Nonparametric designs are attractive because they are easy to understand and implement since the decision rule is intuitive and does not involve complicated calculations. Designs such as the continual reassessment method (O'Quigley, Pepe, and Fisher 1990) and the escalation with overdose control (Babb, Rogatko, and Zacks 1998) are often referred to as parametric designs.

9.2.1 Example: A Traditional 3 + 3 Design

The most widely used design in oncology is the traditional design also known as the standard or 3 + 3 design. According to the 3 + 3 design, subjects are assigned in groups of three starting with the lowest dose with the following provisions:

If only three patients have been assigned to the current dose so far, then:

i. If no toxicities are observed in a cohort of three, the next three patients are assigned to the next higher dose level.

ii. If one toxicity is observed in a cohort of three, the next three patients are assigned to the same dose level.
iii. If two or more toxicities are observed at a dose, the MTD is considered to have been exceeded.

If six patients have been assigned to the current dose, then:

i. If at most one toxicity is observed in six patients at the dose, the next three patients are assigned to the next higher dose level.
ii. If two or more toxicities are observed in six patients at the dose, the MTD is considered to have been exceeded.

The estimated MTD is the highest dose level with observed toxicity rate less than 0.33.

The properties of the 3 + 3 design will be discussed later. To understand this design better we first describe group up-and-down designs.

9.3 Challenges

9.3.1 Scientific Challenges

One of the most difficult issues in Phase II clinical development is dose selection. At this point, there is often a considerable amount of uncertainties regarding any hypothetical dose–response curves. There are two key assumptions:

1. The MTD estimated from Phase I studies is accurate
2. The efficacy is nondecreasing with increasing doses

Even with these two assumptions, the underlying dose–response curve can still take many possible shapes. Under each assumed curve, there are various strategies of allocating doses. For example, in Figure 9.1, the population dose–response curve can be assumed to take a variety of shapes. Curve 1 may represent a projected human population dose–response curve based on mouse models, curve 2 may be the projection from the dog models, and curve 3 may represent that of the rabbit models.

For the first dose ranging study design, it is typical to choose three test doses (low dose, medium dose, high dose) and a placebo (Ting 2006). If we select doses to detect the ascending part of curve 3, then the planned doses should be on the higher range. On the other hand, if we need to select doses to detect the activities of curve 1, then the doses should be chosen on the lower end. Thus, the dose allocation strategy can be very different depending on the underlying assumed dose response curves. Note that the objective of the first dose ranging study in Phase II is to help find a range of doses where the ascending part

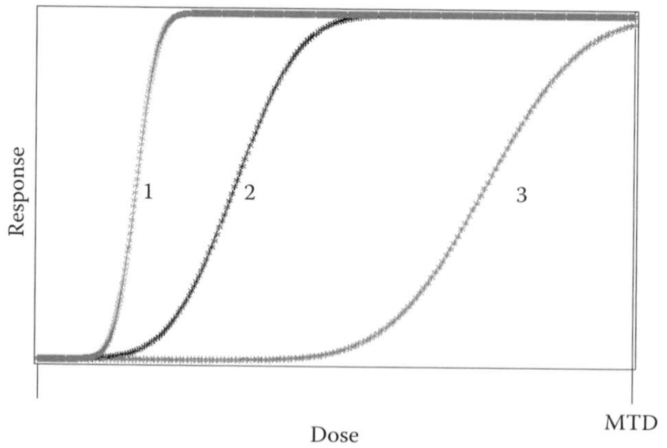

FIGURE 9.1 Several possible dose–response curves.

of the dose response curve is the steepest. Denote this range as the target efficacy dose range (TEDR). One intuitive approach is to start with many doses in the first dose-ranging study so that there is a good chance to capture this TEDR.

In most of the clinical development programs, Phase II clinical trials recruit outpatients for study. When in this situation, it would be very inconvenient if drugs are delivered with flexible dosing (e.g., powder form, liquid, or suspension). In order to encourage patient compliance, test drugs are formulated with fixed strengths in capsules or tablets. This also helps blinding during the study. Hence most of the Phase II studies are carried out based on fixed, preformulated dose strengths. One of the scientific challenges at this point is that clinical scientists hope to include as many doses as possible, but, in practice, there are only a few limited preformulated dose strengths available for testing. Also, adding more doses to the study mounts more difficulties in preparing matching placebos to help blinding the study.

9.3.2 Business Challenges

One of the business challenges at this stage is that statistical hypothesis testing requires a reasonable sample size to compare each test treatment group against placebo. The more doses to be included in the study, the larger the total sample size will be needed. To make things worse, when more groups are compared with placebo, the multiple comparison adjustment makes the alpha for each pairwise comparison smaller; this will translate into even a larger sample size per group. From a business point of view, at this early stage, the sponsor is not sure whether the test drug works or not and, if it works, it is unclear how well it works. Hence a huge investment on a study with such a large sample size is not feasible. This large sample size versus small investment dilemma challenges the entire Phase II clinical development.

In the development of a new drug or new biologics, the entire investment can go as high as $1 billion and the time of development can take up to 10 or more years. This is an expensive cost and a long time to go through. Therefore there is an urge from upper management of sponsors to reduce the cost and to shorten the development time. The current business environment is pushing for "cheaper, faster, and better." When this pressure is applied to the clinical project team, team members tend to speed up the development process. In some cases, this may lead to cutting corners in the Phase II development and causing undesirable consequences.

Another business challenge happens at the end of Phase II, before start of Phase III. At this point, although a lot of efficacy and safety data are available, it may still be uncertain how the drug candidate performs in long-term studies. Upper management in a sponsor company needs to evaluate the entire clinical portfolio, compare various development strategies, before committing to a major Phase III investment for a given drug candidate. This is one of the most critical Go/No Go decisions to be made about progressing or stopping further development for this candidate.

9.4 Objectives

In general, a great number of drug candidates will not meet the stringent scrutiny and be weeded out during the drug development process. The success rate is very low for a nonclinical candidate to successfully pass the Phases I, II, and III selections and eventually be approved by regulatory agencies and be available for general patient use. The most critical challenge in drug development is how to select the best candidate to move forward. Meanwhile, those "not so good" candidates are stopped for development to save investments. Under this circumstance, a successful development strategy is, "To progress a candidate as fast as possible, if this candidate really works, and is safe; and to stop the development of a candidate as early as possible, if it is not safe or efficacious." The question is how to implement such a strategy efficiently during the clinical development process. One way is to consider every clinical trial as a Go/No Go study, and each study is designed to meet a clear No Go criteria. This provides the best opportunity to weed out a bad candidate as early as possible.

The main objectives for Phase I is to understand the PK profile of the drug candidate and to find MTD. In typical clinical development programs, dose selection happens mainly in Phase II. The two major objectives of Phase II are PoC and recommend a few doses for Phase III development. Since Phase II is the first opportunity when patients with the disease are recruited into the trial, this is the first time drug efficacy can be observed in humans. One popular PoC design includes two treatment groups—one high dose group of the test drug and the placebo group. The high dose is close to MTD and it serves as an anchor of the high end of the dose–response curve. If this dose does not deliver efficacy, then this candidate can be stopped for further development. Phase II serves both exploratory and confirmatory purposes. At an earlier stage of Phase II, a wide range of doses are explored. In later Phase II, the interest is in narrowing down the dose range so that one or a few doses can be recommended for Phase III confirmation. Also, Phase II results are used to convince the upper management in a sponsor to commit for major investment in Phase III. The key objectives for Phase III is to confirm the study findings obtained from early Phases, and to demonstrate efficacy and safety of the drug candidate so that regulatory agencies can make a decision to approve or disapprove the drug/biologics for general patient population use.

As stated above, the two major objectives of Phase II are PoC and recommending a few doses for Phase III development. Note that some investigators consider objectives of Phase II to also include establishing the precise minimum effective dose (MinED), characterizing the dose–response relationships (or describing the entire dose–response curves), finding the optimal doses, or understanding the benefit/risk ratio. In fact, these additional objectives are neither realistic, nor desirable at Phase II.

In most of the pharmaceutical industries and bio-tech companies, drugs/biologics are discovered and developed for the general patient population. Hence the dose-selection process is to recommend one or a few doses for the overall patient population use, not for individual patient dosing. If the target dose is for the entire patient population, then the chosen dose cannot be optimal to each individual patient. Therefore, it is not practical to search for an "optimal dose" because an optimal dose is more meaningful to a given individual patient, rather than to the entire patient population.

Although the dose–response curve from Figure 9.1 looks like continuous curves, these are only theoretical curves. In reality, drugs are formulated with discrete dose strengths. In the treatment of chronic diseases, the number of preformulated doses is somewhat limited. From this viewpoint, instead of "characterizing the dose–response relationships," early Phase II studies are designed to help locate the TEDR (the range of doses where the ascending part of the curve is the steepest). Therefore, it is reasonable to consider dose-finding practices as operated under a few fixed dose forms, instead of a continuous dose–response curve. From this point of view, MinED does not have to be a specific number read out from a dose–response model. In practice, MinED can be thought of as a particular preformulated dose strength such that a dose below this strength would not deliver the meaningful population efficacy response. For example, if the test drug is formulated into 10 mg tablets and that 20 mg (2 tablets) were shown to be efficacious, while 10 mg failed to distinguish it from the placebo. Then the MinED, practically, is 20 mg. Suppose a model was applied to the dose–response study, and this model indicates that the MinED is 16.32 mg. In practice, such a MinED is not useful. From the drug development point of view, it is more practical to consider 20 mg as the MinED. Hence the effort to pursue a precise point estimate of MinED may not be necessary.

In most of the drug development programs, benefit/risk ratio is studied after Phase III study results are ready. The benefit-risk discussion is typically covered in the Clinical Overview document in a submission based on the review of the entire clinical database. Hence, to seek clear benefit-risk relationship at Phase II could be premature.

9.5 Pharmacokinetic and Pharmacodynamic

The information used for designing Phase II dose finding studies are mainly from preclinical studies and Phase I trials of the test drug, as well as clinical findings from other drugs of the same class. Preclinical studies establish the mechanism of action of the study drug, provide animal PK and PD properties, also some preliminary pharmacology and toxicity activities based on in vitro and in vivo findings. In some cases, preclinical studies offer certain limitations in drug formulation. These early findings from preclinical experiments are helpful in designing Phase I studies, and in selection of biomarkers or surrogate markers in early clinical trials. Under certain circumstances, drug(s) of the same class as the test drug have already been available on the market. Clinical information observed from these drugs can be useful in designing early Phase trials for the study drug.

Among all the information available before designing the first Phase II dose-finding study, the most critical data are obtained from Phase I PK/PD trials. In these trials, PK can be thought of as what does the human body do to the drug, and PD is what does the drug do to the body. PK and PD are sciences to study the time course of drug concentration in plasma and other tissues of the body. One of the key features obtained from PK analysis is the time profile of the study drug. This information can be used to help determine the frequency of dosing (for example, once a day, twice a day, or every six hours, ...). Additionally, PK profiles obtained from Phase I studies may indicate whether there is dose proportionality, and how the test drug, as well as its metabolites is distributed and eliminated from human body. These results obtained from Phase I studies can help with preliminary dose selection in designing early Phase II trials.

One area where PK information is helpful is on the exposure-response relationship. By studying the exposure-response, scientists can learn about individual dose–response relationship. This can be useful in dose titration studies where each individual receives high or low doses depending on the patient's individual case, instead of a population dose–response relationship. However, because difficulties in interpreting results from dose-titration clinical trials, this type of studies is not commonly used in practice.

Phase I data can also be used to perform PK/PD modeling. With these models, pharmacokenitists can predict time profiles of test drug at different doses, and other characteristics of the test drug. Results obtained from these models can also be useful in designing dose-finding studies.

Among various Phase I clinical trials designed to study the PK/PD properties, one type that can help with Phase II dose finding is the dose proportionality (or linearity) study. As indicated in Cheng, Chow, and Su (2006, p.386), "dose proportionality (or linearity) is arguably the most desirable dose response relationship between dose level and PK responses such as area under the blood or plasma concentration-time curve (AUC) due to its clear interpretation. For example, under the assumption of dose proportionality, we expect to see a doubled AUC if we double the dose. Besides, under the property of dose proportionality (or linearity), the PK responses can be easily predicted with various dose levels."

9.6 Clinical Trial Simulations

Simulation is a useful tool in supporting clinical trial designs. Statisticians often use simulation to help with sample size calculation. In certain complicate designs, the only way to calculate the appropriate sample sizes may be based on simulations. In fact, there are more clinical trial properties can be learned from simulation studies. For classical dose-finding clinical trials, simulations can also be used to evaluate dose–response models, as well as methods for statistical analysis.

Before running a simulation, it is very important for the statistician to understand the objective(s) of this simulation. Note that although the simulations are used to support the protocol design, the objectives of simulations are different from the objectives of the clinical protocol. For example, the objective of the clinical protocol is to study the efficacy and safety of a study drug, while the objective of a simulation could be to help calculate the sample sizes to be used for this protocol. In simple simulation practices, this distinction may not be very critical, however, in some complicated simulations, if the objectives are not clear, lots of effort may not necessarily be directed to address the key question of interest.

All clinical trials are designed with assumptions. Some assumptions are practical, reasonable, and necessary. Some other assumptions can be too strong or unrealistic, and statisticians should carefully evaluate each assumption, and learn and understand the risks behind making each assumption for clinical trial designs. One extreme example can be that the project team assumes the test drug is efficacious and safe. Although in drug development, every team member hopes this to be the case, but this could be an unrealistic assumption. In fact, if this assumption is known to be true, then it is not ethical to run a placebo controlled clinical trial where patients can be exposed to the placebo treatment.

Similarly, simulations are performed based on assumptions. Some assumptions are extrapolations from observed data, some are based on prior experiences of drugs from the same class. In many cases, assumptions are associated with mathematical models being used for simulations. In dose–response modeling, there are various potential model and parameters associate with these models that could be considered. Before incorporating any particular model, or any given set of parameters of the corresponding model, statisticians need to carefully evaluate whether the assumptions behind the selected models and parameters are sensible.

In addition to simulations for sample size calculations, for model comparisons, for selection of analytical methods, simulations can also be applied to study the entire clinical trial. Under this application, a clinical trial simulation protocol need to be prepared. Note this protocol is different from the clinical trial protocol. As mentioned earlier, the objectives of simulation are different from those for the actual clinical trial. Hence the simulation protocol should specify its objectives, evaluation criteria, models to be considered, design options (various sample sizes, number of treatment groups, etc.), analytical methods to be used (multiple comparison procedures or use of dose–response models), interim analysis (IA) strategy in case IA will be performed, as well as other considerations. Only after the simulation protocol is prepared and finalized, then the actual clinical trial simulation can be performed. The major advantage of clinical trial simulation is that this project allows all team members to communicate among each other before the actual trial is designed. Statisticians, clinicians, and pharmocokenitists and other clinical scientists need to meet and discuss various assumptions in designing the study. Of course by the end of simulations, the project team will have a better understanding of various study design features. The major disadvantage of clinical trial simulations is the time delay, and the resource consumption in running these simulations.

The key to a successful simulation, whether it is for a specific purpose like sample size calculation, or for a general purpose such as clinical trial simulation, is to avoid the "garbage in, garbage out" situation. This is because simulation results can only reflect the input characteristics before the simulation. If important features of the clinical trial are not thought of before the simulation, then simulation results cannot provide useful guidance in study design. Hence it is critical to understand the assumptions behind each simulation, and when interpreting simulation results, these assumptions need to be clearly articulated.

9.7 Confirmation Versus Exploration

One important property of a clinical study design is robustness. A robust design refers to a study that is designed with clear objective(s) and only minimum assumptions are required. Every clinical trial starts with a key clinical question. This question is implemented in the study design as the primary objective. The ideal situation is one study that attempts to achieve only one primary objective. Usually there are more than one objective and it is critical to differentiate the primary and the secondary objectives (as well as to differentiate confirmatory objectives and exploratory objectives). Under this circumstance, the study should be designed to address the primary objective. Every study is designed with certain assumptions. In practice, many of these assumptions cannot be verified before the clinical data are observed. If some of the assumptions are not satisfied, the actual study results may not be able to answer the primary question. The most robust design should require the least number of assumptions. Thus, it is very important to understand the assumptions being used for each study design, and to assure that these assumptions are realistic.

In the clinical development process, Phases I and II trials are generally considered as exploratory studies, and Phase III trials are considered as confirmatory. With very few exceptions, most of the

Phases II and III studies are carried out to help making key decisions. For these studies, usually a set of decision criteria is prespecified ahead of time, and then trials are designed to collect clinical data to help with decision making. Meanwhile, each clinical study tends to collect additional data to help scientists learning various clinical properties about the new drug that is being developed. In most of the cases, a Phase II or Phase III clinical trial is designed with at least two purposes: decision making and learning. Trials designed for decision-making purposes are usually called "confirmatory trials." Trials designed for learning are generally called "exploratory trials." However, if most of these trials are used both for confirmatory and for exploratory, it is sensible to design studies considering both properties, in a stepwise fashion—the first step is to confirm the decision and then use the second step to explore (Ting 2008).

In Phase II/III clinical trial designs, the thinking process should be stepwise. The primary objective should be clearly stated up front. If there are secondary objectives, they should also be laid out sequentially in a very explicit fashion. Based on these objectives, studies can be designed to make confirmatory decisions. All additional clinical questions should be considered as exploratory. Hence studies should be designed with confirmatory goals first, and then explore additional clinical questions. It should be a stepwise process in designing these clinical trials.

Statistical methods are widely used in the design and analysis of clinical trials. In the exploratory process, parameter estimation is a fundamental tool to help researchers learn about clinical findings. For this application, point estimates and interval estimates are widely used to help quantify parameters of interest. On the other hand, when the purpose is to confirm, then statistical hypothesis testing procedures are used. Based on the result of a hypothesis test, key clinical decisions can be made regarding the drug candidate under development.

In general, the scientific learning process begins with exploration, knowledge gain from the exploratory findings, generation of new hypothesis, and then experimentation to confirm the hypothesis. After they do more exploration, and learn more, scientists continue this process. However, in designing an individual Phase II or III clinical trial, this thinking process needs to be reversed because each study is designed to address a specific clinical question. This question is formulated as the primary objective of the study. Clinical trials are designed to address this well-defined study objective. Hence this part is a confirmatory step. After the primary objective is achieved, scientists would then explore all available data and see what additional information can be learned from this study.

Based on this way of designing clinical trials, the objectives can be simplified so that a single primary objective is used for the confirmatory purpose. All other objectives can be considered as secondary or even exploratory. The primary objective is then translated into a single statistical hypothesis and the study is powered using this hypothesis. Under this setting, unnecessary assumptions are not required in study design and such a study design tends to be more robust.

9.8 Selection of Type I and Type II Error

The foundation of modern clinical trials is randomization. With this important scientific breakthrough in the twentieth century, clinical evidence obtained from double-blind, randomized, controlled trials can be used to justify new drug approval. Under this setting, one fundamental component of establishing drug efficacy is the statistical hypothesis test. In a placebo-controlled trial, the null hypothesis is that there is no difference in patient response between the test drug and the placebo. Unless there is sufficient evidence to prove otherwise, the observed treatment difference can simply be viewed as a chance finding.

Here "sufficient evidence" is quantified by alpha, the Type I error rate. In practice, the layman statement is that, "If the observed p-value is less than alpha, then patient response from the test drug is significantly different from that of the placebo." In fact, when the observed p-value is less than alpha, the null hypothesis is rejected, and the decision that the test drug is different from placebo could still be a wrong decision. However, the probability that this is a wrong decision is controlled at no more than alpha. Hence the Type I error rate can be interpreted as "the probability of claiming a drug is efficacious when in fact it is not." Note that the consequence of making a Type I error is different at the different stage of new drug development. From the regulatory point of view, once a test drug is approved for marketing, then there can potentially be millions of people taking this drug and in case the drug does not work, and the clinical evidence simply reflects a Type I error, then the undesirable consequence is huge. Therefore, regulatory agencies set the one-sided alpha at 0.025 for each individual study. However, from a sponsor's point of view, the consequence of making a Type I error is to continue investing and develop a test drug that is not efficacious. This is a waste of resources and time, which is a less severe consequence compared with the risk for the regulatory agencies. Consequently the sponsor may be willing to tolerate a higher Type I error rate; for example, one-sided alpha of 0.03, 0.04, 0.05, or could even be higher.

In the classical clinical development programs, Phase I does not involve evaluation of drug efficacy and therefore the Type I error rate for efficacy does not tend to be a major concern at this stage. For Phase III, the results obtained from these clinical trials are for submission purposes. Phase III clinical data need to demonstrate sufficient evidence for regulatory agencies to make approval/rejection decisions. Hence these studies are designed with one-sided alpha of 0.025, and multiplicity adjustments (if necessary) are made so that the experiment-wise Type I error rate is not arbitrarily inflated. For Phase II, protection of Type I error is critical because the sponsor cannot afford to waste the investor's funds and the important drug development time. However, alpha does not have to be set at one-sided 0.025 because the risk of developing a placebo is less serious than in Phase III. In designing a Phase II clinical trial, the project team has the opportunity to discuss the ethical concerns, the budget concerns, and can be flexible about choosing an alpha.

After the clinical results are ready, if the decision is "Go"—continue to the next step of clinical development—then there is a risk of making a Type I error. On the other hand, if the decision is "No Go"—stop further development of this drug candidate—then there is a risk of making a Type II error. The Type II error rate is denoted by beta. Since regulatory agencies do not develop new drugs, Type II error is less of a risk for them. However, for sponsors developing new drugs, the risk of stopping development of a good drug could be very high. In Phase III development, clinical trials are designed with high power (or low beta) so that there is a high probability that the test drug will demonstrate efficacy and will be approved by regulatory agencies. It is typical that Phase III studies are designed with 90% or more power (or, equivalently, 10% or less of making a Type II error). On the other hand, studies designed at Phase II tend to have a power around 80% (or with beta of 0.2).

In designing clinical studies, one typical question a project statistician receives is, "How many subjects will be needed?" Sample size estimation is one of the most critical component in clinical trial design. At this time, the project statistician works with the clinician in order to find out the best study design. In general, sample size is a function of alpha, beta, and delta (the minimally clinically important difference). Typically there are three ways of selecting a delta: (1) based on regulatory requirements, (2) by review of published literatures, or (3) predicted from nonclinical data of the drug candidate under development. Project team members discuss various possible values of delta, and the statistician then works with the project team in order to finalize an agreed quantity. This final delta is then used for sample size estimation. For Phase III studies, the delta is determined using method 1 (based on regulatory requirements), it is often based on the discussion from the end-of-phase II meetings with the FDA.

The other two key inputs to sample size estimation are the Type I and Type II error rates (alpha and beta). In a Phase III study design, one-sided alpha is set at 0.025; beta is chosen to be no more than 0.1. However, for Phase II, the choice of alpha and beta reflects the risks a project team is willing to take. Again, since the budget for a Phase II trial tends to be limited, a study with large sample size may not be acceptable to upper management. One situation can be that the sample size is dictated by the budget, but the project team is willing to take a higher alpha risk or beta risk. Under this circumstance, the project statistician recalculates the sample size so that the total number of subjects to be recruited in the study is within the budget, but some larger alphas or betas are used to reach such a compromised sample size.

At this point, the statistician should clearly articulate the consequences of making a Type I or Type II error to the project team.

Suppose the project team is willing to tolerate a larger alpha. The implication is that after this study is completed, if the clinical results indicate a "Go" decision, then there is a higher probability that the sponsor invests in more resources developing a placebo. On the other hand, if the project team increase beta (or decreases power), then when clinical data indicates the test drug is not efficacious, there is a higher potential of making a Type II error (i.e., stopping the development of a good drug). It is therefore critical for the statistician to discuss with the team at the design stage regarding various risks and help quantify these risks. Once the decision about Type I and Type II errors is made, the corresponding sample size can be determined according to these error rates.

These considerations need to be clearly communicated with the project team so that the Go/No Go criteria can be well spelled out. One very important point is that, although the alpha and beta are negotiable at the design stage, the statistical decision criteria after data readout should be firm. For example, if a Type I error is set at 0.2 in the design stage, then if the observed p-value is 0.21, the statistical conclusion should be "statistically nonsignificant" and if the observed p-value is 0.19, the team can claim "statistical significance." In fact, the final Go/No Go decision may not be purely statistical, but the statistical decision rule should be clear and firm.

9.9 Analysis of Dose-Finding Trials: The MCP-Mod Method

In a typical dose–response clinical trial, a placebo and a few active test doses are studied. Clinical data obtained from these studies can be viewed from two different angles. First, the statistician can perform pairwise comparisons to see if any of these doses is superior to placebo. Second, the statistician can consider parametric models, which include all doses to describe a dose–response relationship. When analyzing data from dose–response studies, statisticians consider two families of common statistical methods—multiple comparison procedures (Tamhane, Hochberg, and Dunnett 1996) and modeling approach (Ruberg 1995).

The multiple comparison procedure (MCP) is usually performed with pairwise comparisons of each test dose against placebo. When pairwise comparisons are made, alpha (the probability of making an experimentwise Type I error) could be inflated and a multiple comparison adjustment needs to be made. For example, in the case of a four-treatment group dose–response design, the three pairwise comparisons are high dose versus placebo, medium dose versus placebo, and low dose versus placebo. The Bonferroni adjustment divides alpha by three, and each pairwise comparison is tested at the alpha/three level. Other MCP adjustments include Dunnett's method, Holm's procedure, closed testing, and many other methods. One of the frequently used procedures in drug development is the gate keeping adjustment (Dmitrienko, Wiens, and Westfall 2006).

An example of the gate-keeping procedure in a four-treatment group dose–response study can be described as follows. The first step is to test the high dose against placebo at alpha. If the null hypothesis is accepted, then stop and claim that none of the test dose is effective. If a p-value less than alpha is observed, then claim that the high dose is significantly different from placebo, and test the medium dose versus placebo at alpha. If a p-value is greater than or equal to alpha, then accept null hypothesis and stop; claim that only the high dose is effective, but none of the lower doses is effective. If the p-value from the second step is less than alpha, then claim that both the high dose and the medium dose are effective, and move to test low dose versus placebo at level alpha. These steps are repeated until a p-value that is greater than alpha, or until all pairwise comparisons to placebo are made.

In general, MCP is very useful in protecting alpha so that it is not arbitrarily inflated. This is extremely important in Phase III studies where regulatory agency will need to make a decision about the study drug.

The other family of methods in analyzing dose–response clinical data is based on the modeling approach. A simple example is to assume that the three test doses and placebo forms a linear dose–response relationship. Based on this model, this four-treatment group study can be analyzed using a linear contrast test, or a simple linear regression, using dose as the regressor. Of course, other models such as Emax, logistic, and many others can also be considered for data analysis. Results obtained from this analysis will help investigators to determine whether there is a linear dose–response or not. Also the coefficient estimated from this model can be used to study various properties of the dose–response relationship. The advantages of using a modeling approach include the following:

- Helps to identify a particular dose of interest, for example, MinED, ED_{90} (a dose with 90% efficacy) and these doses do not necessarily have to be the doses being studied
- Provides confidence intervals on estimated doses
- Avoids multiple testing concerns
- Helps better understanding of dose–response relationship
- Guides planning of future studies

Pinheiro, Bretz, and Branson (2006) propose a method to combine the MCP and the modeling approaches, denoted as the MCP-Mod method, for analyzing dose–response studies. The basic idea is to consider a set of candidate models at the design stage and, then for each model, construct an optimal contrast corresponding to that model. If there is a single candidate model with only a given set of parameters, then the data analysis will be performed with just one contrast. Hence no multiple comparison adjustment is necessary. However, if more than one model is considered to perform the analysis, then multiple comparison adjustment could be applied to these contrasts in order to avoid alpha inflation. Based on hypotheses testing from these contrasts and after MCP adjustment, a single model is selected and this model serves as the dose–response model for data analysis.

Once a dose–response model is determined, this model can be used to estimate target doses of interest and to construct confidence intervals on efficacy responses of these doses. Information obtained from this model helps to design other Phase II studies or Phase III studies. The MCP-Mod is an integrated approach to explore dose–response relationships, while confirming that the study drug is efficacious based on hypothesis testing. Therefore, in designing a dose–response study using MCP-Mod for data analysis, the first step is the confirmatory step, which can be accomplished by the MCP. Then, after the confirmatory step, investigators continue to explore using the Mod step. This analysis method can be considered as an application of the confirm-then-explore thinking paradigm.

9.10 Range of Doses to be Studied

As discussed earlier, drug efficacy can only be studied from patients with the target disease. Hence at the beginning of Phase II, there is no efficacy information to help define the dose range for study. It is desirable to obtain information that helps describing the efficacy and safety dose–response curves. In some cases, studies might be designed to help estimate MaxED, MinED, and possibly to obtain additional information to support MTD. Although estimates regarding MTD should have been available prior to Phase II, more information will be helpful to reconfirm or to adjust MTD estimates obtained from previous trials. If the budget and timeline are permissible, the first dose ranging study should cover a wide dose range in the hope that this study will help identify the doses where most of the activities are. The next study will then be designed to capture the key doses for Phase III confirmation using information obtained from the first study.

Note that nonclinical information on the candidate and perhaps both clinical and nonclinical data from related compounds often provide a minimum drug concentration profile that is expected to be required for efficacy. Together with the PK profile, this provides a dose range that we would want to explore—and possibly a minimum dose expected to have little or no efficacy that we might want to include.

It is important to keep in mind that the dose(s) recommended for the next study (either Phase IIB or Phase III) does not have to be a dose being studied in this current clinical trial. Therefore, the objective of a dose ranging study should not be to characterize the entire dose–response relationship, nor to identify a specific dose that is "optimal." Instead, early Phase II dose ranging studies are designed to help estimate a range of doses where the ascending part of the efficacy dose response curve is the steepest. This range may be considered as the TEDR.

Long-term, large-scale Phase III clinical trials are designed to study one or a few doses for confirmatory purposes. The dose or doses used in a Phase III trial is chosen from TEDR. Because most of the drugs are preformulated with certain dose strengths, the number of doses to be used for Phase III development can be limited. In some cases, the drug is delivered with a device such as an inhaler or a prefilled syringe. The number of doses could further be restricted. In practice, if undesirable effects are observed at a dose in the higher end of TEDR, then lower doses within this dose range may be considered for Phase III development. On the other hand, if there are concerns that the dose at the lower end of TEDR may not deliver ideal efficacy, then higher doses within the range will be used in Phase III. Hence good information about TEDR obtained from Phase II can be very useful in selection of doses for Phase III study design. This is also helpful in the manufacturing and packaging of study medication to be used in Phase III clinical trials.

Dose range in a given clinical study is defined as the high dose divided by the low dose used in the study. For example, in a design with placebo, 500 mg, 750 mg, and 1000 mg of test drug, the dose range is 2 (1000/500). In another design for a different test drug, the doses are placebo, 0.001 mg, 0.01 mg, and 0.1 mg, then the dose range is 100 (0.1/0.001). The second study has a much wider dose range than the first one, although the dose strength is much lower. Regardless where the MTD is (e.g., the MTD could be 0.1 mg, 1 mg, 10 mg, 100 mg, or 1000 mg), the challenges presented in Figure 9.1 is always there—the potential range of active doses can still be very wide. Therefore, the first dose ranging study in Phase II should be designed to cover a wide range. Based on results observed from this study, the project team learns the TEDR—should it be between placebo and low dose? between low and medium dose? between medium and high dose? or a combination of these ranges? Then the team is ready to design the next dose ranging study in order to focus on the range established from the first study. Usually after the two dose ranging studies, one or a few doses can be recommended for Phase III development.

In many cases, when the studied dose range is too narrow in the first dose ranging trial, this study failed to deliver the necessary information for efficacy or safety, and rework will be needed after the study. Costs of rework can be tremendous at times. These may include costs of additional studies and costs of delaying the drug getting to the market, in addition to all the resources wasted in conducting the current study.

In order to help estimate TEDR, a wide dose range should be studied in the first dose ranging trial. One method can be used in selecting doses for this design is known as the binary dose spacing (BDS) approach (Hamlett et al. 2002, p. 859).

If the trial includes two dosing groups and a placebo, then the BDS design identifies a midpoint between the placebo and the MTD and allocates one dose above and another below the midpoint. If the trial includes three dosing groups and a placebo, then the BDS design identifies the high dose as described in the two dose case. A second midpoint is then identified between the placebo and the first midpoint, and a low dose is selected below the second midpoint and the medium dose is selected between the two midpoints. The BDS design iteratively follows this strategy with more dosing groups. The BDS design employs a wide dose range, helps identify the MinED, employs a log-like dose spacing strategy avoiding allocating doses near the MTD (i.e., identifies more doses near the lower end), and is flexible and easy to implement.

Note that the first dose ranging study needs to cover a wide dose range, but this does not have to take a lot of doses. Using the BDS concept, a study with three or four doses can cover a fairly wide dose range. In this situation, with a reasonable total sample size, a wide range of doses can be explored. After the TEDR is identified from the first dose ranging study, the project team uses this information to design the next dose finding study so that one or a few doses can be recommended for Phase III development.

9.11 Other Types of Design

As discussed in the previous sections, the most commonly used design in classical dose-finding studies is double-blind, randomized, placebo-controlled parallel group design. However, in certain situations, other types of design may also be considered. ICH-E4 (1994) discusses the cross-over design, the forced titration design, and the optional titration design.

9.11.1 Cross-Over Dose–Response

A randomized multiple cross-over study of different doses can be successful if drug effect develops rapidly and patients return to baseline conditions quickly after cessation of therapy, if responses are not irreversible (cure, death), and if patients have reasonably stable disease. This design suffers, however, from the potential problems of all cross-over studies: It can have analytic problems if there are many treatment withdrawals; it can be quite long in duration for an individual patient; and there is often uncertainty about carry-over effects (longer treatment periods may minimize this problem), baseline comparability after the first period, and period-by-treatment interactions. The length of the trial can be reduced by approaches that do not require all patients to receive each dose, such as balanced incomplete block designs. The advantages of the design are that each individual receives several different doses so that the distribution of individual dose–response curves may be estimated, as well as the population average curve, and that, compared to a parallel design, fewer patients may be needed. Also, in contrast to titration designs, dose and time are not confounded and carry-over effects are better assessed.

9.11.2 Forced Titration

A forced titration study, where all patients move through series of rising doses, is similar in concept and limitations to a randomized multiple cross-over dose–response study, except that assignment to dose levels is ordered, not random. If most patients complete all doses, and if the study is controlled with a parallel placebo group, the forced titration study allows a series of comparisons of an entire randomized group given several doses of drug with a concurrent placebo, just as the parallel fixed-dose trial does. A critical disadvantage is that, by itself, this study design cannot distinguish response to increased dose from response to increased time on drug therapy or a cumulative drug dosage effect. It is therefore an unsatisfactory design when response is delayed, unless treatment at each dose is prolonged. Even where the time until development of effect is known to be short (from other data), this design gives poor information on adverse effects, many of which have time-dependent characteristics. A tendency toward spontaneous improvement, a very common circumstance, will be revealed by the placebo group, but is nonetheless a problem for this design, as over time, the higher doses may find little room to show an increased effect. This design can give a reasonable first approximation of both population-average dose response and the distribution of individual dose–response relationships if the cumulative (time-dependent) drug effect is minimal and the number of treatment withdrawals is not excessive. Compared to a parallel dose–response study, this design may use fewer patients, and by extending the study duration, can be used to investigate a wide range of doses, again making it a reasonable first study. With a concurrent placebo group this design can provide clear evidence of effectiveness, and may be especially valuable in helping choose doses for a parallel dose–response study.

9.11.3 Optional Titration (Placebo-Controlled Titration to Endpoint)

In this design, patients are titrated until they reach a well-characterized favorable or unfavorable response, defined by dosing rules expressed in the protocol. This approach is most applicable to conditions where the response is reasonably prompt and is not an irreversible event, such as stroke or death.

A crude analysis of such studies, for example, comparing the effects in the subgroups of patients titrated to various dosages, often gives a misleading inverted "U-shaped" curve, as only poor responders are titrated to the highest dose. However, more sophisticated statistical analytical approaches that correct for this occurrence, by modeling and estimating the population and individual dose–response relationships, appear to allow calculation of valid dose–response information. Experience in deriving valid dose–response information in this fashion is still limited. It is important, in this design, to maintain a concurrent placebo group to correct for spontaneous changes, investigator expectations, and so on. Like other designs that use several doses in the same patient, this design may use fewer patients than a parallel fixed-dose study of similar statistical power and can provide both population average and individual dose–response information. The design does, however, risk confounding of time and dose effects and would be expected to have particular problems in finding dose–response relationships for adverse effects. Like the forced titration design, it can be used to study a wide dose range and, with a concurrent placebo group, can provide clear evidence of effectiveness. It too may be especially valuable as an early study to identify doses for a definitive parallel study.

9.12 Example: A True Case Study in Osteoarthritis (OA)

Rofecoxib is a medication developed by Merck for the treatment of rheumatoid arthritis and osteoarthritis (OA). In late 2004, Merck withdrew Rofecoxib from the market because of concerns with excessive cardiovascular events. After this, the drug development environment for any new anti-inflammatory agents became more and more challenging. For every new compound developed to treat OA, both drug safety and efficacy are followed very closely to ensure that the efficacy of this new compound can be well established, while there is no signal of undue safety concern. Therefore in the CDP, after the PoC and early dose ranging studies to demonstrate drug efficacy, large scale, long-term Phase III studies follow to evaluate efficacy, cardiovascular safety, and gastrointestinal (GI) safety.

A true case study (Ting forthcoming) based on clinical development of an OA agent is introduced here as an example. This is a 4-week study where OA patients first go through a screening visit. Then after a wash-out of their on-going OA medication, patients are randomized into this study. Baseline measurements (demographic, medical history, background medications, efficacy, and other data) are collected prior to the first dose of study drug. Thereafter, over the 4-week treatment period, efficacy and safety measurements are continually collected at each visit. Note that at the early stage of clinical development, the length of study is constrained by the time length of animal studies completed in the nonclinical experiments. In this case study, the animal toxicity studies are followed for up to 4 weeks, while the current clinical study is designed with a 4-week study period.

As mentioned earlier, the PoC study needs a high dose to serve as the anchor of the high end of the dose–response curve. With the addition of the requirement of demonstrating long-term drug safety, it is also critical for the new compound to offer doses low enough so that in the Phase III studies, where patients may be exposed to long-term treatment, there is no safety concern at these low doses while patients still experience the treatment benefit of efficacy. Hence it is desirable that in this case study, some low doses of the new compound are explored to help detect a MinED. It becomes of interest to study a wide range of doses (so that the high dose that is close to MTD to help with PoC, and the low dose is low enough to help establish MinED).

Given all the above background, the study is designed with PoC as the primary objective, and the estimation of a MinED as one of the secondary objectives. From a statistical point of view, PoC is achieved with a hypothesis-testing procedure. The null hypothesis is that the test drug is not different from placebo; the alternative hypothesis is that the test drug is efficacious. On the other hand, for finding MinED, this is an estimation process. In the case of estimating a dose–response model, then depending upon the underlying model of interest, there are various parameters that need to be estimated. Based on the estimated range of active doses, further studies can be designed.

In this section, an example is introduced to illustrate how these conditions are considered in designing an early Phase II clinical study to treat patients with OA. In this case, the project team decides to study five parallel dose groups, which cover a wide enough dose range. In addition to these five dose groups, a placebo control and an active control are also used to help confirm the efficacy and explore drug safety.

In most of the early Phase II clinical studies, there is no active control group. Active controls are more likely to be used in Phase III development. The reason to choose an active control in this case study is that, if the results fail to distinguish between placebo and the tested doses, it will be unclear as to whether the test drug is truly ineffective or because there is a very high placebo response. Under this situation, the comparison between an active control and placebo helps the project team to differentiate the two conditions given above: if the active control is clearly superior to placebo, then it can be concluded that the test drug is not efficacious. On the other hand, if the data cannot differentiate between the active control and the placebo, then this study is not informative because it is still unknown as to whether the test drug is beneficial or not. Hence, in this study, the active control is used for reference purposes only.

For this test drug, the MTD was estimated from results observed in previous studies. Furthermore, the formulation group has already prepared tablets with fixed drug strengths. Let the dose at MTD be 100% of the dose strength, and the formulated tablets were prepared at 2.5% and the 12.5% strengths of MTD. Given this, five doses are selected using the BDS approach. In this case study, the doses selected are placebo, 2.5%, 5%, 12.5%, 25%, and 75% of MTD, plus an active control. Based on this design, the dose range is 30 (= 75% ÷ 2.5%). The active control group was selected to be a popular NSAID (nonsteroidal anti-inflammatory drug).

Although osteoarthritis is considered an inflammatory disease, the symptom that brought an OA patient to the doctor is usually joint pain. Hence in clinical studies of OA, the primary measure of efficacy focuses on pain or symptoms related to pain. One of the widely accepted clinical measures for OA is the Western Ontario and McMaster University (WOMAC) Osteoarthritis index (Bellamy et al. 1997). The WOMAC score includes 24 questions, five of these questions relate to the pain domain, two relate to the stiffness domain, and 17 relate to the function domain. In this true case study, the WOMAC pain domain is selected as the primary endpoint for efficacy analysis.

A dose–response model is considered in this case study. Once a model is determined, this model can be used to estimate target doses of interest, the TEDR, and to construct confidence intervals on efficacy responses of selected doses. Information obtained from this model helps to design future Phase II studies or Phase III studies. A linear contrast with discrete doses is proposed to serve as the primary comparison. Here the term "discrete doses" indicate that the designed doses are scaled as 0, 1, 2, 3, 4, and 5, instead of 0%, 2.5%, 5%, 12.5%, 25%, and 75% of MTD. In this linear contrast, the active control is not included in the comparison. As discussed earlier, the NSAID to be used in this study is only for validation purposes, in case the concept is not proven. As such, the proposed linear contrast includes only the five dosing groups plus placebo. In this case study, only one contrast is used and hence there is no MCP adjustment. For a simple linear contrast with discrete doses, the treatment groups are simply ordered from low to high. The placebo response is assumed to be 0, the lowest dose (2.5% of MTD) is assumed to have 20% response, the next lowest dose (5% of MTD) is assumed to have 40% response, the medium dose (12.5% of MTD) is assumed to have 60% of response, the second highest dose (25% of MTD) is assumed to have 80% response, and the high dose (75% of MTD) is assumed to have 100% response. Then the coefficients −5, −3, −1, 1, 3, and 5 are assigned to these treatment groups. Hence the primary hypothesis to be tested is:

$$H_0: -5\mu_0 - 3\mu_1 - \mu_2 + \mu_3 + 3\mu_4 + 5\mu_5 \le 0 \text{ versus } H_A: -5\mu_0 - 3\mu_1 - \mu_2 + \mu_3 + 3\mu_4 + 5\mu_5 > 0,$$

where μ_0 denotes the mean of placebo group,
μ_1 denotes the mean of the 2.5% dose group,

μ_2 denotes the mean of the 5% dose group,
μ_3 denotes the mean of the 12.5% dose group,
μ_4 denotes the mean of the 25% dose group, and
μ_5 denotes the mean of the 75% dose group.

In the case of a dose–response study with k dose groups and placebo, the sample size estimates based on a contrast can be derived as follows (Chang and Chow 2006):

Let μ_i be the population mean for group i, $i = 0, \ldots, k$, where μ_0 is the mean from the placebo group, and let c_i be the corresponding coefficients in the contrast. The null hypothesis of no treatment effect can be written as follows:

$$H_0 : L(\mu) = \sum_{i=0}^{k} c_i\mu_i \leq 0 \,\text{versus}\, H_A : L(\mu) = \sum_{i=0}^{k} c_i\mu_i = \delta > 0.$$

Note that $\sum_{i=0}^{k} c_i = 0$. Under the alternative hypothesis and the condition of homogeneous variance, the sample size per group can be obtained as

$$n = \left[\frac{(z_{1-\alpha} + z_{1-\beta})\sigma}{\delta}\right]^2 \sum_{i=0}^{k} c_i^2,$$

where $z_{1-\alpha}$ and $z_{1-\beta}$ are the corresponding quantile points of a standard normal distribution.

Based on published data, the standard deviation is about four. From the observed placebo response, and the anticipated response from this test drug, possible targeted clinical differences to be considered could be 1.00, 1.25, or 1.50. From such a large standard deviation, and a relatively small delta, the required sample size could be very large. For example, if a pairwise comparison is used, then under one-sided alpha of 0.05, with 90% power, and delta of 1.25, the sample size for each treatment group would be about 176 subjects. For a seven-arm study, this will take a total sample size of 1232 subjects. To power the study using the linear contrast as specified above, the sample size would reduce to 126 per group (882 overall).

Since the test drug is at an early stage of clinical development, and the concept has not been proven, it is difficult to justify a huge budget of 882 subjects in an early Phase II study. Upper management discussed the matter with the project team and decided that they are willing to take a higher risk on alpha, and reduce the sample size to meet the budget constraint. The compromise is that the two-sided alpha can be increased to 0.2 (or one-sided alpha of 0.1) and keep the power at 90%.

For this study, a treatment difference from placebo of approximately 1.25 was selected. A sample size of 97 per treatment group provides estimated power of 90% for one-sided alpha of 0.10 and, with this sample size, the power is over 80% for one-sided alpha of 0.05. A sample size of 100 subjects per treatment group is sufficient to detect differences larger than 1.25 in the mean change from baseline in the WOMAC OA Index Pain Subscale, using the aforementioned linear contrast. Since a single test for linear trend is employed, no adjustment for multiple comparison is needed. If this test is significant at alpha of 0.1 (one-sided), MinED will be estimated.

The final design to study this new OA test drug includes seven treatment groups: placebo, 2.5%, 5%, 12.5%, 25%, and 75% of MTD, plus an NSAID active control. The primary endpoint is the change in WOMAC OA Index Pain Subscale from baseline up to 4 weeks postbaseline, evaluated at a linear contrast with discrete doses. A balanced randomization to recruit 100 OA patients to each treatment group will provide a total of 700 subjects for this study. The one-sided alpha is set at 0.1, with 700 subjects in this study, the power is slightly over 90% using this linear contrast test.

9.13 Summary

In the classical drug development programs, dose finding is one of the most important objectives for Phase II. This chapter focuses on Phase II clinical trial designs and considerations regarding dose finding. Because of its unique role in the clinical development process, Phase II is one of the very challenging stages during new drug research and development. In order to deal with some of these challenges, Phase II studies should be designed with clear and simple objectives, each study design needs to be robust and relies only on minimum but credible and practical assumptions. At the early stage of Phase II, typically two key assumptions are necessary:

1. The MTD estimated from Phase I studies is accurate
2. The efficacy is nondecreasing with increasing doses

Additional assumptions should be minimized. One major objective in the early Phase II is to help estimate the TEDR. In designing clinical trials, the thinking process should be stepwise—confirm first and then explore. Each study needs be designed so that the confirmative objective can be achieved with the prespecified Type I error (alpha). After that, secondary and exploratory objectives can then be studied. Note that in Phase II, both alpha and beta are negotiable at the design stage. Clear communications are needed between the statistician and the project team so that each type of risk is well understood by the team and by the upper management.

With the MCP-Mod method available, statisticians are encouraged to take advantage of this way of thinking in both design and analysis of dose-finding studies. One of the most difficult tasks in designing the first dose-ranging study is to select several doses to be explored. Binary dose spacing (BDS) is a nonparametric method to help allocate study doses and with broad applications. Project teams are encouraged to consider BDS in designing their first dose-ranging studies.

References

Babb, J., Rogatko, A., and Zacks, S. (1998). Cancer Phase I clinical trials: Efficient dose escalation with overdose control. *Statistics in Medicine,* 17: 1103–20.

Bellamy, N., Campbell, J., Stevens, J., Pilch, L., Stewart, C., and Mahmood, Z. (1997). Validation study of a computerized version of the Western Ontario and McMaster Universities VA 3.0 Osteoarthritis Index. *Journal of Rheumatology,* 24: 2413–15.

Chang, M., and Chow, S. C. (2006). Power and sample size for dose–response studies. *Dose Finding in Drug Development,* 220–41. New York: Springer.

Cheng, B., Chow, S. C., and Su, W. L. (2006). On the assessment of dose proportionality: A comparison of two slope approaches. *Journal of Biopharmaceutical Statistics,* 16: 385–92.

Derman, C. (1957). Nonparametric up and down experimentation. *Annals of Mathematical Statistic,* 28: 795–98.

Dixon, W. J., and Mood, A. M. (1954). A method for obtaining and analyzing sensitivity data. *Journal of the American Statistical Association,* 43: 109–26.

Dmitrienko, A., Wiens, B., and Westfall, P. (2006). Fallback tests in dose–response clinical trials. *Journal of Biopharmaceutical Statistics,* 16 (5): 745–55.

Durham, S. D., and Flournoy, N. (1994). Random walks for quantile estimation. In *Statistical Decision Theory and Related Topics V,* eds. S. S. Gupta and J. O. Berger, 467–76. New York: Springer-Verlag.

Durham, S. D., and Flournoy, N. (1995). Up-and-down designs I. Stationary treatment distributions. In *Adaptive Designs,* eds. N. Flournoy and W. F. Rosenberger, 139–57. Hayward, CA: Institute of Mathematical Statistics.

Hamlett, A., Ting, N., Hanumara, C., and Finman, J. S. (2002). Dose spacing in early dose response clinical trial designs. *Drug Information Journal,* 36 (4): 855–64.

ICH-E4. (1994). *Guideline on Dose–Response Information to Support Drug Registration.* Rockville, MD: The U.S. Food and Drug Administration.

Ivanova, A. (2006). Dose-finding in oncology—Nonparametric methods. In *Dose Finding in Drug Development*, 49–58. New York: Springer.

Korn, E. L., Midthune, D., Chen, T. T., Rubinstein, L. V., Christian, M. C., and Simon, R. M. (1994). A comparison of two Phase I trial designs. *Statistics in Medicine,* 13: 1799–1806.

Lin, Y., and Shih, W. J. (2001). Statistical properties of the traditional algorithm-based designs for Phase I cancer clinical trials. *Biostatistics,* 2: 203–15.

O'Quigley, J., Pepe, M., and Fisher, L. (1990). Continual reassessment method: A practical design for Phase I clinical trials in cancer. *Biometrics,* 46: 33–48.

Pinheiro, J. C., Bretz, F., and Branson, M. (2006). Analysis of dose–response studies—Modeling approaches. In *Dose Finding in Drug Development*, 146–71. New York: Springer.

Ratain, M. J., Mick, R., Schilsky, R. L., and Siegler, M. (1993). Statistical and ethical issues in the design and conduct of Phase I and II clinical trials of new anticancer agents. *Journal of National Cancer Institute,* 85: 1637–43.

Rosenberger, W. F., and Haines, L. M. (2002). Competing designs for Phase I clinical trials: A review. *Statistics in Medicine*, 21: 2757–70.

Ruberg, S. J. (1995). Dose response studies II. Analysis and interpretation. *Journal of Biopharmaceutical Statistics*, 5 (1): 15–42.

Storer, B. E. (1989). Design and analysis of Phase I clinical trials. *Biometrics,* 45: 925–37.

Tamhane, A. C., Hochberg, Y., and Dunnett, C. W. (1996). Multiple test procedures for dose finding. *Biometrics*, 52: 21–37.

Ting, N. (2006). General considerations in dose–response study designs. In *Dose Finding in Drug Development*, 1–17. New York: Springer.

Ting, N. (2008). Confirm and explore, a stepwise approach to clinical trial designs. *Drug Information Journal*, 42 (6): 545–54.

Ting, N. (2009). Practical and statistical considerations in designing an early Phase II osteoarthritis clinical trial: A case study. *Communications in Statistics—Theory and Methods*, 38(18): 3282–96.

Tsutakawa, R. K. (1967a). Random walk design in bioassay. *Journal of the American Statistical Association,* 62: 842–56.

Tsutakawa, R. K. (1967b). Asymptotic properties of the block up-and-down method in bio-assay. *The Annals of Mathematical Statistics,* 38: 1822–28.

von Békésy, G. (1947). A new audiometer. *Acta Otolaryngology,* 35: 411–22.

Wetherill, G. B. (1963). Sequential estimation of quantal response curves. *Journal of the Royal Statistical Society B,* 25: 1–48.

10

Improving Dose-Finding: A Philosophic View

Carl-Fredrik Burman
AstraZeneca R&D and Chalmers University of Technology

Frank Miller and Kiat Wee Wong
AstraZeneca R&D

10.1 Introduction

Dose-finding is a trade-off between efficacy and safety. The ultimate goal is to determine the best dose for each patient. However, this goal will never be fully reached. A series of experiments are needed to, hopefully, find a dose that is beneficial to a population of patients. Dose-finding should therefore be seen as an extended scientific process, not as a single clinical trial. Despite this, we will focus on dose-finding in late clinical development, mainly the dose-finding trial in phase IIB but also on the possibility of including two (say) candidate doses in phase III. The design of this late stage clinical program should build firmly on the dose–response information from earlier stages, clinical and preclinical. A key to good dose decisions and to a good design of the development program is to have well thought-through and clearly defined objectives. The optimal design theory can readily be applied to suggest study designs. The answer to what the best design is, however, depends on the study objective, the previously available information, and the study constraints.

In Section 10.2, we will in a relatively nontechnical and brief way describe the dose-finding process, and discuss potential improvements in the later stages of the clinical program, with emphasis on phase IIB. We will for example discuss dose range, dose allocation, adaptive designs, model-based analysis, decision criteria, and sample size.

The theory of optimal study designs will be introduced in Section 10.3, and this theory will be applied to a simple sigmoid dose–response (E_{max}) model where focus is on the drug potency. Modeling of previous data helps for the application of optimal design theory. Adaptive designs can give further improvements of the trial efficacy. We will therefore describe an adaptive dose-finding trial, which extends the previous example by applying optimal design theory also at an interim analysis, thereby redesigning the trial midway. In Section 10.4, it is sketched how adaptive and optimal designs can be applied in more realistic settings. We will discuss multiparameter models, dose limitations, and how to set up criteria for the performance of a trial. We will also complement the adaptivity in dose assignments with adaptivity in sample size.

As Sections 10.3 and 10.4 are concerned with one single effect variable, with no reference to safety, there is a need to deepen the discussion by considering efficacy and safety simultaneously. This will be the topic of Section 10.5. Section 10.6 extends the discussion from a single trial to a program perspective. By viewing phase IIB as input to confirmatory trials, phase IIB sample size determination can be analyzed within a larger frame. It has been suggested to include two or more doses in phase III trials, to get better dose–response information before regulatory approvement decisions and launch. We will therefore contrast designs with two active doses to those containing a single one. The chapter concludes with a brief discussion section.

10.2 Traditional Dose-Finding: Can it be Improved?

10.2.1 The Dose-Finding Process

The dose-finding process begins with preclinical experiments, in vitro and in vivo. Results of animal toxicology trials lead to a definition of a toxicology limit for humans. For most drugs, the first phase I clinical trials are conducted in healthy volunteers and aim at studying tolerability of gradually increased doses, usually starting well below a dose expected to give pharmacodynamic effects. At a maximum, the dose can be increased until the dose corresponding to the toxicology limit based on preclinical data. If there are tolerability problems observed in humans, the highest dose without these problems usually determines an upper limit for the doses that can be tested in later trials. This limit can later be modified in the light of new data. Phase I trials can also study pharmacokinetics (PK) and pharmacodynamics (PD) in healthy volunteers and/or patients. These trials, together with preclinical pharmacology trials and, sometimes, data from other drugs, can give partial information about the dose–response profile of the drug. Sometimes a phase IIA trial in patients is conducted and contributes additional information. The phase IIB clinical trial is, however, the most critical for dose determination. Such trials often include a range of active doses; four to five doses are sometimes said to be the standard but the number may be as low as two and as high as 10 or more. For many drugs, one single dose is chosen for further testing in confirmatory (phase III) trials, based mainly on phase IIB data.

The trial programs vary considerably between indications and between drugs. We will later study the possibility of increasing the number of active doses in phase III from one to two. For some drug classes (e.g., statins, thiazolidinediones, protein pump inhibitors, many blood pressure drug classes), however, it is standard to test more than one dose in phase III and also to market a range of doses. In other areas, dose titration schemes, rather than fixed doses, are studied in the program. For many oncology drugs, on the other hand, one dose is selected already in phase I (see Section 10.5.2).

10.2.2 Traditional Design of a Phase IIB Dose-Finding Study

The most common design for a phase IIB dose-finding study is a randomized parallel study. The patients are randomized to fixed doses that are maintained long enough to allow for dose–response comparison. Nevertheless, an initial forced titration of the dose might be possible if required for safety reasons. The ICH-E4 guideline (1994) states that "including a placebo group ... is desirable but not ... necessary in all cases." Further, "it may also be useful to include one or more doses of an active drug control."

Traditionally, dose-finding trials have often been analyzed by comparing each dose of active treatment separately with placebo (or another control group). The sample size is in many cases chosen to have sufficient power to show superiority of a dose versus placebo with a significance test.

We will now discuss how the design of the phase IIB dose-finding study specifically, and the whole development process with regard to dose-finding in general, can be improved. Some of these ideas are already mentioned in the ICH-E4 guideline (1994) but rarely applied, others were discussed and developed more recently.

10.2.3 Room for Improvement

Dose-finding is a complicated process where each specific drug development project has its own specific circumstances. Thus, there is no single solution that serves all situations. However, it is often possible to improve the process greatly. We will list a number of areas where we believe that alternative approaches hold a potential:

1. Biomarkers
2. Study duration
3. Dose range
4. Optimal designs
5. Adaptive designs
6. Alternative study designs
7. Analysis
8. Exposure-response
9. Sample size
10. Determination of therapeutic dose

In this section we will briefly comment on all these 10 areas. Some of these will be given further attention in the following sections. For example, optimal and adaptive designs are the topics of the next two Sections (10.3–10.4).

1. Biomarkers For many indications, the phase III trials have to be very large and expensive in order to give a reasonable power. That is, it is difficult to prove any placebo-controlled effect on the main variable even in large trials. It is then evident that it would be unrealistic to try to optimize the dose in a smaller phase IIB trial based on the same variable. Thus, biomarkers with better signal-to-noise ratio are often needed in dose-finding trials. The uncertainty in the predictive value of the biomarker has to be considered carefully. Modeling the biomarker-endpoint relation, and the uncertainty therein, is helpful when choosing biomarker, sizing the dose-finding trial, and interpreting phase IIB data before determining if and how to continue into the confirmatory phase. The development of biomarkers (Burzykowski, Molenberghs, and Buyse 2005) is one of the key areas of improvement according to FDA's critical path initiative (see FDA 2004, 2006).

2. Study duration Many drugs do not give full effect on day 1. The lag in effect is often due both to PK and PD. The PK time-course can be modeled relatively easily based on phase I PK data. Normally, PK steady state is reached within a few days. PD lags may be much more serious. In diabetes, it takes months before HbA1c approaches steady state, or rather pseudo steady state, as there is an underlying disease progression. In the area of osteoporosis, a drug that eliminates bone loss could be postulated to reduce the risk of hip fractures. This risk reduction would increase from zero during the first period of drug administration over months and years. Designing phase IIB may involve a decision about treatment duration, where longer trials give more information per patient (better signal-to-noise ratio) but increase cost and overall study time. One option may be to fix a trial stopping date, and allow different treatment durations depending on inclusion date. As treatment duration may be limited by lack of long-term preclinical toxicology data, the potential gains of longer treatment durations should be considered while designing the toxicology study program.

3. Dose range The best trial efficiency is often obtained with a very large dose range. For example, an optimal design with no dose limitations for a 3-parameter E_{max} model (see Section 10.4) has three dose groups, two of which are zero (placebo), and infinity. This, formally optimal, design obviously has to be modified in practice, and it is relatively straightforward to calculate the optimal design given a certain maximal allowed dose, D_{max}. There may be practical limitations (e.g., tablet size) and cost limitations on the available doses. Most importantly, however, the available dose range should be determined based on the benefit-risk of the patients in the trial. For a trial to be ethical, we claim that it should be better for the trial participants to be included in the trial, than to receive standard care. That is, the expected net benefit, given the best available knowledge, should be nonnegative (Lilford 2003; Burman and Carlberg 2009). High doses are excluded as the safety risks outweigh the expected benefits. Placebo and low doses may have to be excluded if they are likely to give suboptimal effects compared to regulatory approved treatment options according to Declaration of Helsinki (WMA 2008). In some instances, the optimal design does not utilize the available dose range; see the examples in Section 10.3. However, it is a common error to choose the dose range too narrow, leading to indistinguishable differences between the doses tested.

4. Optimal designs There is a well-established theory of optimal designs (see Sections 10.3 and 10.4). In order to utilize this theory, it is important to set up criteria for trial performance, to model previous information, and to be clear about which design options are available.

5. Adaptive designs As the best design normally depends on unknown parameters, there is a clear potential value in adaptive dose-finding. In such designs, one learns from previous data at interim analyses and modifies the design in light of this information (Sections 10.3 and 10.4). Wang (2008) gives an example, combining biomarkers (Item **1., Biomarkers**) with adaptive design methodology. She describes a two-stage design and makes use of the prospectively planned genomic or genetic biomarker evaluation in the interim analysis.

6. Alternative designs As an alternative to the parallel-group design, it is sometimes possible to use cross-over (Senn 2002), forced titration or optional titration designs for a study of dose–response; see Sheiner, Hashimoto, and Beal (1991) and ICH-E4 (1994). Such designs can be much more efficient than parallel-group trials, as patients can serve as their own control. A requirement for application of cross-over designs is that the "drug effect develops rapidly and patients return to baseline conditions quickly after cessation of therapy," that "responses are not irreversible (cure, death), and ... patients have reasonably stable disease" (ICH-E4, 1994). A consequence is that cross-over designs are rarely applied in, for example, oncology or in other diseases that typically worsen gradually over time, like Alzheimer disease. They have potential to be applied in, for example, stable pain conditions or in acute pain conditions like migraine that are recurring.

There are risks of bias in cross-over designs, in case the treatment in one period can affect the response in a later period. For example, it is hard to distinguish whether an adverse event is caused by the higher dose in the second treatment period, or rather by the combined duration of the drug exposure in the two treatment periods. This potential bias in cross-over and titration designs is often taken as an argument for not applying these designs in phase IIB. However, we think that the risks are exaggerated and that cross-over designs should be applied more often to dose–response trials. The considerably increased precision in effect estimates would in many situations overwhelm the possible bias. It should be remembered that dose-finding trials belong to a learning phase, and dose determination is primarily done at the sponsor's risk. The use of biomarkers, with uncertain relation to the relevant clinical endpoint, underlines this. Thus, a limited bias may be more acceptable in phase IIB than in the confirmatory trials. In addition, carry-over effects can often be modeled based on pharmacodynamic relationships. This may help to avoid or reduce biases caused by carryover.

Enrichment designs (see, for example, Byas-Smith et al. 1995; Straube et al. 2008) may have potential advantages for dose-finding: In an initial short treatment period in the trial, the patients need to fulfill certain criteria before they are allowed to participate in the dose-finding part. By this, the proportion of nonresponders and AE-related dropouts could be reduced in the longer dose-finding part leading to a better possibility to characterize the dose–response relation. However, a potential drawback is the difficulty to generalize the results to the total population of interest.

7. Analysis The traditional analysis of comparing each dose of active treatment separately with placebo (or other control group) ignores the obvious relation between the dose groups. Doses close to each other can safely be assumed to have similar effects and this can often be utilized in the analysis, leading to greatly improved overall study efficiency. As long as the focus is on proving that the drug works rather than on estimation, there exists robust methods to show an upward trend across doses instead of pairwise testing. One possibility is to apply trend tests based on linear contrasts, see Robertson, Wright, and Dykstra (1988) or Ruberg (1995b). A further option for showing an upward trend is the Bartholomew-test (Bartholomew 1961) based on monotone regression technique. It is notable that the ICH-E4 guideline (1994) for dose-finding trials mentions that "being able to detect a statistically significant difference in pairwise comparisons between doses is not necessary if a statistically significant trend (upward slope) across doses can be established using all the data." Ting (2006, p. 94) confirms this: "In certain situations, a preplanned dose–response test with a positive slope can be considered as one of the pivotal proofs of efficacy trials."

Bretz, Pinheiro, and Branson (2005) have combined testing for efficacy based on linear contrasts with estimation of dose–response according to the best fitting model in a predefined set of candidate models. Building on these results, Pinheiro, Bornkamp, and Bretz (2006) have described how studies with this analysis can be adequately powered and how expert knowledge can be incorporated in the assumptions for power calculation.

Bornkamp et al. (2007) have studied how large the benefits are of model-based analyses. The drawback of an analysis based on a dose–response model is that any model is only an approximation. In many cases, the conclusions are relatively robust to a range of reasonable model assumptions. However, the robustness should better be checked in each particular situation. Model-based approaches make it easier to include a larger number of doses, with smaller sample size per dose. Designs with few doses can be hard to analyze model-based, as the number of parameters can be lower than the number of arms. One interesting alternative is smoothing techniques. Smoothing splines (Kirby, Colman, and Morris 2009), for example, can be applied to dose–response data or a moving average over several doses can be used (Friede et al. 2001). Another approach, which is often very useful, is to utilize previous data and expert assumptions to restrict the model. Based on in vivo data, competitor trials or expert guesses, it may for example, be possible to fix some of the parameters (such as the maximal possible effect) in the model.

8. Exposure-response According to Pinheiro and Duffull (2009), there are two motivations for using drug PK-exposure information: One is that it helps to understand the time course of onset and duration of response. This understanding is for example important when the decision about the right dosing frequency has to be made. Another motivation is that it can explain some of the response variability and by this improve characterization of dose–response with the subdivision into exposure-response-relation and dose-exposure-relation. If PK-exposure is a better predictor than dose for the response, there is the possibility of improving the precision of the dose–response estimates. Hsu (2009) characterizes situations where one gains from applying a PK-response approach. Provided that PK-exposure is the true driving factor for response, he identifies that the advantage of PK-response over dose–response modeling increases with the intrinsic PK variability, as long as the measurement error for PK is low. For dose-finding trials with a reasonably large dose range, however, the extra efficiency from observing PK-data is usually limited.

9. Sample size With increasing sample size in phase IIB follows better precision and larger probability for a good dose selection. Questions about optimal sample size will be discussed in Section 10.6. Although not discussed in this chapter, the choice of biomarker is obviously related to sample size, as is treatment duration.

10. Determination of therapeutic dose The dose-finding problem has often been viewed as the problem of finding a so-called therapeutic window where the drug has sufficient effect and acceptable safety. The statistical problem can then be to estimate the dose interval where the beneficial effect is larger than a constant c_E, while the adverse effect is lower than another constant c_S. Although the therapeutic window concept has some merits, it does not provide a method to find the best dose within the acceptable range. It treats efficacy and safety as two isolated entities and does not attempt to place them on a common scale. In principle, we favor another view, where pros and cons are traded directly against each other (Section 10.5).

10.3 Simple Examples of Optimal and Adaptive Designs

10.3.1 An Example of a Fully Adaptive Design

The effect of a pharmaceutical agent normally increases monotonically with dose. The effect is often limited, in the sense that it tends to a finite maximum as the dose increases. A common dose–response model for such situations is the E_{max} model. With the dose x plotted on a logarithmic scale, this model has an S-shaped dose–response curve, see Figure 10.1. This logarithmic scale is the natural dose scale. The E_{max} model may have up to four parameters, describing potency, placebo effect, maximal placebo-adjusted drug effect, and the steepness of the dose–response curve. In this section, we assume for simplicity that three of these parameters are known. We will consider an E_{max} model with only one parameter for the potency, ED_{50}, which is the dose needed to give 50% of the maximal placebo-adjusted effect. The mean effect f as a function of the dose x is assumed to be:

$$f(x) = \frac{x}{x + ED_{50}}. \quad (10.1)$$

This means that we assume the placebo-effect to be 0 and the maximal effect to be 1. We further assume the observations to be independent and normally distributed with a common variance σ^2. In this, rather unrealistic, situation with only one single parameter in the model, it suffices to have one dose group in a clinical trial to be able to estimate the parameter. With a fixed one-point design, the choice of study dose D is crucial for the efficacy of the trial. Most information is achieved if D equals the potency parameter ED_{50}. As ED_{50} is unknown, the choice of D must be based on an informed guess. Modeling of existing information can here be of considerable value. Figure 10.2 depicts the trial efficiency as a function of the ratio D/ED_{50} (see also Figure 2 in Bretz et al. 2009). The efficiency is here a measure of the amount of

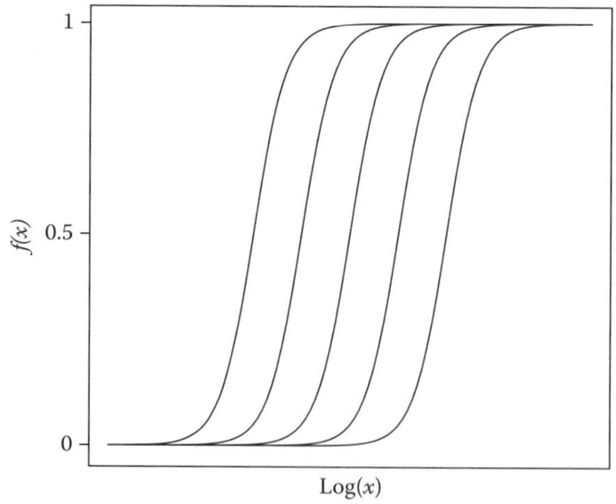

FIGURE 10.1 Illustration of five E_{max} models differing only in potency, x = dose.

information provided by each observation. To attain the same precision in estimating ED_{50}, the sample size thus has to be inversely proportional to the efficiency.

The practical problem is that the most informative study dose cannot be chosen simply because ED_{50} is unknown (and it is in fact the aim of the study to deliver information about the unknown ED_{50}). In the unusual case that trial responses are almost immediate, it could be possible to estimate ED_{50} based on all previous observations, and assign a dose equal to this estimation to the next patient. We assume that there is a restricted dose range $[D_{min}, D_{max}]$ so that the dose for the next patient is taken to be D_{max} in case the estimate is higher than D_{max} (and similarly for D_{min}). This may occur in the beginning of the trial as some observations may be larger than the largest possible mean effect (here 1) or smaller than the smallest possible mean effect (here 0). Figure 10.3 shows a number of simulated trials where each dose is chosen adaptively as described. It is seen that the estimated dose gradually approaches the true

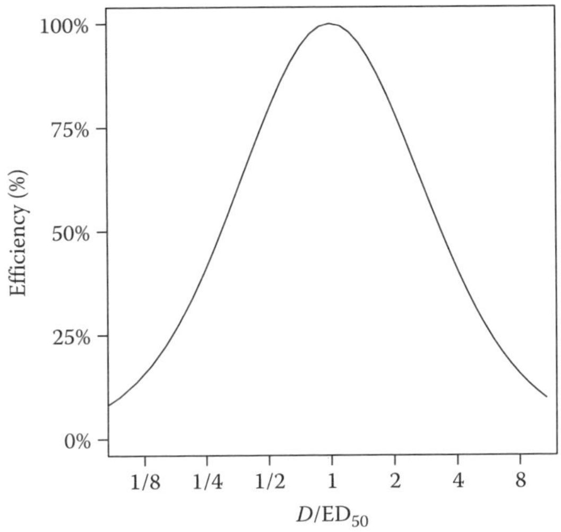

FIGURE 10.2 Efficiency of a single-dose trial as a function of the ratio between the trial dose D and the parameter ED_{50} in a 1-parameter E_{max} model.

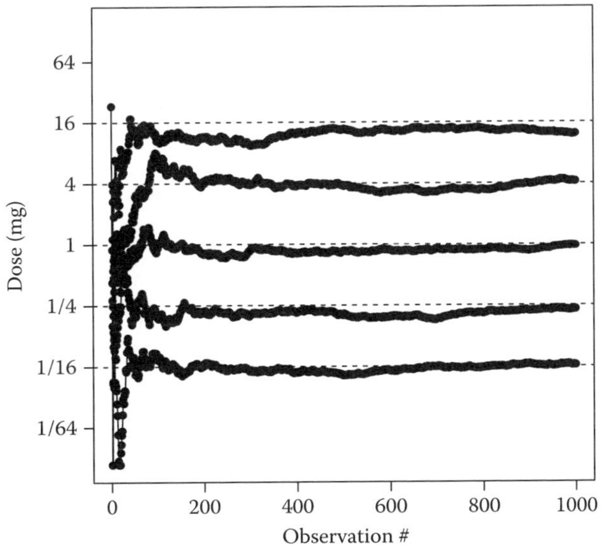

FIGURE 10.3 Simulated doses in five adaptive trials.

ED_{50} value. When compared to the fixed dose design, the adaptive design is much more robust against misspecification of the starting dose.

In the clinical practice, however, it is rarely feasible to implement such a flexible design with adaptations after each patient and possible allocation of the next patient to a huge number of doses. For example Smith et al. (2006) contrast the oral, solid dosage in their study against the intravenous administration of study drug in the ASTIN study. The solid administration made fully flexible dosing less practical for them. Solid doses have to be manufactured prior to the study. Medication-packs, bottles or similar for each dosage need to be prepared and numbered in advance. Further, the primary response variable is usually not measured directly after the first intake of study drug, but several days, weeks or even years later. Also due to this reason, a fully sequential design, adapting based on data from all previous patients, is difficult to apply in most situations.

We discuss in the following Sections 10.3.2 and 10.3.3 more feasible designs for studies in drug development. In Section 10.3.2, we apply optimal design theory in choosing the design for the whole study; that is, we consider a fixed design without adaptation during the study. In Section 10.3.3, we include the additional possibility of adapting the design at an interim analysis.

10.3.2 Optimal Design

The following example illustrates that optimal design theory is a valuable tool for designing dose-finding studies. It also shows how prior knowledge can be incorporated in the computation of the optimal design.

Consider a trial with fixed, nonadaptive design and the one-parameter E_{max} dose–response model Equation 10.1. The optimal design is to observe all patients in the study at dose $x = ED_{50}$. The reason is that $x = ED_{50}$ is the design point that best discriminates between models with different parameter values (see Figure 10.1). In other words, the absolute value of the derivative of f with respect to the parameter $x = ED_{50}$ is maximized by taking $x = ED_{50}$.

For more complex problems, optimal design theory (Atkinson, Donev, and Tobias 2007) provides a useful terminology and apparatus to solve the problems. We will sketch some of this briefly. Transforming the model to the log-dose scale, by defining $y = \log(x)$, gives an expression for the E_{max} model with useful symmetry properties. The model can now be expressed as:

$$f_a(y) = \frac{1}{1+e^{-y+a}},$$

with $a = \log(ED_{50})$. The family of functions f_a for arbitrary parameters a is a family of shifted functions of the same shape as shown in Figure 10.1.

Any fixed size design can be characterized by the number of dose arms k, the log doses $y_1,\ldots,y_k$ and their corresponding randomization ratios, $w_1,\ldots,w_k$, $w_i > 0, \sum_{i=1}^{k} w_i = 1$. Such a design is often written on the form:

$$\xi = \begin{pmatrix} y_1 & y_2 & \cdots & y_k \\ w_1 & w_2 & \cdots & w_k \end{pmatrix}.$$

The asymptotic variance of the least square (LS) estimator for a is proportional to the inverse of the following information matrix (Atkinson, Donev, and Tobias 2007):

$$M(\xi,a) = \sum_{i=1}^{k} w_i \left(\frac{\partial}{\partial a} f_a(y_i)\right)^2 = \sum_{i=1}^{k} w_i \left(\frac{e^{-y_i+a}}{(1+e^{-y_i+a})^2}\right)^2. \quad (10.2)$$

With some elementary calculations, one can show that this expression is maximized for $k_1 = 1$, $w_1 = 1$, $y_1 = a$. This formally proves that the so called locally optimal design (Atkinson, Donev, and Tobias 2007) for estimating a is to perform a study having one dose a for all patients. In their Example 2.7, Braess and Dette (2007) have considered the one-parameter E_{max} model and mention this locally optimal design.

As mentioned before, we cannot directly apply the locally optimal design by performing a study with this design, since we do not know a in advance. Besides the method of sequential allocation described in Section 10.3.1, other methods have been proposed to circumvent this problem. One method is called Bayesian optimal design (sometimes also optimal on average design). The idea is that—even if a is unknown—there is in practice almost always some knowledge about possible values for a and maybe even how likely these are. If this knowledge can be expressed by a probability measure on the possible parameter values (like for example, described from Miller, Guilbaud, and Dette 2007), we can calculate an average information matrix weighted according to this probability measure. The probability measure is called prior knowledge. In this example, we assume that our prior knowledge about the true parameter a is quite vague: the lowest possible dose for ED_{50} is 0.1 mg and the largest possible dose is 2200 mg according to expert judgment. That is, ED_{50} is between $a_{min} = -2.3$ and $a_{max} = 7.7$; that is, on a range of length 10 in the log scale. The experts do not favor any value in this range. Therefore we use the uniform design on the interval $[a_{min}, a_{max}]$ as prior for a. We follow Chaloner and Larntz (1989) or Atkinson, Donev, and Tobias (2007) and define the Bayesian optimal design formally as follows. A design ξ^* is Bayesian optimal with respect to the prior π if and only if ξ^* maximizes:

$$\int \log(M(\xi,a))\,\pi(da). \tag{10.3}$$

Intuitively, one would not use a design with observations for one single dose only, if there is a larger uncertainty about the true a. Indeed, Braess and Dette (2007) have shown that the Bayesian optimal design uses more and more different doses when the prior is a uniform design on an increasing interval. We have numerically calculated the Bayesian optimal design with respect to the prior π in the set of all designs. For this, we have maximized Expression 10.3—with $M(\xi, a)$ from Equation 10.2—for $k = 4$ using MATLAB®. Due to symmetry, $y_1 - a_{min} = a_{max} - y_4$, $y_2 - a_{min} = a_{max} - y_3$ and $w_1 = w_4$, $w_2 = w_3$. We have then shown that this design is indeed Bayesian optimal by using Whittle's (1973) version of an equivalence theorem from Kiefer and Wolfowitz (1960). The design is:

$$\begin{pmatrix} -0.77 & 1.64 & 3.76 & 6.17 \\ 0.284 & 0.216 & 0.216 & 0.284 \end{pmatrix}. \tag{10.4}$$

It has 28.4% of the observations for each of the log-doses −0.77 and 6.17 (corresponding to approximately 0.5 mg and 480 mg) and 21.6% of the observations for each of the log-doses 1.64 and 3.76 (corresponding to approximately 5 mg and 43 mg).

10.3.3 Adaptive Optimal Design

Combining optimal design ideas with adaptive design possibilities we will investigate the following design: In Stage 1, half of the patients are allocated according to the Bayesian optimal design with respect to the prior π, see Equation 10.4. In an interim analysis, ED_{50} is estimated by the LS-estimate $\widehat{ED}_{50}^{(1)}$. In Stage 2, the remaining half of the patients are allocated to $\widehat{ED}_{50}^{(1)}$ (locally optimal design assuming $ED_{50} = \widehat{ED}_{50}^{(1)}$). At the study-end, we calculate the LS-estimate $\widehat{ED}_{50}$ for ED_{50} based on data from both stages.

We compare the performance of this adaptive design and the optimal fixed design by simulations with the true values $a = a_{\min}, a_{\min} + 1, \ldots, a_{\min} + 9, a_{\max}$ on the log-scale, corresponding approximately to 0.1, 0.3, 0.7, 2, 5.5, 15, 40, 110, 300, 810, 2200 mg. As performance metric, we measure the proportion of simulations yielding a value close to the true value. We define close here to have at most a distance of 0.5 on the log-scale to the true value ($|\hat{a} - a| < 0.5$). On the original scale this means that the estimated ED_{50} is at most 65% larger or 39% smaller than the true value. Note that the estimation error of $f_{\hat{a}}(y)$ at all doses y is at most 12.4% of the true maximal drug-effect if $|a - \hat{a}| < 0.5$. This is a reasonable requirement for a good trial outcome.

The simulated study has $n = 500$ patients. In the fixed design, they are all allocated according to the Bayesian optimal design in Equation 10.4. In the adaptive design, only $n_1 = 250$ are allocated according to this design and 250 to the dose estimated at the interim. Due to symmetry reasons, the performance for $a = a_{\min} + s$ is equal to that for $a = a_{\max} - s$, s arbitrary. Therefore, we need to perform simulations for $a_{\min} + 5, a_{\min} + 6, \ldots, a_{\max}$, only.

For the adaptive design, we consider two possibilities to choose the Stage-2-dose: In version 1, all 250 patients in Stage 2 are treated with dose $\widehat{ED_{50}^{(1)}}$, no matter how extreme the estimate is. In Version 2, also one dose is used for all 250 patients in Stage 2. However, the dose $\widehat{ED_{50}^{(1)}}$ is used only, if it is within the interval of possible values according to the prior π; that is, between 0.1 mg and 2200 mg (–2.3 and 7.7 on the log-scale) in our example. If $\widehat{ED_{50}^{(1)}} > 2200$, the Stage-2-dose is 2200, if $\widehat{ED_{50}^{(1)}} < 0.1$, it is 0.1. This means that Version 2 relies on the assumption that ED_{50} has to be between 0.1 and 2200 mg.

Figure 10.4 shows the gain of the adaptive design versus the nonadaptive optimized design: the proportion of simulations yielding a value close to the true value is increased over the whole range of true parameter values ED_{50}. The largest gain for the adaptive design was reported if the true ED_{50} is extreme; that is, here $ED_{50} = 0.1$ or 2200 mg.

It is notable that the optimal design is invariant with regard to shifts on the log-dose scale. This means that we obtain the same design if we consider the uniform prior [–5, 5] on the log-scale except that we have to shift all log-doses with 2.7 units downward.

In order to see if large gains like in Figure 10.4 are obtained for other cases also, we repeated this exercise as above for other prior distributions. As alternative priors, we used the uniform distributions for

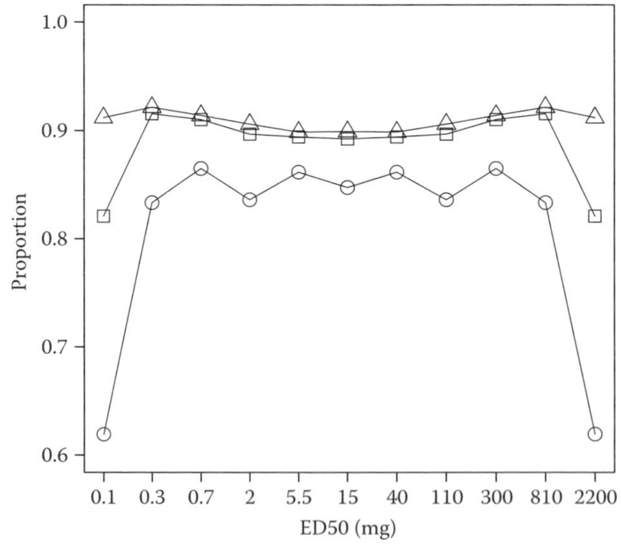

FIGURE 10.4 Proportion of simulations yielding a value close to the true value, defined as $|\hat{a} - a| < 0.5$ for the nonadaptive (circle) and adaptive designs (square and triangle representing Version 1 and Version 2, respectively) based on 10,000 simulations for each true a with length of the prior region = 10.

the unknown parameter a on $[-b, b]$ with $b = 1, 2, \ldots, 6$, where $b < 5$ represents lower uncertainty compared with the example before, $b = 5$ the same uncertainty, and $b > 5$ higher uncertainty. The Bayesian optimal designs for these six cases are as follows.

$$\begin{pmatrix} 0 \\ 1 \end{pmatrix}, \quad \begin{pmatrix} -0.613 & 0.613 \\ 0.5 & 0.5 \end{pmatrix}, \quad \begin{pmatrix} -1.413 & 1.413 \\ 0.5 & 0.5 \end{pmatrix},$$

$$\begin{pmatrix} -2.463 & 0 & 2.463 \\ 0.357 & 0.287 & 0.357 \end{pmatrix}, \quad \begin{pmatrix} -3.47 & -1.06 & 1.06 & 3.47 \\ 0.284 & 0.216 & 0.216 & 0.284 \end{pmatrix},$$

$$\begin{pmatrix} -4.468 & -2.096 & -0.359 & 0.359 & 2.096 & 4.468 \\ 0.236 & 0.172 & 0.092 & 0.092 & 0.172 & 0.236 \end{pmatrix}.$$

Figure 10.5 shows how the performance of the fixed optimal and adaptive design is if the true value is an extreme one ($a = \pm b$). The proportion of simulations yielding a value close to the true value decreases naturally with increasing uncertainty in the prior for a, both for the fixed optimal and the adaptive design. Further, for all priors on $[-b, b]$, $b = 1, 2, \ldots, 6$, the adaptive design performs better than the fixed design.

Let us reflect on the basic idea behind the approach illustrated here: at the beginning of the trial, the design was chosen based on the prior knowledge taking the uncertainty into account (Bayesian optimal design). Then we estimated the unknown parameter and rely afterward on this estimate when we use the locally optimal design in Stage 2. Another possible approach is not to fully rely on the interim estimate but still taking the uncertainty into account. This can be done by calculating the posterior distribution after Stage 1 for the unknown parameter using the Bayes theorem. Then in Stage 2, the Bayesian optimal design according to the posterior distribution could be used. This method was applied for example, by

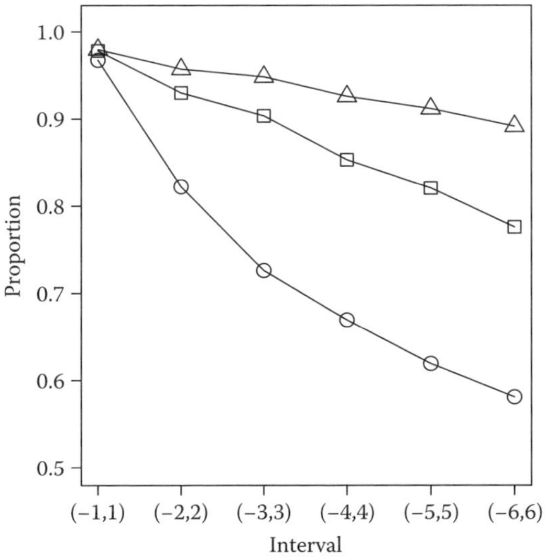

FIGURE 10.5 Proportion of simulations yielding a value close to the true value, defined as $|\hat{a} - a| < 0.5$ for the nonadaptive (circle) and adaptive design (square and triangle representing Version 1 and Version 2, respectively) based on 10,000 simulations for uniform distribution on $[-b, b]$, $b = 1, 2, \ldots, 6$, as prior for a and true extreme $a = \pm b$.

Miller, Guilbaud, and Dette (2007). In a simulation study of Maloney, Karlsson, and Simonsson (2007), both approaches were compared and the performance was quite similar.

10.4 More on Optimal and Adaptive Designs

10.4.1 The Multiparameter Model

In the preceding section, we considered simple models with one unknown parameter. The design minimizing the asymptotic variance of the parameter estimate was defined to be the optimal design. If there are more than one, say p, unknown parameters in the model, there exists no design minimizing the variance of all p parameter estimates at the same time. As a consequence, one has to decide what aspect of the unknown parameter vector is of main interest; that is, to define an optimality criterion. For a statistician in a clinical team it is necessary to choose an optimality criterion based on discussions with the other experts in the team. In this discussion, the team needs to be clear on the objective for study triggering the optimality criterion. Ruberg (1995a) points out that the objective can be quite different in different dose-finding studies.

If one of p parameters in the model is of primary interest, the asymptotic variance of this parameter estimate in the presence of $p - 1$ nuisance parameters can be minimized. This criterion is the so called c-optimality. When it is important to prove that the drug has effect, c-optimality for an appropriate parameter ($E_{\max}$ in the $E_{\max}$-model) or alternatively for a one-dimensional function of the parameter vector corresponding to the maximal effect in the studied dose range, can be used.

If all parameters are of interest, one of several possibilities to define optimality is to minimize the determinant of the asymptotic covariance matrix of the parameter estimates. This criterion is the D-optimality introduced by Wald (1943). A property of this criterion is that it minimizes the asymptotic volume of the confidence ellipsoid for the parameter estimates. If some mild conditions are fulfilled, equivalence theorems from Kiefer and Wolfowitz (1960) for linear models and Whittle (1973) for nonlinear models show that the D-optimal design minimizes the largest variance for any estimate of the effect at a certain dose; that is, the worst-case variance is minimized (equivalence of D- and G-optimality). The use of D-optimality is appropriate if one is generally interested in the nature of the dose–response relationship.

Besides optimality criteria like c- and D-optimality, which are well known from general optimal design theory, there are other optimality criteria applied specifically to dose-finding settings. Nevertheless, the following two criteria (MED and ED_p) can be seen as specific c-optimalities since they are based on nonlinear one-dimensional functions of the parameter vector.

A possible objective used for dose-finding trials is to estimate the minimum effective dose (MED) that is the smallest dose having an effect of at least Δ compared to placebo, where Δ is a clinical relevant difference (see Bretz et al. 2008). A criterion that has been applied to dose-finding trials is to minimize the variability of the MED-estimate. Dette, Haines, and Imhof (2007) derive explicit solutions for locally MED-optimal designs in certain situations.

Instead of the objective to estimate a dose with an effect having a specified absolute difference Δ from placebo, a popular objective is to estimate the effect at a dose having p% of the maximal effect achievable compared to placebo. This dose is the ED_p and we can therefore call the optimality criterion that minimizes the asymptotic variance of the effect at this dose ED_p-optimality. The GADA method in the ASTIN study (Krams, Lees, and Berry 2005) uses ED_{95}-optimality.

MED- and ED_p-optimality are typical choices when the main objective of the study is to choose an optimal dose. It can however be noted that "different groups of people may have a different understanding of what optimal dose means" (Bretz et al. 2008, p. 482).

Besides the problem to define an optimal dose there is the difficulty that during the long development process the definition of the optimal dose may shift: New information about tolerability of the drug or about efficacy of a competing drug might come up. This could affect risk/benefit considerations or requirements for a clinical relevant effect. Motivated by this, Miller, Guilbaud, and Dette (2007) define an objective more robust to a changing environment. They are interested in estimating the effect at all doses in the interesting region of the dose–response curve compared to placebo. The interesting region is defined as all doses up to a maximal dose studied with a true effect of at least δ. The criterion minimizes the average variance for all effect-estimators of doses in the interesting region. This criterion can be called I_L-optimality or, in the special context of dose-finding trials, IntR-optimality.

If a study has multiple main objectives and no single optimality criterion can be chosen, it is possible to combine optimality criteria, see Atkinson, Donev, and Tobias (2007).

Let us consider the $E_{\max}$ model with unknown placebo-effect E_0, unknown maximal possible effect $E_{\max}$, and unknown ED_{50}; that is, the effect function is given by:

$$f(x) = E_0 + E_{\max} \frac{x}{x + ED_{50}}.$$

The locally D-optimal design has three doses: 1/3 of the patients should be allocated to placebo ($x = 0$), 1/3 should receive dose $x = ED_{50}$, and 1/3 should be allocated to a very high dose, theoretically to infinity ($x = \infty$). For the middle dose, $x = ED_{50}$, the same problem occurs as we have discussed for the one-parameter model with known E_0 and $E_{\max}$: We do not know ED_{50} in advance and cannot choose the dose this way. As we did in Section 10.3.2, we can for example determine a Bayesian optimal design for a prior distribution of ED_{50}. If the prior knowledge is quite good (e.g., uniform prior on a small interval), this nonadaptive design is a promising choice. If there is considerable uncertainty around the ED_{50}-parameter, an adaptive design according to the previously described ideas might be a considerable improvement.

The same way of reasoning between locally optimal, Bayesian optimal, and adaptive design can be done if another optimality criterion is used instead of D-optimality. However, the concrete designs will be different. If for example, ED_{50} is the only parameter of interest and the other two parameters are nuisance parameters in the model, the locally c-optimal design for ED_{50} allocates 1/4 of the patients to placebo, 1/2 to dose $d = ED_{50}$, and 1/4 to a very high dose.

As already mentioned in Section 10.2.3 , there is in practice an upper limit for the doses in the trial. The optimal designs need to be adjusted by optimizing over the allowed dose range.

10.4.2 Adaptive Sample Size

When talking about adaptive dose-finding, one thinks in the first instance of adaptively adding or dropping doses or simply choosing the next dose adaptively. However, as generally in adaptive studies, the sample size can also be changed based on interim information. A possibility of changing the sample size is to decide in the interim whether or not to stop the study. An early stop in an interim analysis can be due to a large effect observed (crossing a predefined efficacy boundary and showing by this a drug effect), due to futility (effect observed in the interim is below some boundary, making it unlikely that the drug shows effect in the end), or due to safety problems.

Often, the data available in an interim analysis is too limited to provide sufficient information on safety. As we will see in Section 10.6.1, a further limitation holds especially for dose-finding trials: It is often already challenging to obtain a sufficiently well estimated dose–response curve in the end of the study if the sample size is chosen only to ensure power for proving effect of the drug. One should usually be hesitant before stopping early due to a good observed effect since the information about safety or the dose–response curve is limited at an interim analysis.

On the other hand, it is often a good idea to incorporate the possibility of a futility stop especially if there is already an interim analysis with the aim of choosing doses. In most situations in practice, a drug effect in the target population is not yet established when performing a dose-finding study and hence such a possibility should be implemented. Similarly, it is clear that if unexpected safety problems of sufficient magnitude are apparent in the interim analysis, the study should be stopped as soon as possible. This possibility to stop has ethical advantages (not exposing more patients to a drug with no/low effect or safety problems) and the sponsor company can limit costs and resources.

Several authors have discussed sample size reestimation (SSRE) approaches for confirmatory clinical trials (Bauer and Köhne 1994; Chow and Chang 2006; Chuang-Stein et al. 2006; Friede and Kieser 2006; see also the classification of adaptive designs by Dragalin 2006). In such trials, the planned sample size can be increased (or decreased) based on interim information on effects and/or nuisance parameters like variability. These approaches are in principle also applicable in dose-finding trials, see Bischoff and Miller (2005, 2009) for SSRE based on the observed variance and Wang (2006) for SSRE based on the observed effect using a conditional power approach. An alternative approach, which has similar objectives, is to use a fully Bayesian design, updating the prior at every interim and continuing the trial until a good enough dose can be chosen with sufficient confidence. Using Bayesian decision theory, considering costs and value of information in connection to phase III decisions, the options to stop the trial at a given interim or to continue to collect more data, can be formally compared.

If a dose-finding trial is based on good modeling of available prior information, however, interim data are unlikely to radically change what a reasonable sample size is, unless there are indications that the trial should be prematurely stopped due to safety concerns or futility. Therefore the practical value of these approaches for dose-finding studies, both SSRE and the Bayesian approach with variable sample size, is typically limited to cases with exceptionally large uncertainty about the sample size assumptions. Operational aspects and project timelines may also be a hurdle for implementation of these designs in phase IIB dose-finding trials.

10.5 Dose-Finding: A Trade-Off Between Efficacy and Safety

10.5.1 A Net Benefit Example

We have considered, in the last two sections, the case where there is one single outcome variable upon which we should base the dose decision. Now, in most cases the primary effect is increasing in dose and to obtain the best effect the dose should be very high (technically infinite). In practice, however, there will be factors acting in the opposite direction. Generally, any effective treatment is connected with negative effects and these will likely increase with dose. Thus, the key problem is to strike a balance between trying to increase the positive effects (by increasing the dose) and to decrease negative side effects (by decreasing the dose).

As an example, we take a hypothetic drug with one effect variable and two safety variables. To simplify matters, we make the unrealistic assumptions that we have perfect knowledge of the dose–response curves and that these three variables are the only ones that matter. For further simplification, let us assume that the variables are measured on the same importance scale; that is, it is clear that the overall net benefit is the expected beneficial effect minus the sum of the expected safety effects. [See Burman (2008) for a discussion about importance weighting and uncertainty in dose–response models.]

Figure 10.6 gives the dose–response curve for efficacy (solid curve) as well as for the two safety variables (dotted and dashed curves, respectively). It is seen from the diagram that the net benefit (dot-dashed curve) is positive between approximately 6 mg and 20 mg. That is, in this range the positive effect dominates the safety problems. The E_{max} model, $f(x) = E_0 + E_{max} \cdot x^\gamma / (x^\gamma + \mathrm{ED}_{50}^\gamma)$, is used for all three variables, with $E_0 = 0$. The other parameter values for efficacy are $E_{max} = 1$, $\mathrm{ED}_{50} = 10$, and the Hill coefficient $\gamma = 2$. For safety variable 1, $E_{max} = 0.25$, $\mathrm{ED}_{50} = 0.2$, and $\gamma = 1$. Finally, for safety variable 2, $E_{max} = 5$, $\mathrm{ED}_{50} = 40$, and $\gamma = 3$. The first safety effect in our example is almost constant over the practically interesting dose range. This side effect is tangible already at very low doses. As a result, it is detrimental to the patients to take the drug at low doses. There is a clear safety effect, while the intended effect is low. At high doses, on the other side, safety effect 2 dominates. Thus, too high doses are harmful. Luckily,

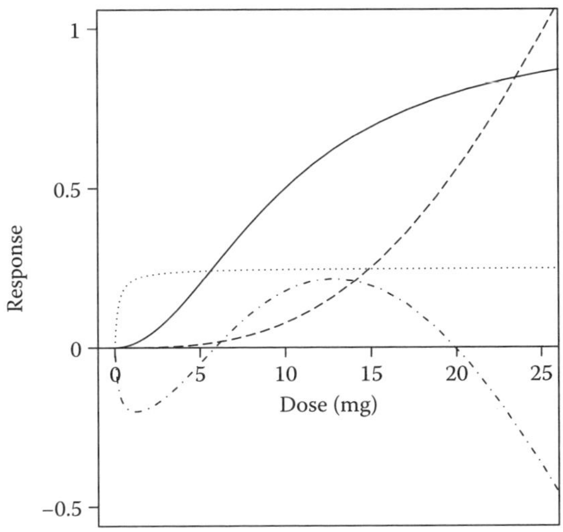

FIGURE 10.6 Dose–response curve for efficacy (solid curve) as well as for the two safety variables (dotted and dashed curves, respectively), and net benefit (dot-dashed curve).

there is a dose interval where the beneficial effect is clearly larger than the first safety effect, and in which the second safety effect is still relatively small. The result is a net benefit that has its maximum at about 13 mg. It should be noted that the maximum is typically flat in the sense that a rather large dose range gives similar net effects. In this example, the beneficial dose range is rather narrow and changing the optimal dose by just a factor two down or up implies only a small positive net effect, and a clear negative net effect, respectively.

There are often considerable variations between patients. Say that the positive effect of a drug is a reduction of the risk of myocardial infarction. Assume that the relative risk is decreased with an equal amount, say with 20%, in all patients. As the baseline risks vary, the absolute risk reduction will be different in different patient groups. Factors as medical history (e.g., earlier myocardial infarctions), age, gender, body weight, and diabetes can easily translate into risk variations in the order of a magnitude even among the patients eligible for treatment with a specific drug. While the positive effects vary a lot according to such prognostic variables, safety variables may have a completely different dependence on patient characteristics. The risk factors for the disease may not affect (much) the risks of safety effects. It is therefore of interest to see how robust the optimal dose is against changes of the positive effect, while keeping the models for the safety effects unaltered.

Figure 10.7 displays the same dose–response curves as Figure 10.6 with the sole modification that the E_{max} for efficacy is increased by a factor five. Despite this large increase of the relative importance of efficacy, the optimal dose increases only by roughly a factor 1.5, from 13 to 20 mg.

10.5.2 Temporal Aspects

There is usually a clear temporal dimension to the effect patterns. It is sometimes possible to learn about emerging adverse effects during the course of the treatment of a patient. The treatment or dose can then be modified to limit the negative effects. The goal of the dose-finding process may not be to find one treatment dose, rather to find a dosing strategy, involving advice on starting dose, monitoring intervals, algorithms for dose adjustments, and so on.

The time dependence of the effects can also mean that early trials with short treatment duration can essentially only give information about some of the important safety or effect variables. For chemotherapy, for example, the most important dose-finding trial is typically conducted already in phase I. Such a trial has tolerability as the key variable and gives no information about the beneficial effect. The

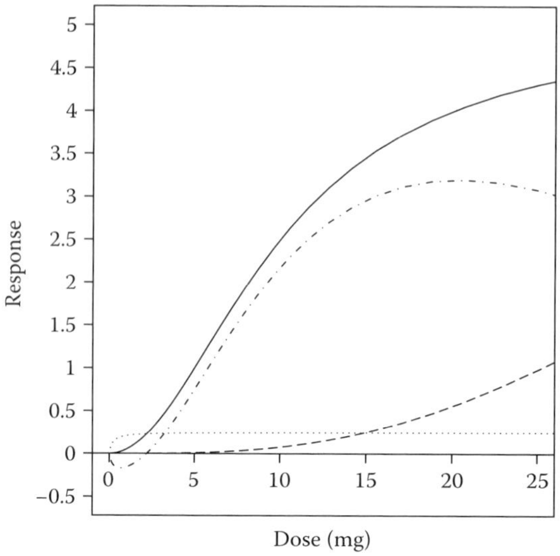

FIGURE 10.7 Modified dose–response curve for efficacy (solid curve) as well as the two safety curves from Figure 10.6 (dotted and dashed curves, respectively), and new net benefit (dot-dashed curve).

idea is that, to get optimal effect, the highest possible dose should be utilized in clinical practice. What is limiting the dose is the tolerability, so the dose is chosen to give the highest level of tolerability problems that is deemed to be acceptable. Dose-finding designs in this situation are discussed for example in Chevret (2006).

It is usually more difficult to obtain safety than efficacy information in early phases, including phase IIB. The question is frequently what dose to bring to confirmatory phase, based on efficacy dose–response data from limited treatment periods but with an unclear safety situation. The safety data from a short trial are certainly useful, and is as always complemented with preclinical data. However, there is always a risk for adverse effects that emerge over long-term or for very serious but relatively infrequent side effects.

Assume that, for example, no drug-induced deaths occur in 1000 patients treated for one month with a new drug. The, somewhat naïve, approach of calculating the 95% confidence interval for drug-induced mortality would lead to the conclusion that the risk is not larger than 3 per mille, or, if the risk is assumed uniform over time, at most 1 in roughly 30 treatment years. For most pharmaceuticals this maximal risk would be clearly unacceptable. Thus, dose-finding data taken alone cannot rule out serious risks, even less determine the optimal dose in case of a dose-dependent serious adverse effect. The conclusion is that we have to rely on indirect indications of safety (such as in vivo trials, pharmacological understanding) when assessing risks at an early stage, and then update this model with phase III and postmarketing data when they become available.

Many clinically valuable pharmaceuticals have important dose-dependent side effects that are difficult to detect in phase IIB trials. Going back to the dose determination, one approach is to try to formalize the uncertainty about safety dose–response. In a fully Bayesian perspective, it is possible to set up a prior distribution for the dose–response of (different) side effects. We can expect that severe problems will be encountered at sufficiently high doses. Our ability of guessing at which doses such problems would occur may, however, be very limited, especially as there is always a risk of safety problems of a kind that was not foreseen. Say that, as an example, a severe adverse effect is anticipated to follow a logistic regression model with dose as the independent variable. We have something close to a vague prior for the location parameter, measured on the log scale. Averaging over different scenarios, it is plausible that the expected safety effect, given the prior, would roughly be linear in the logarithm of the dose. Considering the trade-off between efficacy, which we have reasonable dose–response information about, and safety, this would translate into choosing the dose based on the derivative of the effect with respect to log dose. That is, we go up in dose until a further dose increase by 10%, say, gives only a certain incremental effect. What slope to search for depends on how likely we believe side effects to be.

10.6 Program Design

10.6.1 Designing Phase IIB with the Big Picture in Mind

The most important decision about the dose of a drug is usually taken primarily based on data from the dose-finding trial(s) in phase IIB. One single dose is frequently chosen to enter confirmatory testing in phase III. In this scenario, a choice of a suboptimal dose after phase IIB will be difficult to correct and may lead to ultimate failure of the drug.

In our view, dose selection can mainly be seen as an estimation problem. However, it is common practice to base the sample size of a dose-finding trial only on the power for the test of any positive effect of the drug. In a published simulation study, Bornkamp et al. (2007) concluded that showing a drug-effect is easier than estimating dose–response. The precision of the estimate of a target dose is limited if the sample size is based on the power of proving any positive effect of the drug, even when adaptive designs and more advanced methods of analysis are used. Already Bauer and Kieser (1999, p. 1846) pointed out that "we need larger sample sizes in early trials to get precise enough estimates for assessing … dose–response."

Let us consider a brief example to illustrate the relative difficulty of estimating dose–response compared to showing any positive drug-effect. Assume that we have a normally distributed primary variable. Two doses and placebo are included in a dose-finding trial in order to determine one dose for phase III. The sample size is chosen to have 90% power if the true standardized effect is $\Delta/\sigma = 0.5$ while controlling a one-sided type-I-error of 2.5% (with no multiplicity correction). The sample size per arm is therefore:

$$n = 2\sigma^2 / \Delta^2\left(\Phi^{-1}(\alpha)+\Phi^{-1}(\beta)\right)^2 = 84,$$

where Φ^{-1} is the quantile function of the standard normal distribution. Let us assume that the true effect of the higher dose is indeed $\Delta/\sigma = 0.5$ and the true effect of the lower dose is $\Delta/\sigma = 0.4$. For these true values, it is desirable that the study is able to declare a significant drug effect and that the high dose is chosen for phase III. While power calculation ensures a 90% probability that the study yields a statistical significant advantage of the new drug for the higher dose, there is actually 26% probability that the point estimate of the low dose is better than the estimate of the high dose. If this happens, decision makers will tend to believe these point estimates (even if the length of the confidence intervals point out the uncertainty around them) and will see no need to proceed with the high dose into phase III. Further, it is likely that even if the point estimate of the larger dose is marginally larger compared to the smaller dose, for example, effect size of 0.49 versus 0.47, the lower dose will be preferred hoping for a better safety profile and a better benefit-risk relationship. Hence, there is more than 26% probability to carry the inferior dose into phase III, reducing the probability of success there.

Antonijevic et al. (2010) underlined that it has advantages to put more investments into phase II, having a larger sample size in this phase. This increased both the probability of advancing into phase III, as well as the probability of success in phase III. In their case study, this investment is rewarded in terms of an increased net present value, despite the increased costs for phase II and the slightly shortened period of exclusivity.

10.6.2 Dose Information from Confirmatory Phase

We have seen that the size of phase IIB often is insufficient to give a precise estimate of the optimal therapeutic dose. Given that phase III trials generally are larger, it is natural to consider whether part of the dose selection can be postponed and more than one active dose should be tested in phase III. This strategy has been suggested repeatedly, especially by regulators (e.g., Hemmings 2006).

The conditions are quite different for different drugs. Sometimes, the power for demonstrating efficacy is essentially 100% at the phase III sample sizes that are required to generate sufficient safety information. In such situations, the issue changes to whether safety information on one dose can support registration of another dose. For some indications, there is general agreement that multiple doses are needed on the market and consequently several doses will be tested in phase III. In the common situation, however, when efficacy drives the sample size and the cost of phase III is large, adding a second active dose will lead to considerably higher investment costs.

For this subsection, we will build on a brief example given by Hemmings (2006, Section 2.2.3.2). For a placebo-controlled phase III trial, the sponsor considers whether to test only the dose 400 mg or that dose together with 200 mg. If only 400 mg is tested in phase III and the trial shows a favorable benefit-risk, Hemmings (2006, p. 26–27) says that "this is likely to be perfectly acceptable to the regulator." However, he argues that inclusion of 200 mg in the trial would be beneficial. Let us consider the cost of this alternative. Assume that 10,000 patients are needed to give 80% power for showing that the 400 mg dose is more effective than placebo, given the postulated effect difference Δ. (The type of response variable—survival, dichotomous, continuous, etc.—is irrelevant, as we can assume a normally distributed test variable, supported by the central limit theorem.) One might think that three arms instead of two would increase the sample size by 50%, while giving 80% power for the lower dose in case the higher dose has too many side effects. This presumption would be rash. We have to consider both the true effect of the 200 mg dose and the multiplicity issue. Regulators require that the overall type I error; that is, the familywise error rate (FWER) is controlled at the 5% level (two-sided tests). The most common approach to control the FWER is by Bonferroni correction. Each of the two active doses is then tested against placebo at the 2.5% level (two-sided). To maintain 80% power for the higher dose, the required sample size now increases to 18,165. Assuming that the effect of the lower dose is a fraction k of the assumed effect Δ for the higher dose, the required sample size to give 80% power for the lower dose is $18{,}165/k^2$. That is, if the lower dose preserves $k = 85\%$ of the effect Δ, the required sample size is $18{,}165/0.85^2 = 25{,}142$.

We have demonstrated that inclusion of a second active dose will lead to considerably larger sample sizes in phase III. The extra investment cost and decreased patent life due to a longer trial, may imply that the development of the drug would be seen as a considerably less favorable investment, and may even lead to the premature termination of the project. As two doses in phase III may give better dose information, we should therefore consider whether there are any ways of making this alternative development strategy more attractive. We will consider two approaches: first, alternative multiplicity adjustments. Secondly, in Subsection 10.6.3, to apply an adaptive dose selection during phase III.

Assume that 15,000 patients are equally distributed on the three arms, and that the effects for the high and low doses are Δ and 0.85Δ. Using the Bonferroni correction, the corresponding powers are then 71.2% and 55.6%, respectively. The risk that none of the doses has a significant effect is 19.9%. Table 10.1 compares the performance of the Bonferroni procedure with three alternatives: The first is Holm's procedure, which is a uniform improvement on Bonferroni. The second procedure is the sequential approach, first testing the effect of high dose versus placebo on the full type I error level 5%. If and only if this test is significant, the lower dose can be tested at the same significance level. The third procedure first pools all the data on both active groups and tests the mean effect on active treatment versus placebo. If and only if this test is significant, both the higher dose and the lower dose can be tested at the full level 5%; this follows from the theory of closed testing procedures (Marcus, Peritz, and Gabriel 1976). Included in Table 10.1 is also the unadjusted approach, which does not control the FWER.

The Bonferroni procedure is not to be recommended. The choice between the (unweighted) Holm and sequential procedures depends on the relative importance of showing significant effects of the two doses. The sequential procedure could even be viewed as a weighted Holm procedure with maximal weight on the high dose comparison. In the example of this section, where the efficacy of the lower dose

TABLE 10.1 Power Comparison of Five Multiplicity Approaches for Tests Comparing Active Treatment with Placebo

	Probability of Statistical Significance for			
	High Dose	Low Dose	Any Dose	Both Doses
Unadjusted	80.0%	66.3%	87.6%	58.7%
Bonferroni	71.2%	55.6%	80.1%	46.7%
Holm	74.8%	63.0%	80.1%	57.6%
Sequential	80.0%	58.7%	80.0%	58.7%
Pooled	76.8%	65.4%	84.9%*	58.7%

Notes: The columns give (1) power for the high dose, (2) power for the low dose, (3) power for active treatment, and (4) probability that both doses are statistically significant.

*Note that the pooled procedure is nonconsonant; that is, there can be a statistical significant effect of active treatment (pooled) although none of the separate doses can be claimed to be significant.

is 85% of that of the higher dose, the pooled procedure is arguably the most attractive. However, it does not perform well if there is a large relative difference

10.6.3 Adaptive Dose Selection in Phase III

As indicated in Section 10.6.2, due to limited dose–response information from phase IIB, there are reasons for including more than one dose in phase III, and an adaptive design may decrease the cost of this option. The adaptive phase III trial can start with two or three doses and placebo and in an interim analysis, one or two doses will be chosen and continued together with placebo if the trial is not stopped due to futility.

More radically, it has also been suggested to conduct a seamless phase II/III trial (Maca et al. 2006), instead of both a phase IIB and a phase III trial. Kimani, Stallard, and Hutton (2009) have proposed a phase II/III trial that explicitly considers efficacy and safety simultaneously when adapting dose.

It is more a philosophic question whether a study should be called adaptive phase III or seamless phase II/III. However, no matter what we call it, when the protocol for the study is submitted, the details for the whole study until end of phase III need to be specified, including decision criteria for the interim analysis and the analysis method for the final analysis. It is not possible to change the study population dramatically. The duration of treatment is often shorter in phase IIB than in phase III. In an adaptive trial, however, the treatment duration for all patients has to follow the requirement for phase III. Therefore we prefer adaptive phase III study as the name for the study discussed here. This study could either replace the dose-finding study in phase II postponing the dose-finding to phase III, or it could follow a phase II dose-finding study with an outcome not strongly favoring a specific dose.

To go directly into phase III without any dose–response information from the learning phase should, in our view, be an exceptional case. Note that a requirement for this would also be that there is good confidence in the knowledge of the new drug's profile, especially regarding tolerability. The possibility to add an adaptive phase III trial after a phase II dose-finding study is a more attractive consideration for a larger number of development programs.

The statistical methodology to analyze data from adaptive trials with interim treatment selection controlling for the FWER is well developed. Bauer and Kieser (1999) and Posch et al. (2005) discuss methods based on the combination test approach. Bischoff and Miller (2005) adjust the critical value accounting for treatment selection, SSRE, and early stopping. An adaptive Dunnett procedure was elaborated by König et al. (2008). Stallard and Friede (2008) apply group-sequential testing to adaptive dose-finding designs. Friede and Stallard (2008) compare different methods for significance tests with regard to their statistical properties.

In indications where two phase III trials are a regulatory expectation as basis for drug licensing, the question arises how the second phase III trial should be designed and placed in the program if the first is an adaptive phase III trial. One possibility is to start the second trial after a positive interim analysis with the dose(s) chosen based on Stage I from the first trial. Another possibility is to run two similar adaptive phase III in parallel with alignment of the interim analyses in both studies ensuring that the same dose(s) are chosen in both studies. The first option is more attractive if it is possible to setup the second trial as fast recruiting trial, for example, by having more sites. However, if for example, a long treatment time implies that adding more sites does not decrease the study duration by much, the second option with two aligned adaptive phase III trials seems more appropriate.

10.7 Summary and Discussion

Dose-finding is a multifaceted process. Many information sources contribute to a series of decisions about which doses to investigate further in the different phases of drug discovery and development, and which dose(s) to market. These decisions are currently often ad hoc, rather than model-based using a formal integration of available data under clear assumptions. Although we strongly propose the latter approach, it is clear that models should only be used to support decision makers and not to be trusted blindly.

A key question is how to weigh together the various beneficial and adverse effects of a drug. For example, how much additional efficacy of an increased dose is needed to outweigh a certain increase in the frequency of a side effect? Unless such questions are explicitly stated and discussed, the dose selection thinking process may easily be obscured.

In order to obtain good dose-finding information, it is critical that the experiments are carefully designed. Most importantly, any clinical trial has to be analyzed from an ethical perspective: will the trial participants benefit from taking part in this trial given the proposed design? Next, the efficiency of the trial should be analyzed. Optimal design theory can greatly improve the information value of a trial. However, this theory relies on a number of assumptions. First, the objective of the trial has to be stated in precise terms. That is, the stated objective should not be vague, like "investigating dose–response." It should rather be, for example, "to estimate the dose at which the drug has a 12% effect improvement compared to placebo." There is no universally applicable objective. The objective should be tailored to the specific drug project. Ideally, it should depend on other parts of the program. Secondly, the optimal design generally depends on prior information. As the response is typically nonlinear in dose, a prior guess of, for example, the potency needed to give any idea of which doses to investigate. A formal prior on the parameters makes it possible to calculate a Bayesian optimal design.

The designs of different experiments in the discovery and development program are clearly related. In particular, the size and design of phase IIB and of phase III should not be considered isolated from each other. Including two rather than one active dose in phase III can generate more and better dose response information. However, the increased sample size and need for multiplicity corrections often makes this option intractable. An interesting middle way is to start phase III with two doses or more but, after an interim analysis, conclude it with one. Such adaptive designs are currently widely debated.

References

Antonijevic, Z., Pinheiro, J., Fardipour, P., and Lewis, R. J. (2010). Impact of dose selection strategies used in phase II on the probability of success in phase III. *Journal of Biopharmaceutical Statistics*, to appear.

Atkinson, A. C., Donev, A. N., and Tobias, R. D. (2007). *Optimum Experimental Designs, with SAS*. Oxford: Oxford University Press.

Bartholomew, D. J. (1961). Ordered tests in the analysis of variance. *Biometrika*, 48: 325–32.

Bauer, P., and Kieser, M. (1999). Combining different phases in the development of medical treatments within a single trial. *Statistics in Medicine,* 18: 1833–49.

Bauer, P., and Köhne, K. (1994) Evaluation of experiments with adaptive interim analyses. *Biometrics,* 50: 1029–41.

Bischoff, W., and Miller, F. (2005). Adaptive two-stage test procedures to find the best treatment in clinical trials. *Biometrika,* 92: 197–212.

Bischoff, W., and Miller, F. (2009). A seamless phase II/III design with sample-size re-estimation. *Journal of Biopharmaceutical Statistics,* 19: 595–609.

Bornkamp, B., Bretz, F., Dmitrienko, A., Enas, G., Gaydos, B., Hsu, C. H., König, et al. (2007). Innovative approaches for designing and analyzing adaptive dose-ranging trials. *Journal of Biopharmaceutical Statistics,* 17: 965–95.

Braess, D., and Dette, H. (2007). On the number of support points of maximin and Bayesian D-optimal designs in nonlinear regression models. *Annals of Statistics,* 35: 772–92.

Bretz, F., Branson, M., Burman, C.-F., Chuang-Stein, C., and Coffey, C. S. (2009). Adaptivity in drug discovery and development. *Drug Development Research,* 70: 169–90.

Bretz, F., Hsu, J., Pinheiro, J., and Liu, Y. (2008). Dose finding—A challenge in statistics. *Biometrical Journal,* 50: 480–504.

Bretz, F., Pinheiro, J., and Branson, M. (2005). Combining multiple comparisons and modeling techniques in dose–response studies. *Biometrics,* 61: 738–48.

Burman, C.-F. (2008). Clinical dose–response assessment. In *Encyclopedia of Quantitative Risk Assessment and Analysis,* eds. E. Melnick and B. Everitt. New York: Wiley. Available online at (DOI: 10.1002/9780470061596.risk0616)

Burman, C.-F., and Carlberg, A. (2009). Future challenges in the design and ethics of clinical trials. In *Clinical Trial Handbook,* ed. S. C. Gad. New York: Wiley, 1173–1200.

Burzykowski, T., Molenberghs, G., and Buyse, M. (2005). *The Evaluation of Surrogate Endpoints.* New York: Springer.

Byas-Smith, M. G., Max, M. B., Muir, J., and Kingman, A. (1995). Transdermal clonidine compared to placebo in painful diabetic neuropathy using a two-stage "enriched enrollment" design. *Pain,* 60: 267–74.

Chaloner, K., and Larntz, K. (1989). Optimal Bayesian design applied to logistic regression experiments. *Journal of Statistical Planning and Inference,* 21: 191–208.

Chevret, S. (2006). *Statistical Methods for Dose-Finding Experiments.* Chichester: Wiley.

Chuang-Stein, C., Anderson, K., Gallo, P., and Collins, S. (2006). Sample size re-estimation: A review and recommendations. *Drug Information Journal,* 40: 475–84.

Chow, S. C., and Chang, M. (2006). *Adaptive Design Methods in Clinical Trials.* Boca Raton, FL: Chapman & Hall/CRC.

Dette, H., Haines, L., and Imhof, L. (2007). Maximin and Bayesian optimal designs for regression models. *Statistica Sinica,* 17: 463–80.

Dragalin, V. (2006). Adaptive designs: Terminology and classification. *Drug Information Journal,* 40: 425–35.

FDA. (2004). *Challenge and Opportunity on the Critical Path to New Medical Products.* Rockville, MD: U.S. Food and Drug Administration. Available at http://www.fda.gov/ScienceResearch/SpecialTopics/CriticalPathInitiative/CriticalPathOpportunitiesReports/default.htm

FDA. (2006). *Critical Path Opportunities List.* Rockville, MD: U.S. Food and Drug Administration. Available at http://www.fda.gov/ScienceResearch/SpecialTopics/CriticalPathInitiative/CriticalPathOpportunitiesReports/default.htm

Friede, T., and Kieser, M. (2006). Sample size recalculation in internal pilot study designs: A review. *Biometrical Journal,* 48: 537–55.

Friede, T., Miller, F., Bischoff, W., and Kieser, M. (2001). A note on change point estimation in dose-response trials. *Computational Statistics & Data Analysis,* 37: 219–32.

Friede, T., and Stallard, N. (2008). A comparison of methods for adaptive treatment selection. *Biometrical Journal,* 50: 767–81.

Hemmings, R. (2006). Philosophy and methodology of dose-finding—A regulatory perspective. In *Statistical Methods for Dose-Finding Experiments,* ed. S. Chevret. Chichester: Wiley, 19–57.

Hsu, C.-H. (2009). Evaluating potential benefits of dose-exposure-response modeling for dose finding. *Pharmaceutical Statistics,* 8: 203–15.

ICH guideline E4 (1994). International conference on harmonisation of technical requirements for registration of pharmaceuticals for human use. ICH topic E4: Dose-response information to support drug registration. ICH technical coordination, EMEA, London.

Kiefer, J., and Wolfowitz, J. (1960). The equivalence of two extremum problems. *Canadian Journal of Mathematics,* 12: 363–66.

Kimani, P. K., Stallard, N., and Hutton, J. L. (2009). Dose selection in seamless phase II/III clinical trials based on efficacy and safety. *Statistics in Medicine,* 28: 917–36.

Kirby, S., Colman, P., and Morris, M. (2009). Adaptive modelling of dose-response relationships using smoothing splines. *Pharmaceutical Statistics,* 8: 346–55.

Koenig, F., Brannath, W., Bretz, F., and Posch, M. (2008). Adaptive Dunnett tests for treatment selection. *Statistics in Medicine,* 27: 1612–25.

Krams, M., Lees, K. R., and Berry, D. A. (2005). The past is the future: Innovative designs in acute stroke therapy trials. *Stroke,* 36: 1341–47.

Lilford, R. J. (2003). Ethics of clinical trials from a Bayesian and decision analytic perspective: Whose equipoise is it anyway? *British Medical Journal,* 326: 980–81.

Maca, J., Bhattacharya, S., Dragalin, V., Gallo, P., and Krams, M. (2006). Adaptive seamless phase II/III designs—Background, operational aspects, and examples. *Drug Information Journal,* 40: 463–73.

Maloney, A., Karlsson, M. O., and Simonsson U. S. H. (2007). Optimal adaptive design in clinical drug development: A simulation example. *Quantitative Clinical Pharmacology,* 47: 1231–43.

Marcus, R., Peritz, E., and Gabriel, K. R. (1976). On closed testing procedures with special reference to ordered analysis of variance. *Biometrika,* 63: 655–60.

Miller, F., Guilbaud, O., and Dette, H. (2007). Optimal designs for estimating the interesting part of a dose-effect curve. *Journal of Biopharmaceutical Statistics,* 17: 1097–1115.

Pinheiro, J., Bornkamp, B., and Bretz, F. (2006). Design and analysis of dose-finding studies combining multiple comparisons and modeling procedures. *Journal of Biopharmaceutical Statistics,* 16: 639–56.

Pinheiro, J., and Duffull, S. (2009). Exposure response—Getting the dose right. *Pharmaceutical Statistics,* 8: 173–75.

Posch, M., Koenig, F., Branson, M., Brannath, W., Dunger-Baldauf, C., and Bauer, P. (2005). Testing and estimating in flexible group sequential designs with adaptive treatment selection. *Statistics in Medicine,* 24: 3697–3714.

Robertson, T., Wright, F. T., and Dykstra, R. L. (1988). *Order Restricted Statistical Inference.* Chichester: Wiley.

Ruberg, S. J. (1995a). Dose response studies I: Some design considerations. *Journal of Biopharmaceutical Statistics,* 5: 1–14.

Ruberg, S. J. (1995b). Dose response studies II: Analysis and interpretation. *Journal of Biopharmaceutical Statistics,* 5: 15–42.

Senn, S. (2002). *Cross-Over Trials in Clinical Research.* Chichester: Wiley.

Sheiner, L. B., Hashimoto, Y., and Beal, S. L. (1991). A simulation study comparing designs for dose ranging. *Statistics in Medicine,* 10: 303–21.

Smith, M. K., Jones, I., Morris, M. F., Grieve, A. P., and Tan, K. (2006). Implementation of a Bayesian adaptive design in a proof of concept study. *Pharmaceutical Statistics,* 5: 39–50.

Stallard, N., and Friede, T. (2008). A group-sequential design for clinical trials with treatment selection. *Statistics in Medicine,* 27: 6209–27.

Straube, S., Derry, S., McQuay H. J., and Moore, R. A. (2008). Enriched enrollment: Definition and effects of enrichment and dose in trials of pregabalin and gabapentin in neuropathic pain. A systematic review. *British Journal of Clinical Pharmacology,* 66: 266–75.

Ting, N. (2006). *Dose Finding in Drug Development.* New York: Springer.

Wald, A. (1943). On the efficient design of statistical investigations. *Annals of Mathematical Statistics,* 14: 134–40.

Wang, J. (2006). An adaptive two-stage design with treatment selection using the conditional error function approach. *Biometrical Journal,* 48: 679–89.

Wang, S. J. (2008). Utility of adaptive strategy and adaptive design for biomarker-facilitated patient selection in pharmacogenomic or pharmacogenetic clinical development program. *Journal of the Formosan Medical Association,* 107: S19–S27.

Whittle, P. (1973). Some general points in the theory of optimal experimental design. *Journal of the Royal Statistical Society Series B,* 35: 123–30.

WMA (World Medical Association). (2008). *Declaration of Helsinki* (6th revision). Available at http://www.wma.net/en/30publications/10policies/b3/index.html

11

Adaptive Dose-Ranging Studies

Marc Vandemeulebroecke, Frank Bretz, and José Pinheiro
Novartis Pharma AG

Björn Bornkamp
Technische Universität Dortmund

11.1 Introduction

Clinical drug development aims at developing medical treatments that are both safe and effective, or more generally, have a favorable risk–benefit relation, in a specified indication (ICH E9 1998). This, however, depends on the employed formulation, route of administration, regimen, and perhaps most importantly, dose. Every compound is toxic at excessive doses, and conversely, ineffective at sufficiently low doses. It is well recognized that in the past many drugs have initially been marketed at too high doses, leading to unnecessary safety risks and subsequent dose reductions (FDC Report 1991). Worse even, it is likely that potentially effective compounds could not be made available to patients because wrong doses were investigated in the pivotal trials. The importance of accurate dose–response information, and the frequent lack thereof, has led to the publication of a dedicated guidance on Dose–Response Information to Support Drug Registration by the International Conference of Harmonization (ICH E4 1994). According to this guidance, "assessment of dose–response should be an integral component of drug development."

In its broadest sense, this assessment can cover various types of investigations. Phase I trials that assign different (usually increasing) doses in an algorithmic manner to consecutive small subject groups focus on establishing a maximum tolerated dose (MTD), especially in life-threatening diseases where a certain degree of toxicity can be accepted (see, e.g., Potter 2008 for an overview). Within-subject titration designs can provide suitable dose adjustment options for individual dose optimization in clinical practice (e.g., Vogt, Navis, and de Zeeuw 2005). Exposure–response investigations, directly relating systemic exposure (e.g., AUC or C_{max}) to clinical endpoints, may yield useful additional information (Roy et al. 2010). In this chapter, we focus on another, particularly important type of dose–response investigation, namely, Phase II dose-ranging trials. Here, different doses are applied to different (often parallel) groups of patients, in order to investigate the average dose–response relationship over a certain relevant range of doses. The success of a subsequent Phase III campaign (and thus, of the whole drug development program) often depends critically on the information obtained from such a trial. Dose-finding may be considered a particular application within this type of trial. We will come back to the question of which dose exactly is to be found in this context.

Despite their crucial role in the drug development process, common approaches for dose-ranging trials often have poor statistical properties for some of their main objectives. The power of a particular testing approach for showing a drug effect can be highly dependent on the true dose–response shape (Abelson and Tukey 1963). Even when there is sufficient power for showing a drug effect, the estimation of target doses to be carried into a Phase III program typically lacks the necessary precision (Bornkamp et al. 2007). The inherent problem is the uncertainty about the nature of the dose–response relationship: if we knew it, we could design a powerful and accurate study—but we would not need to conduct it anymore.

Here, adaptive approaches may help. Despite the high level of initial uncertainty, knowledge will emerge as the trial progresses, and the employed methods can be adjusted accordingly. Adaptivity to overcome uncertainty—the idea is appealing. It bears the promise of making the dose-finding phase of a drug development program more informative and efficient. Not surprisingly, it has attracted considerable attention in recent times. A number of different proposals have been put forward to implement this idea in practice. Broadly speaking, these proposals fall into two categories. *Adaptive analysis methods* choose the way the data are analyzed in dependence of this same observed data. For example, a modeling approach may be preceded by a data-driven choice of the model to use. *Adaptive design methods* adjust the way the data are gathered in order to obtain most information. For instance, the allocation scheme may be changed during an ongoing trial to focus on the most relevant dose groups. Methods that adapt the analysis and the design may be counted as a third category or subsumed under the second.

One of the earliest examples of an adaptive analysis method for a dose–response study was presented by Tukey, Ciminera, and Heyse (1985). These authors chose between three different dose metameters (actual dose, log dose, and ordinal dose) depending on which yields the greatest evidence of a drug effect. Capizzi, Survill, and Heyse (1992) refined this method through an appropriate Type I error rate control, taking the correlation between the test statistics into account. A further extension is the multiple trend test discussed in Bornkamp et al. (2007). In the present chapter, we use a method proposed by Bretz, Pinheiro, and Branson (2005) to illustrate some important considerations involved in adaptive analysis methods.

A well-known example of an adaptive design (and analysis) method is the general adaptive dose allocation (GADA) that was employed in the ASTIN trial (Berry et al. 2001; Krams et al. 2003; Grieve and Krams 2005). In this approach, a normal dynamic linear model estimating the dose–response relationship is updated after every patient (using Bayesian methods), each time leading to a possible adaptation in the dose allocation rule for the next patient. The real-time learning about the dose–response and the resulting design adaptations were decisive for the efficiency of the ASTIN trial. In studies where patients are recruited in consecutive cohorts, each interim analysis provides the opportunity to adjust the design for the next cohort. Several authors proposed model-based approaches that use optimal design theory to determine what design makes the next cohort most informative. Dragalin, Hsuan, and Padmanabhan (2007) modeled the dose–response using a sigmoid emax model. They gave analytical expressions for the Fisher information matrix and derived the design for the next cohort such that the expected overall information about all model parameters is maximized. The method can be adapted to other optimization criteria, such as maximizing the expected information about a particular target dose, and also allows switching from one criterion to another (Dragalin et al. 2010). Miller, Guilbaud, and Dette (2007) also used the sigmoid emax model, but their aim was to estimate the "interesting part" of a dose–response curve with the best possible precision. The definition of the interesting part can vary from application to application. Smith (2010) proposed a method for optimizing a weighted combination of multiple objectives, while modeling the dose–response by inverse polynomials. Bornkamp et al. (2010) built on the adaptive analysis method of Bretz, Pinheiro, and Branson (2005) mentioned earlier and extended it by the introduction of adaptive design elements. Later in this chapter, we illustrate some considerations involved in adaptive design methods using this approach. Further proposals include, among others, Hall, Meier, and Diener (2005), Weir, Spiegelhalter, and Grieve (2007), Ivanova, Bolognese, and Perevozskaya (2008), Klingenberg (2009), and Leonov and Miller (2009).

The present chapter is structured as follows. In Section 11.2, we begin with a brief overview of the necessary concepts of (conventional) dose-ranging studies, and we recall two major approaches for their analysis, namely, multiple comparison procedures and modeling. We highlight potential issues that are later addressed by the introduction of adaptive elements. Section 11.3 focuses on the first type of adaptivity: adaptive analyses. A procedure that combines multiple comparisons and modeling into an adaptive analysis technique is presented to illustrate relevant considerations. Adaptive design aspects are the topic of Section 11.4, where this procedure is extended into an adaptive design and analysis approach. This is accomplished by an adaptive implementation of optimal design theory, which we briefly introduce for this purpose. An example based on a real trial planning illustrates the theory throughout Sections 11.3 and 11.4. Section 11.5 concludes the chapter with a short summary.

11.2 Dose-Ranging Studies

In this section, we introduce the main objectives of a dose-ranging study and briefly recall two major approaches that are commonly used to address them. We refer to Bretz et al. (2008) for a more comprehensive discussion of the same topics.

11.2.1 Main Objectives of a Dose-Ranging Study

A dose-ranging study can potentially address a number of questions, and its design will crucially depend on the particular (prespecified!) question(s) in focus. Following Ruberg (1995a, 1995b), the main questions are:

1. Is there any evidence of a drug effect?
2. What doses exhibit a response different from the control response?
3. What is the nature of the dose–response relationship?
4. What is the optimal dose?

Question 1 may be called proof of concept (PoC), and a small, dedicated PoC-study can address it regardless of any dose–response considerations. Alternatively, in the context of a dose-ranging study, an overall test of whether a change in dose leads to a change in response can be performed. A t-test based on a prespecified contrast of the mean responses at different doses is a common way to do this. More specifically, a linear combination of the observed mean responses is built such that its coefficients sum up to zero, and a t-statistic based on this linear combination is used to test the null hypothesis of a flat dose–response. The critical issue is the choice of the contrast coefficients. Broadly speaking, the more the contrast resembles the true pattern of mean responses, the more powerful is the test (Abelson and Tukey 1963). The difficulty arises from the fact that we do not know this pattern.

Question 2 asks for inference about specific doses, usually restricted to those employed in the study. For this, *multiple comparison procedures* offer a large variety of options. The idea is to perform several tests, each aimed at declaring a different dose effective, while strongly controlling the familywise error rate (FWER) through an appropriate adjustment of the individual test levels. Numerous proposals have been put forward in the spirit of this general idea (e.g., Dunnett 1955; Ruberg 1995b; Tamhane, Hochberg, and Dunnett 1996). Again, each procedure's properties are highly dependent on the underlying true dose–response shape.

Question 3 is the first that considers the dose as a continuous (i.e., quantitative, not merely qualitative) factor. It is assumed that dose and response are linked through a functional relationship, and the shape and location of this dose–response curve are investigated. Here, *modeling* is the method of choice. Often, a parametric model is fitted to the observed responses using linear or nonlinear regression techniques.

Subsequent inference is based on the fitted model and is, unlike with multiple comparison procedures, also possible for doses that were not employed in the study. A major difficulty in this context is the choice of the model, and how well it is suited to describe the unknown, true dose–response shape.

Question 4 addresses dose-finding in the strict sense, and it is perhaps the most difficult question to answer. First, one needs to specify what is meant by "optimal dose." Is it the smallest dose that can be proven to produce an average response different from placebo? The largest dose beyond which no further relevant improvement can be achieved? Or the smallest dose that produces a clinically meaningful effect? These concepts may be called minimum detectable dose (MDD; Tamhane et al. 1996), maximum useful dose (MUD; ICH E4 1994), and minimum effective dose (MED; ICH E4 1994: "the smallest dose with a discernible useful effect"), respectively. An MDD can be found by addressing question 2, but it will highly depend on the study design, and in particular, on the sample size. The MUD may be difficult to establish (and practically not relevant) if larger doses cause undesirable side effects. Therefore, the main interest often lies in the MED. For this, one first needs to define what is meant by a useful, or clinically meaningful, effect. Second, in order not to be restricted to the doses employed in the study, it is advisable to estimate the MED based on the model fit from question 3. By consequence, the MED estimation depends on the initial model choice and inherits the aforementioned difficulty of choosing that model well.

Note that question 1 and the shape (but not location) of the dose–response curve in question 3 can in principle be investigated using active doses only, provided that the right dose range is chosen (which would be risky to assume in practice). All other questions require a comparator. Therefore, it is wise to include a comparator (most appropriately, placebo) in any dose-ranging study whenever possible.

11.2.2 Multiple Comparison Procedures

Multiple comparison procedures allow to perform several tests while controlling the FWER in the strong sense (i.e., controlling the probability of falsely rejecting one or more null hypotheses, irrespective of which and how many are true) at a prespecified level α. A simple but conservative example is the Bonferroni correction, where each of K tests is performed at level α/K in order to control the FWER at level α. In the context of question 2, this could be applied to testing each of K doses against placebo. Less conservative procedures were proposed, for example, by Holm (1979) and Hochberg (1988). The fixed-sequence procedure (Maurer, Hothorn, and Lehmacher 1995; Westfall and Krishen 2001) is attractive for its simplicity: each dose is tested against placebo at the full level α, following a prespecified order, as long as significance can be achieved. Here, each test serves as a gatekeeper for all subsequent tests. Under the assumption that the response increases with the dose, it is natural to start with the highest dose and gradually proceed toward lower doses. If, however, this assumption is wrong and the highest dose is not the most effective, the risk is high that effective lower doses are missed. Many more procedures have been proposed based on gatekeeping or related ideas. Yet, the uncertainty about the true dose–response shape remains a limiting factor for the construction of powerful procedures.

A different approach is to exploit the correlation between several single test statistics. For example, Dunnett's test (Dunnett 1955) uses the correlation induced by a common control group when addressing question 2. We apply a similar idea in Section 11.3.1 while addressing question 1. Such approaches require certain distributional assumptions (e.g., normally distributed data), but they tend to perform better than the aforementioned more general methods when these assumptions apply. The stronger the (positive) correlation, the smaller is the penalty that has to be paid for performing multiple comparisons.

11.2.3 Modeling

Multiple comparison procedures allow simultaneous inference about the different doses employed in a study. However, they disregard the fact that these doses are mere choices from a theoretically continuous range of possible doses. What effect will other doses have? It is plausible to assume that similar doses will have a similar effect, or more precisely, that the average relationship between dose and response can be described by a smooth, continuous function. Empirical modeling is the search for such a function that adequately fits the observed data. This function provides the answer to question 3; once it is at hand, further inferences can be derived from it. This is appealing as it allows statements about doses that have not been studied. For example, based on a specified dose–response function, the dose that yields a certain target effect is easily identified by inverse regression. The caveat is that in practice, a parametric model is assumed a priori, and the search for the dose–response function consists in tweaking the model parameters to fit the data as closely as possible (see Pinheiro, Bretz, and Branson 2006, for an overview of commonly used dose–response models and how to use them in practice). Any inference thus depends on the initial choice of the model, and there is typically little certainty in this choice. The method that we present in the next section copes with this problem by choosing the model adaptively.

11.3 Adaptive Analysis of Dose-Ranging Studies

We have highlighted that the performance of any method for analyzing a dose-ranging study will strongly depend on the unknown, true dose–response shape, and on how good our initial assumptions are. It is therefore natural to ask for adaptive analysis methods, that is, methods that adapt the analysis depending on the actual data. To illustrate this idea, we now present an adaptive analysis method proposed by Bretz, Pinheiro, and Branson (2005), which amalgamates elements of multiple comparisons and modeling into an adaptive combination approach. The idea is to perform multiple contrast tests, properly adjusted for multiplicity, for detecting a drug effect, and subsequently to employ modeling techniques to estimate the dose–response relationship and derive a target dose. Proof of concept testing and dose-finding are thus integral parts of the same procedure.

11.3.1 Combining Multiple Comparisons and Modeling into an Adaptive Analysis Approach

Assume that we randomize N patients to k parallel dose groups. The ith group consists of n_i patients, all of whom receive dose d_i (i = 1, …, k; d_1 is placebo; $N = \Sigma_{i=1}^{k} n_i$). We consider a one-way layout for the responses:

$$Y_{ij} = \mu_{d_i} + \varepsilon_{ij},\ \varepsilon_{ij} \overset{\text{iid}}{\sim} \mathcal{N}(0,\sigma^2),\quad i=1,\ldots,k,\ j=1,\ldots,n_i,$$

and we assume that the mean responses per dose group can be expressed as $\mu_{d_i} = f(d_i,\boldsymbol{\theta})$ for some dose–response model f that depends on a parameter vector $\boldsymbol{\theta}$.

Traditional multiple comparison procedures ignore the fact that the μ_{d_i} are linked through the function f. Most modeling techniques, on the other hand, do not address the choice of f; they focus on estimating $\boldsymbol{\theta}$ for a given f. To overcome these limitations, Bretz, Pinheiro, and Branson (2005) proposed to combine both approaches into the following procedure. Software implementing this methodology was developed by Bornkamp, Pinheiro, and Bretz (2009).

In a first step, several candidate dose–response models f_m, $m = 1, \ldots, M$, are specified, covering plausible shapes anticipated for the dose–response relationship. Each f_m is a function of the dose d and depends on a parameter vector $\boldsymbol{\theta}_m$. It is convenient to express f_m in terms of a standardized model f_m^0 such that $f_m(d,\boldsymbol{\theta}_m) = \theta_{m0} + \theta_{m1} f_m^0(d,\boldsymbol{\theta}_m^0)$. The parameters θ_{m0} and θ_{m1} enter the model linearly and determine its location and scale; f_m^0 is a linear or nonlinear function determining its shape. The parameter vector $\boldsymbol{\theta}_m^0$ of the standardized model is chosen a priori, as a best guess. Once the M candidate models have been selected, M contrast test statistics T_m are computed. Each T_m tests the null hypothesis of a flat dose–response, with contrast coefficients $\boldsymbol{c}_m = (c_{m1}, \ldots, c_{mk})'$ that maximize the power of the test if f_m reflects the true dose–response. More precisely,

$$T_m = \frac{\sum_{i=1}^{k} c_{mi} \bar{Y}_i}{S\sqrt{\sum_{i=1}^{k} c_{mi}^2 / n_i}},$$

where $S^2 = (N-k)^{-1}\Sigma_{i=1}^{k}\Sigma_{j=1}^{n_i}(Y_{ij}-\bar{Y}_i)^2$. It can be shown that the optimal contrast coefficients do not depend on θ_{m0} and θ_{m1}; the c_{mi} are proportional to $n_i(\mu_{m,d_i}^0 - \bar{\mu})$, where $\mu_{m,d_i}^0 = f_m^0(d_i, \boldsymbol{\theta}_m^0)$ and $\bar{\mu} = N^{-1}\Sigma_{i=1}^{k}\mu_{m,d_i}^0 n_i$ (Bornkamp 2006). A unique representation is obtained by imposing $\Sigma_{i=1}^{k} c_{mi}^2 = 1$. Under the null hypothesis of a flat dose–response, $(T_1, \ldots, T_M)'$ follows a central multivariate t-distribution with $N - k$ degrees of freedom and correlation matrix $\boldsymbol{R} = (\rho_{ij})$, where

$$\rho_{ij} = \frac{\sum_{l=1}^{k} c_{il} c_{jl} / n_l}{\sqrt{\sum_{l=1}^{k} c_{il}^2 / n_l \sum_{l=1}^{k} c_{jl}^2 / n_l}}.$$

We thus have M correlated test statistics, each maximizing the power if one of the anticipated dose–response shapes is true. Proof of concept is established if any of these statistics is large enough, while addressing multiplicity by exploiting their correlation. More specifically, the null hypothesis of a flat dose–response is rejected if $T_{max} = \max_m T_m$ equals or exceeds the multiplicity-adjusted critical value $q_{1-\alpha}$ determined by the joint distribution of $(T_1, \ldots, T_M)'$. Numerical integration routines such as those implemented in the R package *mvtnorm* (Genz and Bretz 2002, 2009) can be used to compute $q_{1-\alpha}$.

If a flat dose–response cannot be rejected, the procedure stops. Otherwise, all models f_m for which $T_m \geq q_{1-\alpha}$ are declared statistically significant under strong control of the FWER. These models may potentially be used for further inference. In practice, often a single model is selected out of the significant models, although weighted model averaging is also possible. Bretz, Pinheiro, and Branson (2005) did not define a formal selection rule. Rather, any criterion such as the maximum T_m or the minimum AIC or BIC may be used, possibly combined with considerations of numerical stability or any other (even external) information.

Finally, standard modeling techniques are applied to fit the selected model to the observed data and estimate any target dose(s) of interest. Assume that we are primarily interested in the MED, defined as the smallest dose with a benefit of at least, say, $\Delta > 0$ over placebo (given that larger values indicate better outcomes):

$$\text{MED} = \min\{d \in (d_1, d_k]; f(d, \boldsymbol{\theta}) \geq f(d_1, \boldsymbol{\theta}) + \Delta\}.$$

Note that the MED need not exist, especially for large Δ. The restriction to $(d_1, d_k]$ avoids problems that can arise when extrapolating beyond the dose range under investigation. We estimate the MED by the smallest dose that is significantly superior to placebo at some level γ, and for which the predicted response shows a benefit of at least Δ over placebo:

$$\widehat{\text{MED}} = \min\{d \in (d_1, d_k]; f_{m^*}(d, \hat{\boldsymbol{\theta}}_{m^*}) \geq f_{m^*}(d_1, \hat{\boldsymbol{\theta}}_{m^*}) + \Delta, L_{(m^*, d, \gamma)} > f_{m^*}(d_1, \hat{\boldsymbol{\theta}}_{m^*})\},$$

where f_{m*} denotes the selected candidate model, $\hat{\boldsymbol{\theta}}_{m^*}$ the parameter vector estimate based on fitting f_{m*} to the data, and $L_{(m*,d,\gamma)}$ the lower $1-2\gamma$ confidence limit for $f_{m^*}(d,\hat{\boldsymbol{\theta}}_{m^*})$. Bretz, Pinheiro, and Branson (2005) showed that this definition of $\widehat{\text{MED}}$ tends to be less biased than some alternative choices. If no dose qualifies as $\widehat{\text{MED}}$, we conclude that the MED does not exist (in the dose range under investigation).

The MED depends on the true model f, whereas the estimator $\widehat{\text{MED}}$ depends on the selected model f_{m*} and its parameter vector estimate $\hat{\boldsymbol{\theta}}_{m^*}$. In direct model-based approaches, issues of model misspecification may arise at this point. The procedure outlined above addresses this by an adaptive model choice based on the candidate models. This adaptive analysis technique enhances the chances that the fitted model is appropriate. The involved model selection steps are embedded in a rigorous hypothesis testing framework that addresses the associated multiplicity issue up to and including the establishment of proof of concept and the identification of one or more significant models. The impact of the model selection on the precision of the target dose estimates can further be assessed using, for example, bootstrap methods.

11.3.2 Example

To illustrate the methodology from the previous section, we consider an example that is inspired by the design of a real study. A compound is to be investigated for its ability to attenuate dental pain after the removal of two or more impacted third molar teeth. In this setting, it is common to measure the pain intensity on an ordinal scale at baseline and several times after the administration of a single dose. The pain intensity difference from baseline (PID), averaged over several hours after drug administration, may be considered normally distributed and used as primary target variable. We express PID such that larger values indicate better outcomes. The study investigates whether there is a drug effect on PID (PoC step), and if so, how it depends on the dose and what is the MED (estimation step).

As the PoC step requires considerably less subjects than the estimation step (Bornkamp et al. 2007), the study is conducted in two stages. A cohort of 60 patients is treated in the first stage, with 20 patients receiving placebo, 20 patients receiving 50 mg, and 20 patients receiving 200 mg of the investigational drug. PoC is tested at level $\alpha = 0.05$ (one-sided), using the maximum contrast test statistic based on several candidate models as outlined above. If PoC cannot be established, the estimation step is of no interest, and the study stops. Otherwise, a second cohort of 120 patients is treated, with patients being allocated to placebo, 25, 50, 100, 150, or 200 mg in such a way that each dose is administered to 30 patients overall (i.e., in both cohorts together). At the end of the second cohort, the estimation step is carried out, using the model that now yields the maximum contrast test statistic. (Note that this two-stage design is a variation of the general procedure described earlier.) We simplify the estimation by choosing γ large enough to play no practical role. Both study stages are conducted in a randomized and double-blind manner.

The compound is in an early development stage, and no information is available on likely dose–response shapes. In particular, a nonmonotonic dose–response cannot be ruled out. Four candidate models are specified such that a variety of shapes is covered by a parsimonious number of models. Table 11.1 and Figure 11.1 show the standardized versions of these models, where placebo has effect 0 and the maximal effect (over placebo) within the dose range is 1.2 (with the logistic being slightly shifted). An effect of 0.6 (over placebo) is considered minimally clinically relevant, and the MED is defined as the smallest dose that produces this effect. We assume that the variance σ^2 is 1.

First, we calculate key quantities for the PoC test based on Stage 1. The optimal contrasts $\boldsymbol{c}_m$ for the candidate models given in Table 11.1 are (−0.566, −0.226, 0.793)′ for the linear, (−0.799, 0.256, 0.544)′ for the emax, (−0.419, −0.397, 0.816)′ for the logisticl, and (−0.811, 0.324, 0.487)′ for the beta model. Table 11.2 shows the correlation matrix $\boldsymbol{R}$ of the corresponding contrast test statistics. Note that the contrasts are based on the three doses given in Stage 1; the correlations are high when the mean responses *at these doses* follow a similar pattern. The critical value for the maximum contrast test statistic is derived as 1.954.

TABLE 11.1 Candidate and Data-Generating Models Considered in the Example

Model		MED (mg)	Model Used As: Candidate Model	Model Used As: Data-Generating Model
linear	$f(d) = 0.006 * d$	100.0	X	X
emax	$f(d) = 1.32 * d/(20 + d)$	16.7	X	X
logistic1	$f(d) = 1.366238/(1 + \exp((150 - d)/25))$	143.9	X	
logistic2	$f(d) = 1.216281/(1 + \exp((100 - d)/20))$	99.5		X
beta	$f(d) = 4.8 * (d/260) * (1 - d/260)$	38.1	X	X

Notes: All models are standardized such that placebo has effect 0 and the maximal effect (over placebo) within the dose range is 1.2 (with the logistic models being slightly shifted). Candidate models are unique only up to location-scale variants.

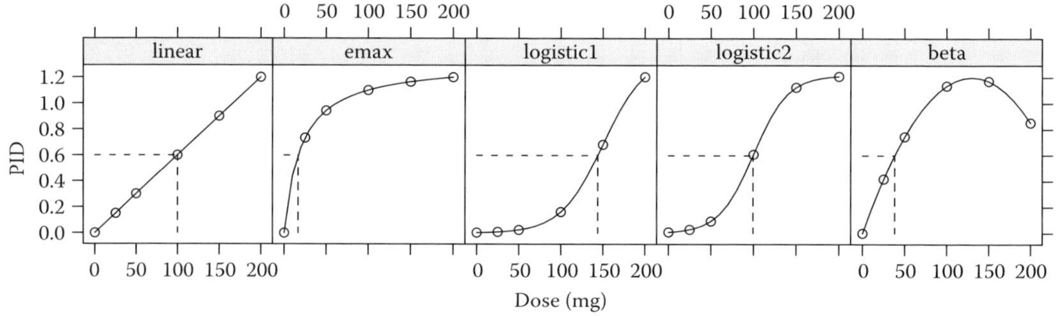

FIGURE 11.1 Models considered in the example, as specified in Table 11.1. Dashed lines indicate the MED and the minimal clinically relevant effect; open dots highlight the responses at the planned doses.

TABLE 11.2 Correlation Matrix ***R*** for the Contrast Test Statistics Based on Stage 1 of the Example, for the Candidate Models Given in Table 11.1

	linear	emax	logistic1	beta
linear	1.000	0.826	0.974	0.771
emax	0.826	1.000	0.677	0.996
logistic1	0.974	0.677	1.000	0.608
beta	0.771	0.996	0.608	1.000

As it accounts for the high correlations, this value is substantially smaller than the value of 2.302 resulting from a simple Bonferroni correction.

Second, we investigate the operating characteristics of the method through simulation. This will allow us, later in Section 11.4.4, to assess what impact it has if we replace the fixed second stage allocation used here by an adaptive allocation. We simulate 10,000 studies under each of five different data-generating dose–response models. Three of them match a candidate model, while one (the logistic) deviates from its candidate, as displayed in Table 11.1 and Figure 11.1. The fifth model (not shown) is a flat dose–response, to verify the Type I error rate control of the PoC step.

In the simulations, the power to establish PoC with the first cohort is at least 98% for the linear, the emax and the logistic2 models, while it is 85.7% for the beta model and 4.7% for the flat model. Thus, the sample size of the first stage provides high power for establishing PoC, and the Type I error

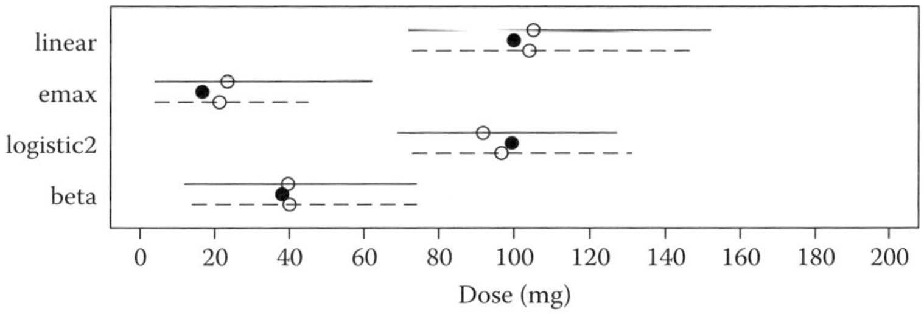

FIGURE 11.2 Simulated MED estimation in the example. Black dot: true MED; open dot: MED estimation, mean over 10,000 studies. Lines extend from the 5th to the 95th percentile. Solid lines: balanced overall sample sizes; dashed lines: adaptive second stage design (see Section 11.4.4).

rate is controlled at level $\alpha = 0.05$. The results of the MED estimation are displayed in Figure 11.2 (solid lines), based on those studies where PoC was achieved. It can be observed that, although the sample size of the first stage is sufficient for the PoC test, the overall sample size is not sufficient for an accurate MED estimation. Especially for the emax model, which is very steep around the MED, this is a reason for concern, since small departures from the true MED lead to largely different effects. Note also that the average bias is most pronounced for the logistic2 model, which deviates from the logistic1 candidate, followed by the emax model, where the MED is rather low and many patients are treated on far higher doses. It may be suspected that this can be improved if we move away from a fixed and balanced patient allocation toward more informative options. This is the topic of the next section.

11.4 Adaptive Design of Dose-Ranging Studies

We have demonstrated how adaptive analysis methods can address some difficulties that are typically encountered in dose-ranging studies due to model uncertainty. However, adaptive analysis methods have a limitation: they are unable to influence where and how the data are gathered. For instance, if emax were the true model in the example from Section 11.3.2, many patients would be treated on too high doses and would contribute relatively little information to the MED estimation. If during a trial there are indications for this type of situation, one may want to change the allocation scheme based on preliminary knowledge of the dose–response shape obtained thus far. Here, adaptive design methods come into play.

Adaptive design methods offer efficient ways to learn about the dose–response through repeated looks at the data being accrued in an ongoing trial. The emerging knowledge can be used to shape the design of the remaining trial parts such that they are most informative with respect to the objective of the trial. In the present section, we illustrate this idea with an approach proposed by Bornkamp et al. (2010). Several alternative approaches have been highlighted in Section 11.1. The proposal of Bornkamp et al. (2010) extends the method of Bretz, Pinheiro, and Branson (2005) presented in Section 11.3.1. Bayesian arguments are used to update and refine the current knowledge of the dose–response at one or more interim analyses. At each interim analysis, optimal design theory is used to determine the most informative design for the next patient cohort, based on the latest knowledge of the underlying dose–response.

In Sections 11.4.1 and 11.4.2, we first introduce essential notions of adaptive designs and optimal design theory (being particularly brief on the former). An adaptive implementation of optimal design concepts then yields the adaptive dose-finding approach by Bornkamp et al. (2010), which we present in Section 11.4.3. In Section 11.4.4, we revisit the example introduced earlier to illustrate the theory with a practical application.

11.4.1 Adaptive Designs

From their beginnings, adaptive designs have been conceived to be able to modify design aspects of an ongoing trial without undermining its validity or integrity. Their predecessors, sequential and group sequential designs, made it possible to stop a trial as soon as its conclusions become evident (e.g., Wald 1947; Jennison and Turnbull 2000). Adaptive designs add the option to adjust, for example, the sample size or the treatment allocation during an ongoing trial. Methods are also available for changes in the study population and many other types of adaptations. This scope is impressive, and it has attracted great attention from industry, academia, and regulatory agencies. Some aspects are still lively debated, but the merit of the general idea is undisputed: to provide a valid framework for useful trial adaptations in clinical development. As the present book is wholly dedicated to this topic, we refrain from a more thorough introduction and refer instead to the overviews by Vandemeulebroecke (2008), Bretz et al. (2009), Wassmer (2010), and the white paper published by PhRMA (2006) as a series of individual articles (including Dragalin 2006).

Despite the by now long-standing history of adaptive designs in general, the idea has only recently begun to be tailored more specifically to dose-ranging studies. We have noted a number of approaches in Section 11.1, among them GADA (Berry et al. 2001; Grieve and Krams 2005), a nonparametric up-and-down design (Ivanova, Bolognese, and Perevozskaya 2008), and several applications of optimal design theory in a model-based setting (Dragalin, Hsuan, and Padmanabhan 2007; Miller, Guilbaud, and Dette 2007; Smith 2010). One particular example of the latter type will be presented in Section 11.4.3. We refer to Dragalin et al. (2010) for an account of an extensive simulation study comparing the performance characteristics of several different adaptive dose-ranging designs in a number of realistic scenarios.

11.4.2 Optimal Designs

Optimal design theory addresses the question of how to design a trial in order to obtain maximal information on the trial's objective. In this context, a design $\xi = (\boldsymbol{x}, \boldsymbol{w})$ consists of several support points $\boldsymbol{x} = (x_1, \ldots, x_k)$ and their nonnegative weights $\boldsymbol{w} = (w_1, \ldots, w_k)$, where $\Sigma_{i=1}^{k} w_i = 1$. In a dose-ranging study, the support points are the employed doses (denoted $d_1, \ldots, d_k$ above), and the weights are the proportions of the total number of patients that are assigned to these doses (note that a weight may be 0). In practice, the sample sizes per dose are rounded to integers. The question is how to allocate the patients, and to which doses, to make the trial most informative.

To answer this question, it is necessary to formalize the trial's objective and define a measure that quantifies how well this objective is attained. Any design that maximizes (or, depending on its orientation, minimizes) this measure is then optimal. Different optimization strategies abound in optimal design theory for a multitude of possible trial objectives. In the interest of the present chapter, we focus on one particular method; we refer to Fedorov (1972) and Atkinson, Donev, and Tobias (2007) for more comprehensive overviews. This method, proposed by Dette et al. (2008), targets the MED estimation and quantifies its accuracy by a first-order approximation of the variance of the MED estimator (defined as in Section 11.3.1) based on one single dose–response model. Since this variance depends on the underlying model and its parameter vector, the sought-after design can only be locally optimal in the sense that it minimizes the MED estimator's variance only for this model and a specified best guess of the model parameters. Again, we face the potential issue of model misspecification. Dette et al. (2008) derived locally optimal designs for several common dose–response models and investigated their robustness against a wrong choice of the model or of its parameters. They found that although some designs cope well with wrong parameter guesses, all are highly sensitive to a wrong model choice.

This leads to the idea of model-robust designs, which perform reasonably well across a range of different models. The concept of candidate models lends itself naturally to this idea. Dette et al. (2008) proposed to minimize a weighted average of the variances of the MED estimators arising from M different candidate models. The weights are chosen a priori and reflect how strongly one believes in each of the candidate models. More specifically, for nonnegative prior weights $\alpha_1, \ldots, \alpha_M$, $\Sigma_{m-1}^{M} \alpha_m = 1$, a Bayesian MED-optimal design is any design $\xi = (\boldsymbol{x}, \boldsymbol{w})$ that minimizes

$$\sum_{m=1}^{M} \alpha_m \ln V_m(\xi, \boldsymbol{\theta}_m),$$

where $V_m(\xi, \boldsymbol{\theta}_m)$ is a first-order approximation of the variance of the MED estimator based on the mth candidate model and parameter vector $\boldsymbol{\theta}_m$. It is Bayesian in the sense that it depends on what can be interpreted as a discrete prior distribution on the M candidate models: the weights $\alpha_1, \ldots, \alpha_M$. In practice, such designs are derived numerically.

Bayesian MED-optimal designs overcome the sensitivity of locally optimal designs to model misspecification. However, they introduce a new element of choice: the prior model weights. An upfront specification of how strongly one believes in the different models will often be difficult, and misspecification of the model weights may be an issue just as much as model misspecification itself. Again, a possible remedy is adaptivity. We can perform interim analyses that provide the opportunity to adjust the model weights, and along with them also the model parameters, during the ongoing trial. This is presented in the next section.

11.4.3 Adaptively Designed Dose-Ranging Studies

In Section 11.3.1, we have outlined a procedure that demonstrates how adaptivity can cope with uncertainty in the analysis of a dose-ranging study. We now extend this procedure by adding adaptive design features to it. More specifically, we apply principles of optimal design theory at one or more interim analyses, each time optimizing the design of the next cohort based on the most up-to-date knowledge of the underlying dose–response. We assume that a grid $\boldsymbol{x}$ of possible doses is at hand (e.g., based on manufacturing constraints), so that we only decide on the allocation of patients to these doses, that is, on the weight vector $\boldsymbol{w}$, for each cohort. We further assume that the number of cohorts and the total sample size of each cohort are fixed.

As before, we start by choosing several candidate dose–response models f_m. However, we now specify prior distributions, rather than only best guesses, for the model parameters. We use a normal-inverse gamma prior for the location and scale parameters and the variance of the response (implying marginal t-distributions for the location and the scale and a marginal inverse-gamma distribution for the variance, cf. O'Hagan and Forster 2004, p. 305–7), and independent (scaled) beta distributions with mode equal to the best guess for the parameters of the standardized models. In addition, we specify nonnegative initial model weights $\alpha_1, \ldots, \alpha_M$, $\Sigma_{m=1}^{M} \alpha_m = 1$, reflecting our a priori beliefs in each of the candidate models. Finally, we choose a patient allocation for the first study cohort based on practical considerations.

After the first cohort, we perform an interim analysis with the aim of optimally designing the next cohort. This is accomplished by updating the model weights and parameter vectors based on the observed data within a Bayesian framework, and then allocating the next cohort such that the weighted average variance of the MED estimators, using the posterior weights and parameters, is minimized. More precisely, the posterior model weights α_m^{post} are proportional to

$$\alpha_m \int p_m(y \mid \boldsymbol{\theta}_m) q_m(\boldsymbol{\theta}_m) d\boldsymbol{\theta}_m,$$

where $p_m(y|\boldsymbol{\theta}_m)$ is the likelihood of $\boldsymbol{\theta}_m$ under the mth model at the observed responses y, and q_m is the density of the prior distribution for $\boldsymbol{\theta}_m$. Posterior estimates $\hat{\boldsymbol{\theta}}_m^{\text{post}}$ for the parameter vectors are derived as those maximizing $p_m(y|\boldsymbol{\theta}_m)q_m(\boldsymbol{\theta}_m)$. The allocation of the next cohort is determined by minimizing

$$\sum_{m=1}^{M} \alpha_m^{\text{post}} \ln V_m(\xi, \hat{\boldsymbol{\theta}}_m^{\text{post}}),$$

where V_m is defined as in Section 11.4.2. Here, $\xi = (\boldsymbol{x}, \boldsymbol{w})$ is the cumulative design; that is, $\boldsymbol{w}$ specifies the partitioning of the total sample size (up to and including the next cohort) to the different doses.

The same steps are repeated at all subsequent interim analyses. Finally, at the end of the trial, the parameter vectors are updated one last time, and the study is analyzed by the procedure outlined in Section 11.3.1.

11.4.4 Example

To illustrate this approach, we revisit the example introduced in Section 11.3.2. There, the analysis after the first cohort had been used to test PoC and trigger the initiation of the second cohort. Now, we take additional advantage of this interim analysis for an optimal allocation of the second cohort based on the current knowledge of the dose–response. The setting is the same as in Section 11.3.2, except that the fixed allocation of the second cohort (balanced overall allocation) is replaced by the adaptive optimal design outlined above. We use uniform prior model weights and weakly informative prior distributions for the model parameters and the variance of the response.

Figure 11.3 shows the average patient allocation to the different doses, based on those studies where PoC was achieved. There is an obvious shift toward smaller doses for the models with a small MED (emax and beta), compared to the balanced allocation. The placebo group is large in all cases, which may be attributed to its role as an anchor of the curve and its involvement in the effect estimation of all other doses. The estimation results are included in Figure 11.2 (dashed lines). Some bias reduction can be observed for the linear, the emax, and most notably for the logistic2 model. The variability (interpercentile range) is somewhat reduced for the linear model, and strongly reduced for the emax model. Overall, the introduction of adaptivity into the design of the second stage has improved the MED estimation.

There is, however, also reason for a word of caution. First, one can ask whether the extent of improvement in this example is meaningful, and whether it is worth the extra logistical effort of the adaptive design. The still rather large variability indicates that it may be worth considering a larger overall sample size. The inclusion of more doses in the first stage or conducting more than one interim analysis could also be explored. Second, the benefit of the adaptive allocation is not always as predictable as it is here for the emax model. For example, the large shift in patient allocation for the beta model seems to have relatively little effect. It would also be interesting to investigate the influence of the model selection before the final fit (e.g., let it depend on the minimum AIC rather than on the maximum contrast test statistic). Third, improving the MED estimation does not imply improving the dose–response estimation. We illustrate this with the mean absolute estimation error, which is averaging the absolute errors occurring in the different simulation runs. This measure can be computed for the estimation not only of the MED, but also of the whole dose–response curve. In the latter case, the absolute error for a

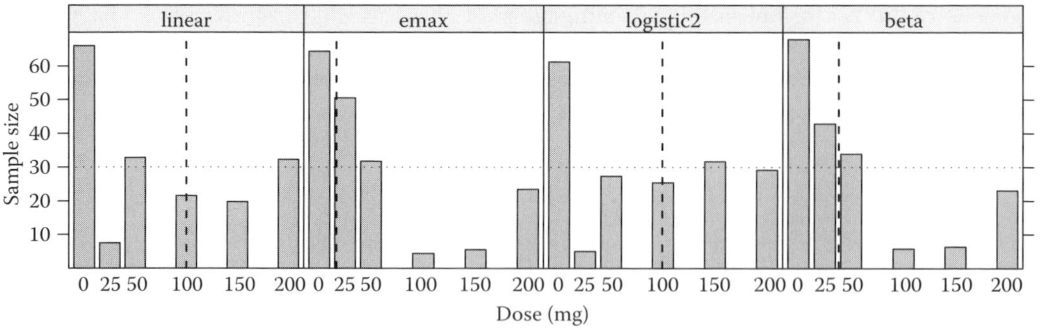

FIGURE 11.3 Average patient allocation to the different doses in the example using the adaptive second stage design (overall, i.e., both cohorts together). Dotted horizontal line: balanced overall sample sizes; dashed vertical lines: MED as given in Table 11.1.

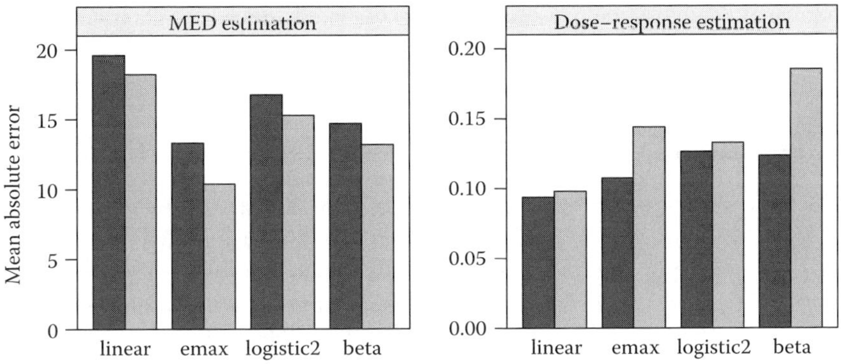

FIGURE 11.4 Mean absolute errors for the estimation of the MED and of the dose–response curve in the example. Black bars: balanced overall sample sizes; gray bars: adaptive second stage design.

particular simulation run is the average across the applied doses of the absolute deviations between the true responses and the predicted responses at these doses (based on the finally fitted model). Figure 11.4 shows the results of this assessment: the improved MED estimation comes at the cost of a less accurate dose–response estimation. Finally, it should be noted that these caveats are not confined to this particular example. Pinheiro et al. (2010) have drawn similar conclusions from a large-scale simulation study. Design adaptations in dose-ranging studies can be of benefit in certain situations, but there is no silver bullet approach that always leads to superior performance.

11.5 Summary

The assessment of the dose–response relationship and the search for an optimal dose are key steps in any drug development program; they can be decisive for its overall success. However, many dose-ranging studies addressing these objectives fail to provide precise and convincing results. One reason may be the desire to proceed to a pivotal trial as quickly as possible, at the risk of selecting a suboptimal dose. Another reason lies in the many aspects of uncertainty that come with the early position of dose-finding in a development program. How shall the dose–response curve be modeled? Where should we expect the relevant dose range? Are there more informative patient allocation schemes than the balanced one? These and similar aspects of uncertainty complicate the design and analysis of dose-ranging studies. Erroneous assumptions can lead to poor statistical properties.

In this chapter, we have demonstrated how this issue can be addressed by the introduction of adaptive elements. This applies to the analysis of a study as well as to its design: both can be adapted depending on emerging knowledge of the dose–response shape. A number of alternative procedures are available for implementing this idea. We have noted several approaches, and have then focused on one of them for the sake of a more concrete presentation of the involved considerations. We emphasize that the key ideas apply much more generally. For example, it is advisable to provide sufficient flexibility to the modeling procedure, be it through the choice of a flexible enough model or through the use of several candidate models. Also, one or more interim analyses can provide valuable opportunities to reduce the initial uncertainty and, for example, to adjust the patient allocation accordingly. In all cases, it is important to cautiously investigate the behavior of the chosen procedure in different scenarios, to be able to weigh its benefits against any possible disadvantages. In doing so, practical considerations such as study conduct logistics should also be taken into account.

In summary, concepts of adaptivity may be well suited to cope with some of the issues typically encountered in dose-finding. Also, some of the caveats that are warranted in confirmatory Phase III trials might be less critical in the learning phase of a development program (cf. Sheiner 1997). A blind belief in the promises of advanced statistical methods is of course never indicated. Yet, further research progress and a more frequent consideration of application—with careful upfront evaluation of each procedure's particular properties—may be able to improve the drug development process as a whole.

Acknowledgment

We would like to thank Ursula Schramm for sharing her clinical expertise with respect to the example.

References

Abelson, R. P., and Tukey, J. W. (1963). Efficient utilization of non-numerical information in quantitative analysis: General theory and the case of simple order. *Annals of Mathematical Statistics*, 34: 1347–69.

Atkinson, A. C., Donev, A. N., and Tobias, R. (2007). *Optimum Experimental Designs, with SAS*. Oxford: University Press.

Berry, D. A., Müller, P., Grieve, A. P., Smith, M., Parke, T., Balazek, R., Mitchard, N., and Krams, M. (2001). Adaptive Bayesian designs for dose-ranging drug trials. In *Case Studies in Bayesian Statistics V. Lecture Notes in Statistics 162,* eds. C. Gatsonis, R. E. Kass, B. Carlin, A. Carriquiry, A. Gelman, I. Verdinelli, and M. West. New York: Springer.

Bornkamp, B. (2006). *Comparison of model-based and model-free approaches for the analysis of dose response studies*. Diploma thesis, University of Dortmund.

Bornkamp, B., Bretz, F., Dette, H., and Pinheiro, J. (2010). Response adaptive dose-finding under model uncertainty. *Submitted.*

Bornkamp, B., Bretz, F., Dmitrienko, A., Enas, G., Gaydos, B., Hsu, C.-H., König, et al. (2007). Innovative approaches for designing and analyzing adaptive dose-ranging trials. *Journal of Biopharmaceutical Statistics,* 17: 965–1032.

Bornkamp, B., Pinheiro, J., and Bretz, F. (2009). MCPMod: An R package for the design and analysis of dose-finding studies. *Journal of Statistical Software,* 29 (7): 1–23.

Bretz, F., Hsu, J., Pinheiro, J., and Liu, Y. (2008). Dose finding—A challenge in statistics. *Biometrical Journal,* 50: 480–504.

Bretz, F., König, F., Brannath, W., Glimm, E., and Posch, M. (2009). Tutorial in biostatistics. Adaptive designs for confirmatory clinical trials. *Statistics in Medicine* , 28: 1181–1217.

Bretz, F., Pinheiro, J., and Branson, M. (2005). Combining multiple comparisons and modeling techniques in dose–response studies. *Biometrics,* 61: 738–48.

Capizzi, T., Survill, T. T., and Heyse, J. F. (1992). An empirical and simulated comparison of some tests for detecting progressiveness of response with increasing doses of a compound. *Biometrical Journal,* 34: 275–89.

Dette, H., Bretz, F., Pepelyshev, A., and Pinheiro, J. (2008). Optimal designs for dose-finding studies. *JASA,* 103: 1225–37.

Dragalin, V. (2006). Adaptive designs: Terminology and classification. *Drug Information Journal,* 40: 425–35.

Dragalin, V., Bornkamp, B., Bretz, F., Miller, F., Padmanabhan, S. K., Patel, N., Perevozskaya, I., Pinheiro, J., and Smith, J. R. (2010). A simulation study to compare new adaptive dose-ranging designs. To appear in *Statistics in Biopharmaceutical Research.*

Dragalin, V., Hsuan, F., and Padmanabhan, S. K. (2007). Adaptive designs for dose-finding studies based on sigmoid E_{max} model. *Journal of Biopharmaceutical Statistics,* 17: 1051–70.

Dunnett, C. W. (1955). A multiple comparison procedure for comparing several treatments with a control. *JASA,* 50:1096–1121.

FDC Report. (1991). FDC Reports from May 6th, 1991. *The Pink Sheet,* 53 (18): 14–15.

Fedorov, V. V. (1972). *Theory of Optimal Experiments.* New York: Academic Press.

Genz, A., and Bretz, F. (2002). Methods for the computation of multivariate *t*-probabilities. *Journal of Computational and Graphical Statistics,* 11: 950–71.

Genz, A., and Bretz, F. (2009). *Computation of Multivariate Normal and t Probabilities.* Lecture Notes in Statistics 195. Heidelberg: Springer.

Grieve, A. P., and Krams, M. (2005). ASTIN: A Bayesian adaptive dose–response trial in acute stroke. *Clinical Trials,* 2: 340–51.

Hall, D. B., Meier, U., and Diener, H.-C. (2005). A group sequential adaptive treatment assignment design for proof of concept and dose selection in headache trials. *Contemporary Clinical Trials,* 26: 349–64.

Hochberg, Y. (1988). A sharper Bonferroni procedure for multiple tests of significance. *Biometrika,* 75: 800–802.

Holm, S. (1979). A simple sequentially rejective multiple test procedure. *Scandinavian Journal of Statistics,* 6: 65–70.

ICH E4. (1994). Dose response information to support drug registration. CPMP/ICH/378/95.

ICH E9. (1998). Statistical principles for clinical trials. CPMP/ICH/363/96.

Ivanova, A., Bolognese, J. A., and Perevozskaya, I. (2008). Adaptive dose-finding based on *t*-statistic for dose–response trials. *Statistics in Medicine,* 27: 1581–92.

Jennison, C., and Turnbull, B. W. (2000). *Group Sequential Methods with Applications to Clinical Trials.* Boca Raton, FL: Chapman & Hall.

Klingenberg, B. (2009). Proof of concept and dose estimation with binary responses under model uncertainty. *Statistics in Medicine,* 28: 274–92.

Krams, M., Lees, K. R., Hacke, W., Grieve, A. P., Orgogozo, J.-M., and Ford, G. A. (2003). Acute Stroke Therapy by Inhibition of Neutrophils (ASTIN). An adaptive dose–response study of UK-279,276 in acute ischemic stroke. *Stroke,* 34: 2543–48.

Leonov, S., and Miller, S. (2009). An adaptive optimal design for the E_{max} model and its application in clinical trials. *Journal of Biopharmaceutical Statistics,* 19: 360–85.

Maurer, W., Hothorn, L. A., and Lehmacher, W. (1995). Multiple comparisons in drug clinical trials and preclinical assays: a-priori ordered hypotheses. In *Biometrie in der chemisch-pharmazeutischen Industrie 6,* ed. J. Vollman. Stuttgart: Fischer.

Miller, F., Guilbaud, O., and Dette, H. (2007). Optimal designs for estimating the interesting part of a dose-effect curve. *Journal of Biopharmaceutical Statistics,* 17: 1097–1115.

O'Hagan, A., and Forster, J. (2004). *Kendall's Advanced Theory of Statistics 2B: Bayesian Inference,* 2nd ed. London: Arnold.

PhRMA. (2006). PhRMA working group on adaptive designs: Full White Paper. *Drug Information Journal,* 40: 421–84.

Pinheiro, J., Bretz, F., and Branson, M. (2006). Analysis of dose–response studies—Modeling approaches. In *Dose Finding in Drug Development,* ed. N. Ting. New York: Springer.

Pinheiro, J., Sax, F., Antonijevic, Z., Bornkamp, B., Bretz, F., Chuang-Stein, C., Dragalin, V., et al. (2010). Adaptive and model-based dose-ranging trials: Quantitative evaluation and recommendations. White Paper of the PhRMA working group on adaptive dose-ranging studies. To appear in *Statistics in Biopharmaceutical Research.*

Potter, D. M. (2008). Phase I studies of chemotherapeutic agents in cancer patients: A review of the designs. *Journal of Biopharmaceutical Statistics,* 16: 579–604.

Roy, A., Hsu, C.-H., Sanil, A., Gillespie, W., and Pinheiro, J. (2010). Value of exposure–response modeling for dose selection and dose–response characterization. *In preparation.*

Ruberg, S. J. (1995a). Dose response studies. I. Some design considerations. *Journal of Biopharmaceutical Statistics,* 5: 1–14.

Ruberg, S. J. (1995b). Dose response studies. II. Analysis and interpretation. *Journal of Biopharmaceutical Statistics,* 5: 15–42.

Sheiner, L. B. (1997). Learning versus confirming in clinical drug development. *Clinical Pharmacology & Therapeutics,* 61: 275–91.

Smith, J. R. (2010). MULTOB: A new multi-objective design approach for use in dose-ranging clinical trials. *Submitted.*

Tamhane, A. C., Hochberg, Y., and Dunnett, C. W. (1996). Multiple test procedures for dose-finding. *Biometrics,* 52: 21–37.

Tukey, J. W., Ciminera, J. L., and Heyse, J. F. (1985). Testing the statistical certainty of a response to increasing doses of a drug. *Biometrics,* 41: 295–301.

Vandemeulebroecke, M. (2008). Group sequential and adaptive designs—A review of basic concepts and points of discussion. *Biometrical Journal,* 50: 541–57.

Vogt, L., Navis, G., and de Zeeuw, D. (2005). Individual titration for maximal blockade of the renin-angiotensin system in proteinuric patients: A feasible strategy? *Journal of the American Society of Nephrology,* 16: 53–57.

Wald, A. (1947). *Sequential Analysis.* New York: Wiley.

Wassmer, G. (2010). Adaptive interim analyses in clinical trials. *Handbook of Adaptive Designs in Pharmaceutical and Clinical Development. Chapter 8 in this book.*

Weir, C. J., Spiegelhalter, D. J., and Grieve, A. P. (2007). Flexible design and efficient implementation of adaptive dose-finding studies. *Journal of Biopharmaceutical Statistics,* 17: 1033–50.

Westfall, P. H., and Krishen, A. (2001). Optimally weighted, fixed sequence and gatekeeper multiple testing procedures. *Journal of Statistical Planning and Inference,* 99: 25–40.

12

Seamless Phase I/II Designs

Vladimir Dragalin
Center for Statistics in Drug Development

12.1 Introduction

The assumptions underlying traditional clinical oncology Phase I designs are that for most cytotoxic agents there is a direct relationship between the dose of a drug, its antitumor effect, and toxicity. Therefore, toxicity and antitumor activity increase with the increasing of the dose of the chemotherapeutic agent and there is a maximum tolerated dose (MTD) that provides clinical activity with acceptable dose-limiting toxicity (DLT). Thus, toxicity has been seen as a surrogate for potentially effective doses. Based on this assumption, the MTD is assumed to be the dose level with the most promising prospects for efficacy. The traditional dose-escalation designs (like 3 + 3, see Ivanova (2006) for a comprehensive overview) are used in Phase I trial to find the MTD of the drug. A Phase II trial is then conducted to determine whether the drug has promising effects at the MTD. With biological agents, acting on highly specific targets expressed in cancer cells, the dose-efficacy and dose-toxicity curves may differ from those for cytotoxic agents, and efficacy may occur at doses that do not induce clinically significant toxicity. For trials involving these targeted therapy agents, occurrence of drug-related biological effects has been suggested as an alternative primary endpoint besides toxicity consideration. The evaluation of such therapies requires specialized trial designs. Instead of conducting a Phase I trial for toxicity and a separate Phase II trial for efficacy, these designs integrate the two phases into one. They are called seamless Phase I/II designs because they combine into a single trial, objectives traditionally addressed in separate trials. However, there is a variety of other circumstances where it is useful to address safety and efficacy simultaneously. Here is just a sample of references with such examples: graft-versus-host disease versus rejection in transplant complications (Gooley et al. 1994); biologic agent IL-12 in malignant melanoma (Thall and Russell 1998); antiretroviral treatment for children with HIV (O'Quigley, Hughes, and Fenton 2001); allogeneic stem cell transplantation for leukemia (Dragalin, Fedorov, and Wu 2008); prevention of venous thrombosis (Dragalin, Fedorov, and Wu 2008), and so on. These designs still require an initial dose-escalation period to designate the admissible doses, but the DLT rates are assessed during this period as well as throughout the trial. This distinguishes them from designs for Phase II dose-ranging studies where patients can be allocated to all available doses from the very beginning of the trial.

Most parts of the proposed designs are mainly concerned with individual ethics: doing what is best for current patients in the trial. The continual reassessment method (CRM) was the first such method that formulates the goal of a dose escalation in Phase I trial as to maximize patient gain (O'Quigley, Pepe, and Fisher (1990)). Thall and Russell (1998) used similar methods to accommodate efficacy and toxicity. Notice however that although these designs rely on a noble intention to maximize individual gain by allocating the patient to the best known dose, the individual ethics may be well compromised by the poor learning about the best dose with such a design.

In contrast, traditional optimal design of experiments, like D-optimal designs (Atkinson and Donev, 1992), are concerned mainly with collective ethics: doing in the dose-finding study what is best for future patients who stand to benefit from the results of the trial. Dragalin and Fedorov (2006) made one of the first attempts to formalize the goal of a dose-finding study as a penalized D-optimal design problem: find the design that maximizes the information (collective (society) ethics) but under the control of the total penalty for treating patients in the trial (individual (all individuals in the trial) ethics).

In this chapter, I will review these various designs from a statistical standpoint. In particular, I will introduce a class of models that can be used in seamless Phase I/II clinical trials in which patient response is characterized by two dependent binary outcomes, one for efficacy, and one for toxicity using a unified notation for easy comparison. Then I will propose a classification of these designs in three large classes and describe some representative designs from each class. It is important to note that this paper is not a review of the extensive literature describing simulated properties of these designs, nor does it present any new simulation studies comparing these designs, nor will it promote a particular design. Instead, this paper should be considered an introduction to the differences and subtleties among the designs from the recent literature. I hope this will help statisticians and investigators in general in Phase I/II clinical trials to understand what design options are available, and what are their strengths and challenges. In Section 12.2, I formulate the seamless Phase I/II study objectives. In Section 12.3, I introduce the parametric models that are used as working models for many of the proposed adaptive designs. In Section 12.4, I describe the nonparametric designs and model-based designs. Finally, in Section 12.5, I draw some conclusions.

12.2 Study Objectives

For seamless Phase I/II designs the outcome in each patient is one of the four possible cases: no efficacy and no toxicity, efficacy without toxicity, no efficacy and toxicity, and efficacy and toxicity. Efficacy may take the form of a usual tumor response (shrinkage), or may be based on a presumed surrogate marker, such as the level of a marker from a blood test or a dichotomized version of several measurements reflecting drug efficacy. Toxicity is usually a DLT. Let $Y \in \{0, 1\}$ indicate occurrence of an efficacy response and let $Z \in \{0, 1\}$ of a toxicity response with 1 for occurrence and 0 for no occurrence. Therefore, a patient outcome is a pair (Y, Z). In some applications, toxicity is fatal and the efficacy response is censored; that is, cannot be observed. In this situation, there are three kinds of outcome possible at each dose level: toxicity, nontoxicity and nonefficacy, and efficacy without toxicity. We will call these toxicity, no response and success, respectively. It is reasonable to assume that the probability of no response decreases monotonically with dose and the marginal probability of toxicity increases monotonically with dose. However, the probability of success may be nonmonotone in dose. Hence, the study objective can be formulated as to find the dose that maximizes the probability of success.

Generally speaking, the goals are to:

1. Limit patient allocation to extreme doses of little interest: keep to a minimum both the number of patients assigned to a toxic dose and the number of patients treated at a dose with low efficacy,
2. Escalate quickly to the correct region of the dose-outcome relationship: safe doses that are close to therapeutic effect, and

3. Accurately determine the MTD and estimate the optimal safe dose (OSD) maximizing the probability of success.

We distinguish two formulations: frequentist and Bayesian.

12.2.1 Frequentist Formulation

Patients have a staggered entry in the trial and are allocated to one of the available doses D from some fixed set of doses $X = \{x_1, x_2,\ldots,x_n\}$. The study objective is based on fixed trial-specific standards for the minimum acceptable response rate q_E and the maximum acceptable toxicity rate q_T. Define $d_E^* z$ as the minimum dose d for which:

$$\Pr(Y=1\,|\,D=d)\geq q_E, \tag{12.1}$$

and d_T^* as the maximum dose d for which:

$$\Pr(Z=1\,|\,D=d)\leq q_T. \tag{12.2}$$

Dose d_E^* is called the minimum effective dose (MED) and d_T^* is called the MTD. The OSD is the dose d^* in the interval $[d_E^*,d_T^*]$ maximizing the probability of success:

$$\Pr(Y=1,Z=0\,|\,D=d).$$

The goals are to select the OSD for Phase II clinical trial, to estimate response and toxicity probabilities at that dose, and to stop the trial early if it becomes unlikely that any dose is safe and effective; that is, $[d_E^*,d_T^*]=\varnothing$.

In case of trinary outcome, one does not have the marginal distribution of efficacy response Y. Therefore, in this case we may define d_E^* as the minimum dose d for which:

$$\Pr(Y=1,Z=0\,|\,D=d)\geq q_E.$$

An alternative way would be to define d_E^* as the minimum dose d for which:

$$\Pr(Y=0,Z=0\,|\,D=d)\leq q_E.$$

12.2.2 Bayesian Formulation

In the Bayesian framework, a parametric model for the dose-outcome relationship is assumed together with a prior distribution for the parameter vector. For example, having a prior for the probability of success and the probability of toxicity at each dose level:

$$\pi_E(d,\theta)=\Pr(Y=1,Z=0\,|\,D=d),$$

$$\pi_T(d,\theta)=\Pr(Z=1\,|\,D=d),$$

we can update the posterior distribution of the parameter θ as the data become available from each successive patient (or cohort of patients), and, consequently, also the posterior distribution for probabilities of success and toxicity at each dose level. Given current data $\mathcal{F}$ a dose d has acceptable efficacy if:

$$\Pr(\pi_E(d,\theta)>q_E\,|\,\mathcal{F})\geq p_E, \tag{12.3}$$

and d has acceptable toxicity if:

$$\Pr(\pi_T(d,\theta) < q_T \mid \mathcal{F}) \geq p_T, \tag{12.4}$$

where p_E and p_T are fixed probability cutoffs and q_E and q_T are as above the minimum acceptable success rate and the maximum acceptable toxicity rate, respectively. A dose d is acceptable if it satisfies both Equations 12.3 and 12.4. The next patient (or cohort) is allocated to the acceptable dose level that maximizes $\Pr(\pi_E(d, \theta) > q_E \mid \mathcal{F})$. When prespecified stopping rules have been met, the OSD is selected according to predefined decision criteria, based on the data from all the patients treated. The goals are to first determine if there is a dose d^* that satisfies Equations 12.3 and 12.4 criteria. If there is such a dose, then an additional goal is to treat a sufficiently large number of patients at acceptable doses to estimate $\pi_E(d^*, \theta)$ and $\pi_T(d^*, \theta)$ with reasonable accuracy.

12.3 Dose–Response Models

One of the most important and often the most difficult part of designing the new model-based seamless Phase I/II trials is choosing the working model (i.e., the functional form) of the dose-outcome curve. It is important that a trained statistician be involved in choosing the mathematical model. And, it is critical that the statistician and clinicians both look at plots displaying this relationship to have a clear understanding of the mathematical model that is being proposed. There are a variety of models to choose from, some of them simpler (with few parameters), others more complex. The art of choosing the right model consists in using a parsimonious model—a model that is simple and requires less information (i.e., fewer patients) to get a more precise estimate of the dose-outcome curve, but flexible enough to accurately depict the true dose-outcome relationship. A thorough simulation study should be conducted to investigate many aspects of the design, including the working model, and to check the sensitivity of design operating characteristics under deviations from the assumptions. We present here a set of such models that have been considered in previous publications or are ready for being used in the new applications.

Define the following probabilities

$$p_{yz}(x) = p_{yz}(x;\theta) = \Pr(Y = y, Z = z \mid D = x), \quad y,z = 0,1.$$

12.3.1 Gumbel Model

In the univariate case, the probability of a response given a dose is expressed as the logistic cumulative distribution function of dose. A natural extension in the bivariate case is to express each of the four cell probabilities as an integral, over the corresponding region of the plane, of a bivariate logistic density function. If the dose x is transformed by the location parameter μ ($\mu_E = ED_{50}$, $\mu_T = TD_{50}$) and scale parameter σ to the standard doses:

$$x_E = \frac{x - \mu_E}{\sigma_E} \quad \text{for efficacy } Y, \text{and} \quad x_T = \frac{x - \mu_T}{\sigma_T} \quad \text{for safety } Z,$$

then individual cell probabilities $p_{yz}(x)$ can be derived:

$$\begin{aligned}
p_{11}(x) &= G(x_E, x_T),\\
p_{10}(x) &= G(x_E, \infty) - G(x_E, x_T),\\
p_{01}(x) &= G(\infty, x_T) - G(x_E, x_T),\\
p_{00}(x) &= 1 - G(x_E, \infty) - G(\infty, x_T) + G(x_E, x_T),
\end{aligned}$$

where $G(y, z)$ is the standard Gumbel distribution function given by:

$$G(y,z) = F(y)F(z)\{1+\alpha[1-F(y)][1-F(z)]\}, \quad -\infty < y,z < +\infty, \tag{12.5}$$

with $|\alpha| < 1$ and:

$$F(y) = \frac{1}{1+e^{-y}},$$

as the standard logistic distribution function. Here $\theta = (\mu_E, \sigma_E, \mu_T, \sigma_T, \alpha)$. A straightforward generalization is to replace $F(\cdot)$ in Equation 12.5 with any distribution function. A further generalization might be to replace the survival function $[1-F(\cdot)]$ in Equation 12.5 with an arbitrary positive nonincreasing function $g(\cdot)$ The latter is so-called Farlie–Gumbel–Morgenstern class of bivariate distributions.

12.3.2 Cox Bivariate Binary Model

Another model for efficacy and toxicity can be adapted from Cox's (1970, p. 107) general model of a bivariate binary response. We can express this as a six parameter model in the following way:

$$p_{11}(x) = \frac{e^{\alpha_{11}+\beta_{11}x}}{1+e^{\alpha_{01}+\beta_{01}x}+e^{\alpha_{10}+\beta_{10}x}+e^{\alpha_{11}+\beta_{11}x}}$$

$$p_{10}(x) = \frac{e^{\alpha_{10}+\beta_{10}x}}{1+e^{\alpha_{01}+\beta_{01}x}+e^{\alpha_{10}+\beta_{10}x}+e^{\alpha_{11}+\beta_{11}x}}$$

$$p_{01}(x) = \frac{e^{\alpha_{01}+\beta_{01}x}}{1+e^{\alpha_{01}+\beta_{01}x}+e^{\alpha_{10}+\beta_{10}x}+e^{\alpha_{11}+\beta_{11}x}}.$$

$$p_{00}(x) = \frac{1}{1+e^{\alpha_{01}+\beta_{01}x}+e^{\alpha_{10}+\beta_{10}x}+e^{\alpha_{11}+\beta_{11}x}}$$

Here $\theta = (\alpha_{11}, \beta_{11}, \alpha_{10}, \beta_{10}, \alpha_{01}, \beta_{01})$. The exponential functions in the model may be replaced by any other smooth strictly increasing positive function of x.

Unlike in the Gumbel model where the marginal probabilities of Y and Z are logistic in dose, in the Cox model marginal probabilities are, in general, neither logistic nor necessarily monotone with respect to dose. Rather, it is the conditional probabilities of response that are logistic in dose:

$$\Pr(Y=1|Z=0;D=x) = \frac{e^{\alpha_{10}+\beta_{10}x}}{1+e^{\alpha_{10}+\beta_{10}x}}.$$

12.3.3 Bivariate Probit Model

Assume V_1 and V_2 follow bivariate normal distribution with zero mean and variance–covariance matrix $\Sigma = \begin{pmatrix} 1 & \rho \\ \rho & 1 \end{pmatrix}$, where ρ can be viewed as the correlation between toxicity and efficacy. This correlation should be specified in advance or treated as an unknown parameter. The correlation can be negative or positive depending on the therapeutic area.

As in Gumbel model, we can define

$$p_{11}(x,\theta) = F(\theta_1^T f_1(x), \theta_2^T f_2(x), \rho)$$
$$= \int_{-\infty}^{\theta_1^T f_1(x)} \int_{-\infty}^{\theta_2^T f_2(x)} \frac{1}{2\pi|\Sigma|^{1/2}} \exp\left\{-\frac{1}{2}V^T\Sigma^{-1}V\right\} dv_1 dv_2,$$

where θ_1 and θ_2 are unknown parameters, T denotes transpose, and $f_1(x) = f_2(x) = (1,x)^T$.

The efficacy $p_{1\bullet} = \Pr(Y = 1|D = x)$ and toxicity $p_{\bullet 1} = \Pr(Z = 1|D = x)$ can be expressed as the marginal distributions of the bivariate normal distribution:

$$p_{1\bullet}(x,\theta) = F(\theta_1^T f_1(x)),$$

and:

$$p_{\bullet 1}(x,\theta) = F(\theta_2^T f_2(x)),$$

where:

$$F(v) = \int_{-\infty}^{v} \frac{1}{\sqrt{2\pi}} \exp(-u^2/2)du.$$

The other probabilities are defined as:

$$\begin{aligned} p_{10}(x,\theta) &= p_{1\bullet}(x,\theta) - p_{11}(x,\theta) \\ p_{01}(x,\theta) &= p_{\bullet 1}(x,\theta) - p_{11}(x,\theta) \\ p_{00}(x,\theta) &= 1 - p_{1\bullet}(x,\theta) - p_{\bullet 1}(x,\theta) + p_{11}(x,\theta). \end{aligned}$$

12.3.4 Continuation-Ratio Bivariate Binary Model

Another bivariate binary model can be used modeling the probability of toxicity and the conditional probability of efficacy given toxicity outcome:

$$\begin{aligned} p_{yz}(d) &= \Pr(Y = y, Z = z \mid D = d) \\ &= \Pr(Z = z \mid D = d) \cdot \Pr(Y = y \mid Z = z; D = d) \\ &= \frac{\exp\left(\frac{d-\mu_T}{\sigma_T} z\right)}{1+\exp\left(\frac{d-\mu_T}{\sigma_T}\right)} \cdot \frac{\exp\left(\frac{d-\mu_E-\omega z}{\sigma_E} y\right)}{1+\exp\left(\frac{d-\mu_E-\omega z}{\sigma_E}\right)}, \qquad y,z \in \{0,1\}. \end{aligned}$$

When $\omega = 0$ the model is equivalent to two independent logistic models. We will see in Section 12.3.6 that these are properties of the well known continuation-ratio model for trinary outcome.

12.3.5 Proportional Odds Model

In order to characterize patient outcome, Thall and Russel (1998) use a trinary ordinal variable U accounting for both efficacy and toxicity:

$$\begin{aligned} \{U = 0\} &= \{Y = 0, Z = 0\}, \\ \{U = 1\} &= \{Y = 1, Z = 0\}, \\ \{U = 2\} &= \{Z = 1\}. \end{aligned}$$

They propose the following proportional odds model for dose–response relationship:

$$logit\{\Pr(U \geq 1 | D = d)\} = \alpha_1 + \beta d,$$
$$logit\{\Pr(U = 2 | D = d)\} = \alpha_2 + \beta d, \tag{12.6}$$

with $\alpha_1 > \alpha_2$ and $\beta > 0$ (here *logit* $(p) = \log\{p/(1-p\})$. This implies:

$$\Pr(Z1 | D = d) = F(\alpha_2 + \beta d),$$

$$\Pr(Y = 1, Z = 0 | D = d) = F(\alpha_1 + \beta d) - F(\alpha_2 + \beta d)$$

$$= \frac{e^{\alpha_1 + \beta d} - e^{\alpha_2 + \beta d}}{[1 + e^{\alpha_1 + \beta d}][1 + e^{\alpha_2 + \beta d}]},$$

$$\Pr(Y = 1 | Z = 0; D = d) = \frac{F(\alpha_1 + \beta d) - F(\alpha_2 + \beta d)}{1 - F(\alpha_2 + \beta d)}$$

$$= \frac{e^{\alpha_1 + \beta d} - e^{\alpha_2 + \beta d}}{1 + e^{\alpha_1 + \beta d}}.$$

Of course, there are several alternatives to the Model 12.6. One may simply change the logit link function with F^{-1} for any c.d.f. F, for example, probit link function or using extreme value c.d.f. $F(x) = 1 - \exp(-\exp(x))$ to obtain the proportional hazards model. Another way is to relax the assumption of proportionality; that is, assume different slope parameters β_1 and β_2. Under these models, one cannot derive the correlation between the efficacy and toxicity responses.

12.3.6 Continuation-Ratio Model

An alternative way of modeling the dose–response in the trinary outcome case is continuation-ratio model in which the logarithm of ratios of probability of a response in each category to the probability of a response in categories from lower levels are assumed linear in dose:

$$\log \frac{\Pr(U = 1 | D = d)}{\Pr(U = 0 | D = d)} = \alpha_1 + \beta_1 d$$

$$\log \frac{\Pr(U = 2 | D = d)}{\Pr(U < 2 | D = d)} = \alpha_2 + \beta_2 d.$$

This implies:

$$\Pr(Z = 1 | D = d) = F(\alpha_2 + \beta_2 d), \tag{12.7}$$

$$\Pr(Y = 1, Z = 0 | D = d) = \frac{e^{\alpha_1 + \beta_1 d}}{[1 + e^{\alpha_1 + \beta_1 d}][1 + e^{\alpha_2 + \beta_2 d}]},$$

$$\Pr(Y = 1 | Z = 0; D = d) = F(\alpha_1 + \beta_1 d),$$

where $F(y)$ is the standard logistic distribution function.

Like in the Cox model, the conditional probability of response given nontoxicity is logistic in dose. Moreover, the marginal distribution of toxicity response is also logistic in dose.

12.3.7 Models Based on Bivariate Discrete Distributions

Braun (2002) proposed the following model for the joint distribution of the binary efficacy and toxicity responses:

$$\Pr(Y=y,Z=z\,|\,D=d) \tag{12.8}$$

$$=K(p_{1\bullet},P_Z,\psi)p_{1\bullet}^{y}(1-p_{1\bullet})^{1-y}p_{\bullet 1}^{z}(1-p_{\bullet 1})^{1-z}\psi^{yz}(1-\psi)^{1-yz},$$

$$(y,z\in\{0,1\},0<\psi<1),$$

where $K=\{\psi p_{1\bullet}p_{\bullet 1}+(1-\psi)(1-p_{1\bullet}p_{\bullet 1})\}^{-1}$ is a normalizing constant and both the marginal probability of efficacy $p_{1\bullet}$ and the marginal probability of toxicity $p_{\bullet 1}$ are two parameter logistic functions of dose. The parameter ψ is constant across all dose levels and governs the association between efficacy and toxicity responses: Y and Z are independent if $\psi = 1/2$ while $\psi > 1/2$ indicates positive association and $\psi < 1/2$ indicates negative association.

12.4 Designs

A large number of adaptive designs have been proposed and evaluated (mostly through extensive simulations) in the past two decades. Candidate designs are usually evaluated on the basis of both relative efficiency—accuracy of the recommended Phase II dose, number of patients, number of cohorts, dose allocations, and relative safety—proportion of underdosed/overdosed patients. They can be classified in three major groups: nonparametric designs, model-based Bayesian designs, and frequentist designs based on theory of optimal designs of experiments.

12.4.1 Nonparametric Designs

12.4.1.1 Model Free Designs

Gooley et al. (1994) investigated dose-escalation designs for Phase I/II clinical trials in bone marrow transplantation. There are actually two forms of toxicity curve here, but because they compete in the same sense that efficacy and toxicity do, we stick to our common notation and take the outcomes no rejection and graft-versus-host-disease (GVHD) to be efficacy and toxicity, respectively, where rejection and GVHD are assumed independent. There are no explicit assumptions about the dose-outcome curves, although all the scenarios considered are monotonic and shaped roughly like logistic response functions. The goal of the trial is to locate acceptable dose values from a (large) discrete set of doses. A dose d is considered acceptable if $\Pr(rejection|D=d) < c_1$ and $\Pr(GVHD|D=d) < c_2$ for c_1, $c_2 > 0$. The approach is to simulate the operating characteristics of a proposed design to determine whether study goals will be adequately met. Design performance metrics are basically the proportion of false positives and false negatives related to the question of whether a dose is acceptable. They also estimate the expected failures for each response curve and the expected sample size. Three designs are considered but the algorithms are quite similar. Initially, between 8 and 10 observations are taken and an up-and-down type of rule is used. If, based on a one-sided 80% confidence interval (CI) for the binomial proportion (based on the data observed so far), $\Pr(rejection) > c_1$ or $\Pr(GVHD) > c_2$ the trial is terminated. The dose is modified if $\Pr(rejection)$ or $\Pr(GVHD)$ is excessive at the current dose. A dose is excessive if the smallest proportion of events at which the lower limit of a one sided $(1-\alpha)$% CI exceeds $c_1 = 0.05$ for rejection or $c_2 = 0.15$ for GVHD.

If the incidence of GVHD is determined to be too high, then the dose is reduced by one level given that rejection is not excessive at this lower dose. Phase II part is restarted. If, however, rejection has already been found to be excessive at this dose then stop the trial and declare that there is no acceptable dose.

If the incidence of rejection is too high, then there is a move up by one dose level as long as it has been concluded that $\Pr(GVHD) < c_2$ so far at this dose. Phase II part is restarted. If, however, GVHD has already been found to be excessive at this dose then stop the trial and declare that there is no acceptable dose. If, in Phase II part, 20 patients have been observed at dose d and no limits for rejection or GVHD have been reached, then the trial terminates and dose d is selected.

The presented operating characteristics describe how often a dose that was acceptable was found to be unacceptable (and why) as well as the reverse scenario. Also estimates of the expected sample sizes and rates for GVHD and rejection were provided. The procedures are completely ad hoc and simulations were run for only three scenarios, so no interesting conclusions can be drawn without comparisons to other methods. It is interesting that Braun (2002) chose to compare his bivariate CRM (bCRM) design only with these methods. Even more interesting is the fact that the bCRM design was not found to be superior, but rather to be roughly as good as Gooley's procedures B and C.

12.4.1.2 Urn Designs

Durham, Flournoy, and Li (1998) proposed a sequential design for maximizing the probability of a favorable response. The problem is formulated with the trinary model in which efficacy is censored if toxicity occurs. Probability of toxicity $\Pr(Z = 1|D = d)$ and probability of efficacy given nontoxicity $\Pr(Y = 1|Z = 0; D = d)$ are assumed to be cumulative distribution functions of dose. Observations are taken from a finite, discrete dose set. However, it is assumed that patient outcome is observed only as success or failure. The goal is to allocate patients as much as possible to the dose with maximal success rate or at doses that have rates close to this. They also seek a sampling procedure with the property that treatment assignments will converge to the global maximum (assuming that it exists)—even when the success curve is not unimodal.

Allocation is according to the following randomized polya urn: The initial urn contains at least one ball to represent each dose and exactly one control ball. At each stage, a ball is drawn with replacement. The patient is allocated to the associated dose and if the outcome is successful, a ball of the same dose is added to the urn. If a failure occurs, no new ball is added. If a control ball is drawn then one new control ball is added. Note that control balls are relevant only to the stopping rule, and that the urn becomes increasingly biased in favor of doses that have been successful. There is a stopping rule when a control ball has been drawn v times. Exact operating characteristics for the urn procedure can be expressed in terms of this stopping variable v.

It is possible to compute expected number of successes and failures for each dose given that v control balls have been drawn. This allows the computation of the expected sample size per dose and hence the expected total sample size. While an optimizing up-and-down procedure is described along with a stochastic approximation scheme (on a continuous dose set); there are no direct comparisons drawn. The one relevant feature seems to be that unimodality is required for the up-and-down and stochastic approximation methods to converge (in some sense) to the dose with the maximal success rate.

In a follow-up publication, Hardwick and Stout (2001) compared these three designs with their unimodal bandit design. The latter has two components: an allocation rule and a curve fitting scheme. The dependencies among the doses were taken into consideration only by the curve fit and not by a joint prior distribution on the dose–response rates. The allocation rule depends on approximations to Gittins indices for the problem in which the bandit arms are independent. The bandit design performed better than all other procedures, with the optimizing up-and-down procedure generally coming in second.

12.4.1.3 Directed Walk Designs

Hardwick, Meyer, and Stout (2003) extended the investigation of different nonparametric (model-free) designs called directed walk designs for dose–response problems with competing failure modes.

They use three dose–response functions: $R(d) = \Pr(Z = 1|D = d), Q(d) = \Pr(Y = 1|Z = 0|D = d)$, and $P(d) = \Pr(Y = 1, Z = 0|D = d)$. It is assumed that both $R(d)$ and $Q(d)$ are nondecreasing in dose and $P(d)$ is unimodal. Moreover, it is assumed that $\Pr(Y = 1|Z = 0|D = d) = \Pr(Y = 1|D = d)$, therefore $P(d) = Q(d)[1 - R(d)]$.

Numerous parametric procedures have been considered in the simulation study along with several nonparametric ones. Dose values are denoted as s_i, $i = 1,\ldots,k$ because they are normalized versions of d_i to fit within (0, 1). For each method, the paper describes how to fit the efficacy function, Q. In each case, the toxicity function R is fit the same way. Let x_j be the number of successes out of m_j trials so far from Q. Then if $q_j = Q(s_j)$, $\hat{q}_j = x_j / m_j, j = 1,\ldots,k$, where k is the number of doses.

The likelihood function is $$\mathcal{L} = \prod_{j=1}^{k} \binom{m_j}{x_j} q_j^{x_j} (1-q_j)^{m_j - x_j}.$$

The following parametric models are used for fitting Q (and similarly R):

1. *Two-parameter logistic with maximum likelihood estimator (MLE):*

$$Q(s) = \frac{\exp(a+bs)}{1+\exp(a+bs)}$$

2. *One-parameter Bayes (CRM)*: $Q(s) = [\{\tan h(3s - 1.5) + 1\}/2]^a$, $\pi(a) = e^{-a}$, $a > 0$, is the prior on a.
3. *Two-parameter Bayes*: Place the following prior distribution on (a, b):

$$\pi(a,b) \propto \prod_{j=1}^{k} \frac{\exp\{\gamma \mu_j m_j (a + bs_j)\}}{\{1+\exp(a+bs_j)\}^{m_j \gamma}},$$

   where μ_k is the prior guess for the probability of response at s_j. The parameter γ is a weight given to the prior, which represents the amount of faith in the prior relative to the data ($\gamma = 0.1$ was used in the simulations).
4. *Convex–concave*: A shape constrained MLE maximizes the likelihood subject to shape assumptions on Q.
5. *Smoothed convex–concave*: Include a term in the likelihood to penalize flatness. The penalized likelihood for Q is proportional to:

$$\prod_{j=1}^{k} \binom{m_j}{x_j} q_j^{x_j} (1-q_j)^{m_j - x_j} \prod_{j=2}^{k} \left(\frac{q_j - q_{j-1}}{s_j - s_{j-1}} \right)^{\lambda},$$

   Here λ is the smoothing parameter, with $\lambda = 0$ corresponding to the unsmoothed MLE ($\lambda = 0.05$ was used in the simulations).
6. *Monotone*: The monotone shape constrained MLE is the weighted least squares monotone regression of $\hat{q}_j$, where $\hat{q}_j$ is weighted by m_j, $j = 1, \ldots, k$.
7. *Smoothed monotone*: The toxicity at each dose is given a beta prior. At each stage, a weighted least squares monotone regression is fit to the posterior distributions, using the posterior mean as the value and the sum of the posterior beta parameters as the weight.

The authors seek designs that behave well along two performance measures—a sampling or ethical error to assess experimental losses and a decision error to predict future losses based on the terminal decision. For a given procedure, let $\xi_n(j)$ be the probability that dose j is selected as best at the end of an experiment of size n. Decision efficiency is a weighted measure of the overall decision quality. Let $p_i = P(s_i)$, $i = 1, \ldots, k$ and $p^* = p_{i^*}$ where dose number i^* is the best dose.

$$\text{Then decision efficiency is given by: } \mathcal{D}_n = \left\{\Sigma_{j=1}^{k} \xi_n(j) p_j\right\} / p^* .$$

The sampling error is the normalized expected loss incurred when sampling from doses other than k^*. Let $\mathbf{E}_n(n_j)$ denote the expected number of observations on dose j in an experiment of size n.

$$\text{Sampling efficiency is given by: } \mathcal{S}_n = \left\{\Sigma_{j=1}^{k} \mathbf{E}_n(n_j) \cdot p_j\right\} / (n \cdot p^*).$$

This is closely related to the well known measure expected successes lost: $np^* - \sum_{j=1}^{k} p_j \mathbf{E}(n_j)$. Note that $p^*\mathcal{S}_n$ is the expected success rate of patients in the experiment, and $p^*\mathcal{D}_n$ is the same rate for subsequent patients if they are given the treatment selected as best.

Some designs require a certain amount of information to form a valid estimator. This is true for MLEs, for example, although not for Bayesian estimators. Thus, depending on the curve fitting method, the first few observations of the directed walk may follow an up-and-down scheme:

$$(Y,Z) = \begin{cases} (1,0), & \text{stay} \\ (0,0), & \text{move up} \\ (\bullet,1), & \text{move down} \end{cases} .$$

Two allocation methods have been considered. First one is the up-and-down design for targeting the optimal dose proposed by Durham, Flournoy, and Li (1998) and further studied by Kpamegan and Flournoy (2001):

At each Stage i, $i = 1,\ldots,n/2$, the rule requires that two consecutive doses be observed. Once the responses at stage i have been observed, allocation for stage $i + 1$ is as follows:

1. Move up to $(j + 1, j + 2)$ if there is a success at dose $j + 1$, a failure at j and $j + 1 < k$.
2. Move down to $(j - 1, j)$ if there is a success at j, a failure at $j + 1$ and $j > 1$.
3. Otherwise, stay at dose levels $(j, j + 1)$.

The second design is the directed walk algorithm or DWA. Assume m subjects have been observed. Given appropriate observations, estimate Q and R using one of the curve estimation routines described above. Determine the dose, $\hat{k}^*$, which has the highest estimated probability of success and move one step toward it. If that same dose was just sampled, then utilize an exploration rule that, while usually reallocating to $\hat{k}^*$, may also indicate a move away from it. To avoid premature convergence to a false maxima with the DWA, an exploration rule is used to force occasional, but infinitely often, sampling at neighbors of the dose in question. As long as the estimators employed are consistent, exploration rules guarantee that the optimal dose will be identified in the limit. Moreover, they are extremely important for problems with small sample sizes to ensure that sampling will eventually occur away from the starting dose region. The exploration rule used for the simulation results forces a move to a neighbor with probability p_{Ei}, $i = 1, \ldots, n$, when three consecutive failures have occurred at the given dose where $\Sigma_{i=1}^{\infty} p_{Ei} = \infty$ and $p_{En} \to 0$ as $n \to \infty$. Whenever a rule indicates sampling at a dose outside the range $\{s_1, \ldots, s_k\}$, the DWA instead samples at the closest endpoint.

Sample size n is fixed, so no additional stopping criteria were considered. Terminal decisions are based on the curve estimation and allocation schemes in play. The final outcome is a choice of the best dose that may be measured empirically or using frequentist or Bayesian estimators.

Estimated values of $\mathcal{D}_n$ and $\mathcal{S}_n$ were obtained via simulation for the DWA, the up-and-down design and equal allocation design. The following three scenarios for dose-outcome have been used for the simulations:

Model 1: $Q(s) = [\{\{\tanh(5s - 3.5) + 1\}/2]^4$; $R(s) = \exp(-2 + 5s)/\{1 + \exp(-2 + 5s)\}$.
Model 2: $Q(s) = \exp(-0.5 + 2s)/\{1 + \exp(-0.5 + 2s)\}$; $R(s) = \exp(-1 + 10s)/\{1 + \exp(-1 + 10s)\}$

Model 3: It is nonparametric. The success curve has approximately the same shape as that of Model 12.2, but both the toxicity and efficacy curves stay away from 0 and 1, making the individual curves harder to estimate.

Data were generated for every combination of the following: three models of probability curves for toxicity and efficacy, total number of patients ($n = 25$ and $n = 50$), and number of dose levels ($D = 6$ and $D = 12$).

The smoothed shape constrained methods performed extremely well compared to the parametric methods—even when the underlying models fit the parametric method in question. Somewhat surprisingly, when averaged over the three models considered, the smoothed monotone method performed the best. This method, along with the two parameter Bayes method, were the only ones to perform well for each of the three scenarios. As expected, both the up-and-down method and equal allocation design performed very poorly. The unsmoothed shape constrained methods were not nearly as good as the smoothed versions.

With respect to large sample properties, a design is considered efficient if $\mathcal{D}_n$ and $\mathcal{S}_n$ converge to 1 as $n \to \infty$. The DWA combined with the curve fitting measure considered in the paper is both decision and sampling efficient. For each method, the simulated analysis of efficiency assumed that the model assumptions for estimating Q and R are met and that F is unimodal. The up-and-down procedure was not comparable to the other procedures.

While it is good to see so many methods compared in a consistent environment, more curve scenarios need to be studied before drawing strong conclusions. Overall, however, it does seem that the smoothed isotonic regression approach works very well. Sensitivity to the prior distributions placed on the success rates for this procedure should be examined.

The DWA itself is fairly straightforward and could be improved in a variety of ways. Allowing dose skipping may prove useful. That was not done in this paper so that the method could be directly compared with random walk methods such as the up-and-down. The authors also note that starting at the middle dose would improve overall results. The inclusion of an exploration rule in the DWA seems to be one of the major contributions in this paper. However, the proposed exploration rule is completely ad hoc and should be adjusted. For example, the rules can be created to ensure more exploratory sampling near the beginning of a trial. Furthermore, more sophisticated rules can be developed to improve or guarantee convergence rates of the sequence of the estimated optimal doses, k_n^* to k^* as $n \to \infty$. On the other hand, there seems to be little interest in large sample behavior for procedures in this clinical trial setting.

12.4.1.4 Repeated SPRT Design

O'Quigley, Hughes, and Fenton (2001) proposed a two-stage dose-finding design with a trinary outcome, assuming separate CRM (one-parameter) models for the toxicity probability $R(d)$ and the probability of efficacy given no toxicity $Q(d)$. They define overall success as efficacy without toxicity, so that $P(d) = Q(d)[1 - R(d)]$ is the probability of success at dose d:

$$R(d) = \Pr(Z = 1 \mid D = d) = \psi(d,a)$$

$$Q(d) = \Pr(Y = 1 \mid Z = 0; D = d) = \phi(d,b)$$

$$P(d) = \Pr(Y = 1, Z = 0 \mid D = d) = \phi(d,b)\{1 - \psi(d,a)\}.$$

Both $\psi(d, a)$ and $\phi(d, b)$ are assumed to be monotonic in d. An acceptable level of toxicity is determined in the first stage, starting with a low toxicity target q that later may be increased, and a sequential probability ratio test (SPRT) differentiating between the hypotheses $H_0 : P(d) < p_0$ and $H_1 : P(d) > p_1$ is used in the second stage to find the dose maximizing $P(d)$.

The design starts with a standard CRM to target some low rate of toxicity. The accumulating information at tested dose levels concerning success is used to test sequentially with an SPRT the above two hypothesis H_0 versus H_1. Inability to conclude in favor of either hypothesis leads to further allocation of patients to the current dose. Conclusion in favor of H_1 leads to termination of the trial and current dose level recommended for next Phase II study. Conclusion in favor of H_0 leads to the current dose level and all lower levels being removed from further allocations. At this point the target toxicity level is changed from q to $q + \Delta$. If none of the dose levels achieve a satisfactory rate of success before the toxicity rate q reached a prespecified threshold q_T, then the whole experiment is deemed a failure as far as the new treatment is concerned.

The design seems to focus on the SPRT that tests whether the success rate at the current dose is $> p_1$ or $< p_0$. There are no optimality properties associated with this test and it is rather ad hoc. The ability to drop doses as well as the option to increase the target toxicity level if efficacy is not observed may be viewed as positive attributes. For consistency purposes, one wonders why the option of adding doses at a higher level is not built into the method since one could go to the highest dose without seeing adequate success while still having observed no toxicities. On the other hand, there are also difficulties associated with dose dropping within the given procedure. It can occur that at some stage we move past argmax $P(d_i)$, $i = 1, \ldots, k$, and then, at some later stage, have observed enough failures to conclude $P(d_i) < p_0$. The rule says to then drop the lower doses and escalate. However, it may be better to move backward and retry lower doses to ensure that potential new successes would not eventually cause the algorithm to stop and conclude H_1. This option seems particularly important in light of the approximate nature of the hypothesis tests.

Ivanova (2003) compared a slight modification of this design with a new version of an up-and-down design and the optimizing design of Kpamegan and Flournoy (2001) in the same setting of trinary outcome. The repeated SPRT design performs better than the new design in the two scenarios where the best doses are d_1 and d_2, and are detected early. The new design yields much smaller median sample size and better, or the same probability of correct selection for the other two scenarios. The optimizing design has the largest sample size in all four scenarios considered, and comparable probability of correct selection.

12.4.2 Bayesian Designs

Bayesian formulation provides a natural framework to incorporate information as it accumulates and make decisions in real-time during the trial. In general, the required elements for the posterior distribution are the parametric model representing the dose-outcome relationship, and a prior distribution for the parameter vector. As the data (Y, Z) become available from each successive cohort of patients, the posterior distribution of the parameters is updated, and the decision criteria are applied how to allocate the next patients and when to stop the trial. In most part, the proposed Bayesian designs are not fully Bayesian and do not rely on formal decision theoretic approach. Rather, the trial is simulated under each of several dose-outcome scenarios as a means to calibrate (fine tune) design parameters to ensure that the design has desirable operating characteristics and perhaps compare its performance to a more traditional design or other competing designs (Chaloner and Verdinelli, 1995).

12.4.2.1 Bivariate CRM

Braun (2002) proposed an extension of the bivariate CRM to seamless Phase I/II trials of two competing outcomes: toxicity and disease progression. His case can be considered in the framework we use here of one toxicity and one efficacy outcome, letting $(1 - Y)$ = disease progression and Z = toxicity. He uses Model 12.8 with:

$$p_{\cdot 1}(d) = F(-3+\beta_1 d)$$

$$p_{1\cdot}(d) = F(-3+\beta_2 d),$$

where $F(\cdot)$ is the logistic distribution function.

The goal of the study is to find the dose that is closest to MTD, where closest is defined via some metric (e.g., Euclidean or weighted Euclidean), and MTD is defined by a pair of maximum tolerable error rates for toxicity (q_T) and disease progression (q_E). Descriptive statistics including probability of correct selection $P(CS)$, percent on nearby doses, expected number of failures of each type, and expected number of patients in the study are used as design performance metrics. Recommendation is to start at best estimate of MTD based on prior information. The allocation rule is as follows:

Assume m subjects have been observed.

1. Update model based on most recent cohort (Bayesian).
2. Calculate one-sided 95% CI for estimated proportion of toxicities (disease progression) so far.
3. If lower bound for the CI is above its respective target rate $q_T(q_E)$ then select dose minimizing metric if it is lower (higher) than current dose. Else move to next lower (higher) dose.
4. Otherwise, calculate metric and allocate next cohort to dose that minimizes it.

The design has a stopping rule:

1. Terminate if procedure suggests moving outside of dose set.
2. Terminate if both CI lower bounds are above their targets.
3. Terminate after M cohorts of size c each; that is, after $n = Mc$ subjects.
4. Select as MTD the dose that minimizes the metric based on the final posterior model.

A simulation study was conducted with the following assumptions $D = 6$; $n = 30$; $q_E = 0.25$; $q_T = 0.30$; $c = 3$; $\psi = 1/3$. Seven curve scenarios are examined and 1000 simulations are carried out. Euclidean metric is used. The bCRM performs best when no dose is acceptable. It tends to be conservative. Otherwise the best performance is obtained when the response curves are steep near the target doses. Starting at the lowest dose increases early termination probability. It seems inadvisable.

Compared to Methods B and C of Gooley et al. (1994), the bCRM seems to perform in between the other two methods and cannot be said to be a better method unless early termination is a highly valued design feature. One main drawback appears to be that the procedure terminates if the bCRM selects a dose outside the range of doses. This seems to extreme.

The other idea proposed here along these lines was to incorporate into the metric a penalty for being on the wrong side of the target. Braun suggests including an indicator function to avoid this entirely, but much better metrics could be proposed. The idea of using the confidence intervals for overall error rates to terminate early or force more conservative dosing makes some sense but is completely ad hoc. This seems a good area for research: How should one constrain the allocation procedure to accommodate generic concerns relating to excessive toxicities?

12.4.2.2 Bayesian Designs Based on Efficacy–Toxicity Trade-Off Contours

Thall and Russell (1998) proposed a strategy for dose-finding and safety monitoring based on efficacy and adverse outcomes in Phase I/II clinical trials. They use a proportional odds model in Equation 12.6 based on a trinary ordinal outcome. In terms of a prior distribution on the parameters (α_1, α_2, β), a variety in Equation 12.9 of response curves from the model were selected. These are intended to represent a reasonable range of shapes for the true curves. A parameter range is then set for each of (α_1, α_2, β) based on the values that defined the sample curves (presumably a clinician is helping with the selection of sample curves). An independent uniform prior is then placed over this range for each parameter.

Authors' goals were: (i) to find a dose that satisfies specific safety and efficacy requirements; (ii) to stop the trial early if it is likely that no dose is both safe and efficacious; and otherwise (iii) to treat as many subjects as possible at the optimal doses and to estimate the rates of these events at the best acceptable dose with a given accuracy. The OSD was selected at the end of the study as the acceptable dose that maximizes the posterior probability $\Pr(\pi_E(d^*, \theta) \geq q_E|\mathcal{F}_n)$.

More specifically,

1. Find d^* from among a set of acceptable doses satisfying the minimum efficacy constraint in Equation 12.3 and the maximum tolerated toxicity constraint in Equation 12.4.
2. Stop early if none of the doses satisfies both criteria in Equations 12.3 and 12.4.
3. Select n, the maximum sample size, so that the posterior $\Pr(q_E - \delta \leq \pi_E(d^*, \theta) \leq q_E + \delta|\mathcal{F}_n)$ given some $\delta > 0$ is sufficiently high.

Probability of selecting each dose as OSD, number treated at each dose, and expected sample size are the design performance metrics. Also shown are probabilities of making each type of incorrect decision such as labeling a dose as toxic or efficacious when it was not. Finally, the probability of correct selection $P(CS)$ is considered over a range of Type I and II errors.

The allocation rule is as follows:

1. Treat in cohorts of size c up to a maximum of n.
2. Start at lowest dose.
3. Never move by more than one level unless all intermediate levels have been sampled previously.
4. If current dose is too toxic and is:
   a Not the lowest dose, then deescalate by one dose.
   b. The lowest dose, then terminate.
5. If current dose is nontoxic but not efficacious, and
   a. The next higher dose level has acceptable toxicity, then move up one dose.
   b. The next higher dose level is too toxic, then terminate.
   c. The current dose is the highest dose, then terminate.
6. If current dose is acceptable, then treat the next cohort at the acceptable dose level with highest efficacy criterion probability; that is, highest $\Pr(\pi_E(d^*, \theta) \geq q_E|\mathcal{F})$.

If any of the following occur, then terminate the trial: 4b, 5b, 5c, or sample size reaches n.

Thall and Cheng (1999) modify the definition of OSD so that, if this criterion $\Pr(\pi_E(d, \theta) \geq q_E|\mathcal{F})$ is very close to the largest value for two or more doses, then the dose among these that maximizes $\Pr(\pi_T(d, \theta) \leq q_T|\mathcal{F})$ is chosen as the best.

As indicated by Thall and Cook (2004), a major limitation of the Thall and Russell (1998) design is that, in cases where all doses have acceptable toxicity but higher dose levels have substantially higher efficacy, it does not escalate to the more desirable doses with high probability. Consequently, in such settings it is likely to fail to select a higher dose level that is safe and provides greater efficacy. They also found that the three-parameter proportional-odds model used by Thall and Russell (1998), while parsimonious, may be overly restrictive in certain cases.

Thall and Cook (2004) propose an alternative design based on explicit trade-offs between π_E and π_T. They use the continuation-ratio model in Equation 12.7 for the trinary outcome case and Gumbel model for the case of two correlated binary endpoints. However, instead of using the efficacy and toxicity criteria in Equations 12.3 and 12.4 to limit the risk of treating patients at a dose with either unacceptably low efficacy or unacceptably high toxicity, they propose the desirability of the pair $(\pi_E(x, \theta), \pi_T(x, \theta))$ in the two-dimensional domain of possible values of (π_E, π_T). A similar approach, but in the frequentist formulation, has been proposed by Dragalin et al. (2008). Doses are selected for successive patient cohorts based on a set of efficacy–toxicity trade-off contours that partition the two-dimensional outcome probability (π_E, π_T) domain. Priors are established by solving for hyperparameters that optimize the fit of the model to elicited mean outcome probabilities.

The main difference to Thall and Russell design is that the selection of the next dose d^* in Step 6 is in terms of the dose desirabilities as the distance of the pair $E(\pi_E(x, \theta), \pi_T(x, \theta))|\mathcal{F})$ to the ideal (1, 0) based on the family of contours generated from the elicited target points. Their simulations show that, under a wide variety of dose-outcome scenarios, the new design is more likely to make correct decisions and, on average, it treats more patients at the more desirable doses.

Zhang, Sargent, and Mandrekar (2006) also use the continuation-ratio model in Equation 12.7 for the trinary outcome case and propose a Bayesian design, called TriCRM, which uses similar allocation rules except in Step 6, the selection of the next dose d^* is maximizing the utility function $\delta_2(x;\theta) = \Pr(Y=1, Z=0|D=x) - \lambda\Pr(Z=1|D=x)$, (where $0 \le \lambda \le 1$ is the relative weight for the toxicity probability), given the prespecified toxicity requirement is satisfied. Their stopping rule terminates the trial after treating at least n_1 patients, provided at least m subjects are treated at the recommended dose level, or a maximum of n_2 subjects are treated, whichever comes first. The TriCRM offers a simple alternative to the Thall and Cook approach with a very intuitive decision criteria.

12.4.3 Adaptive Optimal Designs

An alternative class of model-based designs that use the frequentist formulation of study objective is based on optimal design methods for convex objective functions and cost constraints proposed in Fedorov (1972) and Fedorov and Hackl (1997). However, while these authors considered the static locally optimal designs; that is, designs derived for the whole experiment, these new designs apply similar ideas in adaptive setting. The design working model is one of the models described in Section 12.3 and since these models are nonlinear, the information matrix depends on the values of unknown parameters and the design has to be performed in stages. Initial design is chosen and preliminary parameter estimates are obtained. Then, the next dose is selected from the available range of doses that satisfy the efficacy and toxicity constraints and provide the maximal improvement of the design with respect to the selected criterion of optimality and current parameter estimates. The next available cohort of patients is allocated to this dose. The estimates of unknown parameters are refined given these additional observations. These design-estimation steps are repeated until either the maximum number of patients are enrolled or the set of acceptable doses are empty. Such an approach is efficient from the perspective of both time and patient resources.

The experimental designs are represented by a set of design points (the set of available doses) and a corresponding set of weights representing the allocation proportions to the design points: $\xi = \{x_i, \lambda_i\}_1^k$. An important element in optimal design is the information matrix, say $M(\xi, \theta)$, which is an expression of the accuracy of the θ estimate based on observations at k design points of design ξ. A larger value of M reflects more information (more precision, lower variability) in the estimate. The D-optimal criterion is one of the most popular in determining an optimal design ξ^*. The D-optimal criterion is the determinant of the information matrix that is proportional to the volume of the confidence ellipsoid for θ. However, this criterion is not appropriate for seamless Phase I/II trials because the D-optimal design may require allocating patients to very toxic doses or to doses with very low efficacy. In order to take into consideration these individual ethical concerns, Dragalin and Fedorov (2006) proposed a penalized version of the D-optimal design by using a penalty function that accounts for poor efficacy and high toxicity. More details are provided in this section.

12.4.3.1 Likelihood Function and Information Matrix

The log-likelihood function of a single observation (Y, Z) at dose x is:

$$\ell(\theta | y,z;x) = yz\log p_{11} + y(1-z)\log p_{10} + (1-y)z\log p_{01} + (1-y)(1-z)\log p_{00}.$$

Assume $\{\mathbf{Y},\mathbf{Z}\} = \{y_i, z_i\}_1^N$ are N independent observations at doses $\mathbf{X} = \{x_i\}_1^N$. The corresponding log likelihood function:

$$\ell_N(\theta | \mathbf{Y},\mathbf{Z};\mathbf{X}) = \sum_{i=1}^{N} \ell(\theta | y_i, z_i; x_i),$$

and the maximum likelihood estimate (MLE) of θ is $\hat{\theta}_N = \text{argmax}_\theta \ell(\theta \mid \mathbf{Y}, \mathbf{Z}, \mathbf{X})$. The information matrix is defined as:

$$M_N(\mathbf{X}, \theta) = -E_\theta \left[\frac{\partial^2 \ell(\theta \mid \mathbf{Y}, \mathbf{Z}; \mathbf{X})}{\partial\theta \partial\theta^T} \right] = \sum_{i=1}^{N} \mu(x_i, \theta),$$

where $\mu(x, \theta)$ is Fisher information matrix of a single observation at dose x.

Assume the design region is $\mathcal{X}$. Denote the number of distinct design points by k, and denote the sample size at design point x_i by n_i, $i = 1, \ldots, k$, $\Sigma_i n_I = N$. The experimental designs of interest here are represented by a set of distinct design points and a corresponding set of weights representing the allocations to the design points:

$$\xi = \begin{Bmatrix} x_1, & x_2, & \ldots, & x_k \\ \lambda_1, & \lambda_2, & \ldots, & \lambda_k \end{Bmatrix}, x_1, x_2, \ldots, x_k \in \mathcal{X},$$

where $\lambda_i = n_i/N$ and $\sum_{i=1}^{k} \lambda_i = 1$.

The total normalized information matrix for design ξ is:

$$M(\xi, \theta) = M_N(\mathbf{X}, \theta)/N = \sum_{i=1}^{k} \lambda_i \mu(x_i, \theta).$$

For some common forms of estimates $\hat{\theta}_N$ (e.g., MLE and Bayesian maximum a posteriori), it is known that under rather mild conditions:

$$\lim_{N\to\infty} N\, Cov(\hat{\theta}_N) = D(\xi, \theta),$$

where $D(\xi, \theta) = M^{-1}(\xi, \theta)$ is the asymptotic variance-covariance matrix.

Gumbel model. The Fisher information matrix of a single observation can be written as:

$$\mu(x, \theta) = \frac{\partial \mathbf{p}}{\partial \theta} \nu(\mathbf{p}, \theta) \frac{\partial \mathbf{p}}{\partial \theta^{\mathrm{T}}},$$

where

$$\mathrm{T}\nu(x, \boldsymbol{p}) = \mathbf{P}^{-1} + \frac{1}{1 - p_{11} - p_{10} - p_{01}} ee^{\mathrm{T}}, \quad e^{\mathrm{T}} = (1,1,1),$$

and

$$\boldsymbol{p} = (p_{11}, p_{10}, p_{01})^{\mathrm{T}} \text{ and } \mathbf{P} = \begin{pmatrix} p_{11} & 0 & 0 \\ 0 & p_{10} & 0 \\ 0 & 0 & p_{01} \end{pmatrix}.$$

Direct calculations yield (see details in Dragalin and Fedorov (2006)):

$$\frac{\partial p_{11}}{\partial \mu_E} = -\frac{1}{\sigma_E} F(x_E)[1-F(x_E)]F(x_T)\{1+\alpha[1-2F(x_E)][1-F(x_T)]\},$$

$$\frac{\partial p_{10}}{\partial \mu_E} = -\frac{1}{\sigma_E} F(x_E)[1-F(x_E)] - \frac{\partial p_{11}}{\partial \mu_E}, \quad \frac{\partial p_{01}}{\partial \mu_E} = -\frac{\partial p_{11}}{\partial \mu_E},$$

$$\frac{\partial p_{11}}{\partial \sigma_E} = x_E \frac{\partial p_{11}}{\partial \mu_E}, \quad \frac{\partial p_{10}}{\partial \sigma_E} = x_E \frac{\partial p_{10}}{\partial \mu_E}, \quad \frac{\partial p_{01}}{\partial \sigma_E} = x_E \frac{\partial p_{01}}{\partial \mu_E},$$

$$\frac{\partial p_{11}}{\partial \alpha} = F(x_E)[1-F(x_E)]F(x_T)[1-F(x_T)], \quad \frac{\partial p_{10}}{\partial \alpha} = \frac{\partial p_{01}}{\partial \alpha} = -\frac{\partial p_{11}}{\partial \alpha},$$

and similarly for the partial derivatives with respect to μ_T and σ_T.

Cox model.

$$\mu(x,\theta) = (\mathbf{P} - \boldsymbol{pp}^{\mathrm{T}}) \otimes \mathcal{D}(x),$$

where $\mathcal{D}(x) = \begin{pmatrix} 1 & x \\ x & x^2 \end{pmatrix}$ (see details in Dragalin and Fedorov (2006)).

Probit model. For probit model there are two cases (see details in Dragalin, Fedorov, and Wu (2008)).

Known ρ Let $\theta = (\theta_1, \theta_2) \in R^m$, where $m = m_1 + m_2$, $m_i = dim\{\theta_i\}$, $i = 1, 2$.

The information matrix for a single observation at dose x:

$$\mu(x,\theta) = -E_\theta\left[\frac{\partial^2 \ell(\theta \mid y,z,;x)}{\partial\theta\partial\theta^T}\right] = C_1C_2(P-pp^T)^{-1}C_2^TC_1^T,$$

with

$$C_1 = \begin{pmatrix} \psi(\theta_1^T f_1)f_1 & \mathbf{0} \\ \mathbf{0} & \psi(\theta_2^T f_2)f_2 \end{pmatrix}, \quad C_2 = \begin{pmatrix} F(u_1) & 1-F(u_1) & -F(u_1) \\ F(u_2) & -F(u_2) & 1-F(u_2) \end{pmatrix},$$

$$u_1 = \frac{\theta_2^T f_2 - \rho\theta_1^T f_1}{\sqrt{1-\rho^2}}, \quad u_2 = \frac{\theta_1^T f_1 - \rho\theta_2^T f_2}{\sqrt{1-\rho^2}},$$

$$P = \begin{pmatrix} p_{11} & 0 & 0 \\ 0 & p_{10} & 0 \\ 0 & 0 & p_{01} \end{pmatrix}, \text{ and } p = (p_{11}\ p_{10}\ p_{01})^T,$$

$\psi(v)$ denotes the probability density function of standard normal distribution. Note that in our setting $1 \le \text{rank}\{\mu(x,\theta) \le 2$ and therefore the optimal designs should have at least three support points.

Unknown ρ. When the correlation between toxicity and efficacy ρ is treated as an unknown parameter, the corresponding information matrix for a single observation at dose x becomes:

$$\mu(x,\theta) = \begin{bmatrix} & C_1C_2 & \\ \psi_2 & -\psi_2 & -\psi_2 \end{bmatrix} (P-pp^T)^{-1} \begin{bmatrix} & C_1C_2 & \\ \psi_2 & -\psi_2 & -\psi_2 \end{bmatrix}^T,$$

where $\psi_2 = f(\theta_1^T f_1, \theta_2^T f_2, \rho)$ denotes the probability density function of bivariate normal distribution with means $\theta_1^T f_1$ and $\theta_2^T f_2$, variances 1 and correlation coefficient ρ.

Continuation-Ratio Model Let $\theta = (\alpha_1, \beta_1, \alpha_2, \beta_2)$, $f(t) = e^t/(1 + e^t)^2$ and $F(t) = 1/(1 + e^{-t})$. The Fisher information matrix for a single observation at dose x can be written as:

$$\mu(x,\theta) = \begin{bmatrix} \mu_{up}(x,\theta) & \underline{0} \\ \underline{0} & \mu_{low}(x,\theta) \end{bmatrix},$$

where

$$\mu_{up}(x,\theta) = \frac{f(\alpha_1 + \beta_1 x)}{1 + \exp(\alpha_2 + \beta_2 x)} \mathcal{D}(x)$$

$$\mu_{low}(x,\theta) = f(\alpha_2 + \beta_2 x)\mathcal{D}(x).$$

In case of equal slopes; that is, $\beta_2 = \beta_1$ $\theta = (\alpha_1, \beta_1, \alpha_2)$, the Fisher information matrix for a single observation at dose x can be written as (see details in Fan and Chaloner (2004)):

$$\mu(x,\theta) = f(\alpha_2 + \beta_2 x) \begin{bmatrix} 1 & x & 0 \\ x & x^2 & 0 \\ 0 & 0 & 0 \end{bmatrix}$$

$$+ F(\alpha_1 + \beta_1 x) \begin{bmatrix} 0 & 0 & 0 \\ 0 & x^2 & x \\ 0 & x & 1 \end{bmatrix}.$$

12.4.3.2 Penalized D-Optimal Design

Let the penalty of an observation taken at design point x be defined by the function $\phi(x, \theta)$, which may depend on unknown parameters, and reflects ethical and economical burden associated with that dose. A quite general and flexible penalty function is:

$$\phi(x,\theta;C_E,C_T) = \{p_{10}(x,\theta)\}^{-C_E}\{1 - p_{.1}(x,\theta)\}^{-C_T}, \tag{12.9}$$

that is, lower the probability of success and/or higher the probability of toxicity at the assigned dose, higher the penalty for the taken observation. The parameters C_E, C_T are control parameters that can be used to come up with an appropriate penalty function for given goal of the clinical trial. Then the optimization problem consists in determining a design ξ^* that maximizes the information (as the determinant of the normalized Fisher information matrix) per cost unit:

$$\xi^*(\theta) = \arg\max_{\xi} |\boldsymbol{M}(\xi,\theta)| / \Phi(\xi,\theta), \tag{12.10}$$

where

$$\Phi(\xi,\theta) = \int_X \phi(x,\theta)\xi(dx).$$

The optimization problem is formulated with a restriction on total number of observations N.

Sometime, the experiment has to be run under total cost constraint. For each experiment based on design ξ with N observations, define the total cost:

$$N\Phi(\xi,\theta) = N\int_X \phi(x,\theta)\xi(dx).$$

The optimization problem can be formulated as: for a given total cost C, find the design ξ^* that maximizes the total information:

$$\xi^*(\theta) = \arg\max_{\xi} | NM(\xi,\theta) |, \tag{12.11}$$

in the class of all designs satisfying the total cost constraint:

$$N\Phi(\xi,\theta) \leq C. \tag{12.12}$$

In this case, the optimal design $\xi^*(\theta) = \{w_i, x_i\}_1^k$, will determine $N(\xi^*) = C/\mathcal{F}(\xi^*, \theta)$, and the required number of observations $r_i \approx w_i N(\xi^*)$ will be allocated to x_i. Note that the total cost C is fixed here, not N like in Equation 12.10. It was proved in Dragalin and Fedorov (2006) that these two optimization problems are equivalent.

Pronzato (2008) proposed another optimization problem:

$$\xi^*(\theta) = \arg\max_{\xi} | M(\xi,\theta) |, \tag{12.13}$$

in the class of all designs satisfying:

$$\Phi(\xi,\theta) \leq C. \tag{12.14}$$

Haines, Perevozskaya, and Rosenberger (2003) considered a specific case of penalized optimization problem with:

$$\Phi(x,\theta) = \begin{cases} 1 & \text{if } p_{1\bullet}(x) \geq q_E \text{ and } p_{\bullet 1}(x) \leq q_T \\ \infty & \text{otherwise} \end{cases}, \tag{12.15}$$

where q_E and q_T are prespecified minimum acceptable efficacy response rate and maximum tolerable toxicity rate, respectively.

12.4.3.3 Computation Algorithm for Optimal Designs

The main idea behind the computation algorithm for a general locally optimal design is that at each step of the numerical procedure the sensitivity function $d(x, \xi, \theta)$ defined below in Equation 12.17 is maximized over the design region to determine the best new support point (dose for the next patient). The simplest first-order algorithm for construction of the penalized locally D-optimal design (LDoD) consists of few relatively easy steps:

Step 0. Start with an initial design $\xi_{s_0} = \{x_i, w_i\}_1^n$ with weights $w_i = r_i/s_0$ and $s_0 = \sum_{i=1}^n r_i$. Compute its normalized information matrix $M(\xi_{s0}, \theta)$ and verify its regularity. If this matrix is regular, proceed to Step 1. Otherwise, enrich the initial design.

Step 1. Given design ξ_s, find the next design point:

$$x_{s+1} = \arg\max_{x \in X} d(x, \xi_s, \theta), \tag{12.16}$$

where the sensitivity function is:

$$d(x,\xi,\theta)=\phi^{-1}(x,\theta)\mathrm{tr}\{\mu(x,\theta)\boldsymbol{M}^{-1}(\xi_s,\theta)\}. \tag{12.17}$$

Step 2. Update the design:

$$\xi_{s+1}=(1-\alpha_s)\xi_s+\alpha_s\xi(x_{s+1}),$$

where $\xi(x_{s+1})$ is a design atomized at point x_{s+1}. Here α_s is a predefined sequence of numbers such that $\lim_{s\to\infty}\alpha_s=0$ and $\sum_{s=0}^{\infty}\alpha_s=\infty$. We consider the simple case $\alpha_s = 1/s$. For other choices, see Fedorov and Hackl (1997).

Step 3. Verify the stopping rule. For instance, that:

$$\phi(x_{s+1},\theta)\mathrm{tr}\{\mu(x_{s+1},\theta)\boldsymbol{M}^{-1}(\xi_s,\theta)\}-\Phi^{-1}(\xi_s,\theta)m\le\varepsilon,$$

(here m is the dimension of parameter θ) or simply when the maximum number of iterations, let us say S, is achieved (here ε is a relatively small number). If the stopping rule is satisfied, then stop, otherwise return to Step1.

For the restricted LDoD, Equation 12.16 should be replaced by:

$$x_{s+1}=\arg\max_{x\in[d_E^*,d_T^*]} d(x,\xi_s,\theta).$$

Dragalin and Fedorov (2006) suggested to use this first order algorithm for constructing the locally optimal design for conducting an adaptive design for seamless Phase I/II trial. The implementation of adaptive design typically begins with an initial guess at the unknown parameter and the optimal design. For example, Ivanova (2003) up-and-down design was suggested as an initial design until the first toxicity is encountered. Then, using observations from the first N patients accrued and treated in the trial, an estimate of θ is obtained from the initial design. In the event that the estimator does not exist, we use any reasonable guess at the value of the parameters or continue with the initial design. This value of θ is then used in the sensitivity function in Equation 12.17 and the next dose level is determined as:

$$x_{N+1}=\arg\max_{x\in\mathcal{X}} d(x,\xi_N,\hat{\theta}_N),$$

where $\hat{\theta}_N$ is the maximum likelihood estimator based on the previous N observations. This process is repeated until the total number of patients in the study have been allocated or until there is adequate convergence of the θ estimate or other stopping rules have been obtained. It is possible to implement the adaptive design not only after each patient but also in cohorts of patients either all allocated to the same dose or to several doses. In the latter case, the iteration Step 1 and Step 2 are conducted c times (where c is the cohort size) without changing the value of the $\hat{\theta}_N$.

Asymptotic properties of this adaptive penalized optimal design have been derived in Pronzato (2008). The strong consistency and asymptotic normality of the estimator of model parameters and the convergence of the adaptive design to the locally optimal design are proved under rather general conditions. It may well be argued that asymptotic results are not very relevant in such typically small studies, however, it does provide some theoretical comfort and hints that for small samples things also might work satisfactorily. The latter was shown in Dragalin and Fedorov (2006) by comparing the adaptive penalized D-optimal design with the Ivanova (2003) up-and-down design (see also Padmanabhan, Hsuan, and Dragalin, 2010). For other illustrative examples and simulation results, see Dragalin and Fedorov (2006); Dragalin, Fedorov, and Wu (2008); and Pronzato (2008).

12.5 Conclusion

Biostatisticians dedicated to the discovery and improvement of clinical trial design play a fundamental role in the process of drug development. As in other domains, they generate new designs that are published in statistical journals, using a language typical to the profession but not well understood by their clinical colleagues. Therefore, the transfer of knowledge from statistical research about the design of seamless Phase I/II trials to clinical researchers actually performing these trials tends to be quite slow and the time lags are notable.

Due to their inherent complexity, the operating characteristics of these designs can be assessed only through intensive simulations. It is therefore key to develop a simulation toolbox of such designs, implemented on a unified platform (software) that is sufficiently comprehensive, flexible, and extensible to allow exploration and evaluation of alternative approaches to determine the most appropriate design for a given study. Such a toolbox may facilitate the effective communication between biostatisticians and clinical colleagues and achieve an improved uptake of these innovative experimental designs in clinical trials.

Rogatko et al. (2007, p. 4985) argue that the most effective and fastest way to improve the present situation is a change in the attitude of the gatekeeper—regulatory agencies that "should proactively encourage the adoption of statistical designs that would allow more patients to be treated at near-optimal doses while controlling for excessive toxicity."

References

Atkinson, A. C., and Donev, A. (1992). *Optimum Experimental Designs.* Oxford: Clarendon Press.

Braun, T. (2002). The bivariate continual reassessment method: Extending the CRM to Phase I trials of two competing outcomes. *Controlled Clinical Trials,* 23: 240–56.

Chaloner, K., and Verdinelli, I. (1995). Bayesian experimental design: A review. *Statistical Science,* 10: 273–304.

Cox, D. R. (1970). *The Analysis of Binary Data.* London: Chapman and Hall.

Dragalin, V., and Fedorov, V. (2006). Adaptive designs for dose-finding based on efficacy—Toxicity response. *Journal of Statistical Planning and Inference,* 136: 1800–23.

Dragalin, V., Fedorov, V., and Wu, Y. (2008). Optimal designs for bivariate probit model. *GSK Technical Report 2005-07.* 62 pages.

Dragalin, V., Fedorov, V., and Wu, Y. (2008). Adaptive designs for selecting drug combinations based on efficacy-toxicity response. *Journal of Statistical Planning and Inference,* 138 (2): 352–73.

Dragalin, V., Fedorov, V., and Wu, Y. (2008).Two-stage design for dose-finding that accounts for both efficacy and safety. *Statistics in Medicine,* 27: 5156–76.

Durham, S., Flournoy, N., and Li, W. (1998). A sequential design for maximizing the probability of a favourable response. *Canadian Journal of Statistics,* 26: 479–95.

Fan, S. K., and Chaloner, K. (2004). Optimal designs and limiting optimal designs for a trinomial response. *Journal of Statistical Planning and Inference,* 126: 347–60.

Fedorov, V. V. (1972). *Theory of Optimal Experiments.* New York: Academic Press.

Fedorov, V. V., and Hackl, P. (1997). *Model-Oriented Design of Experiments, Lecture Notes in Statistics 125.* New York: Springer-Verlag.

Gooley, T., Martin, P., Fisher, L., and Pettinger, M. (1994). Simulation as a design tool for Phase I/II clinical trials: An example from bone marrow transplantation. *Controlled Clinical Trials,* 15: 450–62.

Haines, L. M., Perevozskaya, I., and Rosenberger, W. F. (2003). Bayesian optimal designs for Phase I clinical trials. *Biometrics,* 59: 591–600.

Hardwick, J., Meyer, M. C., and Stout, Q. F. (2003). Directed walk designs for dose response problems with competing failure modes. *Biometrics,* 59: 229–36.

Hardwick, J., and Stout, Q. (2001). Optimizing a unimodal response function for binary variables. In *Optimum Design 2000,* eds. A. Atkinson, B. Bogacka, and A. Zhigljavsky, 195–210. The Netherlands: Kluwer Academic Publishers.

Ivanova, A. (2003). A new dose-finding design for bivariate outcomes. *Biometrics,* 59: 1001–7.

Ivanova, A. (2006). Dose-finding in oncology–Nonparametric methods. In *Dose Finding in Drug Development,* ed. N. Ting, 49–58. New York: Springer-Verlag.

Kpamegan, E. E., and Flournoy, N. (2001). An optimizing up-and-down design. In *Optimum Design 2000,* eds. A. Atkinson, B. Bogacka, and A. Zhigljavsky, 211–24. Boston: Kluwer.

O'Quigley, J., Hughes, M., and Fenton, T. (2001). Dose finding designs for HIV studies. *Biometrics,* 57: 1018–29.

O'Quigley, J., Pepe, M., and Fisher, L. (1990). Continual reassessment method: A practical design for Phase 1 clinical trials in cancer. *Biometrics,* 46: 33–48.

Padmanabhan, S. K., Hsuan, F., and Dragalin, V. (2010). Adaptive penalized D-optimal designs for dose finding based on continuous efficacy and toxicity. *Statistics in Biopharmaceutical Research,* 2:182–98.

Pronzato, L. (2008). Asymptotic properties of adaptive penalized optimal design with application to dose-finding. *Technical Report ISRN I3S/RR-2008-19-FR.* University Nice Sophia Antipolis. 33 pages.

Rogatko, A., Schoeneck, D., Jonas, W., Tighiouart, M., Khuri, F. R., and Porter, A. (2007). Translation of innovative designs into Phase I trials. *Journal of Clinical Oncology,* 25: 4982–86.

Thall, P. F., and Cheng, S. C. (1999). Treatment comparisons based on two-dimensional safety and efficacy alternatives in oncology trials. *Biometrics,* 55:746–53.

Thall, P. F., and Cook, J. D. (2004). Dose-finding based on efficacy-toxicity trade-offs. *Biometrics,* 60: 684–93.

Thall, P., and Russell, K. (1998). A strategy for dose-finding and safety monitoring based on efficacy and adverse outcomes in Phase I/II clinical trials. *Biometrics,* 54: 251–64.

Zhang, W., Sargent, D., and Mandrekar, S. (2006). An adaptive dose-finding design incorporating both toxicity and efficacy. *Statistics in Medicine,* 25: 2365–83.

13

Phase II/III Seamless Designs

Jeff Maca
Novartis Pharmaceuticals

13.1 Introduction

One challenge in the development of new and novel medicines is the length of time needed and cost associated with their development as well as the amount of information necessary to demonstrate the benefit of novel medicines. A reasonable goal would include reducing the time needed to collect this information while also increasing the efficiency of the design and analysis. For this reason, there has been much effort in trying to develop clinical trial designs that can improve on both of these aspects. In addition to other clinical trial designs discussed in this book, one possibility is to merge what typically would be separate clinical trials into a single trial. Under proper circumstances, this can reduce the amount of time necessary to complete the overall development process, as well as use the data collected from the trials more efficiently.

Combining studies can be accomplished in other phases as well (see Chapter 12); however, in the later phases of development, there is also great opportunity for benefits over traditional designs. For this chapter, we will assume that there is a selection of a dose (the typical Phase IIb objective), and that this selected dose will be sought for registration and approval. However, because these studies will also be confirmatory in nature, an effort must also be put on maintaining the rigid integrity of the trial, and ensuring that the logistics and implementation are well considered, so that the seamless study can be more efficient than the traditional separate studies.

13.2 General Considerations for Designing a Seamless Phase II/III Study

A seamless Phase II/III study will combine what are traditionally two distinct studies, one for selecting a dose and one for confirming that the selected dose is safe and efficacious, into a single study. This decision is made during the course of the study, and implemented before the study is concluded, or ideally while the study enrollment is still ongoing. Adaptive seamless designs have the potential to yield great benefits for both the sponsor as well as the patients. The ability to run fewer clinical trials and to have less exposure to new medicines is certainly beneficial for both patients and sponsors. Similarly, if the clinical development program can be completed in a shorter timeframe, then novel and helpful medicines can reach the patients who need them sooner. While considering the benefits of seamless designs, however, there is also increased need for careful discussion and planning before such trials can be implemented. Due to the more complex nature of these studies, it is also not possible that every clinical development program could implement a seamless development program. There are many factors that should be considered in the planning stages, and these must be weighed together to decide if a particular development program can use seamless designs to combine Phases II and III. Because they are somewhat complex in their nature, there is no exhaustive list of factors that can be developed, although many key attributes will be discussed here. It is also true that none of these factors alone would prohibit or mandate seamless development, and likewise, a clinical development program cannot be determined to conform or not conform to seamless development. Ideally, if there are multiple development programs ongoing, each program could go through this type of feasibility analysis, and one might find that some clinical programs may be a better fit over another. The process of reviewing programs for this type of development can often be beneficial even if seamless development is not pursued.

The first consideration and possibly the most important is that of the primary endpoint that will be used in the confirmatory setting. In Phase III, these endpoints must be well known and acceptable to health authorities for the approval of the product. In this type of development, the agreement and acceptability of the endpoints must be obtained prior to initiation of the seamless trial. There are cases where there is little experience in a disease area, and primary endpoints are not well understood or accepted. It could even be one of the objectives of the Phase II program to not only select a dose for registration, but also to select the best measure for the efficacy of the drug as the primary endpoint to be used in the Phase III program. This situation would be one scenario that could prohibit seamless development in Phase IIb/III. Therefore, it is essential that the endpoints be well understood and acceptable for seamless development. This would also be true for the case where a surrogate marker would be used for the dose selection. If such a surrogate marker (or early readout of the primary endpoints) will be used, it should be universally accepted as a valid surrogate marker for the primary endpoint.

Another consideration with regard to the endpoint is the length of time that is necessary for a patient to be followed and be able to have a response for the primary endpoint, or the endpoint used for the dose selection. Ideally, this time should be relatively short compared to the time needed to enroll patients into the study. If the time needed to complete this endpoint is short relative to the dose selection endpoint, then enrollment would still be ongoing at the time of the dose selection. Also, enrollment can continue during the dose selection process, as very few patients would be enrolled during this interim period (see Figure 13.1). This quick readout of the primary endpoint allows for a more efficient design, in that the selection can be made sooner, and patients can be allocated to dosage groups more advantageously. However, in some cases, the time required to reach the primary endpoint could be much longer than the expected enrollment period. In this case, enrollment would be completed before the data from the first patient enrolled would be available to contribute to the dose selection process. If this happens, the enrollment period would need to be paused until the dose selection is made, and then restarted once the dose was selected.

If the enrollment is not paused during the dose selection period, then a reasonable question to address is what to do with patients who are enrolled after the last patient recruited for the first stage and before the actual dose selection implementation (the transition period). Ideally, the number of patients enrolled during this time should be a relatively low number. Once the dose has been selected, there are three options for these patients. These patients can either continue with the study until they complete the primary endpoint, they could be switched to the chosen dose, or they can be dropped from the study completely. It would be ideal to keep patients on the dose they were randomized to, so that the dose response could be best understood at the conclusion of the study. However this might not always be

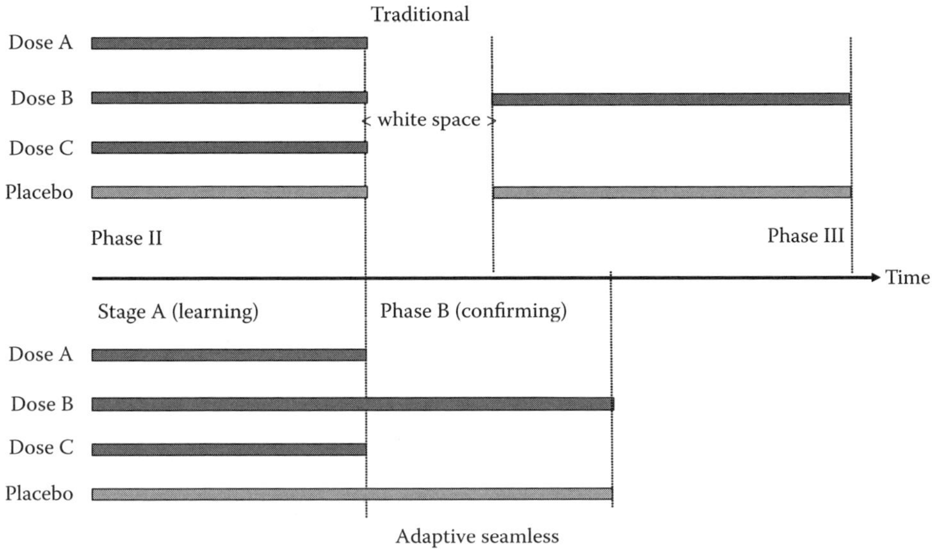

FIGURE 13.1 Enrollment times for development.

possible and those patients on nonselected treatment groups would be switched to the chosen dose, or dropped. If they are switched, these patients will generally not be combined with the patients that were originally randomized to the selected dose, and will be treated as a separate group. These patients will still yield valuable information, such as data that can be incorporated into the safety profile. If none of these options are feasible, then these patients can just be terminated from the study.

When considering a seamless Phase II/III study, then the entire development program should be considered as a seamless development program. It is important to ensure that the entire program can incorporate the seamless design effectively. For example, it must be considered if a second confirmatory trial will be needed (which is usually the case), and how that trial could be initiated based on the dose selection from the seamless trial. One appealing aspect of seamless designs is the ability to reduce the white space between phases, and reduce overall time needed for the product to be registered. However, it must be shown that the second trial could be initiated quickly after the dose selection and completed earlier than if the studies were run separately in the more traditional framework. If it is not possible to reduce the amount of time before a product can be registered, then seeking the use of seamless designs might be reconsidered.

In addition to the issues raised above, the logistics of the study should also be examined. For example, it will be necessary to set up an Interactive voice response system (IVRS) to be used to implement the dose change. This system will need to be established, and the requirements communicated to the IVRS vendor as to what the procedure will be and when the procedure will be used to make the dose selection. Another aspect to consider is whether the final formulation will be available prior to the beginning of the seamless trial. In some development programs, the final formulation is developed during the Phase II portion of the program for use in Phase III. If that is the case, than seamless development could be difficult, as the two pivotal trials could have different formulations and an additional bioequivalence study would be needed.

13.3 Sample Sizes in Seamless Phase II/III Trials

An important consideration for any trial is to ensure that the same size is adequate to achieve the objectives of the trial. For pivotal trials, this quite often implies that the sample size must be determined to ensure that the analysis of treatment effect on the primary endpoint will be considered statistically significant with the desired statistical power given the treatment assumptions. Although other aspects might affect the sample size (i.e., safety endpoints, secondary efficacy endpoints), this is usually a straightforward calculation. However in seamless trials, there are two stages in the study, each with a sample size to calculate. A very natural question becomes how many patients are needed in each stage.

The first stage of the trial will have the objective of selecting a dose. One important consideration that affects the ability to select the desired dose is the true and unknown dose response. For example, if only one of the doses has a substantial beneficial response, it would be rather easy to select this dose, and a relatively smaller sample size would be needed. If there is less differentiation between the doses, then more patients would be needed for the dose selection stage. It should be noted that this is not an aspect that is limited only to seamless development. The same argument might be made for any Phase II trial, however, the objectives of standard Phase II trials are often not framed in that way. However, in order to determine the overall power for the seamless trial, these dose selection probabilities must be determined, which is a beneficial exercise regardless.

The second stage must have a sufficient number of patients such that the trial will have the overall desired power. As previously mentioned, the power will be a function of the dose selection probabilities and the underlying dose response. The most common tool to determine these selection probabilities and overall power is computer simulation. One aspect that makes sample size determination for a seamless Phase II/III trial unique besides the fact that there are two sample sizes to determine, is that there is also not a unique answer to the sample size. For example, if the goal was to have a 90% powered study for a given proposed dose response, it would be possible to have fewer patients in the first stage (which would lower the probability of selecting the most efficacious dose), but could be compensated for by having more patients in the second stage. On the other hand, if the study has a large first stage, then generally the second stage would be smaller.

Other considerations that could drive the sample sizes for each stage might include:

- Fixing a bound on the lowest dose selection probability for the optimal dose (i.e., there must be at least a 75% chance of picking the desired dose).
- Optimizing over the total sample size for the duration of the trial.
- Ensuring data will be sufficient to satisfy the requirements for other endpoints.

Addressing all of these considerations can lead to a design that will have operating characteristics that will satisfy the trial objectives.

It is also advantageous to look at multiple assumptions of the dose response since what may be considered optimal under one dose response might not be considered optimal under another. Once multiple dose responses are investigated and the corresponding desired sample sizes are found, it is likely that there may not be any one set of sample sizes that would be optimal in all cases. Nevertheless, at the end of the exercise, it can be determined that sample size is the most satisfactory over the range of assumptions, and is robust to deviations from the assumed dose response.

13.4 Methodologies

As discussed previously, since these trials would be considered part of the pivotal package for registration, there must be proper analysis methods in place to ensure that the statistical validity of the trial is maintained. Many different methods have been developed to address the analysis of such trials. An important consideration when planning an adaptive seamless trial is understanding what methodology is best suited based on the specific design aspects of the trial.

A seamless Phase II/III trial will have two distinct stages, where the first stage will be selecting a dose(s) and the second stage will continue to gather information on the selected dose(s) and controls. The natural issue is then how to combine the information from both stages of the trial. One choice would be to not combine any information between the two stages and treat them as separate sets of data.

In this framework, this might be referred to as simply a seamless trial, where two separate studies are combined, but still analyzed separately. Purely seamless trials still have the advantage of losing some of the time in between studies (white space). Although it might seem advantageous to always combine information between stages, it could be possible that it is more efficient to not do so. As an example, if the first stage is very small relative to the second stage, any multiplicity penalty or other statistical adjustments required to combine the information could be cause for a less powerful study at the end. As a rule, the power of a purely seamless trial should be calculated for comparison to a seamless trial that attempts to combine data from both stages. If the data between stages are analyzed separately, there is also less concern for bias in the estimates because of the dose selection in the first stage.

However, it is often the case that considerable information is gathered from the first stage, and combining it with the data obtained in the second stage will be more efficient overall in analyzing the benefit of the treatment. If the analysis of data collected from a trial will attempt to combine data between the two stages, then this trial would be an adaptive seamless trial, or an inferentially seamless trial (Maca et al. 2006). There has been considerable research on proper methods to handle this type of statistical analysis in adaptive seamless studies.

Adaptive dose selection trials have been used in some fashion for many years. Many of these designs focused on starting a trial with many treatment arms, and then paring down arms that were not effective enough, or to select the treatment arm that has the maximum efficacy response (Thall, Simon, and Ellenberg 1989). These analysis methods were very specific in the selection rules, and used those selection rules in the analysis methodology. The methodology was further expanded to address time to event type data and more than two stages for the trial (Schaid, Wieand, and Therneau 1990; Stallard and Todd 2003). These types of methods can then be expanded to the more flexible designs and decision processes found in adaptive seamless designs.

The framework that will be discussed here is that of using pairwise comparisons for the analysis of the hypothesis of a treatment effect. This is a natural strategy, given that Phase III trials generally use a statistical hypothesis test to demonstrate efficacy of the drug.

The most straightforward method that would allow for a pairwise comparison framework for the statistical test is the traditional Bonferroni method of splitting the type I error rate (α) by the number of comparisons. For example, if a seamless Phase II/III trial is started with four treatments and a control, the comparison of the selected dose to the control at the conclusion of the trial would be made at $\alpha/4$, even though there is only one treatment comparison to be made. Therefore, the full multiplicity penalty is paid for the treatment selection. This method is usually considered conservative, and might be thought of to be too conservative to consider implementing. However, in many cases, any loss in power compared to other methodologies is minimal. For example, if the number of experimental doses used to begin the study is two or three, there will usually be little gained by using more complicated methods. Furthermore, this method is well understood, straightforward, and easy to implement. This is an advantage as the analysis can be described relatively easily in the protocol and understood. Also, since the full statistical penalty is paid for the dose selection, there is also flexibility in the number of treatment arms that can continue into the second stage. In the example, since four experimental treatment groups begin in the study, and the final test will use $\alpha/4$, this significance level would be valid for testing one or all four treatment comparisons at the end. This flexibility could be useful if there is uncertainty about the dose response, as well as the number of doses that would continue to the second stage. Since the alpha is split for each proposed comparison, it is also useful if there is a plan to do further testing where controlling the familywise error rate is desired. For example, if there are secondary endpoints that need to be tested, then the primary endpoint could be tested at $\alpha/4$, and then further secondary endpoints could be sequentially tested at $\alpha/4$.

Another strategy is to keep the data from the two stages of the trial separate and then combine them at the conclusion of the trial. The idea of combining p-values from independent data to produce a single test was originally considered by Fisher, generally referred to as Fisher's combination test, and was first described for use in the adaptive designs world by Bauer and Köhne (1994). This methodology was further improved on using the inverse normal method of combining p-values, where p-values from independent sets of data can be combined by:

$$C(p_1,p_2)=\sqrt{t_0}\times\Phi^{-1}(1-p_1)+\sqrt{1-t_0}\times\Phi^{-1}(1-p_2).$$

The weight, t_0, is prespecified and is typically the fraction of data included in the first stage, which is:

$$t_0=\frac{n_1}{n_1+n_2}.$$

Since within-stage inferences are computed separately, these types of methods have the added advantage of allowing other adaptations to occur, such as the change of sample size at the interim stage. Therefore, the study could begin with a specific number of treatment groups and then, based on the outcome of that first stage, a dose and sample size could be selected for the second stage. Since all the data are used for the final analysis, and there was a dose selection used, there must also be some way to control the type I error rate. In order to accomplish this, the inverse normal method is often combined with a closed testing strategy. The closed testing procedure would imply that in order to test the pairwise comparison of the chosen dose against the control, all hypotheses containing that dose must also be tested. To test these hypotheses, a testing procedure such as Simes multiple testing procedure could be used.

13.5 Decision Process

One particularly challenging aspect of seamless Phase II/III designs is that the data and analysis pertaining to the dose selection will not generally be available to the clinical team for viewing or discussion. This changes the decision process from a discussion after seeing data to a discussion prior. The dose selection analysis will also be performed by an external decision board, which implies that the decision rule will need to be very specific, and will have little or no involvement from the clinical trial team. Therefore, considerable amount of thought and planning will be necessary to develop the decision rule that can be implemented to select the dose for continuation into the second stage (Gallo 2006).

Computer simulation will be a valuable tool in developing the decision rule. As with the sample size determination, it will be advantageous to understand the decision rule against various dose response scenarios, as well as to try to understand various decision rules. Often, this will be an iterative process in which the sample sizes for the two stages are selected, and then the selection rule is decided upon. Then, after simulating the trial and looking at the operating characteristics of the trial as the result of the simulation, the sample size or decision rule(s) might be adjusted. After looking at various scenarios and possibilities, the overall study could be designed to perform over a wide range of possible dose responses.

13.6 Case Study, Seamless Adaptive Designs in Respiratory Disease

As an example of a seamless adaptive design, consider an example in the development of a product for typical respiratory indication, where forced expiratory volume for 1 second (FEV_1) is the primary measure of efficacy. For this example, assume that there are four experimental doses that are desired to be investigated and two doses will be continued into the second stage. The primary analysis would compare the experimental dose against a placebo treatment group; however, an active control treatment group is also included for comparison. For this indication, the typical endpoint for registration is a change in FEV_1 from baseline after 12 weeks of treatment. However, it is believed that much of the effect could be observed earlier than 12 weeks into the treatment, and hence an early readout of the primary endpoint after 3 weeks of treatment will be used. This is an advantage since if the interim analysis can

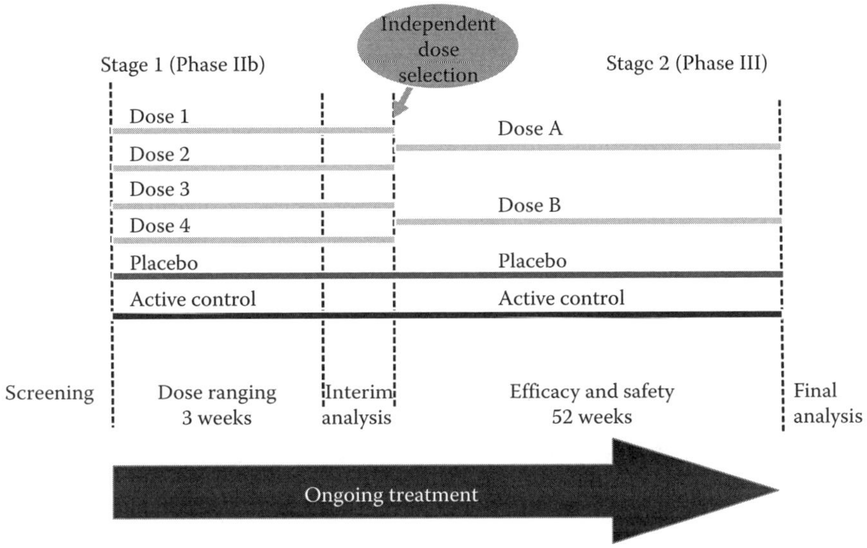

FIGURE 13.2 Design of adaptive seamless Phase II/III design.

be performed quickly, the length of time between enrollment of the last patient for the first stage and the beginning of the second stage will be relatively short and in addition, enrollment could continue through this time. Although the primary endpoint is achieved after 12 weeks of treatment, the patients will be enrolled in the study for 1 year to complete the necessary long-term safety requirements. The overall design for this study can be seen in Figure 13.2.

To design such a study, the next issue would be to determine the sample size, decision rule, and analysis method. One possible decision rule would be to simply choose the treatment groups that demonstrate the highest benefit in efficacy at the interim analysis point. However, another strategy would be to try to choose the lowest doses that still show substantial benefit, which could help alleviate safety concerns. For example, a threshold could be chosen, such that the lowest dose that exceeds the threshold as well as the next highest dose are continued into the second stage. Once this threshold is determined, different dose responses could be hypothesized, and through simulation, the probability of selecting each pair could be determined for different sample sizes for the first stage.

To complete the design of the study, the different analysis methods would also need to be compared. In this situation, where two treatment groups would be selected from the four treatment groups that begin in the study, the Bonferroni adjustment of testing at $\alpha/4$ could be used. This method could be particularly useful since there will be sequential testing against the placebo, active control, and possibly further secondary endpoints. As long as the sample size in the first stage is not considerably smaller than the second stage, there will not be a great loss in power as compared to using a closed testing procedure with the combination of p-values. However, through simulation, the exact powers of both methods, as well as the power of using only the second stage data can be determined. In planning such a study, there would most likely be many different scenarios investigated that might cause changes in the decision rule (for example, the threshold could be modified), or a change in the sample sizes for each stage, until the final design is agreed upon.

13.7 Conclusions

Seamless Phase II/III designs have been a focus of much attention in the design of clinical trials, due to the benefits from the added flexibility that they can bring to a development program. This flexibility can have many benefits including a more efficient use of the data acquired for registration, and the possibility of removing the white space between the programs and reducing the overall time needed for a drug to reach the point of registration. However, careful considerations of the logistics of implementing such a design and the statistical methods needed should be carefully addressed.

References

Bauer, P., and Köhne, K. (1994). Evaluation of experiments with adaptive interim analyses. *Biometrics,* 50: 1029–41.

Gallo, P. (2006). Confidentiality and trial integrity issues for adaptive designs. *Drug Information Journal,* 40: 445–49.

Maca, J., Battacharya, S., Dragalin, V., Gallo, P., and Krams, M. (2006). Adaptive seamless Phase II/III designs—Background, operational aspects, and examples. *Drug Information Journal,* 40: 463–73.

Schaid, D. J., Wieand, S., and Therneau, T. M. (1990). Optimal two stage screening designs for survival comparisons. *Biometrika,* 77: 659–63.

Stallard, N., and Todd, S. (2003). Sequential designs for Phase III clinical trials incorporating treatment selection. *Statistics in Medicine,* 22: 689–703.

Thall, P. F., Simon, R., and Ellenberg, S. S. (1989). A two-stage design for choosing among several experimental treatments and a control in clinical trials. *Biometrics,* 45: 537–47.

14

Sample Size Estimation/Allocation for Two-Stage Seamless Adaptive Trial Designs

Shein-Chung Chow
Duke University School of Medicine

Annpey Pong
Merck Research Laboratories

14.1 Introduction

In clinical trials, it is not uncommon to modify trial and/or statistical procedures during the conduct of clinical trials based on the review of interim data. The purpose is not only to efficiently identify clinical benefits of the test treatment under investigation, but also to increase the probability of success of clinical development. Trial procedures are referred to as the eligibility criteria, study dose, treatment duration, study endpoints, laboratory testing procedures, diagnostic procedures, criteria for evaluability, and assessment of clinical responses. Statistical methods include randomization, study design, study objectives/hypotheses, sample size, data monitoring and interim analysis, statistical analysis plan, and/or methods for data analysis. In this chapter, we will refer to the adaptations (or modifications) made to the trial and/or statistical procedures as the adaptive design methods. Thus, an adaptive design is defined as a design that allows adaptations to trial and/or statistical procedures of the trial after its initiation without undermining the validity and integrity of the trial (Chow, Chang, and Pong 2005). In their recent publication, with the emphasis of the feature of by design adaptations only (rather than ad hoc adaptations), the Pharmaceutical Research Manufacturer Association (PhRMA) Working Group on Adaptive Design refers to an adaptive design as a clinical trial design that uses accumulating data to decide on how to modify aspects of the study as it continues, without undermining the validity and integrity of the trial (Gallo et al. 2006). In many cases, an adaptive design is also known as a flexible design.

The use of adaptive design methods for modifying the trial and/or statistical procedures of on-going clinical trials based on accrued data has been practiced for years in clinical research. Adaptive design methods in clinical research are very attractive to clinical scientists due to the following reasons. First, it reflects medical practice in the real world. Second, it is ethical with respect to both efficacy and safety (toxicity) of the test treatment under investigation. Third, it is not only flexible, but also efficient in the early phase of clinical development. However, it is a concern whether the p-value or confidence interval regarding the treatment effect obtained after the modification is reliable or correct. In addition, it is also a concern that the use of adaptive design methods in a clinical trial may lead to a totally different trial that is unable to address scientific/medical questions that the trial is intended to answer (e.g. EMEA 2002, 2006).

Based on the adaptations employed, commonly considered adaptive design methods in clinical trials include, but are not limited to: (i) an adaptive randomization design, (ii) a group sequential design, (iii) an N-adjustable design or a flexible sample size reestimation design, (iv) a drop-the-loser (or pick-the-winner) design, (v) an adaptive dose finding design, (vi) a biomarker-adaptive design, (vii) an adaptive treatment-switching design, (viii) a hypothesis-adaptive design, (ix) an adaptive seamless trial design, and (x) a multiple adaptive design. Detailed information regarding these adaptive designs can be found in Chow and Chang (2006).

In this chapter, however, we will only focus on the two-stage adaptive seamless trial design, which is probably the most commonly considered adaptive design in clinical research and development. A two-stage seamless adaptive trial design is a study design that combines two separate studies into one single study. In many cases, study objectives and/or study endpoints considered in a two-stage seamless design may be similar but different (e.g., a biomarker versus a regular clinical endpoint). In this case, it is a concern that how the data collected from both stages should be combined for the final analysis. Besides, it is of interest to know how the sample size calculation/allocation should be done for achieving the study objectives originally set for the two stages (separate studies). In this chapter, formulas for sample size calculation/allocation are derived for cases when the study endpoints are continuous, discrete (e.g., binary responses), and time-to-event data assuming that there is a well-established relationship between the study endpoints at different stages.

In the next section, the commonly employed two-stage adaptive seamless design is briefly outlined. Also included in this section is a comparison between the two-stage adaptive seamless design and the traditional approach in terms of type I error rate and power. Sections 14.3.1–14.3.3 provide formulas/procedures for sample size calculation/allocation for testing equality, noninferiority/superiority, and equivalence for a two-stage adaptive seamless design when the study endpoints at different stages are different for continuous endpoints, binary responses, and time-to-event data, respectively. Some major obstacles and challenges regarding sample size calculation when applying adaptive designs in clinical trials especially when there is a shift in patient population due to protocol amendments are discussed in Section 14.4. Some concluding remarks are given in the last section.

14.2 Two-Stage Adaptive Seamless Design

14.2.1 Definition and Characteristics

A seamless trial design is referred to as a program that addresses study objectives within a single trial that are normally achieved through separate trials in clinical development. An adaptive seamless design is a seamless trial design that would use data from patients enrolled before and after the adaptation in the final analysis (Maca et al. 2006). Thus, an adaptive seamless design is a two-stage design that consists of two phases (stages), namely a learning (or exploratory) phase and a confirmatory phase. The learning phase provides the opportunity for adaptations such as to stop the trial early due to safety and/or futility/efficacy based on accrued data at the end of the learning phase. A two-stage adaptive seamless trial design reduces lead time between the learning (i.e., the first study for the traditional approach) and confirmatory (i.e., the second study for the traditional approach) phases. Most importantly, data collected at the learning phase are combined with those data obtained at the confirmatory phase for final analysis.

In practice, two-stage seamless adaptive trial designs can be classified into the following four categories depending upon study objectives and study endpoints at different stages (Chow and Tu 2008):

Category I: Same study objectives and same study endpoints.
Category II: Same study objectives but different study endpoints.
Category III: Different study objectives but same study endpoints.
Category IV: Different study objectives and different study endpoints.

Note that different study objectives are usually referred to dose finding (selection) at the first stage and efficacy confirmation at the second stage, while different study endpoints are directed to biomarker versus clinical endpoint or the same clinical endpoint with different treatment durations. Category I trial design is often viewed as a similar design to a group sequential design with one interim analysis despite that there are differences between a group sequential design and a two-stage seamless design. In this chapter, our emphasis will be placed on Category II designs. The results obtained can be similarly applied to Category III and Category IV designs with some modification for controlling the overall type I error rate at a prespecified level.

In practice, typical examples for a two-stage adaptive seamless design include a two-stage adaptive seamless Phase I/II design and a two-stage adaptive seamless Phase II/III design. For the two-stage adaptive seamless Phase I/II design, the objective at the first stage is for biomarker development and the study objective for the second stage is to establish early efficacy. For a two-stage adaptive seamless Phase II/III design, the study objective is for treatment selection (or dose finding) while the study objective at the second stage is for efficacy confirmation.

14.2.2 Comparison

A two-stage adaptive seamless design is considered a more efficient and flexible study design as compared to the traditional approach of having separate studies in terms of controlling type I error rate and power. For controlling the overall type I error rate, as an example, consider a two-stage adaptive seamless Phase II/III design. Let α_{II} and α_{III} be the type I error rate for Phase II and Phase III studies, respectively. Then, the overall alpha for the traditional approach of having two separate studies is given by $\alpha = \alpha_{II}\alpha_{III}$. In the two-stage adaptive seamless Phase II/III design, on the other hand, the actual alpha is given by $\alpha = \alpha_{III}$. Thus, the alpha for a two-stage adaptive seamless Phase II/III design is actually $1/\alpha_{II}$ times larger than the traditional approach for having two separate Phases II and III studies.

Similarly, for the evaluation of power, let $Power_{II}$ and $Power_{III}$ be the power for Phases II and III studies, respectively. Then, the overall power for the traditional approach of having two separate studies is given by Power = $Power_{II} * Power_{III}$. In the two-stage adaptive seamless Phase II/III design, the actual power is given by $Power = Power_{III}$. Thus, the power for a two-stage adaptive seamless Phase II/III design is actually $1/Power_{II}$ times larger than the traditional approach for having two separate Phases II and III studies.

In clinical development, it is estimated that it will take about 6 months to 1 year before a Phase III study can be kicked off after the completion of a Phase II study. The 6 months to 1 year lead time is necessary due to data management, data analysis, and statistical/clinical report. A two-stage adaptive seamless design could reduce lead time between studies with a well organized planning. At least, the study protocol does not need to resubmit to individual institute review boards (IRBs) for approval between studies if the two studies have been combined into one single trial.

In addition, as compared to the traditional approach for having two separate studies, a two-stage adaptive seamless trial design that combines two separate studies may require less sample size for achieving the desired power to address the study objectives from both individual studies.

14.2.3 Practical Issues

As indicated earlier, a two-stage adaptive seamless trial design combines two separate studies that may use different study endpoints to address different study objectives. As a result, we may have different study endpoints and/or different study objectives at different stages for a two-stage adaptive seamless trial design. This leads to four different kinds of two-stage seamless designs: (i) same study endpoint and same study objective, (ii) same study endpoint but different study objectives (e.g., dose finding versus efficacy confirmation), (iii) different study endpoints (e.g., biomarker versus clinical endpoint) but same study objective, and (iv) different study endpoints and different objectives.

Statistical consideration for the first kind of two-stage seamless designs is similar to that of a group sequential design with one interim analysis. Sample size calculation and statistical analysis for these kinds of study designs can be found in Chow and Chang (2006). For other kinds of two-stage seamless trial designs, standard statistical methods for group sequential design are not appropriate and hence should not be applied directly. In this chapter, statistical methods for a two-stage adaptive seamless design with different study endpoints (e.g., a biomarker versus clinical endpoint or the same clinical endpoint with different treatment durations) but same study objective will be developed. Modification to the derived results is necessary if the study endpoints and study objectives are different at different stages.

One of the questions that are commonly asked when applying a two-stage adaptive seamless design in clinical trials is sample size calculation/allocation. For the first kind of two-stage seamless designs, the methods based on individual *p*-values as described in Chow and Chang (2006) can be applied. However, these methods are not appropriate when different study endpoints are used at different stages. In what follows, formulas and/or procedures for sample size calculation/allocation under a two-stage seamless study design using different study endpoints for achieving the same study objective are derived for various data types including continuous, discrete (binary response), and time-to-event data assuming that there is a well-established relationship between the two study endpoints. In other words, the study endpoint considered at the first stage is predictive of the study endpoint employed at the second stage.

14.3 Sample Size Calculation/Allocation

14.3.1 Continuous Study Endpoints

Without loss of generality, consider a two-stage seamless Phase II/III study. Let x_i be the observation of one study endpoint (e.g., a biomarker) from the ith subject in Phase II, $i = 1, \ldots, n$ and y_j be the observation of another study endpoint (the primary clinical endpoint) from the jth subject in Phase III, $j = 1, \ldots, m$. Assume that x_i's are independently and identically distributed with $E(x_i) = \nu$ and $Var(x_i) = \tau^2$; and y_j's are independently and identically distributed with $E(y_j) = \mu$ and $Var(y_j) = \sigma^2$. Chow, Lu, and Tse (2007) proposed using the established functional relationship to obtain predicted values of the clinical endpoint based on data collected from the biomarker (or surrogate endpoint). Thus, these predicted values can be combined with the data collected at the confirmatory phase to develop a valid statistical inference for the treatment effect under study. Suppose that x and y can be related in a straight-line relationship:

$$y = \beta_0 + \beta_1 x + \varepsilon, \tag{14.1}$$

where ε is an error term with zero mean and variance ς^2. Furthermore, ε is independent of x. In practice, we assume that this relationship is well-explored and the parameters β_0 and β_1 are known. Based on Equation 14.1, the observations x_i observed in the learning phase would be translated to $\beta_0 + \beta_1 x_i$ (denoted by $\hat{y}_i$) and are combined with those observations y_i collected in the confirmatory phase. Therefore, $\hat{y}_i$'s and y_i's are combined for the estimation of the treatment mean μ. Consider the following weighted-mean estimator,

$$\hat{\mu} = \omega\bar{\hat{y}} + (1-\omega)\bar{y}, \tag{14.2}$$

where $\bar{\hat{y}} = (1/n)\Sigma_{i=1}^{n}\hat{y}_i$, $\bar{y} = (1/m)\ \Sigma_{i=1}^{m} y_j$ and $0 \le \omega \le 1$. It should be noted that $\hat{\mu}$ is the minimum variance unbiased estimator among all weighted-mean estimators when the weight is given by:

$$\omega = \frac{n/(\beta_1^2\tau^2)}{n/(\beta_1^2\tau^2)+m/\sigma^2}, \tag{14.3}$$

if β_1, $\tau^2$and σ^2 are known. In practice, τ^2 and σ^2 are usually unknown and ω is commonly estimated by:

$$\hat{\omega} = \frac{n/S_1^2}{n/S_1^2 + m/S_2^2}, \tag{14.4}$$

where S_1^2 and S_2^2 are the sample variances of $\hat{y}_i$'s and y_j's, respectively. The corresponding estimator of μ, which is denoted by:

$$\hat{\mu}_{GD} = \hat{\omega}\bar{\hat{y}} + (1-\hat{\omega})\bar{y}, \tag{14.5}$$

is called the Graybill-Deal (GD) estimator of μ. The GD estimator is often called the weighted mean in metrology. Khatri and Shah (1974) gave an exact expression of the variance of this estimator in the form of an infinite series. An approximate unbiased estimator of the variance of the GD estimator, which has bias of order $O(n^{-2} + m^{-2})$, was proposed by Meier (1953). In particular, it is given as:

$$\widehat{Var}(\hat{\mu}_{GD}) = \frac{1}{n/S_1^2 + m/S_2^2}\left[1 + 4\hat{\omega}(1-\hat{\omega})\left(\frac{1}{n-1} + \frac{1}{m-1}\right)\right].$$

For the comparison of the two treatments, the following hypotheses are considered:

$$H_0: \mu_1 = \mu_2 \qquad v.s. \qquad H_1: \mu_1 \neq \mu_2. \tag{14.6}$$

Let $\hat{y}_{ij}$ be the predicted value $\beta_0 + \beta_1 x_{ij}$, which is used as the prediction of y for the jth subject under the ith treatment in Phase II. From Equation 14.5, the GD estimator of μ_i is given as:

$$\hat{\mu}_{GDi} = \hat{\omega}_i \bar{\hat{y}}_i + (1-\hat{\omega}_i)\bar{y}_i, \tag{14.7}$$

where $\bar{\hat{y}}_i = (1/n_i)\Sigma_{j=1}^{n_i}\hat{y}_{ij}$, $\bar{y}_i = (1/m_i)\Sigma_{j=1}^{m_i} y_{ij}$ and $\hat{\omega}_i = \left[(n_i/S_{1i}^2)/(n_i/S_{1i}^2 + m_i/S_{2i}^2)\right]$ with S_{1i}^2 and S_{2i}^2 being the sample variances of $(\hat{y}_{i1}, \cdots, \hat{y}_{in_i})$ and $(y_{i1}, \cdots, y_{im_i})$, respectively. For Hypotheses 14.6, consider the following test statistic,

$$\tilde{T}_1 = \frac{\hat{\mu}_{GD1} - \hat{\mu}_{GD2}}{\sqrt{\widehat{Var}(\hat{\mu}_{GD1}) + \widehat{Var}(\hat{\mu}_{GD2})}}, \tag{14.8}$$

where

$$\widehat{Var}(\hat{\mu}_{GDi}) = \frac{1}{n_i/S_{1i}^2 + m_i/S_{2i}^2}\left[1 + 4\hat{\omega}_i(1-\hat{\omega}_i)\left(\frac{1}{n_i-1} + \frac{1}{m_i-1}\right)\right],$$

is an estimator of $Var(\hat{\mu}_{GDi})$, $i = 1, 2$. Using arguments similar to those in Section 14.2.1, it can be verified that $\tilde{T}_1$ has a limiting standard normal distribution under the null hypothesis H_0 if Var(S_{1i}^2) and Var(S_{2i}^2) $\rightarrow 0$ as n_i and $m_i \rightarrow \infty$. Consequently, an approximate 100(1 – α)% confidence interval of $\mu_1 - \mu_2$ is given as:

$$\left(\hat{\mu}_{GD1}-\hat{\mu}_{GD2}-z_{\alpha/2}\sqrt{V_T},\ \hat{\mu}_{GD1}-\hat{\mu}_{GD2}+z_{\alpha/2}\sqrt{V_T}\right), \tag{14.9}$$

where $V_T = \widehat{Var}(\hat{\mu}_{GD1})+\widehat{Var}(\hat{\mu}_{GD2})$. Therefore, hypothesis H_0 is rejected if the confidence interval in Equation 14.9 does not contain 0. Thus, under the local alternative hypothesis that $H_1 : \mu_1 - \mu_2 = \delta \neq 0$, the required sample size to achieve a 1 – β power satisfies:

$$-z_{\alpha/2}+|\delta|/\sqrt{Var(\hat{\mu}_{GD1})+Var(\hat{\mu}_{GD2})} = z_\beta.$$

Let $m_i = \rho n_i$ and $n_2 = \gamma n_1$. Then, denoted by N_T the total sample size for two treatment groups is $(1 + \rho)(1 + \gamma)n_1$ with n_1 given as:

$$n_1 = \frac{1}{2}AB\left(1+\sqrt{1+8(1+\rho)A^{-1}C}\right), \tag{14.10}$$

where $A=\left[(z_{\alpha/2}+z_\beta)^2/\delta^2\right]$, $B=\left[\sigma_1^2/(\rho+r_1^{-1})\right]+\left[\sigma_2^2/\gamma(\rho+r_2^{-1})\right]$ and $C = B^{-2}\left\{\left[\sigma_1^2/r_1(\rho+r_1^{-1})^3\right]\right\}+\left[\sigma_2^2/\gamma^2 r_2(\rho+r_2^{-1})^3\right]\}$ with $r_i = \beta_1^2\tau_i^2/\sigma_i^2$, $i = 1, 2$.

For the case of testing for superiority, consider the following local alternative hypothesis that:

$$H_1: \mu_1 - \mu_2 = \delta_1 > \delta.$$

The required sample size to achieve 1 – β power satisfies:

$$-z_\alpha+(\delta_1-\delta)/\sqrt{Var(\hat{\mu}_{GD1})+Var(\hat{\mu}_{GD2})} = z_\beta$$

Using the notations in the above, the total sample size for two treatment groups is $(1 + \rho)(1 + \gamma)n_1$ with n_1 given as:

$$n_1 = \frac{1}{2}DB\left(1+\sqrt{1+8(1+\rho)D^{-1}C}\right), \tag{14.11}$$

where $D = [(Z_\alpha + Z_\beta)^2/(\delta_1 - \delta)^2]$. For the case of testing for equivalence with a significance level α, consider the local alternative hypothesis that $H_1: \mu_1 - \mu_2 = \delta_1$ with $|\delta_1| < \delta$. The required sample size to achieve 1 – β power satisfies:

$$-z_\alpha+(\delta-\delta_1)/\sqrt{Var(\hat{\mu}_{GD1})+Var(\hat{\mu}_{GD2})} = z_\beta.$$

Thus, the total sample size for two treatment groups is $(1 + \rho)(1 + \gamma)n_1$ with n_1 given:

$$n_1 = \frac{1}{2}EB\left(1+\sqrt{1+8(1+\rho)E^{-1}C}\right), \tag{14.12}$$

where $E = [(Z_\alpha + Z_{\beta/2})^2/(\delta - |\delta_1|)^2]$.

14.3.2 Binary Responses

Lu et al. (2009) consider the case where the study endpoint is a discrete variable such as a binary response. Suppose that the study duration of the first stage is cL and the study duration of the second stage is L with $0 < c < 1$. Assume that the response is determined by an underlying lifetime t, and the corresponding lifetime distribution of t for the test treatment is $G_1(t,\boldsymbol{\theta}_1)$ while for the control is $G_2(t,\boldsymbol{\theta}_2)$. If there are n_1 and m_1 randomly selected individuals in the first and second stages for the test treatment, respectively, let r_1 and s_1 be the numbers of respondents observed in the first and second stages for the test treatment, respectively. Similarly, for the control treatment, there are n_2 and m_2 randomly selected individuals for the control treatment. Let r_2 and s_2 be the numbers of respondents observed in the first and second stages, respectively. Based on these observed data, the likelihood functions $L(\boldsymbol{\theta}_i)$ for the test treatment and the control treatment are:

$$L(\boldsymbol{\theta}_i) = G_i^{r_i}(cL,\boldsymbol{\theta}_i)[1-G_i(cL,\boldsymbol{\theta}_i)]^{n_i-r_i}\, G_i^{s_i}(L,\boldsymbol{\theta}_i)[1-G_i(L,\boldsymbol{\theta}_i)]^{m_i-s_i}$$

for $i = 1, 2$; where $i = 1$ represents the test treatment and $i = 2$ represents the control treatment. Assume that the lifetimes under test and control treatments are exponentially distributed with parameters λ_1 and λ_2, respectively. Thus, $G_1(t;\, \boldsymbol{\theta}_1) = G(t,\, \lambda_1)$ and $G_2(t;\, \boldsymbol{\theta}_2) = G(t,\, \lambda_2)$. Then the likelihood functions become:

$$L(\lambda_i) = \left(1-e^{-\lambda_i cL}\right)^{r_i} e^{-(n_i-r_i)\lambda_i cL}\left(1-e^{-\lambda_i L}\right)^{s_i} e^{-(m_i-s_i)\lambda_i L}.$$

Let $\hat{\lambda}_i$ be the maximum likelihood estimate (MLE) of λ_i. Then, for $I = 1, 2$, $\hat{\lambda}_i$ can be found by solving the following likelihood equation:

$$\frac{r_i c}{e^{\lambda_i cL}-1} + \frac{s_i}{e^{\lambda_i L}-1} - (n_i - r_i)c - (m_i - s_i) = 0, \tag{14.13}$$

which is obtained by setting the first order partial derivative $L(\lambda_i)$ with respect to λ_i to zero. Note that the MLE of λ_i exist if and only if r_i/n_i and s_i/m_i do not equal 0 or 1 at the same time. Based on the asymptotic normality of MLE (under suitable regularity conditions), $\hat{\lambda}_i$ asymptotically follows a normal distribution. In particular, as n_i and m_i tend to infinity, the distribution of $(\hat{\lambda}_i - \lambda_i)/\sigma_i(\lambda_i)$ converges to the standard normal distribution where:

$$\sigma_i(\lambda_i) = L^{-1}\left(n_i c^2 (e^{\lambda_i cL}-1)^{-1} + m_i (e^{\lambda_i L}-1)^{-1}\right)^{-1/2}.$$

Let $\sigma_i(\hat{\lambda}_i)$ be the MLE of $\sigma_i(\lambda_i)$. Based on the consistency of MLE, by the Slutsky's Theorem, $(\hat{\lambda}_i - \lambda_i)/\sigma_i(\hat{\lambda}_i)$ follows a standard normal distribution asymptotically. Consequently, an approximate $(1 - \alpha)$ confidence interval of λ_i is given as $\left(\hat{\lambda}_i - z_{\alpha/2}\sigma_i(\hat{\lambda}_i),\ \hat{\lambda}_i + z_{\alpha/2}\sigma_i(\hat{\lambda}_i)\right)$, where $Z_{\alpha/2}$ is the $(1 - \alpha/2)$-quartile of a standard normal distribution. Under an exponential model, comparison of two treatments usually focuses on the hazard rate λ_i. For the comparison of two treatments in pharmaceutical applications, namely, control versus treatment, it is often of interest to study the hypotheses testing of equality, superiority, noninferiority, and equivalence of two treatments. Furthermore, to facilitate the planning of a clinical study, researchers are also interested to determine the required sample size, which would allow the corresponding tests to achieve a given level of power (Chow, Shao, and Wang 2007). For illustration purposes, consider testing the following hypotheses for equality:

$$H_0: \lambda_1 = \lambda_2 \quad vs. \quad H_1: \lambda_1 \neq \lambda_2. \tag{14.14}$$

Let $m_i = \rho n_i$ and $n_2 = \gamma n_1$, $i = 1, 2$. Then the total sample size N_T for two treatments is $(1 + \rho)(1 + \gamma)n_1$, where:

$$n_1 = \frac{(z_{\alpha/2} + z_\beta)^2(\tilde{\sigma}_1^2(\lambda_1) + \tilde{\sigma}_2^2(\lambda_2))}{(\lambda_1 - \lambda_2)^2}, \tag{14.15}$$

$$\tilde{\sigma}_1^2(\lambda_1) = L^{-2}\left(c^2(e^{\lambda_1 cL} - 1)^{-1} + \rho(e^{\lambda_1 L} - 1)^{-1}\right)^{-1},$$

and

$$\tilde{\sigma}_2^2(\lambda_2) = L^{-2}\gamma^{-1}\left(c^2(e^{\lambda_2 cL} - 1)^{-1} + \rho(e^{\lambda_2 L} - 1)^{-1}\right)^{-1}.$$

Similarly, for testing the following hypotheses of superiority, noninferiority, and equivalence,

$$H_0 : \lambda_2 - \lambda_1 \le \delta \quad vs. \quad H_1 : \lambda_2 - \lambda_1 > \delta,$$

$$H_0 : \lambda_2 - \lambda_1 \le -\delta \quad vs. \quad H_1 : \lambda_2 - \lambda_1 > -\delta,$$

$$H_0 : |\lambda_1 - \lambda_2| \ge \delta \quad vs. \quad H_1 : |\lambda_1 - \lambda_2| < \delta,$$

where δ is the corresponding (clinical) superiority margin, noninferiority margin, and equivalence limit, the sample size n_1 is given respectively as:

$$n_1 = \frac{(z_\alpha + z_\beta)^2(\tilde{\sigma}_1^2(\lambda_1) + \tilde{\sigma}_2^2(\lambda_2))}{(\lambda_2 - \lambda_1 - \delta)^2},$$

$$n_1 = \frac{(z_\alpha + z_\beta)^2(\tilde{\sigma}_1^2(\lambda_1) + \tilde{\sigma}_2^2(\lambda_2))}{(\lambda_2 - \lambda_1 + \delta)^2},$$

and

$$n_1 = \frac{(z_\alpha + z_{\beta/2})^2(\tilde{\sigma}_1^2(\lambda_1) + \tilde{\sigma}_2^2(\lambda_2))}{(\delta - |\lambda_2 - \lambda_1|)^2}.$$

14.3.3 Time-to-Event Data

Similar ideas can be applied to derive formulas for sample size calculation/allocation for time-to-event data (Lu et al. 2009). Let t_{ijk} denote the length of time of a patient from entering the trial to the occurrence of some events of interest for the kth subject at the jth stage in the ith treatment, where $k = 1, 2, \ldots, n_{ij}$, $j = 1, 2$, $i = T$ and R. Assume that the study durations for the 1st and the 2nd stage are different, which are given by cL and L respectively, where $c < 1$. Furthermore, assume that t_{ijk} follows a distribution with $G(t,\boldsymbol{\theta}_i)$ and $g(t,\boldsymbol{\theta}_i)$ as the cumulative distribution function and probability density function with parameter vector $\boldsymbol{\theta}_i$, respectively. Then, the data collected from the study can be represented by (x_{ijk}, δ_{ijk}), where $\delta_{ijk} = 1$ indicates that the event of interest is observed and that $x_{ijk} = t_{ijk}$ while $\delta_{ijk} = 0$ means that the event is not observed during the study; that is, x_{ijk} is censored and that $x_{ijk} < t_{ijk}$. In clinical trials, it is not uncommon to observe censored data due to drop-out, loss to follow-up, or survival at the end of the trials. In this chapter, for simplicity, we will only consider the case where censoring is due to survival at the end of trials. Given the observed data, the likelihood function for the test treatment and the control treatment can be obtained as follows:

$$L(\boldsymbol{\theta}_i)=\prod_{j=1}^{2}\prod_{k=1}^{n_{ij}} g^{\delta_{ijk}}(x_{ijk},\boldsymbol{\theta}_i)\left[1-G(x_{ijk},\boldsymbol{\theta}_i)\right]^{1-\delta_{ijk}}, \tag{14.16}$$

for $i = T, R$. In particular, suppose that the observed time-to-event data are assumed to follow a Weibull distribution. Denote the cumulative distribution function (cdf) of a Weibull distribution with λ, $\beta > 0$ by $G(t; \lambda, \beta)$ where $G(t;\lambda,\beta)=1-e^{-(t/\lambda)^{\beta}}$. Suppose that $G(t; \theta_T) = G(t; \lambda_T,\beta_T)$ and $G(t; \theta_R) = G(t; \lambda_R,\beta_R)$; that is, t_{ijk} follows the Weibull distribution with cdf $G(t; \lambda_i,\beta_i)$. Then the likelihood function in Equation 14.16 becomes:

$$L(\lambda_i,\beta_i)=\left(\beta_i\lambda_i^{-\beta_i}\right)^{\sum_{j=1}^{2}\sum_{k=1}^{n_{ij}}\delta_{ijk}} e^{-\sum_{j=1}^{2}\sum_{k=1}^{n_{ij}}\tilde{x}_{ijk}}\prod_{j=1}^{2}\prod_{k=1}^{n_{ij}} x_{ijk}^{(\beta_i-1)\delta_{ijk}}, \tag{14.17}$$

Where $\tilde{x}_{ijk}=\left(x_{ijk}/\lambda_i\right)^{\beta_i}$. Let $l(\lambda_i,\beta_i) = \log(L(\lambda_i,\beta_i))$ be the log-likelihood function. Based on the log-likelihood function, the MLEs of β_i and λ_i (denoted by $\hat{\beta}_i$ and $\hat{\lambda}_i$) can be obtained. Based on the asymptotic normality of MLE (Serfling 1980), for $i = T, R$, $\sqrt{n_{i1}}\left(\hat{\lambda}_i-\lambda_i\right)/\sigma(\lambda_i)$ and $\sqrt{n_{i1}}\left(\hat{\beta}_i-\beta_i\right)/\sigma(\beta_i)$ converge in distribution to a standard normal distribution, where:

$$\Delta_i = E\left[-\frac{\partial^2 l(\lambda_i,\beta_i)}{\partial\lambda_i^2}\right]E\left[-\frac{\partial^2 l(\lambda_i,\beta_i)}{\partial\beta_i^2}\right]-E^2\left[-\frac{\partial^2 l(\lambda_i,\beta_i)}{\partial\lambda_i\partial\beta_i}\right],\ \sigma(\lambda_i)=\left[\frac{n_{i1}}{\Delta_i}E\left(-\frac{\partial^2 l(\lambda_i,\beta_i)}{\partial\beta_i^2}\right)\right]^{1/2} \text{ and}$$

$$\sigma(\beta_i)=\left[\frac{n_{i1}}{\Delta_i}E\left(-\frac{\partial^2 l(\lambda_i,\beta_i)}{\partial\lambda_i^2}\right)\right]^{1/2}.$$

Note that $\sigma(\lambda_i)$ and $\sigma(\beta_i)$ do not depend on n_{ij} for given n_{i2}/n_{i1}. Under the assumption of asymptotic normality of MLE, it can be shown that $\hat{\lambda}_i$ and $\hat{\beta}_i$ are asymptotically normally distributed (EMEA 2002). Thus, formulas for sample size calculation/allocation can be similarly obtained. For illustration purposes, consider testing the following hypotheses of equality between medians:

$$H_0: M_T = M_R \quad vs. \quad H_1:\ M_T \neq M_R, \tag{14.18}$$

where M_i is the median of $G(t; \lambda_i,\beta_i)$, $i = T, R$. Let $\hat{M}_i$ be the MLE of M_i and υ_i be the variance of M_i. Based on the asymptotic normality of $(\hat{\lambda}_i,\hat{\beta}_i)$, $\hat{M}_i$ is approximately normally distributed for sufficiently large n_{ij}. In particular,

$$\left(\hat{M}_i-M_i\right)/\sqrt{n_{i1}^{-1}\upsilon_i}\xrightarrow{d}N(0,1),$$

where

$$\upsilon_i = M_i^2\left[\lambda_i^{-2}\sigma^2(\lambda_i)+\beta_i^{-4}\log^2\left(\log(2)\right)\sigma^2(\beta_i)-2\lambda_i^{-1}\beta_i^{-2}\log\left(\log(2)\right)\sigma(\lambda_i,\beta_i)\right],$$

and

$$\sigma(\lambda_i,\beta_i)=\frac{n_{i1}}{\Delta_i}E\left(\frac{\partial^2 l(\lambda_i,\beta_i)}{\partial\lambda_i\partial\beta_i}\right).$$

Note that $\hat{M}_T$ and $\hat{M}_R$ are independent. Thus, we have:

$$\left[\left(\hat{M}_T-\hat{M}_R\right)-\left(M_T-M_R\right)\right]\Big/\sqrt{n_{T1}^{-1}\upsilon_T+n_{R1}^{-1}\upsilon_R}\xrightarrow{d}N(0,1).$$

Let $\hat{\upsilon}_i$ be the MLE of υ_i with λ_i and β_i replaced by the corresponding MLE. Then, according to the Slutsky's Theorem, the above result also holds if υ_i is replaced by $\hat{\upsilon}_i$. Consequently, $\left(\hat{M}_T-\hat{M}_R\right)\Big/\sqrt{n_{T1}^{-1}\hat{\upsilon}_T+n_{R1}^{-1}\hat{\upsilon}_R}$ is asymptotically distributed as the standard normal distribution under the null hypothesis. Thus, we reject the null hypothesis at an approximate α level of significance if:

$$\left|\hat{M}_T-\hat{M}_R\right|\Big/\sqrt{n_{T1}^{-1}\hat{\upsilon}_T+n_{R1}^{-1}\hat{\upsilon}_R}>z_{\alpha/2}.$$

For sample size calculation/allocation, we first consider the one treatment case; that is, the following hypotheses are considered,

$$H_0: M_T=M_0 \quad v.s. \quad H_1: M_T\neq M_0. \tag{14.19}$$

Based on the asymptotic normality of MLE $\hat{M}_T$, we can then reject the null hypothesis at an approximate α level of significance if $|\hat{M}_T-M_0|/\sqrt{n_{T1}^{-1}\hat{\upsilon}_T}>z_{\alpha/2}$. Since $(\hat{M}_T-M_T)/\sqrt{n_{T1}^{-1}\hat{\upsilon}_T}$ approximately follows the standard normal distribution, the power of the above test under H_1 can be approximated by $\Phi\left(|M_T-M_0|/\sqrt{n_{T1}^{-1}\upsilon_T}-z_{\alpha/2}\right)$, where Φ is the distribution function of the standard normal distribution. Hence, in order to achieve a power of $1-\beta$, the required sample size satisfies $|M_T-M_0|/\sqrt{n_{T1}^{-1}\upsilon_T}-z_{\alpha/2}=z_\beta$. If $n_{T2}=\rho n_{T1}$, the required total sample size N for the two phases is given as $N=(1+\rho)n_{T1}$ where n_{T1} is given by:

$$n_{T1}=\frac{(z_{\alpha/2}+z_\beta)^2\upsilon_T}{(M_1-M_0)^2}. \tag{14.20}$$

Following the above idea, the corresponding sample size to achieve a prespecified power of $1-\beta$ with significance level α can be determined. Hence, the corresponding required sample size for testing hypotheses in Equation 14.19 satisfies the following equation,

$$|M_T-M_R|/\sqrt{n_{T1}^{-1}\upsilon_T+n_{R1}^{-1}\upsilon_R}-z_{\alpha/2}=z_\beta.$$

Let $n_{i2}=\rho_i n_{i1}$ and $n_{R1}=\gamma n_{T1}$. It can be easily derived that the total sample size N_T for the two treatment groups in two stages is $n_{T1}[1+\rho_T+(1+\rho_R)\gamma]$ with n_{T1} given as:

$$n_{T1}=\frac{(z_{\alpha/2}+z_\beta)^2(\upsilon_T+\gamma^{-1}\upsilon_R)}{(M_T-M_R)^2}. \tag{14.21}$$

Similarly, for testing the following hypotheses of superiority, noninferiority, and equivalence,

$$H_0: M_T-M_R\leq\delta \qquad vs \qquad H_1: M_T-M_R>\delta,$$

$$H_0: M_T - M_R \le -\delta \quad vs. \quad H_1: M_T - M_R > -\delta,$$

$$H_0: |M_T - M_R| \ge \delta \quad vs. \quad H_1: |M_T - M_R| < \delta,$$

where δ is the corresponding (clinical) superiority margin, noninferiority margin, and equivalence limit, the sample size n_{T1} is given respectively as:

$$n_{T1} = \frac{(z_\alpha + z_\beta)^2(\upsilon_T + \gamma^{-1}\upsilon_R)}{(M_T - M_R - \delta)^2},$$

$$n_{T1} = \frac{(z_\alpha + z_\beta)^2(\upsilon_T + \gamma^{-1}\upsilon_R)}{(M_T - M_R + \delta)^2},$$

and

$$n_{T1} = \frac{(z_\alpha + z_{\beta/2})^2(\upsilon_T + \gamma^{-1}\upsilon_R)}{(\,|M_T - M_R| - \delta\,)^2}.$$

Note that the above formulas for sample size estimation/allocation are derived based on a parametric approach assuming that the observed data follow a Weibull distribution. Alternatively, we may explore the same problem based on a semiparametric approach under the following Cox's proportional hazard model. Let n_j be total sample size for the two treatments in the jth stage, $j = 1, 2$ and d_j be number of distinct failure times in the jth stage, which are denoted by $t_{j1} < t_{j2} < \ldots < t_{jd_j}$. Furthermore, denote the observation based on the kth subject in the jth stage by:

$$(T_{jk}, \delta_{jk}, z_{jk}(t),\ 0 \le t \le T_{jk}) = (\min(\tilde{T}_{jk}, C_{jk}), I(\tilde{T}_{jk} < C_{jk}), z_{jk}(t),\ 0 \le t \le T_{jk}),$$

where, correspondingly, T_{jk} is the observed time, $\tilde{T}_{jk}$ is time-to-event, δ_{jk} is the indicator for the observed failure, C_{jk} is a censoring time that is assumed to be independent of $\tilde{T}_{jk}$, and $z_{jk}(t)$ is a covariate vector at time t. Let $h(t|z)$ be the hazard rate at time t for an individual with a covariate vector z. The Cox proportional hazard model assumes:

$$h(t\,|\,z(t)) = h(t\,|\,0)e^{b'z(t)},$$

where the baseline $h(t|0)$ is unspecified and b is a coefficient vector with the same dimension as $z(t)$. Thus, the partial likelihood function is:

$$L(b) = \prod_{j=1}^{2}\prod_{k=1}^{d_j} P(\text{observed failure at time } t_{jk}\,|\,R(t_{jk}))$$

$$= \prod_{j=1}^{2}\prod_{k=1}^{d_j} \frac{\exp(b'z_{(jk)}(t_{jk}))}{\sum_{l \in R(t_{jk})} \exp(b'z_l(t_{jk}))},$$

where the risk set $R(t_{jk}) = \{js : \tilde{T}_{js} \ge T_{jk}\}$ is the collection of subjects still on study just prior to t_{jk} in the jth stage. Furthermore, the partial likelihood equation is:

$$U(b)=\sum_{j=1}^{2}\sum_{k=1}^{d_j}\left[z_{(jk)}(t_{jk})-e(b,t_{jk})\right], \tag{14.22}$$

where $e(b,t_{jk})=\{[\Sigma_{l\in R(t_{jk})}\exp(b'z_l(t_{jk}))z_l(t_{jk})]/[\Sigma_{l\in R(t_{jk})}\exp(b'z_l(t_{jk}))]\}$. Thus, the corresponding observed information matrix is given by:

$$I(b)=\sum_{j=1}^{2}\sum_{k=1}^{d_j}\left[\frac{\sum_{l\in R(t_{jk})}\exp(b'z_l(t_{jk}))z_l(t_{jk})z_l'(t_{jk})}{\sum_{l\in R(t_{jk})}\exp(b'z_l(t_{jk}))}-e(b,t_{jk})e'(b,t_{jk})\right]. \tag{14.23}$$

Similarly, the following hypotheses are usually considered for testing equality, superiority/noninferiority, and equivalence by comparing the coefficient vector b:

$$H_0: b=b_0 \quad vs. \quad H_1: b\neq b_0,$$

$$H_0: b\geq\delta \quad vs. \quad H_1: b<\delta,$$

$$H_0: |b| >\delta \quad vs. \quad H_1: |b| <\delta,$$

where δ is the corresponding (clinical) superiority margin ($\delta < 0$), noninferiority margin ($\delta > 0$), and equivalence limit. Define:

$$p_{jk}=n_{Tjk}e^b/(n_{Tjk}e^b+n_{Rjk}),$$

where n_{Tjk} and n_{Rjk} denotes the number of subjects at risk; that is, those who have not failed or censored just prior to the kth observed failure in the jth stage in the test and the control treatment, respectively. It can be verified that sample sizes n_{T1}s for testing the above hypotheses are given respectively as:

$$n_{T1}=\frac{(z_{\alpha/2}+z_\beta)^2}{b^2(p_{T1}p_{R1}u_1+\rho p_{T2}p_{R2}u_2)},$$

$$n_{T1}=\frac{(z_\alpha+z_\beta)^2}{e^\delta(b-\delta)^2K},$$

and

$$n_{T1}=\frac{(z_\alpha+z_{\beta/2})^2}{e^\delta(b-|\delta|)^2K},$$

where

$$K=\frac{p_{R1}p_{T1}u_1}{(p_{R1}+p_{T1}e^\delta)^2}+\frac{\rho p_{R2}p_{T2}u_2}{(p_{R2}+p_{T2}e^\delta)^2}.$$

Note that details regarding the derivation of the above formulas for sample size calculation for testing equality, superiority/noninferiority, and equivalence can be found in Tse, Lu, and Chow (2010).

14.3.4 Remarks

In this chapter, formulas for sample size calculation/allocation for two-stage seamless adaptive designs were derived for continuous, discrete, and time-to-event data for testing hypotheses of equality, superiority, noninferiority, and equivalence under the assumptions that: (1) there is a well-established relationship between different study endpoints at different stages, and (2) the study objectives for both stages are the same. For convenience's sake, formulas for sample size estimation/allocation for continuous, binary, and time-to-event data for testing hypotheses of equality, noninferiority, superiority, and equivalence are summarized in Table 14.1 (continuous endpoints and binary responses) and Table 14.2 (time-to-event-data). Following similar ideas, the derivation of formulas for sample size calculation/allocation for other cases that: (1) the study objectives are different but the study endpoints are the same, and (2) the study objectives and the study endpoints are different is possible and yet complicated.

In practice, it should be noted that such a relationship (i.e., one study endpoint is predictive of the other study endpoint) may not exist. Thus, it is suggested that the relationship be validated based on historical data or the data observed from study. When the study objectives are different at different stages (e.g., dose finding at the first stage and efficacy confirmation at the second stage), the above derived formulas are necessary for controlling the overall type I error rate at α and for achieving the desired powers at both stages.

TABLE 14.1 Formulas for Sample Size Calculation/Estimation for Two-Stage Seamless Adaptive Design with Different Study Endpoints (Continuous Endpoints and Binary Responses)

Hypotheses Testing for	Continuous Endpoint	Binary Response
Equality	$n_1=\frac{1}{2}AB\left(1+\sqrt{1+8(1+\rho)A^{-1}C}\right)$	$n_1=\frac{(z_{\alpha/2}+z_\beta)^2(\tilde{\sigma}_1^2(\lambda_1)+\tilde{\sigma}_2^2(\lambda_2))}{(\lambda_2-\lambda_1)^2}$
Noninferiority ($\delta<0$)	$n_1=\frac{1}{2}BD\left(1+\sqrt{1+8(1+\rho)D^{-1}C}\right)$	$n_1=\frac{(z_{\alpha}+z_\beta)^2(\tilde{\sigma}_1^2(\lambda_1)+\tilde{\sigma}_2^2(\lambda_2))}{(\lambda_2-\lambda_1-\delta)^2}$
Superiority ($\delta>0$)	$n_1=\frac{1}{2}DB\left(1+\sqrt{1+8(1+\rho)D^{-1}C}\right)$	$n_1=\frac{(z_{\alpha}+z_\beta)^2(\tilde{\sigma}_1^2(\lambda_1)+\tilde{\sigma}_2^2(\lambda_2))}{(\lambda_2-\lambda_1+\delta)^2}$
Equivalence	$n_1=\frac{1}{2}EB\left(1+\sqrt{1+8(1+\rho)E^{-1}C}\right)$	$n_1=\frac{(z_{\alpha}+z_\beta)^2(\tilde{\sigma}_1^2(\lambda_1)+\tilde{\sigma}_2^2(\lambda_2))}{(\delta-\lvert\lambda_2-\lambda_1\rvert)^2}$

Note: 1. A, B, C, D, E, and ρ are defined in Section 14.3.1.
2. $\lambda_1, \lambda_2, \tilde{\sigma}_1^2(\lambda_1)$, and $\tilde{\sigma}_2^2(\lambda_2)$ are defined in Section 14.3.2.

TABLE 14.2 Formulas for Sample Size Calculation/Estimation for Two-Stage Seamless Adaptive Design with Different Study Endpoints

Hypotheses Testing for	Weibull Distribution	Cox's Proportional Hazard Model
Equality	$n_1=\frac{(z_{\alpha/2}+z_\beta)^2(\upsilon_T+\gamma^{-1}\upsilon_R)}{(M_T-M_R)^2}$	$n_1=\frac{(z_{\alpha/2}+z_\beta)^2}{b^2(p_{T_1}p_{R_1}u_1+\rho p_{T_1}p_{R_1}u_2)^2}$
Noninferiority	$n_1=\frac{(z_{\alpha/2}+z_\beta)^2(\upsilon_T+\gamma^{-1}\upsilon_R)}{(M_T-M_R-\delta)^2}$	$n_1=\frac{(z_\alpha+z_\beta)^2}{e^\delta(b-\delta)^2K}$ ($\delta<0$)
Superiority	$n_1=\frac{(z_{\alpha/2}+z_\beta)^2(\upsilon_T+\gamma^{-1}\upsilon_R)}{(M_T-M_R+\delta)^2}$	$n_1=\frac{(z_\alpha+z_\beta)^2}{e^\delta(b-\delta)^2K}$ ($\delta>0$)
Equivalence	$n_1=\frac{(z_{\alpha/2}+z_\beta)^2(\upsilon_T+\gamma^{-1}\upsilon_R)}{(\lvert M_T-M_R\rvert-\delta)^2}$	$n_1=\frac{(z_{\alpha/2}+z_{\beta/2})^2}{e^\delta(b-\lvert\delta\rvert)^2K}$

Note: 1. $M_i, \upsilon_i, \gamma, \rho$, and K for i = T, R are defined in Section 14.3.3 ·

14.4 Major Obstacles and Challenges

14.4.1 Instability of Sample Size

In clinical trials, a prestudy power analysis for sample size calculation is often performed based on either: (1) information obtained from pilot studies with limited number of subjects, or (2) purely guess based on the best knowledge of the investigator (with or without scientific justification). The observed data and/or the investigator's best guess could be far deviated from the truth, which may bias the sample size calculation for reaching the desired power for achieving the study objectives. Thus, one of the controversial issues regarding sample size calculation is that how sensitive (robust or stable) the obtained sample size is. Under certain assumptions, sample size for testing hypotheses of equality can be obtained as follows:

$$N_0 = \frac{(z_{\alpha/2} + z_\beta)^2 \sigma^2}{\delta^2},$$

where σ^2/δ^2 is often estimated by sample mean and sample variance from some pilot studies. Let $\theta = \sigma^2/\delta^2$. Then, it can be verified that bias of $\hat{\theta} = s^2/\hat{\delta}^2$ is given by:

$$E(\hat{\theta}) - \theta = 3N_0^{-1}\theta^2\{1 + o(1)\}. \tag{14.24}$$

As a result, sample size obtained based on $\hat{\theta} = s^2/\hat{\delta}^2$ could be substantial and consequently leads to the instability of the sample size calculation. To reduce bias, one may consider using the median of $s^2/\hat{\delta}^2$ such that:

$$P\{s^2/\hat{\delta} \le \eta_{0.5}\} = 0.5.$$

It can be verified that the bias of median estimate is much less as compared to that of Equation 14.18; that is,

$$\eta_{0.5} - \theta = -1.5N_0^{-1}\theta\{1 + o(1)\}. \tag{14.25}$$

Equation 14.25 suggests that a bootstrap-median approach be considered for a stable sample size calculation in clinical trials.

Note that the above discussion indicates that sample size calculation based on limited information obtained from a small pilot study could be rather instable. This discussion also justifies the use of flexible sample size reestimation trial design in clinical trials.

14.4.2 Moving Patient Population

In practice, it is not uncommon to have protocol amendments during the conduct of clinical trials. As a result, it is likely that a shift in patient population may have occurred before and after protocol amendments. Chow, Shao, and Hu (2002) suggests assessing the shift in patient population using the following sensitivity index (Maca et al. 2006):

$$\begin{aligned} |E| &= \left|\frac{\mu}{\sigma}\right| = \left|\frac{\mu_0 + \varepsilon}{C\sigma_0}\right| = \left|\frac{\Delta\mu_0}{\sigma_0}\right| \\ &= |\Delta|\left|\frac{\mu_0}{\sigma_0}\right| = |\Delta||E_0|, \end{aligned} \tag{14.26}$$

where E_0 and E are the effect sizes before and after protocol amendment and $\Delta = (1 + \varepsilon/\mu_0)/C$ is the sensitivity index before and after protocol amendment. When a shift in patient population has occurred, it is recommended to make the following sample size adjustment:

$$N = \min\left\{N_{max}, \max\left(N_{min}, sign(E_0E)\left|\frac{E_0}{E}\right|^a N_0\right)\right\}, \tag{14.27}$$

where N_{min} and N_{max} are the minimum and maximum sample sizes, a is a constant and sign(x) = 1 for x > 0; otherwise sign(x) = −1. Note that it is suggested that a be chosen in the way such that the sensitivity Δ is within an acceptable range.

14.5 Examples

In this section, several examples are considered to illustrate statistical methods described in the previous sections.

Example 1: Continuous response for one treatment:

- Notations (Assumptions)
  - mean effect of Stage 2, $\mu = 1.5$
  - variance at Stage 1, $\tau^2 = 10$
  - variance at Stage 2, $\sigma^2 = 3$
  - the slope of the relationship between the two stages, $\beta_1 = 0.5$
  - $\rho = m/n$, where $n1$ and $m1$ are the sample sizes in Stages 1 and 2, respectively, ($\rho = 4$).
- Hypotheses: H_0: $\mu = \mu_0$ *vs.* H_1: $\mu \neq \mu_0$
- The sample size needed for the first stage to achieve a 80% power at 0.05 level of significance for correctly detecting a difference of $\mu - \mu_0 = 0.5$ is:

$$n = \frac{N_0}{2(\rho + r^{-1})}\left[1 + \sqrt{\frac{8(\rho+1)}{(1+\rho r)N_0}}\right]$$

$$= \frac{94.08}{2(4+1.2)}\left[1 + \sqrt{\frac{8(4+1)}{(1+4\times 0.83)94.08}}\right] = 19.$$

- Then the total sample size is given by:
  $N = (1 + \rho)n = 94.$

Example 2: Binary response for one treatment:

- Notations for one treatment (assumptions)
  - exponential hazard rate, $\lambda_1 = 0.4$
  - the mean life time, $1/\lambda_1 = 2.5$
  - the study duration of Stage 2, $L = 1.73$
  - the study duration of Stage 1 ($cL = 0.69$, i.e., $c = 0.4$)
  - $\rho = m_1/n_1$, where $n1$ and $m1$ are the sample sizes in Stages 1 and 2, respectively. ($\rho = 4$)
- Hypotheses: H_0: $\lambda_1 = \lambda_0$ *vs.* H_1: $\lambda_1 \neq \lambda_0$
- The sample size needed for the first stage to achieve a 80% power at 0.05 level of significance for correctly detecting a difference $\lambda_1 - \lambda_1 = 0.2$ is:

$$n_1 = \frac{(z_{\alpha/2} + z_\beta)^2 \tilde{\sigma}_1^2(\lambda_1)}{(\lambda_1 - \lambda_0)^2} = \frac{(1.96 + 0.84)^2 0.074}{0.2^2} \approx 15.$$

- Then the total sample size is given:
  $N = (1 + \rho)n_1 = 75.$

Example 3 - Binary response for two treatments:

- Notations for two-treatment comparison
  - exponential hazard rate of test treatment $\lambda_1 = 0.15$
  - the mean life time of test treatment, $1/\lambda_1 = 6.67$
  - exponential hazard rate of control treatment, $\lambda_2 = 0.4$
  - the mean life time of control treatment, $1/\lambda_2 = 2.5$
  - the study duration of Stage 2, $L = 1.73$
  - the study duration of Stage 1 ($cL = 0.69$, i.e., $c = 0.4$)
  - $\rho = m_i/n_i, i = 1, 2, r = n_2/n_1$ ($\rho = 3$, and $r = 1$)
- Hypotheses : H_0: $\lambda_1 = \lambda_2$ *vs.* H_1: $\lambda_1 \neq \lambda_2$
- The sample size needed for the first stage under the test treatment to achieve a 80% power at 0.05 level of significance

$$n_1 = \frac{(z_{\alpha/2} + z_\beta)^2 (\tilde{\sigma}_1^2(\lambda_1) + \tilde{\sigma}_1^2(\lambda_1))}{(\lambda_1 - \lambda_0)^2} = \frac{(1.96 + 0.84)^2 0.12}{0.25^2} \approx 15.3$$

- Then the total sample size is given by:

  $N = (1 + \rho)(1 + r)n_1 = 128.$

14.6 Concluding Remarks

In this chapter, formulas for sample size calculation/allocation under a two-stage seamless adaptive trial design that combines two separate studies with different study endpoints but the same study objective are derived assuming that there is a well-established relationship between the two different study endpoints. In practice, a two-stage seamless adaptive trial design that combines a Phase II study for dose finding and a Phase III study for efficacy confirmation is commonly considered (Bauer and Kieser 1999). In this case, the study objectives at different stages are similar but different (i.e., dose finding versus efficacy confirmation). A two-stage seamless adaptive trial means to be able to address both study objectives with the desired power and combine data collected from both stages for a final analysis. In this case, it is a concern how to control the overall type I error rate and achieve the desired powers at both stages. A typical approach is to consider precision analysis at the first stage for dose selection and power the study for detecting a clinically meaningful difference at the second stage (by including the data collected at the first stage for the final analysis). For the precision analysis, the dose with highest confidence level for achieving statistical significance will be selected under some prespecified selection criteria. Some adaptations such as dropping the inferior arms or picking up the best dose, stopping the trial early due to safety and/or futility/efficacy, or adaptive randomization may be applied at the end of the first stage. Although this approach sounds reasonable, it is not clear how the overall type I error rate can be controlled. More research is needed.

From the clinical point of view, adaptive design methods reflect real clinical practice in clinical development. Adaptive design methods are very attractive due to their flexibility and are very useful especially in early clinical development. However, many researchers are not convinced and still challenge its validity and integrity (Tsiatis and Mehta 2003). From the statistical point of view, the use of adaptive methods in clinical trials makes current good statistics practice even more complicated. The validity of the use of adaptive design methods is not well established. The impact of statistical inference on treatment effect should be carefully evaluated under the framework of moving target patient population as the result of protocol amendments (i.e., modifications made to the study protocols during the conduct of the trials). In practice, regulatory agencies may not realize that the adaptive design methods for review and approval of regulatory submissions have been employed for years without any scientific basis. Guidelines regarding the use of adaptive design methods must be developed so that appropriate statistical methods and statistical software packages can be developed accordingly.

References

Bauer, P., and Kieser, M. (1999). Combining different phases in development of medical treatments within a single trial. *Statistics in Medicine*, 18: 1833–48.

Chow, S. C., and Tu, Y. H. (2008). On two-stage seamless adaptive design in clinical trials. *Journal of Formosan Medical Association*, 107 (12): S51–S59.

Chow, S. C., and Chang, M. (2006). *Adaptive Design Methods in Clinical Trials*. Boca Raton, FL: Chapman and Hall/CRC Press, Taylor & Francis.

Chow, S. C., Chang, M., and Pong, A. (2005). Statistical consideration of adaptive methods in clinical development. *Journal of Biopharmaceutical Statistics*, 15: 575–91.

Chow, S. C., Lu, Q., and Tse, S. K. (2007). Statistical analysis for two-stage adaptive design with different study endpoints. *Journal of Biopharmaceutical Statistics*, 17: 1163–76.

Chow, S. C., Shao, J., and Hu, O. Y. P. (2002). Assessing sensitivity and similarity in bridging studies. *Journal of Biopharmaceutical Statistics*, 12: 385–400.

Chow, S. C., Shao, J., and Wang, H. (2007). *Sample Size Calculation in Clinical Research*. 2nd ed. Boca Raton: Chapman Hall/CRC Press, Taylor & Francis.

EMEA. (2002). Point to Consider on *Methodological Issues in Confirmatory Clinical Trials with Flexible Design and Analysis Plan*. The European Agency for the Evaluation of Medicinal Products Evaluation of Medicines for Human Use. CPMP/EWP/2459/02, London, UK.

EMEA. (2006). Reflection paper on *Methodological Issues in Confirmatory Clinical Trials with Flexible Design and Analysis Plan*. The European Agency for the Evaluation of Medicinal Products Evaluation of Medicines for Human Use. CPMP/EWP/2459/02, London, UK.

Gallo, P., Chuang-Stein, C., Dragalin, V., Gaydos, B., Krams, M., and Pinheiro, J. (2006). Adaptive design in clinical drug development—An executive summary of the PhRMA Working Group (with discussions). *Journal of Biopharmaceutical Statistics*, 6: 275–83.

Khatri, C. G., and Shah, K. R. (1974). Estimation of location of parameters from two linear models under normality. *Communications in Statistics*, 3: 647–63.

Lu, Q., Tse, S. K., Chow, S. C., Chi, Y., and Yang, L. Y. (2009). Sample size estimation based on event data for a two-stage survival adaptive trial with different durations. *Journal of Biopharmaceutical Statistics*, 19: 311–23

Maca, J., Bhattacharya, S., Dragalin, V., Gallo, P., and Krams, M. (2006). Adaptive seamless Phase II/III designs—Background, operational aspects, and examples. *Drug Information Journal*, 40: 463–74.

Meier, P. (1953). Variance of a weighted mean. *Biometrics*, 9: 59–73.

Serfling, R. J. (1980). *Approximation Theorems of Mathematical Statistics*. New York: John Wiley & Sons.

Tse, S. K., Lu, Q., and Chow, S. C. (2010). Analysis of time-to-event data under a two-stage seamless trial design in clinical trials. *Journal of Biopharmaceutical Statistics*, 20:705–19.

Tsiatis, A. A., and Mehta, C. (2003). On the inefficiency of the adaptive design for monitoring clinical trials. *Biometrika*, 90: 367–78.

15

Optimal Response-Adaptive Randomization for Clinical Trials

Lanju Zhang
MedImmune LLC

William Rosenberger
George Mason University

15.1 Introduction

15.1.1 Randomization in Clinical Trials

Randomized clinical trials have become the gold standard for modern medical research. Randomization, in the context of a trial with a treatment and a control, is defined as "a process by which all participants are equally likely to be assigned to either the intervention or control group" (Friedman, Furberg, and DeMets 1998, p. 43). Randomization can remove the potential of bias, and also provides a basis to guarantee the validity of statistical tests at the conclusion of the trial.

The definition of Friedman, Furberg, and DeMets (1998) mainly refers to complete randomization or permuted block randomization (Rosenberger and Lachin 2002), which attempts to balance treatment assignments equally among the treatments. Arguments upholding such equal allocation procedures include that they maximize the power of statistical tests and reflect the view of equipoise at the beginning of the trial. The plausibility of these arguments is questioned by Rosenberger and Lachin (2002, p. 169). As they point out, the power of the test is maximized by complete randomization only when responses to two treatments have equal variability. On the other hand, equipoise may not be sustainable through the trial and accruing data may indicate one treatment is performing better than the other, then it may not be ethical to use equal allocation that results in more than necessary participants assigned to the inferior treatment.

In contrast to complete randomization, in adaptive randomization the allocation probability could be unequal for different treatments, and could be changed or updated in the course of randomization. For example, in Efron's biased coin design (Efron 1971), the allocation probability for the next patient to one treatment is smaller if more participants have been randomized to this treatment than the other so far; in other words, the allocation probability depends on imbalance of treatment assignments. The goal of this design is to achieve treatment assignment balance throughout the course of randomization. On the other hand, in the randomized play-the-winner rule (RPW) by Wei and Durham (1978), the allocation probability is updated for the next participants based on the accumulated participant responses so far. The goal of this design is to assign more participants to the better-performing treatment in addressing the ethical issue for equal randomization. Adaptive randomization will reduce to equal randomization if there is no treatment effect or treatment assignment imbalance.

15.1.2 Adaptive Randomization

Adaptive randomization uses accumulated responses, treatment assignments, and/or covariate information in the course of the recruitment to update allocation probability for the next participant so that a specific goal can be achieved; for example, more participants can be assigned to the better performing treatments or treatment assignments can be balanced. There is a vast literature on adaptive randomization. Figure 15.1 presents a schematic classification of methodologies for adaptive randomization. First, adaptive randomization methods can be classified by attributes of clinical trials. For example, adaptive randomization methods for different phases (usually II or III), number of treatments in the trial (two or more than two), or primary endpoints of the trial (binary, continuous, or survival outcomes). Second, adaptive randomization methods can also be classified by different statistical philosophies (Bayesian or frequentist). The next participant is some formulation of the posterior. However, we will make the distinction that statistical methods for adaptive randomization without explicit prior specification as the frequentist method. Finally, adaptive randomization methods can be classified by the scope of adaptation: restricted randomization, response-adaptive randomization, covariate adaptive randomization, and covariate-adjusted response-adaptive (CARA) randomization. For the definition of these concepts, readers are referred to Hu and Rosenberger (2006).

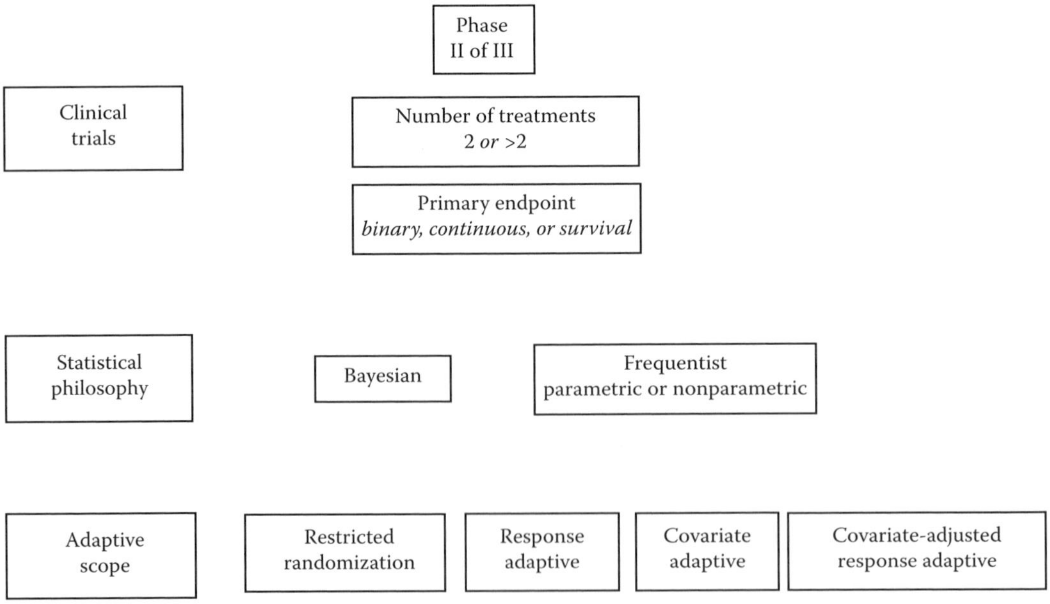

FIGURE 15.1 Classification of adaptive randomization in clinical trials.

Methodologies of adaptive randomization for different combinations of these classifiers could be very different. For example, Bayesian methods are mainly used in Phase II trials with flexibility in number of treatments and primary endpoints for response-adaptive randomization. On the other hand, some response-adaptive randomization methods (e.g., optimal response-adaptive randomization to be discussed below) for two treatments can be very difficult to generalize to more than two treatments (Tymofyeyev, Rosenberger, and Hu 2007).

For a review of Bayesian adaptive randomization, see Thall and Wathen (2007). Bayesian methods are often applied in Phase II trials for dose response studies. Restricted randomization and covariate adaptive randomization have been discussed extensively in Rosenberger and Lachin (2002). In this chapter, we will focus on the frequentist approach to response-adaptive randomization and CARA randomization for Phase III trials with all three types of endpoints.

15.1.3 Balance, Ethics, and Efficiency

Randomization in clinical trials has multiple objectives. Balance across treatment groups is considered essential for comparability with respect to unknown or uncontrollable covariates. Efficiency is critical in sample size determination and thus the cost of the trial. Ethics is a necessary consideration for all medical research involving human beings. The interplay among these objectives could be compatible, but more often they are in conflict. Rosenberger and Sverdlov (2008) give an insightful schematic description on situations where they are in conflict in Phase III clinical trials. In this chapter, we will focus response-adaptive randomization where ethics and efficiency are of central concern. In this regard, Hu and Rosenberger (2003) present an explicit formulation to evaluate the relationship between these two goals. We will discuss more of this point later.

15.1.4 Response-Adaptive Randomization

In response-adaptive randomization, the allocation probability for the next participant is updated using accumulated responses so that by the end of recruitment more participants will be allocated to the better performing treatment arm. Response adaptive randomization could be conducted with or without covariate adjustment, as in Figure 15.1 and Hu and Rosenberger (2006).

There are several approaches to response-adaptive randomization. One intuitive and heuristic approach is through urn models. Different colors of balls in the urn correspond to different treatment arms. One updates the urn composition based on available participant outcomes and randomizes participants to a treatment according to the color of a ball drawn randomly from the urn. Typical urn models include the randomized play-the-winner (Wei and Durham 1978) and the drop-the-loser (Ivanova 2003). Urn models are extensively studied in Hu and Rosenberger (2006). Another approach is procedures based on the optimal allocation. In this approach, a target allocation proportion is derived from some optimization problem, then a randomization procedure is utilized to actualize the allocation proportion in randomization of clinical trials. Recently Zhang and Yang (2010) discuss an approach that has both heuristic and optimal allocation elements. We will focus on the optimal allocation approach in this chapter.

In this chapter we will take a three-step paradigm for response-adaptive randomization: optimization, implementation, and inference. By optimization, we will discuss how to derive optimal allocations using formal optimization criteria. By implementation, we will discuss how to implement various randomization procedures to target the optimal allocation proportion. By inference, we will discuss issues related to data analysis following response-adaptive randomization.

This chapter is organized as follows. Section 15.2 discusses the optimization step and presents optimal allocation for various scenarios. Section 15.3 discusses the implementation step and presents different randomization procedures. Section 15.4 discusses the inference step and presents properties of maximum likelihood method for response-adaptive randomization trials. We conclude in Section 15.5.

15.2 Optimization

In response-adaptive randomization, there is a trade-off between ethical consideration (skewing to the better performing treatment arm) and preservation of power of the statistical test. A large skewing to the better performing treatment often leads to significant loss of test power, which is evidently impractical. To balance these contradictory objectives, Jennison and Turnbull (2000, Chapter 17) propose to use a constrained optimization problem to define the optimal allocation proportion. The objective function will be some metric that is a function of parameters of the response distributions and the constraint will be a function of power. We will see various forms of this optimization problem in the following.

Unless specifically stated otherwise, we will assume there are two treatments in the trial. Let n_i, $i = 1, 2$ denote the number of participants to be randomized to treatment i and $n = n_1 + n_2$. Let $\rho = n_1/n$ be the desired allocation proportion for treatment 1.

15.2.1 Binary Outcomes

Suppose X_i, $i = 1, 2$ is the response of participants randomized to treatment i. Then $X_i \sim$ *Bernoulli* (p_i) where p_i is the successes probability for treatment i. Let $q_i = 1 - p_i$. We will consider testing the hypotheses:

$$H_0 : p_1 - p_2 = 0 \text{ vs } H_a : p_1 - p_2 \neq 0.$$

The standard textbook statistic for testing the hypotheses is Wald test:

$$\frac{\hat{p}_1 - \hat{p}_2}{\sqrt{\frac{\hat{p}_1(1-\hat{p}_1)}{n_1} + \frac{\hat{p}_2(1-\hat{p}_2)}{n_2}}},$$

where $\hat{p}_i$ is the maximum likelihood estimate (MLE) of p_i.

To define an optimal allocation proportion, Rosenberger et al. (2001) consider the following optimization problem:

$$\begin{cases} \min n_1 q_1 + n_2 q_2 \\ s.t. \dfrac{p_1(1-p_1)}{n_1} + \dfrac{p_2(1-p_2)}{n_2} \equiv C_0 \end{cases}, \tag{15.1}$$

where C_0 is a constant.

This amounts to minimizing the total expected failures with a constraint that the variance of $\hat{p}_1 - \hat{p}_2$ being held constant. The solution is the following allocation proportion:

$$\rho_{b1} = \frac{\sqrt{p_1}}{\sqrt{p_1} + \sqrt{p_2}},$$

where the subscript b indicates this allocation proportion is for binary outcomes (same convention is used for continuous and survival outcomes in the following sections). Note that ρ_{b1} is often referred to as the RSIHR allocation proportion, as an acronym of the author name initials of Rosenberger et al. (2001).

In Equation 15.1 one can also minimize the total sample size n, leading to Neyman allocation:

$$\rho_{b2} = \frac{\sqrt{p_1 q_1}}{\sqrt{p_1 q_1} + \sqrt{p_2 q_2}},$$

which can be interpreted in another way; that is, given the sample size, ρ_{b2} will result in the maximum power of the test.

Zhang and Yang (2010) point out that there is a gap between statistical tests covered in the literature (mainly Wald test) and tests used in practice. For example, for binary outcomes, Wald test is rarely used in practice. However, the power constraint in optimization in Equation 15.1 is based on the Wald test. Zhang and Yang (2010) derive an optimal allocation derived from Equation 15.1 where the constraint is replaced with:

$$\bar{p}(1-\bar{p})\left(\frac{1}{n_1} + \frac{1}{n_2}\right) = C_0,$$

where $\bar{p} = (n_1 p_1 + n_2 p_2)/n$. This test is a special case of Farrington and Manning (1990). However, the closed form solution is rather complicated and will be not presented here.

15.2.2 Continuous Outcomes

Now let us entertain continuous outcomes. There are many response-adaptive randomization designs proposed for continuous outcomes, for instance, Bandyopadhyay and Biswas (2001) and Atkinson and Biswas (2005). However, these designs are not based on an optimal allocation approach. Zhang and Rosenberger (2006) proposed a continuous analog of RSIHR allocation for binary case. They extensively evaluate available allocation proportions for normally distributed outcomes. In the following, we will give some of these allocation proportions.

Suppose we want to compare two treatments with normally distributed responses $X_1 \sim N(\mu_1, \sigma_1^2)$ and $X_2 \sim N(\mu_2, \sigma_2^2)$, respectively. We assume that a smaller response, is more desirable to participants. First, similar to binary case, the Neyman allocation proportion, which maximizes power of the test for a given size n, can be given as $\rho_{c1} = \sigma_1/(\sigma_1 + \sigma_2)$.

Since a small response is desirable, the total expected response from all participants should be minimized, leading to the following optimization problem:

$$\begin{cases} \min\limits_{n_1/n_2} & \mu_1 n_1 + \mu_2 n_2 \\ \text{s.t.} & \dfrac{\sigma_1^2}{n_1} + \dfrac{\sigma_2^2}{n_2} \equiv C_0 \end{cases}. \tag{15.2}$$

Solving this problem yields:

$$\rho = \frac{\sqrt{\mu_2}\,\sigma_1}{\sqrt{\mu_2}\,\sigma_1 + \sqrt{\mu_1}\,\sigma_2}. \tag{15.3}$$

When $\mu_1 < \mu_2$, there are possible values of σ_1 and σ_2 that makes n_1/n_2 less than 1. While this may maximize power for fixed expected treatment failures, it is not appropriate to allocate more participants to the inferior treatment. Define $r = \sigma_1\sqrt{\mu_2}/\sigma_2\sqrt{\mu_1}$ and:

$$s = \begin{cases} 1 & \text{if } (\mu_1 < \mu_2 \text{ and } r > 1) \text{ or } (\mu_1 > \mu_2 \text{ and } r < 1), \\ 0 & \text{otherwise.} \end{cases} \tag{15.4}$$

They modify the allocation as follows:

$$\rho_{c2} = \begin{cases} \dfrac{\sigma_1\sqrt{\mu_2}}{\sigma_1\sqrt{\mu_2}+\sigma_2\sqrt{\mu_1}} & \text{if } s=1, \\ \dfrac{1}{2} & \text{otherwise.} \end{cases} \quad (15.5)$$

Note that there are two limitations in ρ_{c2}. On the one hand, if μ_i is close to zero or negative, this optimal allocation proportion is not well defined. In that case, one might use some transformation, such as $exp(\mu_i)$. On the other hand, this allocation proportion is derived assuming a smaller response is more desirable. If a larger response is more desirable, then one cannot maximize the total expected response to obtain a solution. An alternative is to minimize $n_1 f(\mu_1) + n_2 f(\mu_2)$ for some function f (e.g., $f(x) = exp(-x)$). However, these alternatives are not explored in the paper.

Biswas and Mandal (2004) generalized the binary optimal allocation for normal responses in terms of failures. Specifically, they minimize:

$$n_1\Phi\left(\frac{\mu_1 - C}{\sigma_1}\right)+n_2\Phi\left(\frac{\mu_2 - C}{\sigma_2}\right),$$

instead of $n_1\mu_1 + n_2\mu_2$ in Equation 15.2, where C is a constant and $\Phi(\cdot)$ is the cumulative density function of standard normal distribution. This amounts to minimizing the total number of participants with response greater than C. The corresponding optimal allocation proportion is given by:

$$\rho_{c3} = \frac{\sqrt{\Phi(\frac{\mu_2 - C}{\sigma_2})}\sigma_1}{\sqrt{\Phi(\frac{\mu_2 - C}{\sigma_2})}\sigma_1 + \sqrt{\Phi(\frac{\mu_1 - C}{\sigma_1})}\sigma_2}.$$

15.2.3 Survival Outcomes

There is limited literature on response-adaptive randomization in clinical trials with survival outcomes. Yao and Wei (1996) use the RPW for dichotomized survival times. Rosenberger and Seshaiyer (1997) use the logrank test statistic as a mapping of the treatment effect for skewing the randomization probability. The first attempt to derive an optimal allocation utilizing survival times with consideration of censoring is Zhang and Rosenberger (2007). Both exponential and Weibull models are considered. In the following we will introduce the optimal allocation for exponential case only.

Suppose participants randomized to treatment $k = 1, 2$ have a survival time T_k following an exponential distribution with parameter θ_k. The participants also are subject to an independent right censoring scheme. Let (t_{ik}, δ_{ik}), $i = 1, \ldots, n_k$ be a random sample, where t_{ik} is a survival time and $\delta_{ik} = 1$ if the ith participant assigned to treatment k is not censored, and a censoring time and $\delta_{ik} = 0$ if the participant is censored.

To test H_0: $\theta_1 = \theta_2$, we use the following statistic:

$$Z = \frac{\hat{\theta}_1 - \hat{\theta}_2}{\sqrt{\frac{\hat{\theta}_1^2}{r_1} + \frac{\hat{\theta}_2^2}{r_2}}} \sim N(0,1),$$

where $r_k = \sum_{i=1}^{n_k} \delta_{ik}$ is the total deaths from treatment k. To derive the optimal allocation in this case, assume that $\varepsilon_k = E(\delta_{ik})$ is the same for all $i = 1, \ldots, n_k$. Then $E(r_k) = n_k E(\delta_{ik}) = n_k \varepsilon_k$. Minimizing the total expected hazard, we have the following problem,

$$\begin{cases} \min\limits_{n_1} & n_1\theta_1^{-1}+(n-n_1)\theta_2^{-1} \\ s.t. & \theta_2^2/(n_1\varepsilon_1)+\theta_2^2/((n-n_1)\varepsilon_2)=C_0. \end{cases}$$

So the solution is:

$$\frac{n_1}{n_2} = \frac{\theta_1^{3/2}\varepsilon_2^{1/2}}{\theta_2^{3/2}\varepsilon_1^{1/2}}. \tag{15.6}$$

Accordingly, the allocation rule is given by,

$$\rho_{s1} = \frac{\sqrt{\theta_1^3\varepsilon_2}}{\sqrt{\theta_1^3\varepsilon_2}+\sqrt{\theta_2^3\varepsilon_1}}. \tag{15.7}$$

One can also minimize other ethical cost to obtain other allocation proportions, such as those considered for continuous outcomes (Zhang and Rosenberger 2006). For instance, if we minimize the total number of participants $n_A + n_B$ above, we will obtain Neyman allocation, given by:

$$\rho_{s2} = \frac{\theta_1\sqrt{\varepsilon_2}}{\theta_1\sqrt{\varepsilon_2}+\theta_2\sqrt{\varepsilon_1}}.$$

We can also dichotomize the survival times; that is, a survival time less than some threshold c is considered to be a failure. Then we can minimize, as in Biswas and Mandal (2004), $n_1(1-e^{-c/\theta_1})+n_2(1-e^{-c/\theta_2})$, and obtain the following allocation proportion:

$$\rho_{s3} = \frac{\theta_1\sqrt{\varepsilon_2(1-e^{-C/\theta_2})}}{\theta_1\sqrt{\varepsilon_2(1-e^{-C/\theta_2})}+\theta_2\sqrt{\varepsilon_1(1-e^{-C/\theta_1})}}.$$

where ρ is the proportion of participants to be randomized to treatment 1.

For a particular censoring scheme, we are able to determine the explicit form of ε_k. Here we consider the censoring scheme used in Rosenberger and Seshaiyer (1997). In their paper the trial has a duration D. Participant arrival times follow independent uniform distribution on $[0, R]$. Independently, participants are subject to a censoring time C that has a uniform distribution on $[0, D]$. The survival time T_k of a participant allocated to treatment $k = 1, 2$ follows an exponential distribution with parameter θ_k. Let $Z_k = \min\{T_k, C, D - R\}$. Define $W_k = 1$ if $Z_k = T_k$ and 0 otherwise. Then it is shown that:

$$\varepsilon_k = E(W_k) = \Pr(W_k = 1) = 1 - \frac{\theta_k}{D} + e^{-D/\theta_k}\frac{\theta_k}{DR}(e^{R/\theta_k}(2\theta_k - R) - 2\theta_k).$$

Therefore we can obtain the explicit allocation proportion defined in the above equations for ρ_{sj}, $j = 1, 2, 3$.

Optimal allocations for Weibull model of survival times can be found in Zhang and Rosenberger (2007).

15.2.4 More than Two Treatments

Optimal allocation proportions for trials with more than two treatments are more difficult to determine than for two treatments. This is largely due to the fact that solving the optimization problem, as in the previous sections, for more than two treatments is not a straightforward generalization. Tymofyeyev, Rosenberger, and Hu (2007) are the first attempt to such generalizations to $K \geq 3$ treatments for binary outcomes. Specifically, consider comparing $K \geq 3$ binomial distributions with parameters (n_k, p_k), $k = 1, \ldots, K$, by testing the following hypotheses:

$$H_0 : \boldsymbol{p}_c = \boldsymbol{0} \text{ versus } H_A : \boldsymbol{p}_c \neq \boldsymbol{0}, \tag{15.8}$$

where $p_c = (p_1 - p_K, \ldots, p_{K-1} - p_K)$ is the contrast comparing a control (treatment K) to other treatments.

A generalization of Equation 15.1 results in the following optimization problem,

$$\begin{cases} \min \sum_{k=1}^{K} n_k q_k \\ s.t.\ p'_c \Sigma_n^{-1} p_c \equiv C_0, \\ \quad n_k / n \geq B, \end{cases} \tag{15.9}$$

where Σ_n is the variance covariance matrix of maximum likelihood estimator of p_c, $n = \sum_{k=1}^{K} n_k$, $q_k = 1 - p_k$ and $B \in [0, 1/K]$ is a constant. The constant B in the second constraint is a lower bound for the proportion n_k/n to ensure an explicit control of the feasibility region of the problem. This is a well-defined optimization problem and the existence of a unique solution is proved. However, the difficulty lies in finding an explicit form of the solution. An explicit solution to the problem for Neyman allocation is found in Tymofyeyev, Rosenberger, and Hu (2007). However, no explicit form solution is worked out for Problem 15.9. Instead, a numerical solution with a smoothing technique is used in their evaluation of the properties of the allocation proportion.

When $K = 3$ Jeon and Hu (2009) solved optimization Problem 15.9 obtaining a solution with closed form. The solution is rather complicated and will not be presented here.

For continuous outcomes, Zhu and Hu (2009) solved Problem 15.9 with a closed form solution for exponentially distributed responses and $K = 3$. The solution is also complicated and will not be presented here. Although they claim that their method applies to other continuous outcomes, no closed-form solution is given for most commonly used distribution–normal distribution.

In many cases, the overall Hypothesis 15.8 may not be the main interest. Instead, multiple comparisons are conducted after the overall test. The least significant difference (LSD) test is discussed in Tymofyeyev, Rosenberger, and Hu (2007), restricted to case of $K = 3$. Optimal allocation derived with a constraint on the power of multiple comparisons is unknown.

15.2.5 Optimal Allocation for Covariate-Adjusted Response-Adaptive Randomization

In the previous subsections, we discussed optimal allocation for response-adaptive randomization in clinical trials with binary, continuous, or survival outcomes. More than two treatments are also considered. In this subsection, we consider situations where important covariates exist and have to be adjusted.

Covariates have been considered in restricted randomization (Rosenberger and Lachin 2002). Balancing treatment assignments across important covariates allows for valid comparison of treatment effect. In clinical trials, there might be a treatment and covariate(s) interaction. For example, treatment 1 may be better than treatment 2 for female participants and worse than treatment 2 for male participants. In this case, different optimal allocation proportions are called for in female and male participants.

A simple way to address this issue is to stratify the participant population according to these covariates and apply response-adaptive randomization in each stratum. This approach was used in Tamura et al. (1994). Rosenberger, Vidyashankar, and Agarwal (2001) and Bandyopadhyay, Biswas, and Bhattacharya (2007) consider CARA randomization procedures for the binary case. Atkinson and Biswas (2005) consider such procedures for normal responses using D_A-optimal designs. Note that no optimal allocation is discussed in these papers. Rosenberger and Sverdlov (2008) compare some covariate-adjusted versions of optimal allocation for binary outcomes.

15.3 Implementation

An optimal allocation proportion gives the desirable proportion of participants to be randomized to a treatment. All the allocation proportions derived so far are dependent on unknown parameters. A randomization procedure is needed to determine the actual value of the allocation proportion before randomizing the next participant. For example, a natural way is to replace the unknown parameters with their estimate based on available responses. If the MLE is used, then the procedure is called sequential maximum likelihood estimate (SMLE) procedure (Melfi, Page, and Geraldes 2001).

In the following, we will first discuss randomization procedures that can target a specific allocation proportion.

15.3.1 Real-Valued Urn Models

Urn models are mentioned at the beginning of the chapter. Typically an urn model is used in clinical trials with binary outcomes and can only target one proportion $q_2/(q_1 + q_2)$ in two-treatment case. Yuan and Chai (2008) develop a real-valued urn model that can be applied to other outcomes and target any allocation proportion.

In the usual urns, suppose the initial composition is $A = (\alpha_1, \ldots, \alpha_K)$, corresponding to K treatment arms respectively. Each time the composition is updated by adding a given number of balls $B = (\xi_1, \ldots, \xi_K)$; B depends on the participants, responses in response-adaptive randomization. Therefore, in the usual urn models, A and B can only take whole numbers. In real-valued urns, A and B can take any nonnegative real values. By careful designing of the functional relationship between B and participant responses, Yuan and Chai (2008) show that any allocation proportion can be targeted. The closed form variance of N_k/n can be evaluated, where N_k is the number of participants randomized to treatment k, a random quantity for each trial. This procedure can be applied to all types of outcomes.

15.3.2 The Doubly Biased Coin Design Procedures

Hu and Zhang (2004) propose the doubly biased coin design (DBCD), of which the SLME procedure is a special case. For two-treatment case, one randomizes the next participant to treatment 1 with probability $g(N_{1j}/j,\hat{\rho})$ after j participants have been allocated. The allocation function $g(x, y)$ is defined as:

$$g(x,y)=\begin{cases} 0 & \text{if } x=1 \\ \dfrac{y(\frac{y}{x})^{\gamma}}{y(\frac{y}{x})^{\gamma}+(1-y)(\frac{1-y}{1-x})^{\gamma}} & \text{if } 0<x<1 \\ 1 & \text{if } x=0, \end{cases}$$

where $\gamma \geq 0$ is a tuning parameter controlling the degree of randomness of the procedure. When $\gamma = 0$, it becomes the SMLE procedure. Note that this function can be generalized to the case of $K \geq 3$ treatments (Hu and Zhang 2004). The closed form variance of N_k/n can also be evaluated in most cases. This procedure can be applied to all types of outcomes and is very well studied in the literature.

15.3.3 Efficient Randomized Adaptive Design (ERADE)

Hu, Zhang, and He (2009) propose the following allocation function:

$$g(x,y) = \begin{cases} \gamma & \text{if } x > y \\ y & \text{if } x = y \\ 1-\gamma(1-y) & \text{if } x < y, \end{cases}$$

where $0 \leq \gamma < 1$ is the tuning parameter for degree of randomness. When $\gamma = 0$, this procedure is deterministic. A larger γ leads to a more random procedure. Also note that when $\rho = 1/2$, this procedure becomes Efron's biased coin design (Efron 1971).

15.3.4 D_A-Optimal Procedure

Atkinson and Biswas (2005) proposed a response-adaptive randomization procedure based on D_A-optimal design. The design is first derived from D_A-optimality criterion for estimating a conflict of interest, traced back to Atkinson (1982). They propose a modification so that the procedure can target any allocation proportion. However, the asymptotic distribution of N_k/n is not available.

15.3.5 Performance Evaluation of Optimal Response-Adaptive Randomization Procedures

What should one consider when choosing an optimal allocation or a procedure? Hu and Rosenberger (2003) present a template that relates power of the test, the allocation proportion, and the variability of N_k/n. This template allows one to compare asymptotic properties of different randomization procedures targeting the same allocation proportion, or compare asymptotic properties of different allocation proportions using the same randomization procedure. Hu, Rosenberger, and Zhang (2006) further give a lower bound of the variance of N_k/n for a given allocation proportion and define the asymptotically best randomization procedure to be the one by which variance of N_k/n attains its lower bound.

Hu and Rosenberger (2003) and Rosenberger and Hu (2004) use the template comparing different allocation proportions for binary outcomes. The RSIHR is shown to be the best in balancing preservation of power of the test and reduction of number of treatment failures. Zhang and Yang (2009) evaluate the performance of the optimal allocation based on Farrington and Manning test. They also compare family of allocations by Zhang and Biswas (2007) using Fisher's exact test by simulation. Zhang and Rosenberger (2006) evaluate different optimal allocations for continuous outcomes using the DBCD procedure. Their results indicated that the ρ_{c2} should be used if a smaller outcome is more desirable and the outcomes are positive. Otherwise, ρ_{c3} can be used. Different optimal allocations for survival outcomes are evaluated in Zhang and Rosenberger (2007).

A basic requirement for a response-adaptive randomization procedure is consistency. In other words, $N_k/n \to \rho_k$ as $n \to \infty$, where ρ_k is the target allocation proportion for treatment k. The first three response-adaptive randomization procedures presented above meet this requirement. Furthermore, Hu, Rosenberger, and Zhang (2006) can be used to evaluate whether a randomization procedure is asymptotically best for an allocation proportion. The ERADE procedure has been shown to be asymptotically best.

Another point to consider is start-up of the randomization process. Since all response-adaptive randomization procedures are dependent on estimation of unknown procedures, many propose first randomizing a given number of participants with equal allocation, then start the response-adaptive randomization process (e.g., Section 15.5.2 Regularization of Atkinson and Biswas 2005). A natural question is how many participants should be allocated before start-up of response-adaptive randomization. An alternative is to adjust the estimator of the MLE. For example, one could estimate p_1 with $(N_1 + 0.1)/(n + 0.2)$ and start response-adaptive randomization from the very first participants.

15.4 Inference

Data analysis following a response-adaptive randomization can be conducted using MLE (Chapter 11 of Rosenberger and Lachin 2002; and Chapter 3 of Hu and Rosenberger 2006). Correlation among responses due to dependence of treatment assignments on accumulated responses has to be accounted for. In general, if the parameter space is open, the distributions are from an exponential family and the allocation proportions N_k/n converge almost surely to a constant between 0 and 1, then the MLEs are strongly consistent and asymptotically follow a normal distribution. The asymptotic variance can be obtained as the inverse of the Fisher's information matrix, which must take the optimal allocation ρ into account. Therefore the usual tests (e.g., Wald test) can be routinely applied. One should be aware that maximum likelihood estimators are biased. Coad and Ivanova (2001) derive the bias of $\hat{p}_k$ for the binary case. However, the MLE bias for other cases has not been addressed in the literature.

In practice, most late phase clinical trials employ group sequential monitoring so that the trial can be stopped early if safety risk is intolerably high for the investigation treatment, or there is reliable evidence concluding that the investigation drug is superior (inferior, or noninferior) to the control in terms of efficacy (Jennison and Turnbull 2000). There is little work in the literature combining response-adaptive randomization with sequential monitoring. Recently, Zhu and Hu (2010) consider the DBCD procedure with group sequential monitoring using an α-spending function to control the type I error rate. They show that, under mild regularity conditions, the standardized (Wald) test statistic asymptotically follows a standard Brownian motion under the null hypothesis. Therefore the sequence of the test statistics at the interim and final looks constitute a canonical joint distribution as defined in Jennison and Turnbull (2000). It follows that all group sequential methods can be readily applied in conjunction with response-adaptive randomization.

From the logistic point of view, updating the allocation probability after each response of a participant is available is cumbersome, if not impossible. Advancement in technology, such as electronic data capture, has lowered this hurdle. Response-adaptive randomization combined with group sequential design, where the allocation probability is updated only after each interim look, has been considered in Jennison and Turnbull (2000) and Karrison, Huo, and Chappell (2003). However, little is known about how the procedures discussed in this chapter could be applied in group sequential trials.

15.5 Conclusion

In this chapter we take a three-step paradigm; that is, optimization, implementation, and inference, for response-adaptive randomization in clinical trials. Other issues related to response-adaptive randomization, such as staggered entry and delayed response, are not covered in this chapter, but can be found in Hu and Rosenberger (2006). It is the authors' hope that these optimal allocations with appropriate randomization procedures will expedite the practical application of response-adaptive randomization.

References

Atkinson, A. C. (1982). Optimal biased coin designs for sequential clinical trials with prognostic factors. *Biometrika,* 69: 61–67.

Atkinson, A. C., and Biswas, A. (2005). Bayesian adaptive biased coin designs for clinical trials with normal responses. *Biometrics,* 61: 118–25.

Bandyopadhyay, U., and Biswas, A. (2001). Adaptive designs for normal responses with prognostic factors. *Biometrika,* 88: 409–19.

Bandyopadhyay, U., Biswas, A., and Bhattacharya, R. (2007). A covariate adjusted two-stage allocation design for binary responses in randomized clinical trials. *Statistics in Medicine,* 26: 4386–99.

Biswas, A., and Mandal, S. (2004). Optimal adaptive designs in Phase III clinical trials for continuous responses with covariates. In *m0Da 7-Advances in Model-Oriented Design and Analysis*, eds. A. Di Bucchianico, H. Lauter, and H. P. Wynn, 51–58. Heidelberg: Physica-Verlag.

Coad, D. S., and Ivanova, A. (2001). Bias calculations for adaptive urn designs. *Sequential Analysis,* 20: 229–39.

Efron, B. (1971). Forcing a sequential experiment to be balanced. *Biometrika,* 58: 403–17.

Farrington, C. P., and Manning, G. (1990). Test statistics and sample size formulae for comparative binomial trials with null hypothesis of non-zero risk difference or non-unity relative risk. *Statistics in Medicine,* 9: 1447–54.

Friedman, L. M., Furberg, C. D., and DeMets, D. L. (1998). *Fundamentals of Clinical Trials.* New York: Springer-Verlag.

Hu, F., and Rosenberger, W. F. (2003). Optimality, variability, power: Evaluating response-adaptive randomization procedures for treatment comparisons. *Journal of American Statistical Association,* 98: 671–78.

Hu, F., and Rosenberger, W. F. (2006). *The Theory of Response-Adaptive Randomization in Clinical Trials.* New Jersey: Wiley.

Hu, F., Rosenberger, W. F., and Zhang, L. X. (2006). Asymptotically best response-adaptive randomization procedures. *Journal of Statistical Planning and Inference,* 136: 1911–22.

Hu, F., and Zhang, L. X. (2004). Asymptotic properties of doubly adaptive biased coin design for multitreatment clinical trials. *Annals of Statistics,* 32: 268–301.

Hu, F., Zhang, L. X., and He, X. (2009). Efficient randomized adaptive designs. *Annals of Statistics*, 37: 2543–60.

Ivanova, A. (2003). A play-the-winner type urn model with reduced variability. *Metrika,* 58: 1–13.

Jennison, C., and Turnbull, B. W. (2000). *Group Sequential Methods with Applications to Clinical Trials.* Boca Raton, FL: Chapman and Hall/CRC.

Jeon, Y., and Hu, F. (2010). Optimal adaptive designs for binary response trials with three treatments. *Statistics in Biopharmaceutical Research.* To appear.

Karrison, T. G., Huo, D., and Chappell, R. (2003). A group sequential, response-adaptive design for randomized clinical trials. *Controlled Clinical Trials,* 24: 506–22.

Melfi, V. F., Page, C., and Geraldes, M. (2001). An adaptive randomized design with application to estimation. *The Canadian Journal of Statistics,* 29: 107–16.

Rosenberger, W. F., and Hu, F. (2004). Maximizing power and minimizing treatment failures in clinical trials. *Clinical Trials,* 1: 141–47.

Rosenberger, W. F., and Lachin, J. L. (2002). *Randomization in Clinical Trials, Theory and Practice.* New York: Wiley.

Rosenberger, W. F., and Seshaiyer, P. (1997). Adaptive survival trials. *Journal of Biopharmaceutical Statistics,* 7: 617–24.

Rosenberger, W. F., Stallard, N., Ivanova, A., Harper, C., and Ricks, M. (2001). Optimal adaptive designs for binary response trials. *Biometrics,* 57: 173–77.

Rosenberger, W. F., and Sverdlov, O. (2008). Handling covariates in the design of clinical trials. *Statistical Science,* 23: 404–19.

Rosenberger, W. F., Vidyashankar, A. N., and Agarwal, D. K. (2001). Covariate-adjusted response-adaptive designs for binary response. *Journal of Biopharmaceutical Statistics,* 11: 227–36.

Tamura, R. N., Faries, D. E., Andersen, J. S., and Heiligenstein, J. H. (1994). A case study of an adaptive clinical trial in the treatment of out-patients with depressive disorder. *Journal of the American Statistical Association,* 89: 768–76.

Thall, P. F., and Wathen, K. S. (2007). Practical Bayesian adaptive randomization in clinical trials. *European Journal of Cancer,* 43: 859–66.

Tymofyeyev, Y., Rosenberger, W. F., and Hu, F. (2007). Implementing optimal allocation in sequential binary response experiments. *Journal of the American Statistical Association,* 102: 224–34.

Yao, Q., and Wei, L. J. (1996). Play the winner for Phases II and III clinical trials. *Statistics in Medicine,* 15: 2413–23.

Yuan, A., and Chai, G. X. (2008). Optimal adaptive generalized Polya urn design for multi-arm clinical trials. *Journal of Multivariate Analysis,* 99: 1–24.

Wei, L. J., and Durham, S. (1978). The randomized play-the-winner rule in medical trials. *Journal of the American Statistical Association,* 73: 840–43.

Zhang, L., and Biswas, A. (2007). Optimal failure-success response-adaptive designs for binary responses. *Drug Information Journal,* 41: 709–18.

Zhang, L., and Rosenberger, W. F. (2006). Response-adaptive randomization for clinical trials with continuous outcomes. *Biometrics,* 62: 562–69.

Zhang, L., and Rosenberger, W. F. (2007). Response-adaptive randomization for clinical trials with survival outcomes: The parametric approach. *Journal of the Royal Statistical Society C,* 53: 153–65.

Zhang, L., and Yang, H. (2010). Practical considerations for optimal response-adaptive randomization in clinical trials with binary outcomes. Submitted.

Zhu, H., and Hu, F. (2009). Implementing optimal allocation in sequential continuous response experiments. *Journal of Statistical Planning and Inference,* 139: 2420–30.

Zhu, H., and Hu, F. (2010). Sequential monitoring of response-adaptive randomized clinical trials. *Annals of Statistics.* To appear.

16

Hypothesis-Adaptive Design

Gerhard Hommel
Universitätsmedizin Mainz

16.1 Introduction

Adaptive designs are usually applied when changes of the experimental design after an interim analysis are intended. Common examples are modification of the sample size, but also changes of the setup of the trial, the test procedure, or the inclusion criteria. When multiple hypotheses are to be tested, the same modifications are possible. The question arises as to whether it would even be possible to change the position or the structure of the hypotheses themselves, given a multiple test problem. The result could be a change of the weights or of the hierarchy of the hypotheses. Of course, this type of action has been applied for a long time in practice, though without fixed decision rules. From the statistical point of view, this has been strongly advised against, since the result is nearly always an excessive number of falsely positive decisions. Therefore, it is not surprising that a positive result could often not be repeated.

In the following, it will be shown that an adaption of hypotheses is nevertheless possible in a formally correct way. However, it is problematic because of other reasons: the danger of a manipulation is substantially enlarged, complicated logistic problems occur (in particular for controlled clinical trials), and if the initial knowledge is too low, the price to be paid for hypothesis adaptions is very high.

In the next sections, we will first describe the historical development of multiple testing in adaptive designs based on the fundamental paper by Bauer (1989a) regarding a global test. Then we consider genuine multiple test procedures (MTPs) for important special cases, such as dropping endpoints, or treatment groups. In a methodological section, the basic technique is presented, which is essentially the combination of the closure test with methods of adaptive designs. It follows that it is not only possible to reduce the system of hypotheses, but also to change the valuation of hypotheses and even to include new hypotheses. The problems connected with this freedom are elucidated in the next section, in particular from the regulatory standpoint. Finally, some other aspects are mentioned, such as dependence of hypotheses and test statistics, estimation and confidence intervals, and the control of the false discovery rate (FDR).

16.2 Definitions and Notions

Let there be given a parameter space Θ and $n \geq 1$ (null) hypotheses $H_1,\ldots,H_n$ with $H_i \subset \Theta$, $\varnothing \neq H_i \neq \Theta$, for all $i \in N$, where $N = \{1,\ldots,n\}$. As usual, a probability distribution P_θ on a sample space is given for all $\theta \in \Theta$.

The global hypothesis is $H_0 = \cap\{H_i : i \in N\}$.

We denote by s the number of the stages of the trial (often we will consider $s = 2$ stages).

For each hypothesis and each stage, p-values are determined after the respective stage. These p-values are denoted by:

$$p_{ij}, i \in N, j = 1,\ldots,s.$$

For each $i \in N$, it is assumed that the p_{ij} are either independent and uniformly distributed on the unit interval under H_i or satisfy the p-clud condition (Brannath, Posch, and Bauer 2002); that is, their distribution is stochastically larger than or equal to the uniform distribution, given the p_{ij} of earlier stages.

16.3 Global Tests with Adaptive Designs

Already the first publications by Bauer (1989a, 1989b) use a formulation in the context of a multiple test problem, though conclusions are only made for the global hypothesis H_0.

The first paper (Bauer 1989b) concerns the planning of s consecutive trials. An "s, k, α decision rule" defines stopping criteria with the possibility of early rejection of H_0 or early termination due to futility. The nominal significance level α_* for a single trial is determined over the binomial distribution. Though not yet explicitly mentioned, the possibility exists to change the test of H_0 within each trial, based on suitable tests of the H_i, $i \in N$; for example, one can choose a test for any H_i.

The second paper (Bauer 1989a) has become fundamental for the development of adaptive designs. Also there, the problem has been formulated for multiple tests (even for an infinite number of hypotheses), but the conclusions can only be made in a global way, as in Bauer (1989b). It is assumed that an arbitrary level α test for combining n independent p-values is specified in advance. Then, a selective test procedure is possible; that is, after each stage one can choose the H_i that will be tested in the next stage. The argument is again that a p-value for an H_i is also a p-value for H_0. As an example for combining p-values, Fisher's (1932) combination test is used:

$$\text{Reject } H_0 \text{ if } \prod_{j=1}^{s} p_j \leq c_{s,\alpha} = \exp[-\frac{1}{2}\chi^2_{2s}(1-\alpha)],$$

where the p_j are the p-values obtained by the test used in stage j.

The continuation of this idea was made in Bauer and Köhne (1994), still in the multiple context. It was observed that one could stop with rejection of H_0 already after $t < s$ stages when $\prod_{j=1}^{t} p_j \leq c_{s,\alpha}$ (nonstochastic curtailing). Moreover, by introduction of the bound $\alpha_0 < 1$ with the possibility of stopping for futility, one also obtains an improved bound $\alpha_1 > c_{s,\alpha}$ for early stop with rejection.

The publications mentioned so far are already relevant when only one hypothesis is at hand ($n = 1$), since design changes are possible anyway. The first formulation where a proper multiple test problem is imperative has been made in Bauer and Röhmel (1995), who investigated a dose–response relationship. After an interim analysis one can change the dose(s) used in earlier steps. However, only a global statement can be made; in Section 16.3 of the paper by Bauer and Röhmel, a thorough discussion is performed about the potential conclusions when H_0 has been rejected.

16.4 Multiple Tests

The first attempt to obtain multiple decisions under control of the multiple level α was made by Hommel (1989), who obtained a rather conservative solution. Bauer and Köhne (1994), Section 2.4, describe a closed test strategy for $s = 2$ stages using Fisher's combination test as follows. Let:

- H_1 = the hypothesis of the first stage;
- $H_{(2)}$ = the hypothesis selected for the second stage (it might be any of the hypotheses H_i, $i \in N$, based on the results of the first stage).

We write for short $p_1 = p_{11}$ and $p_2 = p_{(2)2}$. Intuitively, one would apply the closure test as follows:

- If H_0 cannot be rejected (since $p_1 > \alpha_0$ or $p_1 p_2 > c_{2,\alpha}$), retain also $H_1 \cap H_{(2)}$ and stop.
- Otherwise, reject $H_1 \cap H_{(2)}$ and continue.
- Reject H_1 if $p_1 \le \alpha$ (this includes a rejection after the first stage since $\alpha_1 < \alpha$).
- Reject $H_{(2)}$ if the second stage is reached (i.e., $\alpha_1 < p_1 \le \alpha_0$) and $p_2 \le \alpha$.

However, the probability of a type I error may be exceeded, as one can see by the following example (Bauer and Köhne, 1994): Start with a true null hypothesis H_1. If $\alpha_1 < p_1 \le \alpha$, proceed to an H, which is not true and can be rejected with probability 1. For $p_1 > \alpha$, proceed to a true H_i (e.g., test H_1 again). Then the probability of committing a type I error is greater than α since it is already exhausted by the event $p_1 \le \alpha$.

The reason that a formal application of the closure test does not work here, is that the choice of the second hypothesis is a random variable, dependent on the result of the first stage. We consider now publications where the closure test is applied correctly.

Tang and Geller (1999) have described how the closure test can be performed within a group-sequential (nonadaptive) design; different stopping criteria are considered.

Kieser, Bauer, and Lehmacher (1999) apply the closure test for the case of multiple endpoints and an adaptive design. They consider two situations: (1) an a priori order of the endpoints, and (2) the Bonferroni-Holm procedure for all endpoints. For both situations, it is possible to drop endpoints after an interim analysis either because their hypotheses can already be rejected or because of futility (provided $\alpha_0 < 1$).

Bauer and Kieser (1999) applied the closure test for comparisons of $n \ge 2$ treatments with a control and an adaptive design with two stages. Of course, after an interim analysis one can make design changes (in particular a reassessment of the sample sizes), but one can also drop nonpromising treatments. When one can reject at least one hypothesis after an interim analysis, one can stop, but it is also possible to continue with the remaining treatments.

Lehmacher, Kieser, and Hothorn (2000) considered multiple testing problems for dose–response analysis under the assumption of ordered alternatives. They formulated a general construction rule for combining multiple and sequential procedures.

Hellmich (2001) additionally considered the case of all pairwise comparisons when interim analyses are performed in order to exclude treatments. He described, based on results by Follmann, Proschan, and Geller (1994) that problems may occur when pure group-sequential designs are applied. These problems can be overcome when using adaptive designs in the sense of Bauer and Köhne (1994).

16.5 General Methodology

16.5.1 The Closure Test

We describe the closure test (Marcus, Peritz, and Gabriel 1976) in the modified version by Hommel (1986).

Given n (null) hypotheses $H_1,\ldots,H_n$, one defines for each nonempty $I \subseteq N = \{1,\ldots,n\}$ an intersection hypothesis:

$$H_I = \bigcap\{H_i : i \in I\}.$$

Further, one has to find for all I a local level α test Φ_I; that is,

$$P_\theta(H_I \text{ rejected by } \Phi_I) \leq \alpha \text{ for all } \theta \in H_I.$$

The MTP is defined as follows:

$$\text{Reject an } H_I \text{ if } H_J \text{ is rejected by all } \Phi_J \text{ with } J \supseteq I.$$

Hence, one obtains decision rules in particular for the given hypotheses $H_i = H_{\{i\}}$, $i \in N$.

First assume that the free combination condition is satisfied; that is, each combination of true and false null hypotheses can occur within Θ (Holm 1979). Then the MTP is coherent; that is, when a hypothesis H_I is rejected, all hypotheses implying it (all $H_J \subseteq H_I$) must also be rejected. Furthermore, the MTP controls the multiple level α; that is, the probability of rejecting at least one true null hypothesis is less than or equal to α, irrespective of which and how many null hypotheses are true. Control of the multiple level is often denoted as "control of the familywise error rate (in the strong sense)" (Hochberg and Tamhane 1987, p. 3).

In practical applications, the free combination condition is often not satisfied. Nevertheless, control of the multiple level is still guaranteed, although the procedure need not be coherent (Hommel 1986).

It is often useful to define the local tests Φ_I by means of p-values p_I having the property that $P_\theta(p_I \leq c) \leq c$ for all $\theta \in H_I$ and all c with $0 \leq c \leq 1$. Then the result of the MTP for an H_I, $I \subseteq N$, can be defined by means of an adjusted p-value $\text{apv}_I = \max\{p_J : J \supseteq I\}$; that is, H_I is rejected by the MTP when $\text{apv}_I \leq \alpha$. For the adjusted p-values of the given hypotheses, we write for short apv_i instead of $\text{apv}_{\{i\}}$.

Example: The Φ_I are often chosen as local Bonferroni tests; that is, H_I is rejected if $p_i \leq \alpha/|I|$ for at least one $i \in I$ (the p_i are p-values for the test of H_i, and $|I|$ denotes the number of indices in I). The resulting closure test is the sequentially rejective procedure by Holm (1979), using the stepwise bounds α/n, $\alpha/(n-1),\ldots,\alpha/2$, α. The adjusted p-values for this procedure are easy to compute, see for example, Wright (1992).

16.5.2 The Closure Test for Adaptive Designs

In principle, the closure test can also be applied as described above to adaptive designs. The crucial problem is to find suitable tests Φ_I resp. p-values p_I. For simplicity of notation, we will describe the method for the special case of $s = 2$ stages; that is, one interim analysis. For this case, we need local p-values p_{Ij} for each $I \subseteq N$ and each stage ($j = 1, 2$) satisfying the p-clud condition (see Section 16.2) under H_I. With this notion, the p-values of Section 16.2 can also be written as $p_{ij} = p_{\{i\}j}$.

Furthermore, we need a conditional error function $A_I(x)$, for all $x \in [0, 1]$, which is nonincreasing in x and has the property:

$$\int_0^1 A_I(x) f_{\theta I}(x)dx \leq \alpha \text{ for all } \theta \in H_I,$$

where $f_{\theta I}(.)$ is either the density of the random variable p_{I1}, for given θ, or the uniform density.

The conditional error function determines the significance level for the second stage, given the interim test result of the first stage. The result of the first stage is often presented as a realization of a standard normal random variate (e.g., Proschan and Hunsberger 1995); for our purposes, it is easier to consider it after a transformation into a p-value.

We define:

$$\alpha_{1I} = \begin{cases} \sup\{x : A_I(x) = 1\}, & \text{if } A_I(0) = 1 \\ 0 & \text{otherwise} \end{cases},$$

and

$$\alpha_{0I} = \begin{cases} \inf\{x : A_I(x) = 0\}, & \text{if } A_I(1) = 0 \\ 1 & \text{otherwise} \end{cases}.$$

α_{1I} and α_{0I} determine stopping rules as usual for the test of H_I.

Using the conditional error function, the local test Φ_I is defined as follows:

$$\text{Reject } H_I \text{ if either } p_{I1} \le \alpha_{1I} \text{ or } (\alpha_{1I} < p_{I1} \le \alpha_{0I} \text{ and } p_{I2} \le A_I(p_{I1})).$$

The most common examples for the choice of A_I are based on Fisher's combination test (Bauer and Köhne 1994), on the inverse normal combination function (Lehmacher and Wassmer 1999), or on the procedure of Proschan and Hunsberger (1995).

16.5.3 Remarks

1. It should be emphasized that the choice of all $A_I(.)$ and consequently of α_{0I} and α_{1I} has to be fixed for all H_I at the beginning of the study.
2. It is often sufficient to choose all $A_I(x)$ identically to an $A(x)$; then one has the same α_0 and α_1 for all Φ_I. However, there are also good reasons to choose them differently: for the test of a single hypothesis $H_i = H_{\{i\}}$ it can be useful to choose a small $\alpha_{0\{i\}}$, whereas for testing an intersection of many hypotheses, it would be better to choose α_{0I} large (or even equal to 1) in order to make the stopping rule not too restrictive.
3. One can also apply the closure test strategy for unplanned interim analyses as described by Müller and Schäfer (2004). Then for each H_I, a conditional rejection error probability has to be determined that determines the significance level for the remaining part of the study.
4. Again, it is often useful to define Φ_I over a suitably constructed p-value p_I (see Brannath, Posch, and Bauer 2002). For this approach, it is necessary to define a whole class of conditional rejection functions (see also Vandemeulebroecke 2006). This p-value is often called the overall p-value. However, it should not be confounded with the p-values used in each stage for the test of the overall (global) hypothesis H_0.

Using the p_I, one can also determine adjusted p-values $\text{apv}_I = \max\{p_J : J \supseteq I\}$ for an adaptive design. It should be emphasized that it would be incorrect to first compute adjusted p-values $\text{apv}_{Ij} = \max\{p_{Jj} : J \supseteq I\}$ for each stage and then to combine them using a conditional error function, since then closure test arguments are no longer valid.

16.6 Applications

In this section we refer mainly to the paper by Hommel (2001). Again, we restrict ourselves to $s = 2$ stages.

16.6.1 Reduction of the Set of Initial Hypotheses

In the first stage, the local level α tests of H_I leading to p_{I1} can be based on the whole set of hypotheses $H_1,\ldots,H_n$. The simplest example are local Bonferroni tests with $p_{I1} = \min\{1;|I|\cdot\min\{p_{i1} : i \in I\}\}$. After the interim analysis, some hypotheses H_i may be excluded from further consideration because they can already be rejected. For this aim, one needs $\text{apv}_i \leq \alpha$; that is, $p_{I1} \leq \alpha_{1I}$ for all I with $i \in I$. Other hypotheses may be excluded because of futility; this is satisfied for all i that are elements of at least one I with $p_{I1} > \alpha_{0I}$. Of course, exclusion of hypotheses with nonrejection is always possible. Denote the set of indices of excluded hypotheses by E ($E \subseteq N$ can also be empty). For the second stage, only intersection hypotheses H_I with $I \cap E = \varnothing$ are of interest. Consequently, the respective local tests of H_I leading to p_{I2} must include only the hypotheses H_i with $i \in I \setminus E$. Using local Bonferroni tests, one then obtains $p_{I2} = \min\{1;|I \setminus E| \cdot \min\{p_{i2} : i \in I \setminus E\}\}$.

By Bauer and Kieser (1999) this principle has been applied to the elimination of treatments compared with a control. As local tests for an H_I to be applied, the authors propose Dunnett tests, Tukey tests, or tests considering an order relation, as the Bartholomew or Jonckheere test. An extensive review of methods using adaptive treatment selection is given in Posch et al. (2005). This methodology plays an important role for adaptive seamless designs that have been proposed in the last years for drug development (see for example Bretz et al. 2006). The aim is to integrate Phases IIb and III within a single clinical trial; in the first stage usually different doses of a drug are included from which one or few are forwarded into the Phase III stage.

The reduction of multiple endpoints has been described by Kieser, Bauer, and Lehmacher (1999). In particular, one can find there the use of local Bonferroni tests leading to the Bonferroni-Holm procedure with an instructive example. Though the formal idea for applying the closure test is relatively clear, the authors explicitly show the complicated structure of the decision tree for the simple case $n = s = 2$ in a flow chart. It should be noted that dropping an endpoint can lead to problems when data for this endpoint are collected in further stages. When these data contradict an early rejection, an interpretation problem arises, though the rejection is formally correct.

16.6.2 Reweighting

Westfall, Krishen, and Young (1998) considered the situation of performing two subsequent studies with the same set of multiple endpoints. They proposed using the results of the first study in order to choose suitable weights for the endpoints within the second study. By this means, adequate sample sizes for the second study can be determined and the power can be improved.

The same strategy is possible for a two-stage study with an adaptive interim analysis. Again, arbitrary multiple testing problems can be treated. At the beginning, the local tests for producing the p_{I1} (usually with equal weighting) and the corresponding conditional error functions have to be fixed. After the interim analysis, one can determine suitable weights $w_1,\ldots,w_n \geq 0$ with $\sum_{i=1}^{n} w_i \leq 1$ for the null hypotheses (e.g., corresponding to endpoints). For Bonferroni tests, one obtains as local p-values for index sets I with $\sum_{i\in I} w_i > 0$:

$$p_{I2} = \min\{1;(\sum_{i\in I} w_i)\cdot\min\{p_i/w_i : i \in I, w_i > 0\}\}$$

It is even possible to choose different weights within each intersection hypothesis (at each stage), see Hommel, Bretz, and Maurer (2007). This may be particularly useful when a gatekeeping strategy is applied together with an adaptive design.

Since choosing weights equal to 0 for certain i is permitted, the case of eliminating hypotheses is covered with this strategy.

16.6.3 A Priori Ordered Hypotheses

Similarly to the allocation of weights, one can also determine a complete order of the hypotheses with respect to their importance (cf. Bauer et al. 1998). This order can be a natural one in the sense that testing a hypothesis is only of interest if another hypothesis has been rejected. It can also be determined by the importance of the objectives to be investigated, or it is given by the expected power of the tests under consideration. We write:

$$H_1 \succ H_2 \succ \ldots \succ H_n,$$

which means that H_1 is more important than H_2, H_2 is more important than H_3, and so on. The sequentially rejective test procedure rejects H_i (at level α) if all H_k with $k \leq i$ are rejected at level α. A proof that this procedure controls the multiple level α can be performed by means of the closure test, using the test of the front hypothesis H_f as a local level α test of an H_I, where $f = \min I$; that is, H_f is the most important one among the hypotheses H_i, $i \in I$.

Consider now a study with an adaptive interim analysis, where an a priori order was chosen for the first stage; that is, the local tests are based on $p_{I1} = p_{f1}$, with $f = \min I$. If the same order is also maintained in the second stage, one obtains a procedure described by Kieser, Bauer, and Lehmacher (1999). However, it is not necessary to continue with the order chosen for the first stage. For example, one can choose another a priori order, can choose weights, or can leave out hypotheses. If another a priori order is chosen based on the results of the first stage, then the front hypothesis may be changed; that is, $p_{I2} = p_{g2}$, where g is the index of the revised most important hypothesis among the H_i, $i \in I$, and may differ from f. It should be emphasized that a combination test of H_I must combine p_{f1} and p_{g2}; that is, it requires p_{I1} according to the original order.

A motivating example for this strategy was described in Kropf et al. (2000). An explicit description for the algorithm was given by Hommel and Kropf (2001) and for another example by Hellmich and Hommel (2004).

16.6.4 Inclusion of New Hypotheses

The boldest method of applying a hypothesis-adaptive design is a reverse strategy as in Section 16.6.1, namely to include new hypotheses after the interim analysis. This means that some hypotheses, say all H_i with $i \in E$, are excluded at the beginning, but can be included after the interim analysis. Hence, for $I \not\subseteq E$, the p_{I1} are based only on the tests of H_i, $i \notin E$ (for $I \subseteq E$ one can predetermine tests for H_I in the first stage that may become important for the combination test). After the interim analysis, one can (but need not) include some of the H_i, $i \in E$, and one can also exclude some of the H_i with $i \notin E$.

For illustration, consider the situation of $n = 2$ hypotheses H_1, H_2 where it has been decided to include only H_1 in the first stage. The possible local tests leading to p_{Ij} in stage j ($j = 1,2$) are the following:

- $I = \{1\}$ One determines a suitable combination test since H_1 may also be important in the second stage.
- $I = \{2\}$ If data for testing H_2 are available in the first stage, one can again determine a suitable combination test. If insufficient data are expected, one can decide in the planning Phase that information of the first stage will be completely ignored. This leads to a degenerate combination test using only a potential p-value p_{22} from the second stage; that is, a conditional rejection function $A_{\{2\}}(x) \equiv \alpha$ is used.
- $I = \{1, 2\}$ Since H_1 is the only important hypothesis in the first stage, it is reasonable to choose $p_{I1} = p_{11}$. After the interim analysis, one can choose the test leading to p_{I2} adaptively. This may be $p_{I2} = p_{12}$ (H_1 remains the front hypothesis), or $p_{I2} = p_{22}$ (a reversal of the a priori order), any (weighted) combination of the test results in the second stage, or a specific multiple test.

From a technical point of view, it is even possible to include completely new hypotheses that do not belong to the predetermined pool of hypotheses $H_1,\ldots,H_n$. This is formally correct since the closure test also controls the multiple level α for infinite sets (for all thinkable sets) of hypotheses. Formally, if we consider an intersection hypothesis H_I with $I = I_1 \cup I_2$, where $I_1 \subseteq N$ and I_2 consists of indices of new hypotheses, then one has to choose $p_{I1} = p_{I_1 1}$ and $A_I(x) = A_{I1}(x)$ for $I_1 \neq \varnothing$, anyway. For $I_1 = \varnothing$ it is mandatory to choose $p_{I1} = p_{I_2 1} \equiv 1$, and therefore the best choice for $A_I(x)$ is to set it identically to α (as described in the illustration above for $I = \{2\}$). In order to reject any of the new hypotheses H_k, $k \notin N$, one obtains as a necessary condition that $p_{k2} \leq \min\{A_I(p_{I1}) : I \subseteq N\}$; when $p_{I1} > \alpha_{0I}$ for only one $I \subseteq N$, no rejection of any new hypothesis is possible.

The problem of adding new treatments in a study, as well as the serious penalty to be paid, has also been described by Posch et al. (2005).

16.7 How Much Freedom Should be Allowed?

The application of adaptive designs is very attractive for researchers, because one obtains the freedom to react when the initial assumptions are imprecise or even wrong. However, this freedom also implies the possibility of manipulating the results. Of course, such a manipulation will not be committed intentionally by a serious researcher, but unintentional manipulation is also made easier, since researchers are convinced of their ideas or sponsors are mainly interested in obtaining positive results. Many researchers still undervalue the problems that can occur with an adaption without fixed rules and how rapidly the danger of a falsely positive result can increase. Moreover, each interim analysis requires additional logistics, leading to more danger of manipulation. At the beginning of each scientific work where an adaption is intended, it is therefore indispensable to formulate a written protocol containing the aims of the study and the conditions where an adaptation may be performed. In order to ensure credibility and scientific integrity, this protocol should be deposited at an independent authority. When, in addition to modifications of the design, even a change of the objectives of the study may be possible, such a protocol and additional careful planning are all the more necessary.

When the formulation of the study aims is still too vague, one should advise against an adaptive design and rather recommend performing a pilot study. In any case, a change of the objectives causes additional penalty costs; this has been illustrated drastically in particular when new hypotheses might be included (see end of Section 16.6).

A change in priorities also usually leads to a substantial loss in power. This was shown by Kieser (2005) in a simulation study. He considered the situation of two endpoints (corresponding to two hypotheses) where the first endpoint was considered as the more promising one. Using an adaptive design with one interim analysis, the following strategies were compared:

- Choice of an a priori order that remained unchanged after the interim analysis;
- Change of the a priori order if the interim result for endpoint two is more promising than for endpoint one;
- Change of the a priori order only if the interim result for endpoint two is clearly more promising than for endpoint one (more careful strategy);
- Unweighted Bonferroni-Holm procedure with no change after the interim analysis (as in Kieser, Bauer, and Lehmacher 1999); and
- Weighted Bonferroni-Holm procedure (with weights $\frac{2}{3}$ for endpoint one and $\frac{1}{3}$ for endpoint two), with no change, equally.

The results showed clear superiority of both Bonferroni procedures when the expected power for both endpoints was similar. But also when the power for endpoint one was clearly higher than for endpoint two, both Bonferroni procedures often attained the power of the procedures based on the a priori order. The concept of this simulation study was extended by Duncker (2007), by considering still more careful strategies, in particular the use of weights ($\frac{2}{3}$, $\frac{1}{3}$) instead of a complete order. He could show that the use of weights can lead to a slight gain in power for certain situations; nevertheless the Bonferroni–Holm procedure with no change is recommended because of its robustness against violations of the initial assumptions.

It is of special importance to maintain scientific integrity when a study with an adaptive design is concerned with medical products for human use. Regulatory authorities were very wary of adaptive designs at the beginning of methodical research; however, nowadays they have recognized the advantages for certain types of design changes, as modification of the sample size or of the randomization ratio after an interim analysis. In a reflection paper by EMEA (2007), these advantages are acknowledged, but also the prerequisites, problems, and pitfalls of adaptive designs are critically discussed. Design changes are only recommended when clear justification is given. Modifications of hypotheses are automatically connected with the problem of multiplicity (see the points to consider by EMEA 2002) and are discussed much more sceptically:

- The change of a primary endpoint is considered to be very difficult to justify since primary endpoints are chosen to describe a clinically relevant treatment effect. At best, one could use feasibility or recent external knowledge as arguments. It is emphasized that the clinical benefit is essential regarding endpoint choice and not the possibility to differentiate between experimental groups.
- Dropping a treatment arm is considered useful, but very careful planning is deserved. When different dose groups are included, it is stressed that "… the mere rejection of the global hypothesis … is not usually sufficient …"; then a multiple testing procedure has to be incorporated.
- When the aims of the trial are to show superiority as well as noninferiority, it is recommended to plan showing noninferiority; it might be possible to switch to superiority in the interim analysis. It is generally considered unacceptable to change the objective from superiority to noninferiority.

16.8 Further Aspects

16.8.1 More than Two Stages

All methods described in Sections 16.5 and 16.6 can be directly extended to designs with $s > 2$ stages, although the notation will become still more technical. One can either define multistage combination tests for the combination of more than two p-values (Lehmacher and Wassmer 1999), or one can choose the number of interim analyses adaptively over recursive combination tests (Brannath, Posch, and Bauer 2002). For both methods, the principle of combining the techniques of the closure test and of adaptive designs will be maintained.

16.8.2 Logical Relations of Hypotheses

In Section 16.5 we have considered the modification of the closure test (Hommel 1986). The reason was that it would be easier to argue with procedures that use Bonferroni adjustments. When the free combination condition is satisfied (as for the case of multiple endpoints), this modification is identical to the usual closure test (Marcus, Peritz, and Gabriel 1976; Hochberg and Tamhane 1987). Otherwise the modified procedure can be improved, since it is not necessary to consider all index sets leading to intersection hypotheses. Consequently, if $H_I = H_J$ for different index sets I, J, one can choose the same local tests $\Phi_I = \Phi_J$ and therefore the same conditional rejection function $A_I = A_J$. The most prominent example for utilizing such a logical relationship is the comparison of multiple treatment arms (see Bauer and Kieser 1999). For multiple doses, it is often possible to assume monotonicity of the response leading to a further reduction of the set of intersection hypotheses.

Improvements of the usual Bonferroni–Holm procedure are described by Shaffer (1986) and Hommel and Bernhard (1999) and can also be applied in connection with adaptive designs.

16.8.3 Correlations of Test Statistics

The advantage of the Bonferroni adjustment is that control of the α level is guaranteed for arbitrary correlations among the test statistics. However, the adjustment may become very conservative, in particular when the tests are highly positively correlated. Therefore it is desirable to find more specific tests exhausting the level α. An important aspect for a MTP is also that the local tests are well matched. This can be achieved when consonant test procedures are used (see Hommel, Bretz, and Maurer 2007). Improvements to Bonferroni type procedures can then be made using resampling methods (Westfall and Young 1993). It should be noted that it nevertheless can occur when a procedure that is consonant for a one-stage procedure is not completely consonant in the case of an adaptation (Duncker 2007).

16.8.4 Two-Sided Tests

When the p-values to be used for an adaptive design with one hypothesis are based on one-sided tests, the interpretation of a significant result is straightforward. When the test problem is two-sided (as demanded in pharmaceutical studies), it is often recommended to perform two one-sided tests each at the level $\alpha/2$.

For the case of stepwise MTPs, the problem is more complex (even without any interim analysis) since it is not ensured that, in general, directional errors (type III errors) are controlled together with control of type I errors (cf. Finner 1999). Nevertheless, one should recommend the use of two one-sided tests in the same manner as above whenever possible. Mostly it can be expected that the additional errors caused by directional decisions are negligible.

16.8.5 Confidence Intervals and Point Estimates

An important regulatory requirement is that the results of a study are not only presented by means of p-values and significance statements, but that also satisfactory estimates and confidence intervals for the treatment effects are available. When only one hypothesis has to be tested, an extensive methodology for constructing point and interval estimates after the application of an adaptive design has been developed; for an overview see Brannath, König, and Bauer (2006). Based on the approach by Müller and Schäfer (2001), more general methods for constructing confidence intervals have been developed by Mehta et al. (2007) and Brannath, Mehta, and Posch (2009).

For multiple testing problems together with an adaptive design, one can apply the same methods for finding point estimates, and also for confidence intervals when it is sufficient to guarantee the confidence level for each hypothesis (treatment effect) separately. However, when simultaneous confidence intervals are desired; that is, the (simultaneous) probability of covering all true parameters is at least $1 - \alpha$, a satisfactory solution is possible for one-step MTPs at most. When the closure test is applied, one obtains stepwise procedures, in general. Then one obtains the well-known problem that the test decisions and the statements on the respective parameters do not correspond in a straightforward manner. Therefore, using conservative confidence intervals which include all parameters for which the corresponding null hypothesis cannot be rejected is usually recommended. For example, when the Bonferroni–Holm procedure has been applied, one constructs confidence intervals based on the nonstepwise Bonferroni test. Posch et al. (2005) describe how a respective construction can be performed when after an interim analysis treatment arms can be eliminated; a generalization of this idea to arbitrary hypothesis-adaptive designs is possible.

In two recent publications (Guilbaud 2008; Strassburger and Bretz 2008) it has been shown how one can obtain simultaneous confidence intervals corresponding to the decisions of certain MTPs. However, the form of these intervals is not very informative, as a rule, and the authors of these papers themselves discuss this construction very critically.

16.8.6 Many Hypotheses

When a large number of hypotheses is investigated, it is often not advisable to control the multiple level α. An error rate that can be controlled instead is the FDR. The FDR is the expected value of the ratio V/R, where V is the number of all erroneously rejected null hypotheses, and R is the number of all rejected hypotheses.

The most common applications are gene expression or gene association studies. It is very desirable to perform these studies in more than one stage, such that many nonpromising hypotheses (genes or SNPs) can be excluded in early stages. A solution to this problem has been worked out for a two-stage design under the constraint of a fixed budget by Zehetmayer, Bauer, and Posch (2005). In a subsequent publication, Zehetmayer, Bauer, and Posch (2008) found a solution for optimizing multistage designs where the number of stages as well as the allocation of cases/genes to the different stages can be varied. Both publications consider control of the multiple level as well as the FDR.

Victor and Hommel (2007) addressed the same problem for control of the FDR, but without a fixed budget and with the possibility of early rejections. They considered in particular the bounds of the explorative Simes procedure (Benjamini and Hochberg 1995), since it is uncertain at the interim analysis which bound will be used at the end of the study.

16.9 Closing Remarks

We have seen several possibilities for performing adaptations of hypotheses, such as change of weights or of an order, elimination, and even inclusion of new ones. From the technical point of view, one has to combine the concepts of the closure test principle with the methods of adaptive designs. It has also been demonstrated that the correct use of this technique may be connected with severe penalties: one can expect a substantial loss in power when the initial assumptions or objectives are too vague. The most crucial problem in practice is, however, that it is more difficult to perform such studies in a scientifically proper and convincing way. Because of the danger of (intentional or unintentional) manipulation, it is indispensable to formulate a careful protocol at the beginning of a study. For applications in the medical field, it must be agreed fully that regulatory authorities view hypothesis modifications very sceptically. Already for adaptive designs without a change of hypotheses one needs careful planning; this requirement is much more essential when even the objectives may be modified or changed.

Acknowledgment

I wish to thank Andreas Faldum for his careful review of the manuscript.

References

Bauer, P. (1989a). Multistage testing with adaptive designs. *Biometrie und Informatik in Medizin und Biologie*, 20: 130–36.

Bauer, P. (1989b). Sequential tests of hypotheses in consecutive trials. *Biometrical Journal*, 31: 663–76.

Bauer, P., and Kieser, M. (1999). Combining different phases in the development of medical treatments within a single trial. *Statistics in Medicine*, 18: 1833–48.

Bauer, P., and Köhne, K. (1994/1996). Evaluation of experiments with adaptive interim analyses. *Biometrics*, 50: 1029–41. Correction *Biometrics*, 52: 380.

Bauer, P., and Röhmel, J. (1995). An adaptive method for establishing a dose-response relationship. *Statistics in Medicine*, 14: 1595–1607.

Bauer, P., Röhmel, J., Maurer, W., and Hothorn, L. (1998). Testing strategies in multi-dose experiments including active control. *Statistics in Medicine*, 17: 2133–46.

Benjamini, Y., and Hochberg, Y., (1995). Controlling the false discovery rate: A practical and powerful approach to multiple testing. *Journal of the Royal Statistical Society,* B57: 289–300.

Brannath, W., König, F., and Bauer, P. (2006). Estimation in flexible two stage designs. *Statistics in Medicine,* 25: 3366–81.

Brannath, W., Mehta, C. R., and Posch, M. (2009). Exact confidence bounds following adaptive group sequential tests. *Biometrics,* 65: 539–46.

Brannath, W., Posch, M., and Bauer, P. (2002). Recursive combination tests. *Journal of the American Statistical Association,* 97: 236–44.

Bretz, F., Schmidli, H., König, F., Racine, A., and Maurer, W. (2006). Confirmatory seamless phase II/III clinical trials with hypotheses selection at interim: General concepts. *Biometrical Journal,* 48: 623–34.

Duncker, J. W. (2007). Änderung der Zielgröße einer klinischen Studie nach einer Zwischenauswertung. Mainz: PhD Thesis.

EMEA. (2002). Points to consider on *Multiplicity Issues in Clinical Trials.* The European Agency for the Evaluation of Medicinal Products. Committee for proprietary medicinal products (CPMP). London, UK.

EMEA (2007). Reflection paper on *Methodological Issues in Confirmatory Clinical Trials Planned with an Adaptive Design.* European Medicines Agency. Committee for medicinal products for human use (CHMP), London, UK.

Finner, H. (1999). Stepwise multiple test procedures and control of directional errors. *Annals of Statistics,* 27: 274–89.

Fisher, R. A. (1932). *Statistical Methods for Research Workers.* London: Oliver & Boyd.

Follmann, D. A., Proschan, M. A., and Geller, N. L. (1994). Monitoring pairwise comparisons in multi-armed clinical trials. *Biometrics,* 50: 325–36.

Guilbaud, O. (2008). Simultaneous confidence regions corresponding to Holm's step-down and other closed-testing procedures. *Biometrical Journal,* 50: 678–92.

Hellmich, M. (2001). Monitoring clinical trials with multiple arms. *Biometrics,* 57: 892–98.

Hellmich, M., and Hommel, G. (2004). Multiple testing in adaptive designs—A review. In *Recent Developments in Multiple Comparison Procedures. IMS Lecture Notes—Monograph Series.* eds. Y. Benjamini, F. Bretz, and S. Sarkar, 47: 33–47. Beachwood, Ohio: Institute of Mathematical Statistics.

Hochberg, Y., and Tamhane, A. C. (1987). *Multiple Comparison Procedures.* New York: Wiley.

Holm, S. (1979). A simple sequentally rejective multiple test procedure. *Scandinavian Journal of Statistics,* 6: 65–70.

Hommel, G. (1986). Multiple test procedures for arbitrary dependence structures. *Metrika,* 33: 321–36.

Hommel, G. (1989). Comment on Bauer, P.: Multistage testing with adaptive designs. *Biometrie und Informatik in Medizin und Biologie,* 20: 137–39.

Hommel, G. (2001). Adaptive modifications of hypotheses after an interim analysis. *Biometrical Journal,* 43: 581–89.

Hommel, G., and Bernhard, G. (1999). Bonferroni procedures for logically related hypotheses. *Journal of Statistical Planning and Inference,* 82: 119–28.

Hommel, G., Bretz, F., and Maurer, W. (2007). Powerful short-cuts for multiple testing procedures with special reference to gatekeeping strategies. *Statistics in Medicine,* 26: 4063–73.

Hommel, G., and Kropf, S. (2001). Clinical trials with an adaptive choice of hypotheses. *Drug Information Journal,* 35: 1423–29.

Kieser, M. (2005). A note on adaptively changing the hierarchy of hypotheses in clinical trials with flexible design. *Drug Information Journal,* 39: 215–22.

Kieser, M., Bauer, P., and Lehmacher, W. (1999). Inference on multiple endpoints in clinical trials with adaptive interim analyses. *Biometrical Journal,* 41: 261–77.

Kropf, S., Hommel, G., Schmidt, U., Brickwedel, J., and Jepsen, M. S. (2000). Multiple comparisons of treatments with stable multivariate tests in a two-stage adaptive design, including a test for non-inferiority. *Biometrical Journal,* 42: 951–65.

Lehmacher, W., Kieser, M., and Hothorn, L. (2000). Sequential and multiple testing for dose-response analysis. *Drug Information Journal,* 34: 591–97.

Lehmacher, W., and Wassmer, G. (1999). Adaptive sample size calculations in group sequential trials. *Biometrics,* 55: 1286–90.

Marcus, R., Peritz, E., and Gabriel, K. R. (1976). On closed testing procedures with special reference to ordered analysis of variance. *Biometrika,* 63: 655–60.

Mehta, C. R., Bauer, P., Posch, M., and Brannath, W. (2007). Repeated confidence intervals for adaptive group sequential trials. *Statistics in Medicine,* 26: 5422–33.

Müller, H. H., and Schäfer, H. (2001). Adaptive group sequential designs: Combining the advantages of adaptive and classical group sequential approaches. *Biometrics,* 57: 886–91.

Müller, H. H., and Schäfer, H. (2004). A general statistical principle for changing a design any time during the course of a trial. *Statistics in Medicine,* 23: 2497–2508.

Posch, M., König, F., Branson, M., Brannath, W., Dunger-Baldauf, C., and Bauer, P. (2005). Testing and estimation in flexible group sequential designs with adaptive treatment selection. *Statistics in Medicine,* 24: 3697–3714.

Proschan, M. A., and Hunsberger, S. A. (1995). Design extensions of studies based on conditional power. *Biometrics,* 51: 1313–24.

Shaffer, J. P. (1986). Modified sequentially rejective multiple test procedures. *Journal of the American Statistical Association,* 81: 826–31.

Strassburger, K., and Bretz, F. (2008). Compatible simultaneous lower confidence bounds for the Holm procedure and other Bonferroni-based closed tests. *Statistics in Medicine,* 27: 4914–27.

Tang, D. I., and Geller, N. L. (1999). Closed testing procedures for group sequential clinical trials with multiple endpoints. *Biometrics,* 55: 1188–92.

Vandemeulebroecke, M. (2006). Two-stage adaptive tests: Overall p-values and new tests. *Statistica Sinica,* 16: 933–51.

Victor, A., and Hommel, G. (2007). Combining adaptive designs with control of the false discovery rate—A generalized definition for a global *p*-value. *Biometrical Journal,* 49: 94–106.

Westfall, P. H., Krishen, A., and Young, S. S. (1998). Using prior information to allocate significance levels for multiple endpoints. *Statistics in Medicine,* 17: 2107–19.

Westfall, P. H., and Young, S. S. (1993). *Resampling-Based Multiple Testing.* New York: Wiley.

Wright, S. P. (1992). Adjusted p-values for simultaneous inference. *Biometrics,* 48: 1005–13.

Zehetmayer, S., Bauer, P., and Posch, M. (2005). Two stage designs for experiments with a large number of hypotheses. *Bioinformatics,* 21: 3771–77.

Zehetmayer, S., Bauer, P., and Posch, M. (2008). Optimized multi-stage designs controlling the false discovery or the family-wise error rate. *Statistics in Medicine,* 27: 4145–60.

17

Treatment Adaptive Allocations in Randomized Clinical Trials: An Overview

Atanu Biswas
Indian Statistical Institute

Rahul Bhattacharya
West Bengal State University

17.1 Introduction

In any clinical trial, reasonable allocation of subjects to treatments under consideration is often the most challenging task. Most of the early clinical experiments adopted arbitrary schemes for treatment assignment. Randomization, the systematic procedure of assigning subjects to different treatments, was contributed by Sir R. A. Fisher (1935) in the context of assigning treatments to plots in agricultural experiments. However, in a clinical trial's scenario the purpose of randomization is to produce groups similar with respect to all risk factors that might affect the outcome of interest, apart from the treatments. Randomization provides a degree of trade-off between balance, ensuring that the desired proportion of subjects per treatment arm is approximately achieved, and nonpredictability, ensuring that clinicians referring subjects for enrollment cannot dictate the next assignment.

Adaptive designs are data driven randomization procedures, where the stopping rule may be data-driven (see Dragalin 2006) and/or assignment of any entering subject is based on the information on treatment assignments and/or covariates of the subjects allocated so far. We may restrict our discussion within the framework of double-blinded trials (see Matthews 2006). For a formal description of different randomization schemes, we introduce the following notations. Consider a clinical trial of n patients, each of whom is to be assigned to either of the t competing treatments. Let δ_{kj} and X_{kj} be respectively the treatment indicator (= 1 if treatment k is applied, = 0 otherwise) and response that would be observed if treatment k was assigned to the jth subject, $k = 1, 2, \ldots, t, j = 1, 2, \ldots$, and in addition, let $\mathbf{Z}_j$ denote the corresponding vector of covariate information. Let $\mathcal{T}_n$, $\mathcal{X}_n$, and $\mathcal{Z}_n$ denote, respectively, the information (i.e., a σ-algebra) contained in the first n treatment assignments, responses, and covariates and in addition, let $\mathcal{F}_n$ denote the totality of all response, allocation, and covariate information up to the nth subject plus the covariate information of the (n + 1)th subject. Then any randomization scheme can be defined by the conditional expectation

$$E(\delta_{kn} \mid \mathcal{F}_{n-1}),\ n \geq 1, k = 1, 2, .., t.$$

Depending on the nature of the allocation strategy and following Hu and Rosenberger (2006), we have the following classification of randomization procedures:

- Complete Randomization:

$$E(\delta_{kn} \mid \mathcal{F}_{n-1}) = E(\delta_{kn});$$

- Restricted Randomization:

$$E(\delta_{kn} \mid \mathcal{F}_{n-1}) = E(\delta_{kn} \mid \mathcal{T}_{n-1});$$

- Response-adaptive randomization:

$$E(\delta_{kn} \mid \mathcal{F}_{n-1}) = E(\delta_{kn} \mid \mathcal{T}_{n-1}, \mathcal{X}_{n-1});$$

- Covariate-adaptive randomization:

$$E(\delta_{kn} \mid \mathcal{F}_{n-1}) = E(\delta_{kn} \mid \mathcal{T}_{n-1}, \mathcal{Z}_n);\ \text{ and}$$

- Covariate-adjusted response-adaptive randomization:

$$E(\delta_{kn} \mid \mathcal{F}_{n-1}) = E(\delta_{kn} \mid \mathcal{T}_{n-1}, \mathcal{X}_{n-1}, \mathcal{Z}_{n+1}).$$

However, depending on the allocation probability, Chow and Chang (2006) identified the following randomization rules: conventional randomization (allocation probability remains fixed throughout the trial), treatment-adaptive randomization (allocation probabilities are updated on the basis of allocation history), covariate-adaptive randomization (allocation probabilities are modified based on the cumulative information on treatment allocations and covariates), and response-adaptive randomization (allocation probabilities are set on the basis of the available response information). Throughout the current work, we consider randomization schemes allowing the current allocation probability to depend on the accumulated information on treatment assignments and/or covariates and we use the phrase, treatment-adaptive allocation, to refer such a procedure.

Treatment adaptive designs are becoming popular in the context of real life applications. For example, in the recently concluded first joint workshop on Adaptive Designs in Confirmatory Clinical Trials organized by the European Medicines Agency (EMA 2008) in collaboration with the European Federation of Pharmaceutical Industries and Associations, Robert Hemmings (MHRA & SAWP) presented real life experience from the SAWP of the CHMP, based on approximately 15–20 Scientific Advice applications with adaptive designs in confirmatory trials. See the report on the EMEA–EFPIA Workshop on Adaptive Designs in Confirmatory Clinical Trials (EMEA/106659/2008). PharmaED's workshop, Adaptive Trial Designs, Maximizing the use of Interim Data Analysis to Increase Drug Development Efficacy and Safety in Philadelphia during September 10–11, 2007, had an in-depth preconference workshop, Lessons Learned from the Field: Design, Planning and Implementation, on more than 300 Adaptive Trials. These are indicators of the growing popularity of adaptive designs in real life applications of the pharmaceutical industries.

In Section 17.2, we discuss several requirements of an allocation design. In Section 17.3, we provide a review of the existing treatment adaptive allocation designs without covariates. Designs in the presence of covariates are discussed in Section 17.4. Finally Section 17.5 ends with some concluding remarks.

17.2 Requirements of an Allocation Design: A Clinician's Perspective

Randomization plays an important role in clinical research. An appropriately randomized trial not only produces a truly representative sample of the target patient population under the study, but also provides a basis for valid statistical inference. Ensuring balance and unpredictability of treatment assignments are the basic requirements of any randomization procedure and in this vein, we provide below a brief discussion on these issues that will help us to judge the effectiveness of each treatment-adaptive allocation. Moreover, we also provide the principles of inference following any treatment-adaptive randomization scheme. Dragalin (2006) defined "Adaptive Design" as a multistage study design that uses accumulating data to decide how to modify aspects of the study without undermining the validity and integrity of the trial. Dragalin (2006) discussed several terminologies in this context that include validity, integrity, allocation rule, sampling rule, stopping rule, decision rule, sample size reassessment, flexible design, optimal design, conditional power, seamless Phase II/III designs, and so on. Adaptive seamless Phase II/III design is then elaborated by Maca et al. (2006).

17.2.1 Treatment Imbalance

Treatment-adaptive allocations are usually considered to balance the difference between the observed number of allocations to different treatments. Lack of balance could result in a decrease in statistical power for detecting a clinically meaningful difference and consequently makes the validity of the trial questionable. In fact, randomization and balance are in conflict, in general the more randomized the sequential design the less likely it is to be balanced when stopped at an arbitrary time point. Thus, it becomes necessary to examine the possibility of imbalance for any randomization procedure. For a formal development, consider a two treatment trial with $N_k(j) = \sum_{i=1}^{j} \delta_{ki}$ denoting the observed number of allocation to treatment k among the first j subjects, $k = 1, 2, j = 1, 2, \ldots$. Then, for an n subject trial, possible treatment imbalance can be measured by the absolute value of D_n, where $D_n = N_1(n) - N_2(n)$. Investigation of the properties of $|D_n|$ could reveal whether these imbalances compromise the statistical requirements.

In the presence of covariate information it is desired to ensure balance between treatment groups with respect to known covariates. The possibility of covariate imbalance introduces a type of experimental bias, called accidental bias (see Efron 1971). It is a measure of the bias caused by an unobserved covariate in estimating the treatment effect. However, such a bias may be vulnerable in small studies, but the possibility of accidental bias becomes negligible for large studies. Comprehensive details regarding the accidental bias can be found in Rosenberger and Lachin (2002).

17.2.2 Selection Bias

Lack of concealment of allocation in randomized clinical trials result in the preferential enrollment of specific subjects into one treatment arm over the other(s). For example, patients more likely to respond may be enrolled only when the next assignment is known to be made to the active treatment, and patients less likely to respond may be enrolled only when the next treatment to be assigned is known to be the control. The great clinical trialist Chalmers (1990) was convinced that the most essential requirement for a good clinical trial must be that the clinician, deciding the randomization, must have no clue as to which treatment is more likely to be selected. Such predictability of the randomization leads to what is known in literature as selection bias. It arises when, subconsciously or otherwise, an experimenter attempts to beat the natural flow of randomization by assigning a subject to a treatment that the investigator feels best suited (Karlowski et al. 1975; Byington, Curb, and Mattson 1985; Deyo et al. 1990). For example, a sympathetic nurse coordinator tries to assign a favorite subject to the new therapy with a view that the new therapy will be more effective than the placebo. Selection bias can be thought of as simple as guessing the outcome of a throw of a coin. Consequently, Smith (1984) points out that wrong guesses are more frequent than the right choices and hence elimination of selection bias should be the primary requirement for the success of a clinical trial. Thus, every randomization procedure should be evaluated in the light of the ability to control the selection bias.

We adopt a simple model suggested by Blackwell and Hodges (1957) and Lachin (1988a) and assess the potential selection bias due to a wrong guess of treatment assignments by investigators. The model assumes that guessing the randomization sequence, the experimenter will attempt to assign each subject on the treatment, believed best for the subject. The Blackwell–Hodges (1957) model also assumes independence of treatment assignment and responses; that is, the model is inappropriate for response adaptive randomization schemes. Table 17.1 represents the Blackwell–Hodges model for selection bias where each patient is assumed to have an equal chance of being assigned to either the test drug or the placebo.

Thus for a n subject trial, the expected sample size for both the test drug and the placebo is $n/2$. Then, the total potential selection bias for evaluation of the treatment effect introduced by the investigator is represented as the (expected) difference between the observed sample means according to the treatment assignments guessed by the investigator. If G_n is the total number of correct guesses in an n subject trial, then selection bias can be measured by the expected bias factor, $E(F_n) = E[G_n - (n/2)]$, the difference between the expected number of correct guesses and the number expected by chance. The expected difference thus can be expressed as the product of the investigator's bias in favor of the test drug, times the expected bias factor $E(F_n)$. Blackwell and Hodges (1957) showed that the optimal strategy for the experimenter is to guess a treatment for an incoming subject if the number of allocations to that treatment is the lowest up to that point of time. In a tied situation, the experimenter guesses with equal probability. This is called convergence strategy. A variation can be found in Stigler (1969), where the Blackwell–Hodges model is described in terms of a minimax strategy and consequently arrived at his proportional convergence strategy.

17.2.2.1 Analysis Following Randomization

After the responses are observed, the question of carrying out inference naturally arises. However, there is a fundamental difference between a simple randomization model and the treatment adaptive randomization model. The simple randomization model assumes that the subjects under study are a random sample from a well defined population and consequently the respective responses may be considered to be independently and identically distributed under treatment equivalence. However, this model is often questionable in clinical trials as patients enter the trial in a nonrandom fashion. Moreover, under

TABLE 17.1 Blackwell–Hodges Diagram for Selection Bias

	Random Assignment	
Investigator's Guess	Test Drug	Placebo
Test drug	a	$\frac{n}{2}-b$
Placebo	$\frac{n}{2}-a$	b
Expected sample size	$\frac{n}{2}$	$\frac{n}{2}$

Source: Blackwell, D., and Hodges, J. L. *Annals of Mathematical Statistics,* 28, 449–60, 1957.

a simple randomization model the likelihood is identical with that under a nonrandomized procedure (Rosenberger and Lachin 2002), and hence a likelihood based analysis would ignore the underlying randomization mechanism completely. Fortunately, permutation tests or randomization tests, originally proposed by Fisher (see e.g., Basu 1980), provides the basis for an assumption-free statistical test of the treatment equivalence. The null hypothesis of a permutation test is that the assignment of treatment 1 versus treatment 2 had no effect on the responses of the n subjects randomized under the study. Therefore, under a null hypothesis of randomization, the set of observed responses are assumed to be a set of deterministic values that are unaffected by the treatment and hence the observed difference between the treatment groups depends only on the adopted method of randomization. Thus, for any given sequence of treatment assignments, the value and the associated probability of the selected test statistic is entirely defined by the observed sequence of responses and treatments and the particular randomization scheme adopted. It is, therefore, possible to enumerate all possible sequences of treatment assignments, test statistic values, together with their associated probability of selection as determined by the particular randomization scheme, and hence the exact null distribution of the test statistic. We note that under a simple randomization model, all possible treatment assignments have the same probability $(1/2)^n$, but these probabilities vary under a treatment adaptive randomization model. The sum of the probabilities of those randomization sequences whose test statistic values are at least as extreme as what was observed is clearly the probability of obtaining a result at least as extreme as the one that was observed; that is, precisely the p-value of the unconditional permutation test. A very small p-value indicates rejection of the null hypothesis of no difference among the treatments. Linear rank tests (Lehmann 1986), Wilcoxon rank-sum test and log rank tests are often used for the purpose. However, enumeration of all possible permutations becomes practically impossible for moderate sample sizes, and for further description on implementation we refer to Rosenberger and Lachin (2002) and Dirienzo (2000). Permutation tests (Fisher 1935; Pitman 1937, 1938) can also be carried out for such purposes.

17.3 Treatment Adaptive Allocations: Without Covariates

Now we are at a position to discuss different allocation designs together with their performances in fulfilling the requirements of a clinical trial. However, the most commonly employed randomization procedure in clinical trials is the simple random allocation, where at each step, treatment allocation probabilities (not necessarily 1/2 to either treatment) remain fixed independently of the earlier response and/or allocation history. If the trial size n is known in advance, exactly $n/2$ subjects are selected at random and given one of the treatments, and the rest assigned to the other. The procedure is called fixed random allocation. However, in most of the trials the trial size is not known a-priori and the subjects are assigned sequentially to one of the treatment groups with a fixed allocation probability. To achieve equal fraction to each treatment, an equal probability for each treatment arm is usually considered and the resulting procedure is termed complete randomization. Equal allocation probability removes selection bias completely. It is ethical in the sense of equal toxicity (Lachin 1988b). However the major disadvantage is that, at any point of randomization, including the end, there could be a substantial imbalance, though in the long run the allocation is exactly balanced. Moreover, a randomization technique forcing balance can make a test more powerful than the complete randomization (Baldi Antognini 2008). The relevance of mentioning these randomization procedures is due to their easy implementation in real clinical trials, though the procedures are far from a treatment adaptive allocation. See Wei (1988) and Rosenberger and Lachin (2002) in the context of permutation test for adaptive allocation.

17.3.1 Random Allocation Rule

To overcome the possibility of severe treatment imbalance of complete randomization, various randomization procedures have been developed imposing the restriction of exact balance of the final allocation. We start with the random allocation rule (RAR) of Lachin (1988b; also known as Lachin's urn model) where it is assumed that the investigator has control over the total number of subjects to be randomized. For a two treatment trial, the rule can be best described by the allocation probability

$$E(\delta_{1j} \mid \mathcal{T}_{j-1}) = \begin{cases} \dfrac{\dfrac{n}{2} - N_1(j-1)}{n-(j-1)} & \text{for } j \geq 2, \\ \dfrac{1}{2} & \text{for } j = 1. \end{cases}$$

The above can also be described in terms of an urn model as follows. Consider an urn containing $n/2$ white and the same number of black balls. Each time a patient enters a ball is drawn, its color noted and not returned to the urn. If the ball drawn is white, the subject is assigned Treatment 1; otherwise Treatment 2 is given to the subject. The procedure continues until the urn is exhausted. However, one can immediately find some drawbacks in RAR. First, once $n/2$ subjects have been assigned to one treatment arm, all further treatment assignments become absolutely predictable and hence leads to selection bias. Secondly, there could be significant treatment imbalances at any intermediate point of the trial. Although the procedure results in a perfect balance after all subjects are randomized, the maximum imbalance occurs when half of the treatment allocations are completed. With $r(>0)$ as the size of the imbalance, the maximum imbalance can be approximated by $2\{1-\Phi[(2r/n)\sqrt{n-1}]\}$.

17.3.2 Truncated Binomial Design

Another way of achieving balance over the treatment allocation is to use a truncated binomial design (TBD) after Blackwell and Hodges (1957), where the subjects are allocated randomly to a treatment by tossing a coin until one treatment has been assigned half the times. The allocation probability at any intermediate stage of the trial can be expressed as

$$E(\delta_{1j} \mid \mathcal{T}_{j-1}) = \begin{cases} 0 & \text{if } \dfrac{N_1(j-1)}{n} = \dfrac{1}{2}, \\ \dfrac{1}{2} & \text{if } \max\left\{\dfrac{N_1(j-1)}{n}, \dfrac{N_2(j-1)}{n}\right\} < \dfrac{1}{2}, \\ 1 & \text{if } \dfrac{N_2(j-1)}{n} = \dfrac{1}{2}, \end{cases}$$

with n even. As the tail of the randomization sequence is entirely predictable, selection bias exists. Moreover, there can be moderate treatment imbalance during the course of the trial, though unconditionally $E(\delta_{1j}) = 1/2$, for any j. For further mathematical deductions, we refer to Rosenberger and Lachin (2002).

17.3.3 Permuted Block Design

Both RAR and TBD can result in severe imbalances at any intermediate time point during the trial. Permuted Block Design (PBD), introduced by Hill (1951), is a way to control the imbalance during the randomization through blocking. For the PBD, B blocks, each containing $b = (n/B)$ subjects are used, where n is the prespecified trial size with B and b both positive integers. For a two treatment trial, within each block $b/2$ subjects are assigned to each treatment. RAR or TBD is most commonly used within each block to ensure balance. In practice, the possible $b!/[(b/2)!(b/2)!]$ arrangements of length b with two symbols (each symbol represents a distinct treatment) are prepared in advance, one of these arrangements is randomly selected and accordingly the b participants are randomized to two treatments. The minimum block size commonly chosen in clinical trials is two, which leads to an alternative assignment of the two treatments.

The advantage of blocking is that balance between the number of subjects in each group is ensured during the course of the trial. The imbalance at any stage can not exceed $b/2$. In the extreme situation, $B = (n/B)$ and every pair randomized is balanced. The potential drawback is that within each block after a certain stage the allocation becomes deterministic and hence leads to selection bias. For example, if $b = 4$ and the first two assignments are known to be made to Treatment 1, then the last two assignments are essentially to Treatment 2. However, the last assignments within each block are always predictable and this results in selection bias for every bth randomized subject. The degree of unpredictability is greater for smaller block sizes. For example, with block size 2, knowledge of the block size and the first allocation in a block predicts with certainty the next assignment. Thus, in general, a trial using PBD for randomization should have a large enough block size to guard against predictability.

A variation of PBD is to allow the block size to vary. In fact, after each block of randomization sequences, the next block size is randomly selected from a set of feasible choices. Random block sizes make it difficult to determine the starting and ending of the allocation sequence and hence ensures some amount of unpredictability. However, Rosenberger and Lachin (2002) noted that random blocks virtually provide no reduction in selection bias.

17.3.4 Biased Coin Designs

Biased coin designs allocate a subject, with probability greater than 1/2, to the treatment arm that had previously been assigned fewest subjects. These methods provide a significant reduction in predictability over the other allocation designs.

17.3.4.1 Efron's Biased Coin Design

Efron (1971) developed the biased coin design to balance the treatment allocation between the treatment arms. The corresponding allocation probability can be expressed as

$$E(\delta_{1j} \mid \mathcal{T}_{j-1}) = \begin{cases} \frac{1}{2} & \text{if } D_{j-1} = 0, \\ p & \text{if } D_{j-1} < 0, \\ 1-p & \text{if } D_{j-1} > 0, \end{cases}$$

for some known $p \in (1/2, 1]$. Thus at any stage, the treatment arm with the lowest number of subjects is preferred for the allocation of any incoming subject. Efron (1971) abbreviated the above by BCD(p); for $p = 1/2$ we get the complete randomization and with $p = 1$ we have the PBD with block size 2. However Efron's personally favorite choice for p was 2/3. The marginal allocation probability for any subject to either treatment is exactly 1/2. Moreover $|D_n|$, the absolute imbalance is even or odd according as n is even or odd and hence the minimum imbalance for even n is zero and it is one for odd n. Applying the theory of random walk it is established that

$$\lim_{n\to\infty} P(|D_{2n}| = 0) = \frac{2p-1}{p}, \text{ and}$$

$$\lim_{n\to\infty} P(|D_{2n+1}| = 1) = \frac{2p-1}{p^2}.$$

As $p \to 1$, perfect balance is achieved but the resulting procedure becomes deterministic.

As a modification over Efron's BCD, Soares and Wu (1982) proposed the big stick rule by imposing a bound on the degree of imbalance. With c as the prespecified degree of imbalance, the rule can be described by

$$E(\delta_{1j} \mid \mathcal{T}_{j-1}) = \begin{cases} \frac{1}{2} & \text{if } |D_{j-1}| < c, \\ 0 & \text{if } D_{j-1} = c, \\ 1 & \text{if } D_{j-1} = -c, \end{cases}$$

A similar type of allocation, using the proportionate degree of imbalance instead of absolute imbalance, can be found in Lachin et al. (1981). In the sequel, combining the aspects of both the big stick rule and the Efron's BCD, Chen (1999) developed the biased coin design with imbalance tolerance BCDWIT(p, c), where

$$E(\delta_{1j} \mid \mathcal{T}_{j-1}) = \begin{cases} \frac{1}{2} & \text{if } D_{j-1} = 0, \\ 0 & \text{if } D_{j-1} = c, \\ 1 & \text{if } D_{j-1} = -c, \\ p & \text{if } 0 < D_{j-1} < c, \\ 1-p & \text{if } -c < D_{j-1} < 0, \end{cases}$$

A comprehensive detailed account on the asymptotic and balancing properties of the procedure can be found in Chen (1999).

17.3.4.2 Friedman–Wei's Urn Design

In Efron's BCD(p), p remains fixed throughout the trial regardless of the degree of imbalance and hence modifying the role of p, Wei (1977, 1978a) developed an urn biased randomization procedure, where the allocation probabilities are updated according to the degree of imbalance using an urn. The allocation procedure is actually a modified version of Friedman's (1949) urn model; modified with an aim to use the model for treatment assignments in sequential clinical trials. The resulting procedure can be described as below: Consider an urn containing α white balls and α black balls, two colors of balls representing the two treatment types. For the randomization of an incoming subject, a ball is drawn, its color noted and replaced to the urn. The corresponding treatment is assigned and β balls of opposite color are added to the urn. The procedure is repeated for each incoming subject, where α and β may be any reasonable positive integers. Addition of balls skew the urn composition in favor of the treatment under represented so far, and hence the allocation probability is updated in accordance to the existing treatment imbalance. Denoting the procedure by $UD(\alpha, \beta)$, mathematically we can express it as:

$$E(\delta_{1j} \mid \mathcal{T}_{j-1}) = \begin{cases} \dfrac{\alpha + \beta N_2(j-1)}{2\alpha + (j-1)\beta} & \text{for } j \geq 2, \\ \dfrac{1}{2} & \text{for } j = 1. \end{cases}$$

Clearly $UD(\alpha, 0)$ is nothing but complete randomization. Using the theory of stochastic processes, with $D_0 = 0$ and $n \geq d \geq 1$, Wei (1977) established that

$$P(|D_{n+1}|=d\pm 1 \,\|\, D_n|=d)=\frac{1}{2}\mp\frac{d\beta}{2(2\alpha+n\beta)},$$

and

$$P(|D_{n+1}|=1 \,|\, |D_n|=0)=1.$$

Thus $UD(\alpha, \beta)$ forces the trial to be more balanced when several imbalance occurs. For a relatively small trial using $UD(\alpha, \beta)$, a near balance is ensured. However, $UD(\alpha, \beta)$ behaves like complete randomization for moderately large trials. In addition, it is also shown in Wei (1978b) that as $n \to \infty$,

$$\sqrt{n}\left(\frac{N_1(n)}{n}-\frac{1}{2}\right)\to\mathcal{N}\left(0,\frac{\alpha+\beta}{4(3\beta-\alpha)}\right)$$

in distribution, provided $\alpha < 3\beta$. Consequently the probability of imbalance of degree r can be approximated by $2\left\{1-\Phi\left(r\sqrt{[(3\beta-\alpha)/n(\alpha+\beta)]}\right)\right\}$.

17.3.4.3 Ehrenfest Urn Design

Ehrenfest urn design, proposed by Chen (2000), is a randomization procedure in the sequel to enforce balance. The procedure starts with two urns U_1 and U_2, representing two treatments; Treatments 1 and 2, and w balls, equally distributed in the urns. For possible randomization of an entering subject, a ball is drawn at random from w balls. If the ball came from U_k, treatment k is assigned and the ball is replaced in the other urn, $k = 1, 2$, and the procedure is repeated for each arriving subject. Thus, the total number of balls are kept constant throughout the trial. For the design, denoted by EUD(w), we have

$$E(\delta_{1j} \,|\, \mathcal{T}_{j-1})=\frac{1}{2}-\frac{N_1(j)-N_2(j)}{w} \quad \text{for every } j\geq 1.$$

By the properties of Ehrenfest process, Chen (2000) analyzed the design analytically and established that $E[N_1(n)/n] = 1/2$ for any n; that is, the expected imbalance vanishes at any intermediate stage. Chen (2000) also compared EUD(w) with the biased coin design and the BCDWIT and concluded that EUD(w) is more effective than the biased coin design in terms of the imbalance, though the improvement was not uniform.

Recently, Baldi Antognini (2004) has extended the EUD(w) by introducing the Ehrenfest-type urns, generated by suitable extensions of the Ehrenfest process. The first extension, called asymmetric Ehrenfest design and denoted by AED(w, p), consists in putting the ball drawn in U_1 with probability p independently of the urn from which it has been drawn. Another extension consists in assuming that the probability of replacing the selected ball is based on the so called Brillouin term; that is, it depends on both the current number of balls in the urns and the values of two real parameters α_1 and α_2, representing correlation, in some sense, between adding the ball to the urn and the existing number of balls in it at each stage. The procedure is called the Ehrenfest–Brillouin design (see Baldi Antognini 2004) and denoted by EBD(w; α_1, α_2). These designs are very flexible, since they can be designed to achieve almost sure convergence to any given target proportion of allocations and can also be generalized to the case of multiple treatments. A detailed analysis of the convergence properties can be found in Baldi Antognini (2004).

17.3.4.4 Generalizations

As a simple extension of $UD(\alpha, \beta)$, Wei (1978a) developed an adaptive BCD, where for some decreasing function f, symmetric about 0,

$$E(\delta_{1j} \mid \mathcal{T}_{j-1}) = f\left(\frac{N_1(j-1)-N_2(j-1)}{j-1}\right),$$

and also established that the procedure is asymptotically balanced. In the sequel, Smith (1984) introduced another generalization, a generalized biased coin design (GBCD), where for some function ϕ,

$$E(\delta_{1j} \mid \mathcal{T}_{j-1}) = \phi(N_1(j-1), N_2(j-1)) = \phi(j-1).$$

Choosing the allocation function ϕ appropriately, a large class of allocation designs like Efron's BCD, Wei's adaptive BCD, and Chen's EUD(w), among the others can be unified. For example, Efron's BCD(p) is obtained through

$$\phi(j) = \begin{cases} \frac{1}{2} & \text{if } N_1(j) = N_2(j), \\ p & \text{if } N_1(j) < N_2(j), \\ 1-p & \text{if } N_1(j) > N_2(j), \end{cases}$$

whereas, the choice $\phi(j) = 1/2 - [\beta(N_1(j) - N_2(j))/(4\alpha + j\beta)]$, leads to $UD(\alpha, \beta)$. In addition, Smith (1984) also proposed the allocation function $\phi(j) = \{N_2(j)\}^\rho/[\{N_1(j)\}^\rho + \{N_2(j)\}^\rho]$, for some nonnegative parameter ρ. For $\rho = 1$, we get UD(0, 1), and the procedure reduces to complete randomization with $\rho = 0$. But Smith favored to choose $\rho = 5.0$. A reasonable multitreatment extension of these procedures can be found in Wei, Smythe, and Smith (1986). A recent generalization of Efron's biased coin design, called the adjustable BCD, can be found in Baldi Antognini and Giovagnoli (2004). At each step of the adjustable BCD, the probability of selecting the under represented treatment is a decreasing function of the current imbalance. The rule can be expressed as

$$E(\delta_{1j} \mid \mathcal{T}_{j-1}) = F(D_{j-1}),$$

where F is a nonincreasing function on [0, 1] such that for all x, with $F(x) + F(-x) = 1$, and hence, the approach to balance becomes stronger with the progress of the trial. Adjustable BCD includes simple randomization, Efron's BCD(p), the big stick rule, BCD with imbalance tolerance and the EUD(w), among others as special cases. Baldi Antognini and Giovagnoli (2004) investigated the performance of the adjustable BCD and compared it with the existing coin designs in terms of imbalance and predictability, both numerically and asymptotically. Moreover, Baldi Antognini (2008) also established that the adjustable BCD is uniformly more powerful than any other coin designs whatever the trial size may be. With notations introduced in Sections 17.2.1 and 17.2.2, a comparison of the expected proportional imbalance $E(|D_n|/n)$ and the expected proportional bias $E(F_n/n)$ under the convergence strategy for different randomization procedures can be found in Figure 17.1. We, in addition, compare the variabilities of the observed allocation proportions to treatment 1 for $n = 60$. Figure 17.2 exhibits the relevant comparison through a box plot.

17.4 Treatment Adaptive Allocations: With Covariates

For adjustment of baseline covariates there is the EMEA guidelines. Committee for Proprietary Medical Products (CPMP) prepared a detailed report on the points to consider on adjustment for baseline

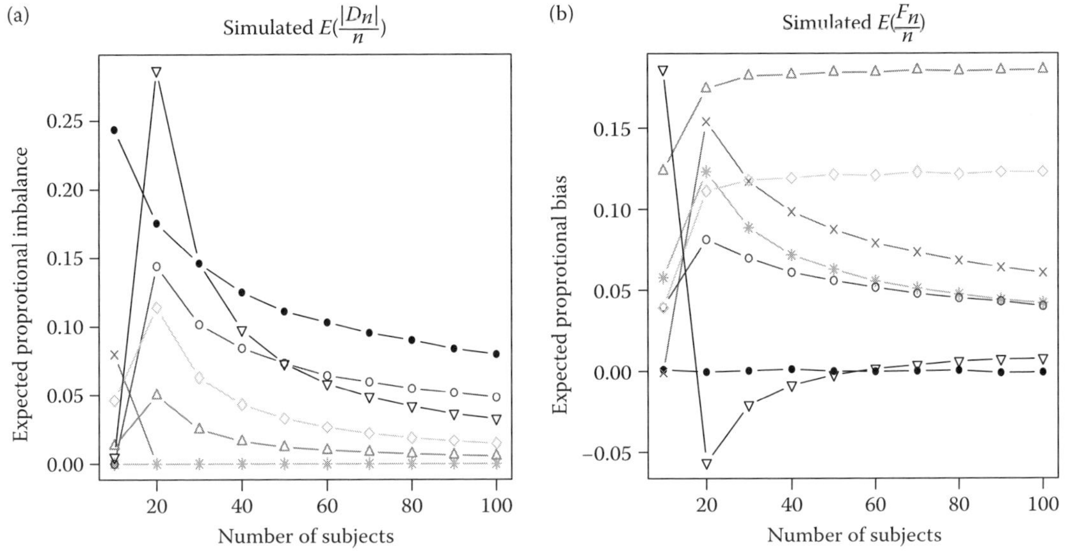

FIGURE 17.1 Comparison of CR [•], RAR [×], TBD [*], UD(1,1)[○], BCD (2/3)[◊], EUD (4) [Δ], and BCDWIT(2/3,4)[∇] procedures.

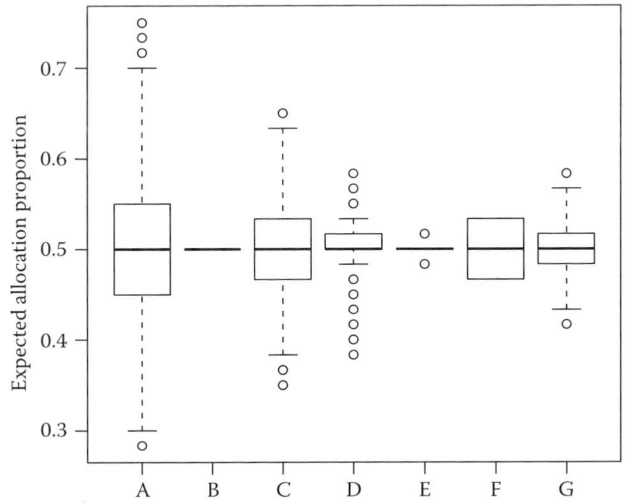

FIGURE 17.2 Comparison of variability of simulated allocation proportions among the A: CR, B: RAR, C: UD (1,1), D: BCD (2/3) , E: EUD (4), F: BCDWIT (2/3,4) and G: Smith's (ρ = 5).procedures.

covariates (CPMP/EWP/2863/99, 2003). See the paper by Grouin, Day, and Lewis (2004) in this context. Treatment adaptive allocation in the presence of covariates is a complicated exercise. Stating from the work of Senn (1994), covariate balancing received attention of authors in different directions. See Campbell, Elbourne, and Altman (2004) and the recent work by Hansen and Bowers (2008), and the references therein, in this context.

17.4.1 Stratified Randomization

The discussion of the previous section ignored the possibility of any covariate information, but in practice, there are many covariates, such as age, sex, disease history, and many others that may influence the patients' responses. The accuracy and reliability of the trial can be seriously challenged by the heterogeneity caused by these covariates. Such a heterogeneity is controlled by forming what is known as strata. The use of strata in clinical trials is motivated from the concept of blocking (Fisher 1935) in agricultural field experiments. The idea is that, if a covariate causes heterogeneity, then the patients are stratified into several homogeneous groups; that is, strata, with respect to the covariate. Randomization of patients to the treatment is then performed independently within the strata and termed stratified randomization. Generally, a PBD is used within each stratum to ensure balance and the resulting procedure is known as a stratified blocked randomization.

However, stratified randomization requires that covariate information be measured at least at the time of randomization. For example, the National Institute of Neurological Disorders and Stroke rt-PA stroke study group (1995) suspected that the time from the onset of stroke to the beginning of treatment of rt-PA may have a significant impact on neurologic improvement as assessed by the National Institute of Health Stroke Scale (NIHSS). Consequently, the study considered two strata of patients based on the time (in minutes) from the onset to the start of the treatment, namely 0–90 minutes and 91–180 minutes. However, with multiple covariates, several groups are formed for each covariate and a stratum is formed by selecting one group from each covariate. The total number of strata is, therefore, the product of the number of groups corresponding to each covariate. The advantage of stratification is to keep the variability of patients within strata as small as possible and the between-strata variability as large as possible so that precise inference on the treatment effect can be made and also to prevent imbalance with respect to important covariates. However, stratification should be used only to a limited extent, especially for small trials where it is the most useful, otherwise stratification will produce many empty or partly filled strata making the implementation difficult (see Chow and Liu 2004 for details).

17.4.2 Covariate-Adaptive Randomization

A stratified randomization procedure, though widely applied, is not treatment adaptive by nature. Moreover, as separate randomization is run for each strata, a stratified randomization procedure cannot control covariate imbalance between the treatment groups. As a result, an entirely different procedure, called covariate-adaptive randomization has been suggested, where the allocation probability is updated taking the covariate information and treatment assignments together.

17.4.2.1 Zelen's Procedure

We start with the Zelen's rule, where an entering subject is initially placed in the appropriate stratum and the prevailing treatment imbalance within the strata is determined; if the imbalance exceeds a certain threshold, the subject is assigned to the treatment arm having fewer number of subjects. Clearly, Zelen (1974) ignored stratification. To be specific, suppose we have s strata and $N_{ik}(n)$ denote the number of subjects on treatment k among the n subjects of stratum i, $i = 1,2,\ldots,s$, $k = 1,2$. An incoming subject (say, the $(n + 1)$th) of the ith stratum is randomized according to the schedule if $|N_{i1}(n) - N_{i2}(n)| < c$, for some integer c; otherwise will be assigned to the treatment with the fewer number of subjects. Zelen proposed to vary c among the Choices 2, 3, or 4.

17.4.2.2 Pocock–Simon Model

A similar type of randomization scheme can be found in Pocock and Simon (1975), of course taking into account the existing stratification. For a detailed description of the model, we assume two treatments (Treatments 1 and 2), I covariates with n_i categories for the ith covariate and hence $s = \Pi_{i=1}^{I} n_i$ number of strata. In addition, for any incoming subject, we define covariate coordinate $(r_1, \ldots, r_I)$, where r_j denotes the category to which he/she will be placed according to his/her jth covariate value, $j = 1, 2,\ldots, I$. Let $N_{ijk}(n)$ be the number of subjects in category j of the ith covariate on treatment k after n subjects have been allocated; $i = 1,2,\ldots, I; j = 1,2,\ldots,n_i$, and $k = 1,2$. Suppose the $(n + 1)$th incoming subject has covariate coordinate $(r_1,\ldots,r_I)$, then his/her allocation is decided on the basis of the weighted imbalance measure $D(n)=\Sigma_{i=1}^{I} w_i\left\{N_{ir_i1}(n)-N_{ir_i2}(n)\right\}$, where the weights w_i are to be chosen depending on the relative importance of the covariates. Here $D(n) < 1/2$ indicates that Treatment 2 has been favored so far among the subjects with covariate coordinate $(r_1,\ldots,r_I)$, and hence with high probability, the $(n + 1)$th subject should be assigned to Treatment 1, and vice-versa if $D(n)$ exceeds 1/2. Pocock and Simon (1975) suggest assigning the $(n + 1)$th subject to

$$\text{Treatment 1 with probability } p \text{ if } D(n)<\tfrac{1}{2}$$

$$\text{Treatment 2 with probability } p \text{ if } D(n)>\tfrac{1}{2}$$

$$\text{Treatment 1 with probability } \tfrac{1}{2} \text{ if } D(n)=\tfrac{1}{2},$$

where $p = (c^* + 1)/3$ and $c^* \in [1/2,1]$.

Note that for $c^* = 1$, we have Efron's BCD type rule, and with $c^* = 2$, the procedure reduces to the Taves's (1974) deterministic minimization method. In fact, with a biased coin twist for added randomization, a number of procedures can be generated from these. One such rule can be found in Efron (1980) with an application to a clinical trial in ovarian cancer research.

Extension of the procedure to multitreatment trials can also be found in Pocock and Simon (1975). Considering a reasonable weighted sum, set of allocation probabilities p_k, $k = 1,2,\ldots,t$, with p_k as the assignment probability for the kth treatment, was determined. Pocock and Simon (1975) suggest to assign the $(n + 1)$th subject with covariate coordinate $(r_1,\ldots r_I)$ to treatment k with probability

$$p_k = c^* - \frac{2(tc^* - 1)}{t(t+1)}, \quad k = 1,2,..,t.$$

17.4.2.3 Wei's Marginal Urn Design

If the number of covariates results in a large number of strata with comparatively small stratum sizes, use of separate urns for each stratum could result in treatment imbalance within strata. With a view to reduce imbalance, Wei (1978a) proposed the marginal urn design. For the description of the procedure, we use the notations introduced in the Pocock–Simon Model above. Instead of using s urns, he suggested using the urn with maximum imbalance to perform randomization each time. For each category j of covariate i, let there be a corresponding urn U_{ij}, which initially contains two types of balls, representing two treatment types, equal in number. Suppose the incoming subject has covariate coordinate $(r_1, \ldots, r_I)$. To achieve balance in the numbers of subjects randomized to each treatment group within each category of each covariate, we select, with highest probability, the urn from $\left\{U_{ir_i}, i=1,2,..,I\right\}$ showing the greatest imbalance in the numbers of subjects randomized to each treatment group so far and use it to generate the treatment assignment for the entering subject. Suppose that the urn U_{mr_m} is selected, then a ball is drawn from it with replacement. The treatment represented by the color of the ball, is assigned and β_i balls of the opposite color are added to U_{ir_i}, $i = 1, 2, \ldots, I$. Wei (1978b) called this procedure a marginal urn design as it tends to balance treatment assignments within each category of each covariate marginally, and hence also jointly (Rosenberger and Lachin 2002).

17.4.2.4 Imbalance Minimization Procedure

This procedure, developed by Birkett (1985), is an alternative to stratified randomization when a large number of covariates influences the response. Under the imbalance minimization method, the covariate coordinate of an entering subject is determined first. The subject is then tentatively assigned to each treatment group and a summary measure of the resulting treatment imbalance is calculated. The sum of the absolute values of the excess number of subjects receiving one treatment than the other for every category of each covariate is used as a summary measure. Comparing the two measures, the final allocation is made to the group minimizing the imbalance measure. This method is sometimes called minimization as it minimizes the imbalance in the distribution of covariates. According to Birkett (1985), the procedure would help to gain in power.

17.4.2.5 Optimal Design Driven Allocations

Most of the procedures discussed so far are developed with an aim to balance treatment allocation across strata. However, an entirely different but relevant approach may be to determine the allocation fraction by minimizing the variance of the estimated treatment difference assuming the presence of covariates. Begg and Iglewicz (1980) and Atkinson (1982) used the optimum design theory (Silvey 1980) to develop allocation designs. For a detailed description, we consider a multitreatment clinical trial and sequential entrance of subjects. The arriving subjects are to be randomized to one of the t treatments taking into account their respective covariate values. The data, perhaps after transformation, are to be analyzed using the linear model

$$E(\mathbf{Y}_n) = X_n\gamma = Z_n\alpha + F_n\beta,\ Disp(\mathbf{Y}_n) = \sigma^2 I_n,$$

where $\mathbf{Y}_n$ is vector of responses, Z_n is the $n \times t$ matrix of treatment indicators (i.e., with one zero entry per row), α is the $t \times 1$ vector of treatment effects and F_n is the $n\times\overline{q-1}$ matrix of covariates for the first n subjects. Let $\mathbf{f}_{n+1}$ be the known covariate and Z_{n+1} be the fictitious allocation vector for the next entering; that is, $(n + 1)$th subject. In optimum design theory based allocations, the task is to determine Z_{n+1} in such a way that the variability of estimated α (or some convenient linear function of it) is minimized. Atkinson (1982) considered minimization of the variability of estimated $A^T\gamma$. Since β is the vector of nuisance parameters, he considered

$$A^T = (C^T\ \ O),$$

to reflect interest in contrasts of treatment parameters, where C is a $\overline{t-1}\times t$ contrast matrix. If only $t'(< t - 1)$ specific contrasts are of interest, C can be modified accordingly. Then one possible criterion is Sibson's (1974) D_A optimality. Since with n subjects in the trial, the dispersion matrix of the estimated $A^T\gamma$ is expressed as $\sigma^2 A^T(X_n^TX_n)^{-1}A$, D_A optimum design minimizes the generalized variance $|A^T(X_{n+1}^TX_{n+1})^{-1}A|$, where X_{n+1} is formed by augmenting with X_n the row $\mathbf{x}_{n+1}^T(j) = (\mathbf{z}^T(j)\ \mathbf{f}_{n+1}^T)$ provided treatment j is allocated and hence $\mathbf{z}(j)$ has its jth element unity and all other elements 0. However, in the sequential construction of these designs, the allocation of the $(n + 1)$th subject is made to treatment k if the maximum of the directional derivatives

$$d_A(j,\mathbf{f}_{n+1}) = \mathbf{x}_{n+1}^T(j)(X_n^TX_n)^{-1}A\{A^T(X_n^TX_n)^{-1}A\}^{-1}A^T(X_n^TX_n)^{-1}\mathbf{x}_{n+1}(j), j = 1,..,t,$$

occurs at $j = k$. However, the resulting design is deterministic and consequently Atkinson (1982) suggests to assign the $(n + 1)$th subject to treatment j with probability

$$\pi_A(j|\mathbf{f}_{n+1}) = \frac{d_A(j,\mathbf{f}_{n+1})}{\sum_{k=1}^{t} d_A(k,\mathbf{f}_{n+1})}, j = 1,..,t.$$

For $t = 2$ treatments, without any covariate information, the above reduces to

$$\pi_A(j) = 1 - \frac{\{N_j(n)\}^2}{\{N_1(n)\}^2 + \{N_2(n)\}^2}, j = 1,2,$$

that is, Smith's (1984) allocation function corresponding to $\rho = 2$.

Atkinson (1999a, 1999b) compared his rule to Efron's BCD, complete randomization and stratified blocked randomization in terms of the simulated variance of the estimated treatment effect taking normally distributed covariate and concluded that the less randomized the design the smaller the variance, but the greater the potential biases. In addition, Atkinson (1999b) formulated an ingenious method of comparing the performance of various sequential designs. The D_A efficiency of some n subject design X_n (i.e., with X_n as the design matrix) relative to the optimum design $\tilde{X}_n$ is defined by

$$\mathcal{E}_n = \left\{ \frac{|A^T(\tilde{X}_n^T \tilde{X}_n)^{-1} A|}{|A^T(X_n^T X_n)^{-1} A|} \right\}^{1/s},$$

with s as the number of estimated linear combinations in the trial. Another efficiency measure can be loss; introduced by Burman (1996) and measured by

$$\mathcal{L}_n = n(1 - \mathcal{E}_n).$$

Here $\mathcal{L}_n$ is a random variable, depending on the pattern of covariates and randomness of the rule. Designs forcing more balance are expected to have lower values of $\mathcal{L}_n$ in the long run. By means of a simulation study, Atkinson (2002) concluded that the loss approaches the informative asymptotic value quickly and hence the efficiencies of all the designs tend to unity. Thus, designs with little randomness in the allocation have small loss but large selection bias; that is, given the knowledge of previous allocations and the covariate of the entering subject, there is a high probability of correctly guessing the next treatment allocation. However, Atkinson relied on the normal linear model based responses, though many clinical trials result in binary or survival outcomes.

17.4.2.6 Bayesian Allocation Designs

Most of the sequential optimum designs provide a method of balancing the trial as early as possible and hence minimizes loss. However, Bayesian methods can be applied to have better performance in terms of bias and loss (Atkinson 2002) and also to skew the allocation reasonably in the long run. Ball, Smith, and Verdinelli (1993) introduced a Bayesian BCD to provide a balance between randomization and design efficiency. However, these designs provide equal allocation to all treatment arms in the long run. Atkinson and Biswas (2005) extended the approach to derive a skewed allocation, which, in the long run, assigns p_j fraction of subjects to treatment j, $j = 1,2,\ldots,t$. They consider minimization of the utility

$$U = U_V - \eta U_R,$$

where the contribution of U_V is to provide precise estimates whereas U_R induces randomness. η is the trade-off coefficient between the two aspects. Considering,

$$U_V = \sum_{j=1}^{t} \pi_B(j)\phi_j, \text{ and}$$

$$U_R = \sum_{j=1}^{t} \pi_B(j) log\left\{\frac{\pi_B(j)}{p_j}\right\},$$

with ϕ_j is a measure of information from applying treatment j, they maximized the utility U and obtained the required allocation probability $\pi_B(j)$ for treatment j as

$$\pi_B(j) = \frac{p_j \exp(\phi_j/\eta)}{\sum_{j=1}^{t} p_j \exp(\phi_j/\eta)}.$$

In addition they have also worked out the expression for sequential D_A optimal designs. Assuming a multivariate normal prior for the treatment parameter α, the posterior distribution of α was worked out and taking $\phi_j = -log\,|X_{n+1}^T X_{n+1}|$, Atkinson and Biswas (2005) obtained the conditional allocation probability for the $(n + 1)$th subject with covariate vector $\mathbf{f}_{n+1}$ to receive treatment j as

$$\pi_B(j\,|\,\mathbf{f}_{n+1}) = \frac{p_j\{1 + d_A(j, \mathbf{f}_{n+1})\}^{1/\eta}}{\sum_{j=1}^{t} p_j\{1 + d_A(j, \mathbf{f}_{n+1})\}^{1/\eta}}.$$

Comparing the performance of the classical and Bayesian skewed designs, Atkinson and Biswas (2005) arrived at the conclusion that the Bayesian designs forces balance over covariates at the early stage of the trials allowing gradually increasing randomness in the allocation. A further discussion on the topic can be found in Atkinson, Donev, and Tobias (2007).

17.5 Concluding Remarks

In the present chapter we reviewed and discussed the pros and cons of the various treatment adaptive designs available in the literature. We compared the performances of the various individual designs in terms of their variability. Of course we included the designs with covariates also in our discussion.

The basic objective of treatment adaptive designs is to achieve balance in allocation, to get better and more precise estimates. For a multitreatment scenario the design might change if the treatment contrast(s) under interest varies. That is not taken care of in the designs other than the optimal designs.

One related area of interest might be the response-adaptive designs where the responses also play a serious role to determine the allocation pattern. See the book-length discussion of Hu and Rosenberger (2006) in this context. The details are beyond the scope of this present chapter.

Acknowledgment

The authors wish to thank the referee for careful reading and some helpful comments.

References

Atkinson, A. C. (1982). Optimum biased coin designs for sequential clinical trials with prognostic factors. *Biometrika,* 69: 61–67.

Atkinson, A. C. (1999a). Optimum biased-coin designs for sequential treatment allocation with covariate information. *Statistics in Medicine,* 18: 1741–52.

Atkinson, A. C. (1999b). Bayesian and other biased-coin designs for sequential clinical trials. *Tatra Mountains Mathematical Publications,* 17: 133–39.

Atkinson, A. C. (2002). The comparison of designs for sequential clinical trials with covariate information. *Journal of the Royal Statistical Society A,* 165: 349–73.

Atkinson, A. C., and Biswas, A. (2005). Bayesian adaptive biased-coin designs for clinical trials with normal responses. *Biometrics,* 61: 118–25.

Atkinson, A. C., Donev, A. N., and Tobias, R. D. (2007). *Optimum Experimental Designs, with SAS.* New York: Oxford University Press Inc.

Baldi Antognini, A. (2004). Extensions of Ehrenfest's urn designs for comparing two treatments. In *moDa 7—Advances in Model-Oriented Design and Analysis,* eds. A. Di Bucchianico, H. Läuter, and H. P. Wynn, 21–28. Heidelberg: Physica-Verlag.

Baldi Antognini, A. and Giovagnoli, A. (2004). A new " biased coin design" for the sequential allocation of two treatments. *Journal of Royal statistical Society Series C,* 53: 651–64.

Baldi Antognini, A. (2008). A theoretical analysis of the power of biased coin designs. *Journal of Statistical Planning and Inference,* 138: 1792–98.

Ball, F. G., Smith, A. F. M., and Verdinelli, I. (1993). Biased coin designs with a Bayesian bias. *Journal of Statistical Planning and Inference,* 34: 403–21.

Basu, D. (1980). Randomization analysis of experimental data: The Fisher randomization test. *Journal of the American Statistical Association,* 75: 575–95.

Begg, C. B., and Iglewicz, B. (1980). A treatment allocation procedure for sequential clinical trials. *Biometrics,* 36: 81–90.

Birkett, N. J. (1985). Adaptive allocation in randomised controlled trials. *Controlled Clinical Trials,* 6: 146–55.

Blackwell, D., and Hodges, J. L. (1957). Design for the control of selection bias. *Annals of Mathematical Statistics,* 28: 449–60.

Burman, C. F. (1996). *On Sequential Treatment Allocations in Clinical Trials.* Goteborg: Department of Mathematics.

Byington, R. P., Curb, J. D., and Mattson, M. E. (1985). Assessment of double-blindness at the conclusion of the beta-blocker heart attack trial. *Journal of American Medical Association,* 263: 1733–83.

Campbell, M. K., Elbourne, D. R., and Altman, D. G. (2004). Consort statement: Extension to cluster randomised trials. *British Medical Journal,* 328: 702–8.

Chalmers, T. C. (1990). Discussion of biostatistical collaboration in medical research by Jonas H. Ellenberg. *Biometrics,* 46: 20–22.

Chen, Y. P. (1999). Biased coin design with imbalance tolerance. *Communications and Statistics-Stochastic Models,* 15: 953–75.

Chen, Y. P. (2000). Which design is better? Ehrenfest urn versus biased coin. *Advances in Applied Probability,* 32: 738–49.

Chow, S. C., and Chang, M. (2006). *Adaptive Design Methods in Clinical Trials.* Boca Raton, FL: Chapman & Hall/CRC.

Chow, S. C., and Liu, J. P. (2004). *Design and Analysis of Clinical Trials.* Hoboken, NJ: John Wiley & Sons, Inc.

CPMP. (2003). Points to consider on *Adjustment for Baseline Covariates* (CPMP/EWP/2863/99). London: EMEA.

Deyo, R. A., Walsh, N. E., Schoenfeld, L. S., and Ramamurthy, S. (1990). Can trials of physical treatments be blinded: The example of transcutaneous electrical nerve stimulation for chronic pain. *American Journal of Physical Medicine & Rehabilitation*, 69: 6–10.

Dirienzo, A. G. (2000). Using urn models for the design of clinical trials. *Sankhya B*, 62: 43–69.

Dragalin, V. (2006). Adaptive designs: Terminology and classifications. *Drug Information Journal*, 40: 425–35.

Efron, B. (1971). Forcing a sequential experiment to be balanced. *Biometrika*, 58: 403–17.

Efron, B. (1980). Randomizing and balancing a complicated sequential experiment. In *Biostatistics Casebook*, eds R. G. Miller, B. Efron, B. W. Brown, and L. E. Moses. New York: Wiley, 19–30.

European Medicines Agency. (2008). *Report on the EMEA-EFPIA Workshop on Adaptive Designs in Confirmatory Clinical Trials (EMEA/106659/2008)*. London, March 12, 2008.

Fisher, R. A. (1935). *The Design of Experiments*. Edinburgh: Oliver and Boyd.

Friedman, B. (1949). A simple urn model. *Communications in Pure and Applied Mathematics*, 2: 59–70.

Grouin, J.-M., Day, S., and Lewis, J. (2004). Adjustment for baseline covariates: An introductory note. *Statistics in Medicine*, 23: 697–99.

Hansen, B. B., and Bowers, J. (2008). Covariate balance in simple, stratified and clustered comparative studies. *Statistical Science*, 23: 219–36.

Hill, A. B. (1951). The clinical trial. *British Medical Bulletin*, 71: 278–82.

Hu, F., and Rosenberger, W. F. (2006). *The Theory of Response Adaptive Randomization in Clinical Trials*. New York: Wiley Interscience.

Karlowski, T. R., Chalmers, T. C., Frenkel, L. D., Kapikian, A. Z., Lewis, T. L., and Lynch, J. M. (1975). Ascorbic acid for the common cold: A prophylactic and therapeutic trial. *Journal of American Medical Association*, 231: 1038–42.

Lachin, J. M. (1988a). Statistical properties of randomization in clinical trials. *Controlled Clinical Trials*, 9: 289–311.

Lachin, J. M. (1988b). Properties of simple randomization in clinical trials. *Controlled Clinical Trials*, 9: 312–26.

Lachin, J. M., Marks, J., Schoenfield, L. J., and The Protocol Committee and The NCGS Group. (1981). Design and methodological considerations in the National Cooperative Gallstone Study: A multi-center clinical trial. *Controlled Clinical Trials*, 2: 177–230.

Lehmann, E. L. (1986). *Nonparametrics: Statistical Methods Based on Ranks*. San Francisco: Holden-Day.

Maca, J., Bhattacharya, S., Dragalin, V., Gallo, P., and Krams, M. (2006). Adaptive seamless phase II/III designs—Background, operational aspects, and examples. *Drug Information Journal*, 40: 463–73.

Matthews, J. N. S. (2006). *An Introduction to Randomized Controlled Clinical Trials*, 2nd ed. London: Edward Arnold.

National Institute of Neurological Disorders and Stroke rt-PA Stroke Group. (1995). Tissue plasminogen activator for acute ischemic stroke. *New England Journal of Medicine*, 333: 1581–87.

Pitman, E. J. G. (1937). Significance tests which may be applied to samples from any population. *Royal Statistical Society Supplement*, 4: 119–30 and 225–32 (Parts I and II).

Pitman, E. J. G. (1938). Significance tests which may be applied to samples from any population. Part III. The analysis of variance test. *Biometrika*, 29: 322–35.

Pocock, S. J., and Simon, R. (1975). Sequential treatment assignment with balancing for prognostic factors in the controlled clinical trials. *Biometrics*, 31: 103–15.

Rosenberger, W. F., and Lachin, J. L. (2002). *Randomization in Clinical Trials: Theory and Practice*. New York: Wiley.

Senn, S. J. (1994). Testing for baseline balance in clinical trials. *Statistics in Medicine*, 13: 1715–26.

Sibson, R. (1974). DA-optimality and duality. In *Progress in Statistics, Vol.2—Proceedings of the 9th European Meeting of Statisticians, Budapest*, eds J. Gani, K. Sarkadi, and I. Vincze. Amsterdam: North-Holland.

Silvey, S. D. (1980). *Optimum Design*. London: Chapman & Hall.

Smith, R. L. (1984). Sequential treatment allocation using biased coin designs. *Journal of the Royal Statistical Society B,* 46: 519–43.

Soares, J. F., and Wu, C. F. J. (1982). Some restricted randomization rules in sequential designs. *Communications in Statistics-Theory and Methods,* 12: 2017–34.

Stigler, S. M. (1969). The use of random allocation for the control of selection bias. *Biometrika,* 56: 553–60.

Taves, D. R. (1974). Minimization: A new method of assigning patients to treatment and control groups. *Clinical Pharmacology & Therapeutics,* 15: 443–53.

Wei, L. J. (1977). A class of designs for sequential clinical trials. *Journal of the American Statistical Association,* 72: 382–86.

Wei, L. J. (1978a). The adaptive biased-coin design for sequential experiments. *Annals of Statistics,* 9: 92–100.

Wei, L. J. (1978b). An application of an urn model to the design of sequential controlled clinical trials. *Journal of the American Statistical Association,* 73: 559–63.

Wei, L. J., Smythe, R. T., and Smith, R. L. (1986). K-treatment comparisons with restricted randomization rules in clinical trials. *Annals of Statistics,* 14: 265–274.

Wei, L. J. (1988). Exact two-sample permutation tests based on the randomized play-the-winner rule. *Biometrika,* 75: 603–6.

Zelen, M. (1974). The randomization and stratification of patients to clinical trials. *Journal of Chronic Diseases,* 28: 365–75.

18

Integration of Predictive Biomarker Diagnostics into Clinical Trials for New Drug Development

Richard Simon
National Cancer Institute

18.1 Introduction

Clinical trials of new oncology drugs have traditionally been conducted with broad patient populations to avoid discrepancies between the population tested and the population eventually treated with the drug. This approach has, however, resulted in treating many patients who do not benefit. For example, less than 10% of women with estrogen receptor positive breast cancer that has not spread to the axillary lymph nodes require or benefit from cytotoxic chemotherapy although most have traditionally received such drugs. Over-treatment results in a substantial number of adverse events and expense for treatment of patients who receive no benefit. In oncology, accumulating understanding of genomic differences among tumors of the same primary site indicates that most molecularly targeted agents are likely to benefit only the patients whose tumors are driven by deregulation of the targeted pathways. Availability of improved tools for characterizing tumors biologically makes it increasingly possible to predict whether a particular tumor will be responsive to a particular treatment (Paik, Taniyama, and Geyer 2008). Today many cancer drugs are being developed with companion diagnostics that identify the patients who are good candidates for treatment. Successful prospective codevelopment of a drug and companion diagnostic, however, presents many new challenges. In this chapter we will address some of the issues in the design of clinical trials for new treatments and diagnostic tests that provide both reliable tests of the overall null hypothesis and also provide reliable indication of which patients benefit from the new treatment.

18.2 Terminology

Predictive markers are pretreatment measurements that provide information about which patients are likely or unlikely to benefit from a specific treatment. For example, HER2 amplification is a predictive classifier for benefit from herceptin. The presence of a mutation in the KRAS gene identifies patients with colorectal cancer who are unlikely to benefit from anti-EGFR antibodies.

Although our objective here is to discuss the use of predictive markers in clinical trial design, we should start by clarifying the distinction between predictive markers and prognostic markers. Prognostic markers are pretreatment measurements that provide information about long-term outcome for patients who are either untreated or who receive standard treatment. Prognostic markers often reflect a combination of intrinsic disease factors and sensitivity to standard therapy. Although there is a huge literature of prognostic factors in oncology, few are actually measured in practice (Pusztai 2004). Prognostic factors are rarely used unless they help with therapeutic decision making. Unfortunately, most prognostic factor studies are conducted without a clear intended medical use driving patient selection and analysis. On the contrary, most prognostic factor studies are conducted using a convenience sample of heterogeneous patients whose tissues are available (Simon and Altman 1994).

Predictive and prognostic biomarkers are quite different from the more traditional endpoint biomarkers. Traditionally, the term biomarker referred to a measurement that tracks the pace of a disease; increasing as the disease progresses and decreasing as it regresses. Although there are many potential uses for such biomarkers in early clinical development of new drugs, our focus here will be on baseline biomarkers. Since validation or qualification only has meaning in terms of fitness for the intended use, the criteria for validation of endpoint biomarkers should not be mistakenly applied to prognostic or predictive biomarkers. The validation of prognostic and predictive biomarkers, although demanding, is often much more feasible than the validation of biomarkers as surrogate endpoints.

In this chapter we will refer to three different types of validation for prognostic and predictive biomarkers. When there is a gold standard measurement, analytical validity means that the test is accurate relative to the gold standard. Otherwise, analytical validity means that the test is reproducible and robust. It should be robust with regard to assay performance and with regard to tissue handling. Clinical validity means that the test result correlates with a clinical endpoint. This correlation can often be established in a retrospective study. For example, a test for predicting response to a chemotherapy regimen may be clinically validated using data from a single arm Phase II study of patients who received that regimen. Clinical validation of a test is often accompanied by calculating the sensitivity of the test for identifying responders and the specificity of the test for identifying nonresponders and examination of the receiver operating characteristic curve that relates estimated sensitivity and specificity as the threshold of positivity is varied. The third type of validation is establishing medical utility for a biomarker. Medical utility means that use of the test results in improved outcome for patients compared to not using the test. Medical utility requires that the test is actionable and that the outcome measure reflects patient benefit. Establishing medical utility usually requires a prospective clinical trial.

We will use the term classifier to refer to a diagnostic test that translates one or more biomarker measurements to a set of predicted categories. For example, with a prognostic classifier the categories may refer to low risk of tumor recurrence, moderate risk of recurrence, and high risk of recurrence. With a predictive classifier the categories may refer to patients most likely to benefit from the new regimen and less likely to benefit. A gene expression based classifier may involve measurement of the expression of many genes, but it is a discrete indicator of two or more classes and can be used for selecting or stratifying patients in a clinical trial just like a classifier based on a single gene or protein. Validating a gene expression based classifier means evaluating whether the classifier, as a composite entity, is fit for its intended use. It does not mean determining whether the individual gene components are prognostic or predictive in a new study.

18.3 Development of Predictive Biomarkers

In oncology, most predictive biomarkers successfully used to date have been based on single protein or single gene measurements that are closely linked to the mechanism of action of the drug. In some cases, the target of the drug is known but it is not clear how to best measure the essentiality of the target to the pathogenesis of a specific tumor. For example, with trastuzumab, over-expression of the HER2 protein was initially used as the biomarker for selecting patients but this was later replaced by amplification of the HER2 gene. In the development of the small molecule inhibitors of the EGFR gene in lung cancer, there was considerable uncertainty about whether over-expression of the protein, amplification of the gene, mutation of the gene, or some combination of these would be an appropriate predictive biomarker. Small molecule kinase inhibitors generally have multiple targets and this can considerably complicate the development of an appropriate predictive biomarker. Although monoclonal antibodies are generally very specific for a single target, over-expression of the target of the drug may not itself be a useful biomarker. A drug may inhibit its target but unless that target is driving tumor growth and invasion, inhibition of the target will not result in effective treatment. For example, with the anti-EGFR antibodies in colorectal cancer, expression of the target and lack of a KRAS mutation turned out to be a much better predictive marker than expression of the target alone.

In general, unless the biology of drug–disease interaction is well understood, it can be very difficult to develop a good candidate predictive biomarker. In some cases investigators are attempting to develop gene expression signatures as predictive biomarkers. The individual genes included in the signature are not the biomarkers, but rather a score or classification based on a model that includes expression levels of multiple genes is viewed as a single biomarker. A substantial literature of machine learning models has been developed, mostly for predicting a binary endpoint based on a large number of genes (Dudoit and Fridlyand 2003). Dupuy and Simon (2007) have discussed the care that is needed in establishing clinical validity of such models and the flaws that are so prevalent in the literature resulting from use of highly biased resubstitution estimates and estimates based on incomplete cross-validation for these $p > n$ problems.

For developing a predictive classifier of patients likely to benefit from a new drug, one can perform gene expression profiling of patients on Phase II trials of the drug and compare the expression profiles of responders to those of nonresponders in order to identify the differentially expressed genes and train a completely specified predictive classifier. Dobbin et al. (Dobbin and Simon 2007; Dobbin, Zhao, and Simon 2008) have developed methods for planning the number of cases needed to effectively develop such a classifier and indicated the need for generally having at least 20 cases in each of the response classes considered. Obtaining at least 20 responders may necessitate performing larger Phase II studies. Pusztai, Anderson, and Hess (2007) indicated the problems that may arise with having too few responders for such analyses.

If a diagnostic is to be codeveloped with a drug, the Phase II studies must be designed to evaluate the candidate assays available, to select one, and then to perform analytical validation of the robustness and reproducibility of the assay prior to launching the Phase III trial. This can be very challenging. Kamb et al. (2007, p. 118) said: "Barring breakthroughs in patient selection methods or a windfall of imatinibs, the 'all comers' clinical development approach remains a valid—if frustrating and expensive—route to drug approval." Sawyers (2008, p. 548) has stated, "One of the main barriers to further progress is identifying the biological indicators, or biomarkers, of cancer that predict who will benefit from a particular targeted therapy." This increases the complexity of drug development, although it has potential benefits for patients and for controlling medical expenses. However, it requires that an effective predictive biomarker be identified and a test for it analytically validated prior to the launch of the Phase III pivotal clinical trials of the drug.

18.4 Phase II Designs for Oncology Trials

Several authors have introduced new Phase II clinical trial designs for use early in the evaluation of the drug with a candidate predictive biomarker. Pusztai, Anderson, and Hess (2007) proposed a design based on Simon's optimal two-stage single arm Phase II design (Simon 1989). In the first stage, patients are accrued without restriction based on the companion biomarker. If a sufficient number of first stage responses are observed, second stage accrual continues, unrestricted by the biomarker. In this case, the end of trial analysis may address how the responses observed related to biomarker status. If however, an insufficient number of first stage responses are seen, then a new two-stage accrual plan is initiated with eligibility restricted to marker positive patients. The objective is to assure that the drug is not discarded as inactive based on a trial that may have very few marker positive patients.

Jones and Holmgren (2007) introduced an adaptive modification of Simon's optimal two-stage design for use with a candidate binary predictive biomarker. Initially n_- biomarker negative patients and n_+ biomarker positive patients are treated with the single agent. If the level of response is insufficient in either stratum, then the trial terminates. If the level of response is sufficient in both strata, then an additional n_{un} patients are accrued, unrestricted by biomarker status. If the level of responses is sufficient for the positive stratum but not for the negative stratum, then an additional m_+ biomarker positive patients are accrued. The authors set the decision criteria and sample sizes to satisfy error criteria while limiting the accrual of excessive numbers of patients.

An additional design that might be considered in the early development of a drug with several (K) candidate binary biomarkers is the following. In the first stage, patients are accrued based on broad eligibility criteria and unrestricted with regard to any marker status. The first stage might even include patients with tumors of different primary sites. The sample size for the first stage (N_1) should be chosen large enough so that there will be an adequate number of marker positive responders if the marker prevalence is at least π and the response rate for marker positive patients is at least p^*. For example, with $\pi = 0.20$ and $p^* = 0.25$, and a first stage of 80 patients, one would expect 16 marker positive patients and four responders. During the second stage, patients are accrued based on their marker status. N_2 patients positive for marker k are accrued for each marker k for which the number of first stage responses is at least r^*. The values of N_1, N_2, and r^* can be optimized to satisfy error constraints. This design is flexible in employing multiple candidate biomarkers, but it could accrue a substantial number of patients in the first stage who are negative for all markers.

For a more fully adaptive approach one might jointly model p_{k-} and p_{k+}, the response probabilities for patient negative and positive for marker k, respectively. Let joint priors for (p_{k-}, p_{k+}) be specified and denoted by $f(p_{k-}, p_{k+})$. These priors will be independent for different markers and will often be identical. The posterior will be written $f((p_{k-}, p_{k+})|D)$ after observing data D. The joint prior for marker k is updated with regard to the number of responders and nonresponders for patients positive for marker k and for patients negative for marker k. At any point, a new patient with biomarker vector $\underline{x}$ is considered for entry, one computes the probability of response with regard to the posterior distribution of the parameters at that point for each of the K models. Let $p_k(x_k|D)$ denote the predictive probability of response for a patient with marker k value x_k; that is, $x_k = 0$ meaning negative and $x_k = 1$ meaning positive. For a patient with $x_k = 1$ for example, the predictive probability can be written as follows if the joint prior distribution is discrete

$$p_k(x_k = 1 | D) = \sum_{(p_{k-}, p_{k+})} p_{k+} f(p_{k-}, p_{k+} | D).$$

Similarly,

$$p_k(x_k = 0 | D) = \sum_{(p_{k-}, p_{k+})} p_{k-} f(p_{k-}, p_{k+} | D).$$

If the predictive probability of response is less than a specified value ε for all K models, then the patient would not be treated on the study. Accrual can also be terminated when sufficient information about responsc and its relationship to the markers has been obtained. Since the design of Phase III trials may be influenced critically by the selection of a predictive biomarker, Phase II sample sizes larger than those traditionally used should be considered.

With this Bayesian approach, care in specification in the joint priors is required. Independent convenience priors may not be appropriate. One reasonable simple approach is to use a rectangular grid prior based on low, intermediate, and high values for p_{k-} and p_{k+}. The grid point with low values for both p_{k-} and p_{k+} corresponds to low activity of marker negative and marker positive patients. The grid point with low p_{k-} value and high p_{k+} value corresponds to low activity of marker negative patients but high activity of marker positive patients. This grid prior would be easily updated. A Bayesian approach in which randomization weights are adaptively modified is described by Zhou et al. (2008).

18.5 Clinical Trial Designs Incorporating Predictive Biomarkers

The standards for evaluating effectiveness of a new drug are well established. Ideally one would like a randomized clinical trial that establishes that treatment of a defined selection of patients with the new drug results in improved clinical outcome than for the control group. Since clinical outcome for cancer patients is usually measured by survival or progression/recurrence free survival, a randomized control group is usually essential. The role of the predictive biomarker for evaluating the new drug is in refining the definition of the target population.

There is considerably less clarity about what constitutes appropriate validation of a predictive biomarker test. As described previously, three levels of validation can be distinguished. Analytical validation of the test does not even require specimens from patients who have received the drug in question. For drugs used in regimens for treating patients with metastatic disease where individual patient response can be assessed, clinical validation can be based on Phase II data from a single arm trial in which all patients receive the new drug. The evaluation involves estimating the positive and negative predictive values for identifying patients who respond to the new regimen. With such data ROC curves can be generated and a test cut-point selected.

Medical utility generally means that use of the test results in patient benefit compared to treatment according to the standard of care. If the diagnostic enables the identification of a subset of patients for whom a new drug provides improved clinical outcome (e.g., prolongs survival) compared to a randomized standard care control group, then one might argue that use of the diagnostic in conjunction with the new regimen provides patient benefit. Establishing the medical utility of a companion diagnostic will generally be based on the same Phase III pivotal trials used to establish the effectiveness of the new drug. Medical utility of a companion diagnostic means that it enables the physician to identify patients as belonging to the target population who benefit from the new drug and that test negative patients are less likely to benefit from the drug. The calculation of positive predicted value (PPV), negative predicted value (NPV) and ROC curves do not usually play a role in this analysis as they generally do not reflect the nature of the time-to-event endpoint and the randomized control group. In the following sections we will review some designs for Phase III pivotal trials that utilize new drugs and companion diagnostics. Some of these designs have also been discussed by Sargent et al. (2005) and Pusztai and Hess (2004). Some of the designs incorporate both test positive and test negative patients and hence are somewhat self-contained in their ability to provide evidence that the former patients benefit from the new drug and the latter patients do not. The enrichment designs described below incorporate only test positive patients. Those designs are for situations where there is either a strong biological rationale for excluding test negative patients from the development or compelling Phase II evidence that test negative patients will not benefit from the new drug.

18.6 Enrichment Designs

The objective of a Phase III pivotal clinical trial is to evaluate whether a new drug, given in a defined manner, has medical utility for a defined set of patients. Pivotal trials test prespecified hypotheses about treatment effectiveness in specified patient population groups. The role of a predictive biomarker classifier is to specify the population of patients. The process of classifier development may be exploratory and subjective, but the use of the classifier in the pivotal trial must not be.

With an enrichment design, a diagnostic test is used to restrict eligibility for a randomized clinical trial of a regimen containing a new drug to a control regimen. This approach was used for the development of trastuzumab in which patients with metastatic breast cancer whose tumors expressed HER2 in an immunohistochemistry test were eligible for randomization. Simon and Maitournam (2005, 2006; Maitournam and Simon 2005) studied the efficiency of this approach relative to the standard approach of randomizing all patients without measuring the diagnostic. They found that the efficiency of the enrichment design depended on the prevalence of test positive patients and on the effectiveness of the new treatment in test negative patients. When fewer than half of the patients are test positive and the new treatment is relatively ineffective in test negative patients, the number of randomized patients required for an enrichment design is often dramatically smaller than the number of randomized patients required for a standard design. This was the case for trastuzumab. Simon and Maitournam (2005, 2006) also compared the enrichment design to the standard design with regard to the number of screened patients. Zhao and Simon have made the methods of sample size planning for the design of enrichment trials available online at http://linus.nci.nih.gov/brb/. The web based programs are available for binary, survival/disease-free survival, or uncensored quantitative endpoints. The planning takes into account the performance characteristics of the tests and specificity of the treatment effects. The programs provide comparisons to standard nonenrichment designs based on the number of randomized patients required and the number of patients needed for screening to obtain the required number of randomized patients.

The enrichment design is particularly appropriate for contexts where there is such a strong biological basis for believing that test negative patients will not benefit from the new drug and that including them in would be unethical. In many situations, the biological basis is strong but not compelling. On the one hand, we recognize that understanding of the molecular targets of the drug are sometimes flawed. On the other hand, we do not really want to be including test negative patients in clinical trial to show that a treatment that we do not believe will work for them actually does not work. This is particularly true when the drug has adverse effects. The enrichment design does not provide data on the effectiveness of the new treatment compared to control for test negative patients. Consequently, unless there is preliminary data or compelling biological evidence that the new drug is not effective in test negative patients, the enrichment design may not be adequate to support approval of the test as a medical device. Consequently, designs that include both test positive and test negative patients should be considered.

18.7 Designs that Include Both Test Positive and Test Negative Patients

When test positive and test negative patients are included in the randomized clinical trial comparing the new treatment to a control, it is essential that an analysis plan be predefined in the protocol for how the predictive classifier will be used in the analysis and that the trial be sized for the specific analysis plan. It is not sufficient to just stratify the randomization with regard to the classifier without specifying a complete analysis plan. In fact, the main importance of stratifying the randomization is that it assures that only patients with adequate test results will enter the trial.

It is important to recognize that the purpose of this design is to evaluate the new treatment in the subsets determined by the prespecified classifier. The purpose is not to modify the classifier. If the classifier is a composite gene expression based classifier, the purpose of the design is not to reexamine the contributions of each component. If the classifier is modified, then an additional Phase III trial may be needed to evaluate treatment benefit in subsets determined by the new classifier. In moving from post hoc correlative science to reliable predictive medicine, it is important to separate the data used for developing classifiers from the data used for testing treatment effects in subsets determined by those classifiers. The process of classifier development can be exploratory, but the process of evaluating treatments should not be. In the following sections we will describe a variety of analysis strategies and relate these strategies to sample size planning.

18.7.1 Analysis of Test Negatives Contingent on Significance in Test Positives

The simplest analysis plan would consist of separate comparisons of the new treatment to the control in the test positive and test negative patients. In cases where a-priori one does not expect the treatment to be effective in the test negative patients unless it is effective in the test positive patients, one might structure the analysis in the following manner: test treatment versus control in test positive patients using a threshold of significance of 5%. If the treatment difference in test positive patients is not significant, do not perform statistical significance test in negative patients. Otherwise, compare treatment to control in the test negative patients using a threshold of statistical significance of 5%. This sequential approach controls the overall Type I error at 5%.

With this analysis plan, the number of test positive patients required are the same as for the enrichment design, say n_E. When that number of patients are accrued, there will be approximately n_E/prev total patients and approximately $n_- =$ (1-prev) n_E/prev test negative patients where prev denotes the proportion of test positive patients. One should make sure that the n_E is large enough that there are a sufficient number of test negative patients for analysis. With a time-to-event endpoint like survival or disease-free survival, the planning will be somewhat more complex. For example, suppose we wish to have 90% power in the test positive patients for detecting a 50% reduction in hazard for the new treatment versus control at a two-sided 5% significance level. This requires about 88 events of test positive patients. At the time that there are E_+ events in test positive patients, there will be approximately

$$E_- = E_+\left(\frac{\lambda_-}{\lambda_+}\right)\left(\frac{1-\text{prev}}{\text{prev}}\right), \tag{18.1}$$

events in the test negative group where the symbols λ_- and λ_+ denote the event rates in the test negative and test positive control groups at the time that there are E_+ events in the test positive group. If the ratio of lamda's is about 1, and the prevalence of test positive patients is 0.25, then when E_+ is 88 E_- will be approximately 264. This will provide approximately 90% power for detecting a 33% reduction in hazard at a two-sided significance level of 5%. In this case, the trial will not be delayed compared to the enrichment design, but a large number of test positive patients will be randomized, treated and followed on the study rather than excluded as for the enrichment design. If the proportion of test positive patients were 0.50 instead of 0.25, then at the time that there are 88 events in test positive patients there will be only about 88 events in test negative patients. Hence one will not have 90% power for detecting a 33% reduction in hazard in test negative patients; one will only have 90% power for detecting a 50% reduction. It is possible that at that time a futility analysis in the test negative patients will indicate that there is unlikely to be a medically important treatment effect in test negative patients. If the futility analysis does not support such a conclusion, however, one should continue to follow test negative patients and perform the final analysis at a time when there are substantially more events. This may necessitate increasing the accrual period of the trial.

18.7.2 Analysis Determined by Interaction Test

The traditional approach to the two-way analysis of variance problem is to first test whether there is a significant interaction between the effect of one factor (treatment versus control) and the second factor (test negative and positive). The interaction test is often performed at a threshold above the traditional

5% level. If the interaction test is not significant, then the treatment effect is evaluated overall, not within levels of the second factor. If the interaction test is significant, then treatment effect is evaluated separately within the levels of the second factor (e.g., test positive and test negative classes). This is similar to the test proposed by Sargent et al. (2005). In the example described above with 88 events in test positive patients and 264 events in test negative patients, the interaction test will have approximately 93.7% power at a one-sided significance level of 0.10 for detecting an interaction with 50% reduction in hazard for test positive patients and no treatment effect in test negative patients. If the treatment reduces the hazard by 33% in test negative patients, the interaction test has little power, but that is fine because the overall analysis of treatment effect will be appropriate in that circumstance. The power of the test of interaction is not highly sensitive to the proportion of patients that test positive because the power of the interaction test for survival data is approximately:

$$\Phi\left\{\frac{\delta_+ - \delta_-}{\sqrt{4/E_+ + 4/E_-}} - k_{1-\alpha_I}\right\}. \tag{18.2}$$

Where E_+ and E_- denote the numbers of events in the test positive and test negative patients at the time of analysis, δ_+ and δ_- denote the log-hazards of treatment effect in test positive and test negative patients, Φ denotes the standard Gaussian distribution function, and $k_{1-\alpha_I}$ denotes the $100(1-\alpha_I)$th percentile of the standard Gaussian distribution.

Computer simulations indicate that with 88 test positive patients and 264 test negative patients, the two-stage design with $\alpha_I = 0.10$ detects a significant interaction and a significant treatment effect in test positive patients in 88% of replications when the treatment reduces hazard by 50% in test positive patients and is ineffective in test negative patients. If the treatment reduces hazard by 33% in both test positive and test negative patients, the interaction is nonsignificant and the overall treatment effect is significant in 87% of cases. In this latter case, the interaction test is falsely significant and the treatment effect in test positive cases is significant in an additional 10% of cases. So the overall power is 97% in this case, because 88 + 264 events is a larger sample size than one would traditionally require for detecting a uniform 33% reduction in hazard.

If one were planning a trial to detect a uniform 33% reduction in hazard with 90% power and 5% two-sided significance level, one would require approximately 256 events. If 25% of the cases were test positive and the test were not prognostic, then at time of analysis there would be approximately 64 events in test positive cases and 192 events in test negative cases. If the treatment reduces hazard by 33% in both test positive and test negative patients, the interaction is nonsignificant and the overall treatment effect is significant in approximately 81% of cases. The interaction test is falsely significant and the treatment effect in test positive cases is significant in an additional 10% of cases. So the overall power is 90% with the two-stage interaction analysis plan, If the treatment reduces hazard by 50% in test positive cases and is ineffective in test negative cases, then the interaction is significant and the treatment effect in test positive cases is significant in 76% of replications. So even if the trial is sized for detecting a uniform 33% reduction in hazard, the two-stage analysis plan will have approximately 76% power for detecting a substantial treatment effect restricted to the test positive patients.

Sizing the trial to have high power for obtaining an interaction significant at a 5% significance level may require a substantially increased sample size compared to sizing the trial for adequately evaluating treatment effects separately in the marker positive and marker negative groups. Some statisticians believe that establishing the validity of the predictive biomarker requires such significance, but for a prospective trial of a predictive biomarker one expects that the treatment effect will differ qualitatively based on marker level. This context is quite different from the post hoc analysis settings in which demonstrating statistical significance at a 5% level as a justification for subset analysis has been required. Requiring treatment of a sufficient number of marker negative patients in order to obtain an interaction significant at a 5% level may in some cases not be feasible, or even ethical. When the event rates in the marker negative and marker positive groups are equal, then Equation 18.1 becomes

$$E_- = E_+\left(\frac{1-\text{prev}}{\text{prev}}\right). \tag{18.3}$$

If the trial is sized to have power $1 - \beta_+$ at a one sided significance level α_+ for testing the hypothesis that the treatment is ineffective in marker positive patients against the alternative that the treatment effect in marker positive patients has value δ_+^*, then the number of events required in marker positive patients are

$$E_+ = 4\left\{\frac{k_{1-\alpha_+} + k_{1-\beta_+}}{\delta_+^*}\right\}^2.$$

From Equation 18.3, the total number of events observed are

$$E_{\text{total}} = \frac{4}{\text{prev}}\left\{\frac{k_{1-\alpha_+} + k_{1-\beta_+}}{\delta_+^*}\right\}^2. \tag{18.4}$$

If alternatively the study is sized to have power $1 - \beta_I$ at a one sided significance level α_I for testing the hypothesis that there is no interaction against the alternative that the treatment effect has value δ_+^* in marker positive patients and value 0 in marker negative patients, then the number of required events in marker positive patients can be obtained from Equation 18.2 as

$$E_+^I = \frac{4}{(1-\text{prev})}\left\{\frac{k_{1-\alpha_I} + k_{1-\beta_I}}{\delta_+^*}\right\}^2, \tag{18.5}$$

and the total events required (using Equation 18.3) is

$$E_{\text{total}}^I = \frac{4}{\text{prev}(1-\text{prev})}\left\{\frac{k_{1-\alpha_I} + k_{1-\beta_I}}{\delta_+^*}\right\}^2. \tag{18.6}$$

Consequently,

$$\frac{E_+^I}{E_+} = \frac{1}{1-\text{prev}}\left\{\frac{k_{1-\alpha_I} + k_{1-\beta_I}}{k_{1-\alpha_+} + k_{1-\beta_+}}\right\}^2, \tag{18.7}$$

and also

$$\frac{E_{\text{total}}^I}{E_{\text{total}}} = \frac{1}{1-\text{prev}}\left\{\frac{k_{1-\alpha_I} + k_{1-\beta_I}}{k_{1-\alpha_+} + k_{1-\beta_+}}\right\}^2. \tag{18.8}$$

Traditionally one would have $\alpha_+ = 0.025$ and $\beta_+ = 0.10$ so $k_{0.975} = 1.96$ and $k_{0.90} = 1.28$. If $\alpha_I = 0.05$ and $\beta_I = 0.10$, then the squared factor in Equation 18.7 and Equation 18.8 equals 0.815. Testing for interaction requires approximately 63% more events if the prevalence of marker positivity is 0.5, approximately 22% more events if the prevalence is 0.33, but only about 9% more events if the prevalence is 0.25.

18.7.3 Fallback Analysis Plan

Simon and Wang (2006) proposed an analysis plan in which the new treatment group is first compared to the control group overall. If that difference is not significant at a reduced significance level such as 0.04, then the new treatment is compared to the control group just for test positive patients. The latter comparison uses a threshold of significance of 0.01, or whatever portion of the traditional 0.05 not used by the initial test. This design was intended for situations where it was expected that the new treatment would be broadly effective; the subset analysis being a fallback option.

Suppose that the trial is planned for having 90% power for detecting a uniform 33% reduction in overall hazard using a two-sided significance level of 0.03. Then 297 events are required instead of the 256 events needed for a similar trial based on a two-sided significance threshold of 0.05. If, however, the overall test of treatment effect is not significant at the 0.03 level, the test positive subset will include approximately 75 events if only 25% of the patients are test positive and the event rates in the two groups are equal. In that case, the test of treatment effect performed at the two-sided 0.02 level for the test positive patients has power 0.75 for detecting a 50% reduction in hazard. By delaying the treatment evaluation in the test positive patients power 0.80 can be achieved when there are 84 events and power 0.90 can be achieved when there are 109 events in the test positive subset.

Song and Chi (2007) and Wang, O'Neill, and Hung (2007) have proposed a refinement of the significance levels used that takes into account the correlation between the test of overall treatment effect and the treatment effect within the test positive subset. The critical value for the subset test defined by Song and Chi (2007), however, depends on the results for the overall analysis. The requirement that a test in a subset be conditional on significance overall is a statistical tradition to protect against false claims from post hoc subset analysis and this seems inappropriate for clinical trials with a focused primary analysis plan involving a predictive biomarker.

18.7.4 Max Test Statistic

An analysis plan can also be constructed based on use of a test statistic that indicates whether the strongest evidence of treatment effectiveness occurs in the test positive patients or for the overall group. Let the estimated treatment effects for test positive and test negative patients be denoted $\hat{\delta}_+$ and $\hat{\delta}_-$, respectively. They have variances approximately $4/E+$ and $4/E_-$, respectively. An overall estimate of treatment effect $\hat{\delta}$ having variance 1 can be constructed as a weighted average of these subset specific estimates with the weights equal to the proportion of events in the subsets. Then a test statistic

$$z_{\max} = \max\left\{\hat{\delta}, \frac{\hat{\delta}_+}{\sqrt{4/E_+}}\right\},$$

indicates the strongest evidence of treatment effectiveness. The critical value for assessing the statistical significance of $z_{\max}$ can be determined based on the approximate bivariate null distribution of the two components, or based on permutation of the treatment group labels of the cases.

With 88 test positive cases and 264 test negative cases, the statistical power of the $z_{\max}$ test is 86.7% if the new treatment reduces the hazard by 50% in test positive cases and is ineffective for test negatives. The statistical power is 95.1% if the new treatment reduces the hazard by 33% for both test positive and test negative cases. If the trial were planned for a total of only 256 events, 64 test positive and 192 test negative, then the statistical power is 70% if the new treatment reduces the hazard by 50% in the test positive cases and is ineffective for the test negatives, and 83.9% if the new treatment reduces hazard

33% uniformly. These are based on a two-sided statistical significance level of 5%. The power of the z_{max} test does not appear superior to that based on a preliminary test of interaction. The interaction approach also has the advantage of providing a clearer basis for either focusing on the overall population or the test positive subset.

18.8 Adaptively Modifying Types of Patients Accrued

Wang, O'Neill, and Hung (2007) proposed a Phase III design comparing a new treatment to a control that starts with accruing both test positive and test negative patients. An interim analysis is performed evaluating the new treatment in the test negative patients. If the observed efficacy for the control group exceeds that for the new treatment group and the difference exceeds a futility boundary, then accrual of test negative patients terminates and accrual of additional test positive patients are substituted for the unaccrued test negative patients until the originally planned total sample size is reached. Wang, O'Neill, and Hung (2007) show computer simulations that indicate this design has greater statistical power than nonadaptive approaches, but their design accrues many more test positive patients and may require a much longer trial.

The concept of curtailing accrual of test negative patients based on an interim futility analysis can be implemented, however, without the extension of trial duration resulting from substitution of test positive for test negative patients to achieve a prespecified total sample size. The trial may be planned for specified numbers of test positive and test negative patients in order to provide adequate power for separate analysis of the two subsets. For example, the tests could be powered to detect a 50% reduction in hazard in test positive patients and a 33% reduction in test negative patients. If an interim analysis indicates futility for the test negative patients, then accrual of test negative patients may cease without affecting the target sample size or analysis for the test positive patients. This approach can be useful if the time to observing a patient's endpoint is rapid relative to the accrual rate. For many oncology Phase III trials using survival or disease-free survival, however, most of the patients would be accrued before a meaningful futility analysis based on sufficient events could be conducted. An additional limitation is the conservativeness of futility boundaries. Wang, O'Neill, and Hung (2007) require that the futility boundary be in the region in which the observed efficacy is greater for the control group than for the new treatment group. Consequently, even if the new treatment is completely ineffective in the test negative subset, the futility analysis will be successful less than half of the time.

18.9 Biomarker Adaptive Threshold Design

Jiang, Freidlin, and Simon (2007) reported on a biomarker adaptive threshold design for situations where a predictive index is available at the start of the trial, but a cut-point for converting the index to a binary classifier is not established. With their design, tumor specimens are collected from all patients at entry, but the value of the predictive index is not used as an eligibility criteria. Jiang, Freidlin, and Simon (2007) described two analysis plans. The first begins with comparing outcomes for all patients receiving the new treatment to those for all control patients. If this difference in outcomes is significant at a prespecified significance level α_1 (e.g., .03) then the new treatment is considered effective for the eligible population as a whole. Otherwise, a second stage test is performed using significance threshold $\alpha_2 = 0.05 - \alpha_1$. The second stage test involves finding the cut-point b for the predictive index that leads to the largest treatment versus control treatment effect when restricted to patients with predictive index above b. Let $S(b)$ denote the partial log likelihood for the treatment effect when restricted to patients with predictive index above b. Let $b^* = \arg\max(S(b))$; that is, the cut-point resulting in the largest treatment effect, and let $S^* = S(b^*)$, be the largest observed treatment effect. Jiang, Freidlin, and Simon (2007) evaluated the statistical significance of S^* by randomly permuting the labels of which patients were in the new treatment group, and which were controls and determining the maximized partial log likelihood for the permuted data. This is done for thousands of random permutations. If the value S^* is beyond the $1 - \alpha_2$th percentile of this null distribution created from the random permutations, then the second stage test is considered significant. They also describe construction of a confidence interval for the optimal cut-point b using a bootstrap resampling approach. Jiang, Freidlin, and Simon (2007) also described an alternative analysis plan that does not employ a first stage comparison of the treatment groups overall and provides sample size considerations for the two analysis plans.

18.10 Multiple Biomarker Design

The global testing approach used by Jiang, Freidlin, and Simon (2007) can be extended beyond the context of selecting the best threshold for a single biomarker score to Phase III trials started with multiple (K) binary biomarkers. Let B_k denote the subset of patients positive for marker k, for $k = 1,2, \ldots, K$. The first stage analysis compares outcome for the two treatment groups overall for all randomized patients using a threshold of significance $\alpha_1 < 0.05$. If the null hypothesis is not rejected in the first stage, then the second analysis uses a significance level of $0.05 - \alpha_1$ In the second stage of analysis, the log likelihood of treatment effect (S_k) is computed for the subset B_k of patients positive for marker k. This is done for each marker. Then $k^* = \text{argmax}\{S_k, k = 1,2, \ldots, K\}$ and $S^* = S_{k^*}$. The null distribution of S^* is generated by permuting the treatment labels and repeating the calculations and the $0.05 - \alpha_1$ quantile of the null distribution is used as the critical value for claiming statistical significance. If the result is significant at that level, one claims that patients positive for marker k^* benefit from the new treatment. Stability of k^* under bootstrap sampling can be studied.

18.11 Adaptive Signature Design

For codevelopment of a new drug and companion diagnostic it is best to have the candidate diagnostic completely specified and analytically validated prior to its use in the pivotal clinical trials. This is difficult, however, and in some cases is not feasible, particularly with multigene expression based classifiers.

Freidlin and Simon (2005) proposed a design for a Phase III trial that can be used when no classifier is available at the start of the trial. The design provides for development of the classifier and evaluation of treatment effects in subsets determined by the classifier in a single trial. The analysis plan of the adaptive signature design is structured to preserve the principal of separating the data used for developing a classifier from the data used for evaluating treatment in subsets determined by the classifier, although both processes are part of the same clinical trial.

The analysis plan described by Freidlin and Simon (2005) is in two parts as for several of the designs previously described. At the conclusion of the trial the new treatment is compared to the control overall using a threshold of significance of α_1 that is somewhat less than the total 0.05. A finding of statistical significance at that level is taken as support of a claim that the treatment is broadly effective. At that point, no biomarkers have been tested on the patients, although patients must have tumor specimens collected to be eligible for the clinical trial. If the overall treatment effect is not significant at the α_1 level then a second stage of analysis takes place. The patients are divided into a training set and testing set. Freidlin and Simon (2005) used a 50-50 split, but other proportions can be employed. The data for patients in the training set is used to define a single subset of patients who are expected to be most likely to benefit from the new treatment compared to the control. Freidlin and Simon (2005) indicated methods for identifying a subset of patients whose outcome on the new treatment is better than the control. They use machine learning methods based on screening thousands of genes for those with expression values that interact with treatment effect. When that subset is explicitly defined, the new treatment is compared to the control for the testing set patients with the characteristics defined by that subset. The comparison of new treatment to control for the subset is restricted to patients in the testing set in order to preserve the principle of separating the data used to develop a classifier from the data used to test treatment effects in subsets defined by that classifier. The comparison of treatment to control for the subset uses a threshold of significance of $0.05 - \alpha_1$ in order to assure that the overall chance of a false positive conclusion does not exceed 0.05. These thresholds can be sharpened using the method of Wang, O'Neill, and Hung (2007).

Friedlin and Simon (2005) proposed the adaptive signature design in the context of multivariate gene expression based classifiers. The size of Phase II databases may not be sufficient to develop such classifiers before the initiation of Phase III trials (Pusztai and Hess 2004; Dobbin and Simon 2007; Dobbin, Zhao, and Simon 2008). Freidlin and Simon (2005) showed that the adaptive signature design can be effective for the development and use of gene expression classifiers if there is a very large treatment effect in a subset determined by a set of signature genes. The power of the procedure for identifying the subset is limited, however, by having to test the treatment effect at a very stringent significance level in subset patients restricted to the testing set not used for classifier development.

The analysis strategy used by the adaptive signature design can be used more broadly than in the context of identifying de novo gene expression signatures as described by Freidlin and Simon (2005). For example, it could be used when several gene expression signatures are available at the outset and it is not clear what to include in the final statistical testing plan. It could also be used with classifiers based on a single gene but several candidate tests for measuring expression or deregulation of that gene. For example, the focus may be on EGFR but there may be uncertainty about whether to measure over-expression at the protein level, point mutation of the gene, or amplification of the gene. In these settings with a few candidate classifiers, a smaller training set may suffice instead of the 50-50 split used by Freidlin and Simon (2005).

The adaptive signature design provides a clear illustration of the distinction between the traditional approach of post hoc correlative studies and a clear separation between development of a classifier and the testing of subsets determined by the classifier. For registration trials, however, it has some clear limitations. One is the limited statistical power for the subset analysis described above. The other is the fact that the test used for the subset analysis may not have been analytically validated prior to its use in the clinical trial.

18.12 Conclusions

Developments in cancer genomics and biotechnology are improving the opportunities for development of more effective cancer therapeutics and molecular diagnostics to guide the use of those drugs. These opportunities can have enormous benefits for patients and for containing health care costs. One of the greatest opportunities is developing predictive biomarkers of the patients who require treatment and are likely to benefit from specific drugs. Codevelopment of drugs and companion diagnostics adds complexity to the development process however. Traditional post hoc correlative science paradigms do not provide an adequate basis for reliable predictive medicine. New paradigms are required for separating biomarker development from evaluation. New clinical trial designs are required that incorporate prospective analysis plans that provide flexibility in identifying the appropriate target population in a manner that preserves overall false positive error rates. This chapter has attempted to describe some of these approaches.

References

Dobbin, K., and Simon, R. (2007). Sample size planning for developing classifiers using high dimensional DNA expression data. *Biostatistics,* 8: 101–17.

Dobbin, K. K., Zhao, Y., and Simon, R. M. (2008). How large a training set is needed to develop a classifier for microarray data? *Clinical Cancer Research,* 14: 108–14.

Dudoit, S., and Fridlyand, J. (2003). Classification in microarray experiments. In *Statistical Analysis of Gene Expression Microarray Data,* ed. T. Speed. Boca Raton, FL: Chapman & Hall/CRC.

Dupuy, A., and Simon, R. (2007). Critical review of published microarray studies for cancer outcome and guidelines on statistical analysis and reporting. *Journal of the National Cancer Institute,* 99: 147–57.

Freidlin, B., and Simon, R. (2005). Adaptive signature design: An adaptive clinical trial design for generating and prospectively testing a gene expression signature for sensitive patients. *Clinical Cancer Research*, 11: 7872–78.

Jiang, W., Freidlin, B., and Simon, R. (2007). Biomarker adaptive threshold design: A procedure for evaluating treatment with possible biomarker-defined subset effect. *Journal of the National Cancer Institute*, 99: 1036–43.

Jones, C. L., and Holmgren, E. (2007). An adaptive Simon two-stage design for Phase 2 studies of targeted therapies. *Contemporary Clinical Trials*, 28: 654–66.

Kamb, A. Wee, S. Lengauer, C. (2007). Why is cancer drug discovery so difficult. *Nature Reviews Drug Discovery* 6: 115–120.

Maitournam, A., and Simon, R. (2005). On the efficiency of targeted clinical trials. *Statistics in Medicine*, 24: 329–39.

Paik, S., Taniyama, Y., and Geyer, C. E. (2008). Anthracyclines in the treatment of HER2-negative breast cancer. *Journal of the National Cancer Institute*, 100: 2–3.

Pusztai, L. (2004). Perspectives and challenges of clinical pharmacogenomics in cancer. *Pharmacogenomics*, 5 (5): 451–54.

Pusztai, L., Anderson, K., and Hess, K. R. (2007). Pharmacogenomic predictor discovery in Phase II clinical trials for breast cancer. *Clinical Cancer Research*, 13: 6080–86.

Pusztai, L., and Hess, K. R. (2004). Clinical trial design for microarray predictive marker discovery and assessment. *Annals of Oncology*, 15: 1731–37.

Sargent, D. J., Conley, B. A., Allegra, C., and Collette, L. (2005). Clinical trial designs for predictive marker validation in cancer treatment trials. *Journal of Clinical Oncology*, 23 (9): 2020–27.

Sawyers, C. L. (2008). The cancer biomarker problem. *Nature*, 452: 548–52.

Simon, R. (1989). Optimal two-stage design for Phase II clinical trials. *Controlled Clinical Trials*, 10: 1–10.

Simon, R., and Altman, D. G. (1994). Statistical aspects of prognostic factor studies in oncology. *British Journal of Cancer*, 69: 979–85.

Simon, R., and Maitournam, A. (2005). Evaluating the efficiency of targeted designs for randomized clinical trials. *Clinical Cancer Research*, 10: 6759–63.

Simon, R., and Maitournam, A. (2006). Evaluating the efficiency of targeted designs for randomized clinical trials: Supplement and Correction. *Clinical Cancer Research*, 12: 3229.

Simon, R., and Wang, S. J. (2006). Use of genomic signatures in therapeutics development. *The Pharmacogenomcs Journal*, 6: 1667–73.

Song, Y., and Chi, G. Y. H. (2007). A method for testing a prespecified subgroup in clinical trials. *Statistics in Medicine*, 26: 3535–49.

Wang, S. J., O'Neill, R. T., and Hung, H. M. J. (2007). Approaches to evaluation of treatment effect in randomized clinical trials with genomic subset. *Pharmaceutical Statistics*, 6: 227–44.

Zhou, X., Liu, S., Kim, E. S., Herbst, R. S., and Lee, J. J. (2008). Bayesian adaptive design for targeted therapy development in lung cancer—a step toward personalized medicine. *Clinical Trials*, 5: 181–93.

19

Clinical Strategy for Study Endpoint Selection

Siu Keung Tse
City University of Hong Kong

Shein-Chung Chow
Duke University School of Medicine

Qingshu Lu
University of Science and Technology of China

19.1 Introduction

In clinical trials, it is important to identify the primary response variables that will be used to address the scientific and/or medical questions of interest. The response variables, also known as the clinical endpoints, are usually chosen during the planning stage of the study protocol in order to achieve the study objectives. Once the response variables are chosen, the possible outcomes of treatment are defined and the corresponding information would be used to assess the efficacy and safety of the test treatment under study (Paul 2000). For evaluation of the efficacy and safety of a test treatment, a typical approach is to test whether there is a statistically significant difference between the test treatment and an active control or a placebo control. If a statistically significant difference is observed, the trial is powered to have a high probability of correctly detecting a clinically meaningful difference if such a difference truly exists (Chow and Liu 2004). As a result, in practice, a prestudy power analysis for sample size estimation is usually performed to ensure that the trail with the intended sample size will have a desired power, say 80%, for addressing the scientific/medical questions of interest. Note that a prestudy power analysis for sample size estimation is often performed based on some required information such as the clinically meaningful difference of interest, variability associated with the observed response, significance level, and the desired power provided by the investigator (Chow, Shao, and Wang 2008).

Sample size estimation is often carried out based on an appropriate statistics under a valid study design and hypotheses. Different study designs and testing hypotheses may result in different sample size requirements for achieving a desired power for correctly detecting a clinically meaningful difference of interest to the investigator. However, in many clinical studies, it is not uncommon that the sample size of a clinical study is determined based on expected absolute change from baseline of a primary study endpoint but the collected data are analyzed based on relative change from baseline (e.g., percent change from baseline) of the primary study endpoint, or based on the percentage of patients who show some improvement (i.e., responder analysis). The definition of a responder could be based on either absolute change from baseline or relative change from baseline of the primary study endpoint. It is very controversial in terms of the interpretation of the analysis results, especially when a significant result is observed based on a study endpoint (e.g., absolute change from baseline, relative change from baseline, or the responder analysis) but not based on the other study endpoint (e.g., absolute change from baseline, relative change from baseline, or responder analysis). In practice, it is then of interest to explore how an observed significant difference of a study endpoint (e.g., absolute change from baseline, relative change from baseline, or responder's analysis) can be translated to that of the other study endpoint (e.g., absolute change from baseline, relative change from baseline, or responder's analysis). An immediate impact on the assessment of treatment effect based on different study endpoints is the power analysis for sample size calculation. For example, sample size required in order to achieve the desired power based on the absolute change could be very different from that obtained based on the percent change, or the percentage of patients who show an improvement based on the absolute change or relative change at the α level of significance.

As an example, consider a clinical trial for evaluation of possible weight reduction of a test treatment in female patients. Weight data from 10 subjects are given in Table 19.1: mean absolute change and mean percent change from pretreatment are 5.1 lbs and 4.8%, respectively. If a subject is considered a responder if there is weight reduction by more than 5 lbs (absolute change) or by more than 5% (relative change), the response rates based on absolute change and relative change are given by 40 and 30%, respectively. Thus, it should be noted that sample sizes required for achieving a desired power for detecting a clinically meaningful difference, say, by an absolute change of 5.5 lbs and a relative change of 5.5%, for the two study endpoints would not be the same. Similarly, the required sample sizes are also different using the response rates based on absolute change and relative change. Related discussion can be found in Chow, Tse, and Lin (2008).

As discussed above, sample sizes required for achieving a desired power for detecting a clinically meaningful difference at the 5% level of significance may be very different depending upon: (i) the choice of study endpoint, and (ii) the clinically meaningful difference.

In clinical trials, for a given primary response variable, commonly considered study endpoints include: (i) measure based on absolute change; (ii) measure based on relative change; (iii) proportion of responders based on absolute change; and (iv) proportion of responders based on relative change. We will refer these study endpoints as the derived study endpoints because they are derived from the original data collected from the same patient population. In practice, it will be more complicated if the intended trial is to establish noninferiority of a test treatment to an active control (reference) treatment. In this case, sample size calculation will also depend on the size of the noninferiority

TABLE 19.1 Weight Data from 10 Female Subjects

Pretreatment	Posttreatment	Change	Relative Change (%)
100	96	4	4.0
95	85	10	10.5
110	105	5	4.5
100	98	2	20.0
150	143	7	4.7
96	90	6	6.3
160	155	5	3.1
130	126	4	3.1
123	120	1	2.4
100	93	7	7.0
Mean = 116.4	111.1	5.1	4.8

margin, which may be based on either absolute change or relative change of the derived study endpoint. For example, based on responder's analysis, we may want to detect a 30% difference in response rate or to detect a 50% relative improvement in response rate. Thus, in addition to the four types of derived study endpoints, there are also two different ways to define a noninferiority margin. Thus, there are many possible clinical strategies with different combinations of the derived study endpoint and the selection of noninferiority margin for assessment of the treatment effect. To ensure the success of the intended clinical trial, sponsor will usually carefully evaluate several clinical strategies for selecting the type of study endpoint, clinically meaningful difference, and noninferiority margin during the stage of protocol development. Some strategies may lead to the success of the intended clinical trial (i.e., achieve the study objectives with the desired power), while some strategies may not. A common practice for the sponsor is to choose a strategy to their best interest. However, regulatory agencies such as the U.S. Food and Drug Administration (FDA) may challenge the sponsor as to the inconsistent results. This has raised the following questions. First, which study endpoint is telling the truth regarding the efficacy and safety of the test treatment under study? Second, how to translate the clinical information among different derived study endpoints since they are obtained based on the same data collected from the same patient population. These questions, however, remain unanswered thus far.

In this chapter, we attempt to provide some insight to the above issues. In particular, the focus is to evaluate the effect to the power of the test when the sample size of the clinical study is determined by an alternative clinical strategy based on different study endpoint and noninferiority margin. In the next section, model and assumptions for studying the relationship among these study endpoints are described. Section 19.3 provides a comparison of different clinical strategies for endpoint sections in terms of sample size and the corresponding power. A numerical study is given in Section 19.4 to provide some insight regarding the effect to the different clinical strategies for endpoint selection. A brief concluding remark is presented in the last section.

19.2 Model Formulation and Assumptions

Suppose that there are two test treatments, namely: a test treatment (T) and a reference treatment (R). Denote the corresponding measurements of the ith subject in the jth treatment group before and after the treatment by W_{1ij} and W_{2ij}, respectively, where $j = T, R$ corresponds to the test and the reference treatment, respectively. Assume that the measurement W_{1ij} is lognormal distributed with parameters μ_j and σ_{1j}^2; that is, $W_{1ij} \sim \text{lognormal}(\mu_j, \sigma_j^2)$. Let $W_{2ij} = W_{1ij}(1 + \Delta_{ij})$, where Δ_{ij} denotes the percentage change after receiving the treatment. In addition, assume that Δ_{ij} is lognormal distributed with parameters $\mu_{\Delta j}$ and $\sigma_{\Delta j}^2$; that is, $\Delta_{ij} \sim \text{lognormal}(\mu_{\Delta j}, \sigma_{\Delta j}^2)$. Thus, the difference and the relative difference between the measurements before and after the treatment are given by $W_{2ij} - W_{1ij}$ and $(W_{2ij} - W_{1ij})/W_{1ij}$, respectively. In particular, $W_{2ij} - W_{1ij} = W_{1ij}\Delta_{ij} \sim \text{lognormal}(\mu_j + \mu_{\Delta j}, \sigma_j^2 + \sigma_{\Delta j}^2)$ and $(W_{2ij} - W_{1ij})/W_{1ij} \sim \text{lognormal}(\mu_{\Delta j}, \sigma_{\Delta j}^2)$. To simplify the notations, define X_{ij} and Y_{ij} as $X_{ij} = \log(W_{2ij} - W_{1ij})$, $Y_{ij} = [(W_{2ij} - W_{1ij})/W_{1ij}]$. Then, both X_{ij} and Y_{ij} are normally distributed with means $\mu_j + \mu_{\Delta j}$ and $\mu_{\Delta j}$, $i = 1, 2, \ldots, n_j$, $j = T, R$, respectively (Johnson and Kotz 1970).

Thus, possible derived study endpoints based on the responses observed before and after the treatment as described earlier include:

i. X_{ij}, the absolute difference between before treatment and after treatment responses of the subjects;
ii. Y_{ij}, the relative difference between before treatment and after treatment responses of the subjects;
iii. $r_{Aj} = \#\{x_{ij} > c_1, i = 1, \ldots, n_j\}/n_j$, the proportion of responders, which is defined as a subject whose absolute difference between before treatment and after treatment responses is larger than a prespecified value c_1; and

iv. $r_{Rj} = \#\{y_{ij} > c_2,\ i = 1, \ldots, n_j\}/n_j$, the proportion of responders, which is defined as a subject whose relative difference between before treatment and after treatment responses is larger than a prespecified value c_2.

To define notation, for $j = T, R$, let $p_{Aj} = E(r_{Aj})$ and $p_{Rj} = E(r_{Rj})$. Given the above possible types of derived study endpoints, we may consider the following hypotheses for testing noninferiority with noninferiority margins determined based on either absolute difference or relative difference:

i. The absolute difference of the responses:

$$H_0:\ (\mu_R - \mu_{\Delta R}) - (\mu_T - \mu_{\Delta T}) \geq \delta_1 \quad \text{vs.} \quad H_1: (\mu_R - \mu_{\Delta R}) - (\mu_T - \mu_{\Delta T}) < \delta_1. \tag{19.1}$$

ii. The relative difference of the responses:

$$H_0:\ \mu_{\Delta R} - \mu_{\Delta T} \geq \delta_2 \quad \text{vs.} \quad H_1: \mu_{\Delta R} - \mu_{\Delta T} < \delta_2. \tag{19.2}$$

iii. The difference of responders' rates based on the absolute difference of the responses:

$$H_0:\ p_{AR} - p_{AT} \geq \delta_3 \quad \text{vs.} \quad H_1: p_{AR} - p_{AT} < \delta_3. \tag{19.3}$$

iv. The relative difference of responders' rates based on the absolute difference of the responses:

$$H_0:\ \frac{p_{AR} - p_{AT}}{p_{AR}} \geq \delta_4 \quad \text{vs.} \quad H_1: \frac{p_{AR} - p_{AT}}{p_{AR}} < \delta_4. \tag{19.4}$$

v. The absolute difference of responders' rates based on the relative difference of the responses:

$$H_0:\ p_{RR} - p_{RT} \geq \delta_5 \quad \text{vs.} \quad H_1: p_{RR} - p_{RT} < \delta_5. \tag{19.5}$$

vi. The relative difference of responders' rate based on the relative difference of the responses:

$$H_0:\ \frac{p_{RR} - p_{RT}}{p_{RR}} \geq \delta_6 \quad \text{vs.} \quad H_1: \frac{p_{RR} - p_{RT}}{p_{RR}} < \delta_6. \tag{19.6}$$

For a given clinical study, the above are the possible clinical strategies for assessment of the treatment effect. Practitioners or sponsors of the study often choose the strategy to their best interest. It should be noted that current regulatory position is to require the sponsor to prespecify what study endpoint will be used for assessment of the treatment effect in the study protocol without any scientific justification.

In practice, however, it is of particular interest to study the effect to power analysis for sample size calculation based on different clinical strategies. As pointed out earlier, the required sample size for achieving a desired power based on the absolute difference of a given primary study endpoint may be quite different from that obtained based on the relative difference of the given primary study endpoint. Thus, it is of interest to clinician or clinical scientist to investigate this issue under various scenarios. In particular, the following settings are often considered in practice:

	Settings					
Strategy used for	1	2	3	4	5	6
Sample size determination	19.1	19.2	19.3	19.4	19.5	19.6
Testing treatment effect	19.2	19.1	19.4	19.3	19.6	19.5

There are certainly other possible settings besides those considered above. For example, Hypotheses 19.1 may be used for sample size determination but Hypotheses 19.3 are used for testing treatment effect. However, the comparison of these two clinical strategies would be affected by the value of c_1, which is used to determine the proportion of responders. However, in the interest of a simpler and easier comparison, the number of parameters are kept as minimal as possible. Details of the comparison of the above six settings are given in the next section.

19.3 Comparison of the Different Clinical Strategies

19.3.1 Results for Test Statistics, Power, and Sample Size Determination

Note that X_{ij} denotes the absolute difference between before treatment and after treatment responses of the ith subjects under the jth treatment, and Y_{ij} denotes the relative difference between before treatment and after treatment responses of the ith subjects under the jth treatment. Let $\bar{x}_{.j} = 1/n_j \sum_{i=1}^{n_j} x_{ij}$ and $\bar{y}_{.j} = 1/n_j \sum_{i=1}^{n_j} y_{ij}$ be the sample means of X_{ij} and Y_{ij} for the jth treatment group, $j = T, R$, respectively.

Based on normal distribution, the null hypothesis in Equation 19.1 is rejected at a level α of significance if

$$\frac{\bar{x}_{.R} - \bar{x}_{.T} + \delta_1}{\sqrt{\left(\frac{1}{n_T} + \frac{1}{n_R}\right)\left[\left(\sigma_T^2 + \sigma_{\Delta T}^2\right) + \left(\sigma_R^2 + \sigma_{\Delta R}^2\right)\right]}} > z_\alpha. \tag{19.7}$$

Thus, the power of the corresponding test is given as

$$\Phi\left(\frac{(\mu_T + \mu_{\Delta T}) - (\mu_R + \mu_{\Delta R}) + \delta_1}{\sqrt{(n_T^{-1} + n_R^{-1})\left[\left(\sigma_T^2 + \sigma_{\Delta T}^2\right) + \left(\sigma_R^2 + \sigma_{\Delta R}^2\right)\right]}} - z_\alpha\right), \tag{19.8}$$

where $\Phi(.)$ is the cumulative distribution function of the standard normal distribution. Suppose that the sample sizes allocated to the reference and test treatments are in the ratio of ρ, where ρ is a known constant. Using these results, the required total sample size for the test the Hypotheses 19.1 with a power level of $(1-\beta)$ is $N = n_T + n_R$, with

$$n_T = \frac{(z_\alpha + z_\beta)^2(\sigma_1^2 + \sigma_2^2)(1 + 1/\rho)}{\left[(\mu_R + \mu_{\Delta R}) - (\mu_T + \mu_{\Delta T}) - \delta_1\right]^2}, \tag{19.9}$$

$n_R = \rho n_T$ and z_u is $1 - u$ quantile of the standard normal distribution.

Note that y_{ij}'s are normally distributed. The testing statistic based on $\bar{y}_{.j}$ would be similar to the above case. In particular, the null hypothesis in Equation 19.2 is rejected at a significance level α if

$$\frac{\bar{y}_{T.} - \bar{y}_{R.} + \delta_2}{\sqrt{\left(\frac{1}{n_T} + \frac{1}{n_R}\right)\left(\sigma_{\Delta T}^2 + \sigma_{\Delta T}^2\right)}} > z_\alpha. \tag{19.10}$$

The power of the corresponding test is given as

$$\Phi\left(\frac{\mu_{\Delta T}-\mu_{\Delta R}+\delta_2}{\sqrt{(n_T^{-1}+n_R^{-1})(\sigma_{\Delta T}^2+\sigma_{\Delta R}^2)}}-z_\alpha\right). \tag{19.11}$$

Suppose that $n_R = \rho n_T$, where ρ is a known constant. Then the required total sample size to test Hypotheses 19.2 with a power level of $(1-\beta)$ is $(1+\rho)n_T$, where

$$n_T=\frac{(z_\alpha+z_\beta)^2(\sigma_{\Delta T}^2+\sigma_{\Delta R}^2)(1+1/\rho)}{[(\mu_R+\mu_{\Delta R})-(\mu_T+\mu_{\Delta T})-\delta_2]^2}. \tag{19.12}$$

For sufficiently large sample size n_j, r_{Aj} is asymptotically normal with mean p_{Aj} and variance $[p_{Aj}(1-p_{Aj})]/n_j$ $j = T, R$. Thus, based on Slutsky Theorem (Serfling 1980), the null hypothesis in Equation 19.3 is rejected at an approximate α level of significance if

$$\frac{r_{AT}-r_{AR}+\delta_3}{\sqrt{\frac{1}{n_T}r_{AT}(1-r_{AT})+\frac{1}{n_R}r_{AR}(1-r_{AR})}}>z_\alpha. \tag{19.13}$$

The power of the above test can be approximated by

$$\Phi\left(\frac{p_{AT}-p_{AR}+\delta_3}{\sqrt{n_T^{-1}p_{AT}(1-p_{AT})+n_R^{-1}p_{AR}(1-p_{AR})}}-z_\alpha\right). \tag{19.14}$$

If $n_R = \rho n_T$, where ρ is a known constant. Then, the required sample size to test Hypotheses 19.3 with a power level of $(1-\beta)$ is $(1+\rho)n_T$, where

$$n_T=\frac{(z_\alpha+z_\beta)^2[p_{AT}(1-p_{AT})+p_{AR}(1-p_{AR})/\rho]}{(p_{AR}-p_{AT}-\delta_3)^2}. \tag{19.15}$$

Note that, by definition, $p_{Aj}=1-\Phi\left[c_1-(\mu_j+\mu_{\Delta j})/\sqrt{\sigma_j^2+\sigma_{\Delta j}^2}\right]$, where $j = T, R$. Therefore, following similar arguments, the above results also apply to test Hypotheses 19.5 with p_{Aj} replaced by $p_{Rj} = 1 - \Phi[(c_2-\mu_{\Delta j})/\sigma_{\Delta j}]$and δ_3 replaced by δ_5.

The hypotheses in Equation 19.4 are equivalent to

$$H_0:\ (1-\delta_4)p_{AR}-p_{AT}\geq 0 \quad \text{vs.} \quad H_1:(1-\delta_4)p_{AR}-p_{AT}<0. \tag{19.16}$$

Therefore, the null hypothesis in Equation 19.4 is rejected at an approximate α level of significance if

$$\frac{r_{AT}-(1-\delta_4)r_{AR}}{\sqrt{\frac{1}{n_T}r_{AT}(1-r_{AT})+\frac{(1-\delta_4)^2}{n_R}r_{AR}(1-r_{AR})}}>z_\alpha. \tag{19.17}$$

Using normal approximation to the test statistic when both n_T and n_R are sufficiently large, the power of the above test can be approximated by

$$\Phi\left(\frac{p_{AT}-(1-\delta_4)p_{AR}}{\sqrt{n_T^{-1}p_{AT}(1-p_{AT})+n_R^{-1}(1-\delta_4)^2 p_{AR}(1-p_{AR})}}-z_\alpha\right). \qquad (19.18)$$

Suppose that $n_R = \rho n_T$, where ρ is a known constant. Then the required total sample size to test Hypotheses 19.10, or equivalently 19.16, with a power level of $(1 - \beta)$ is $(1 + \rho)n_T$, where

$$n_T = \frac{(z_\alpha+z_\beta)^2[p_{AT}(1-p_{AT})+(1-\delta_4)^2 p_{AR}(1-p_{AR})/\rho]}{\left[p_{AT}-(1-\delta_4)p_{AR}\right]^2}. \qquad (19.19)$$

Similarly, the results derived in Equations 19.17 through 19.19 for the Hypotheses 19.4 also apply to the hypotheses in Equation 19.6 with p_{Aj} replaced by $p_{Rj} = 1 - \Phi[(c_2 - \mu_{\Delta j})/\sigma_{\Delta j}]$and δ_4 replaced by δ_6.

19.3.2 Determination of the Noninferiority Margin

Based on the results derived in Section 19.3.1, the noninferiority margins corresponding to the tests based on the absolute difference and the relative difference can be chosen in such a way that the two tests would have the same power. In particular, Hypotheses 19.1 and 19.2 would give the power level if the power function given in Equation 19.8 is the same as that given in Equation 19.11. Consequently, the noninferiority margins δ_1 and δ_2 would satisfy the following equation

$$\frac{(\sigma_T^2+\sigma_{\Delta T}^2)+(\sigma_R^2+\sigma_{\Delta R}^2)}{\left[(\mu_T+\mu_{\Delta T})-(\mu_R+\mu_{\Delta R})+\delta_1\right]^2} = \frac{(\sigma_{\Delta T}^2+\sigma_{\Delta R}^2)}{\left[(\mu_{\Delta T}-\mu_{\Delta R})+\delta_2\right]^2}. \qquad (19.20)$$

Similarly for Hypotheses 19.3 and 19.4, the noninferiority margins δ_3 and δ_4 would satisfy the following relationship

$$\frac{p_{AT}(1-p_{AT})+p_{AR}(1-p_{AR})/\rho}{(p_{AR}-p_{AT}-\delta_3)^2} = \frac{p_{AT}(1-p_{AT})+(1-\delta_4)^2 p_{AR}(1-p_{AR})/\rho}{\left[p_{AR}-(1-\delta_4)p_{AT}\right]^2}. \qquad (19.21)$$

For Hypotheses 19.5 and 19.6, the noninferiority margins δ_5 and δ_6 satisfy

$$\frac{p_{RT}(1-p_{RT})+p_{RR}(1-p_{RR})/\rho}{(p_{RR}-p_{RT}-\delta_5)^2} = \frac{p_{RT}(1-p_{RT})+(1-\delta_6)^2 p_{RR}(1-p_{RR})/\rho}{\left[p_{RR}-(1-\delta_6)p_{RT}\right]^2}. \qquad (19.22)$$

Results given in Equations 19.20, 19.21, and 19.22 provide a way of translating the noninferiority margins between endpoints based on the difference and the relative difference. In the next section, we will present a numerical study to provide some insight how the power level of these tests would be affected by the choices of different study endpoints for various combinations of parameters values.

19.4 A Numerical Study

In this section, a numerical study was conducted to provide some insight about the effect to the different clinical strategies.

TABLE 19.2 Sample Sizes for Noninferiority Testing Based on Absolute Difference and Relative Difference ($\alpha = 0.05$, $\beta = 0.20$, $\rho = 1$)

	$(\mu_R + \mu_{\Delta R}) - (\mu_T + \mu_{\Delta T}) = 0.20$									$(\mu_R + \mu_{\Delta R}) - (\mu_T + \mu_{\Delta T}) = 0.30$								
$\sigma_T^2 + \sigma_R^2$	1.0			2.0			3.0			1.0			2.0			3.0		
$\sigma_{\Delta T}^2 + \sigma_{\Delta R}^2$	1.0	1.5	2.0	1.0	1.5	2.0	1.0	1.5	2.0	1.0	1.5	2.0	1.0	1.5	2.0	1.0	1.5	2.0
Absolute difference																		
$\delta_1 = 0.50$	275	344	413	413	481	550	550	619	687	619	773	928	928	1082	1237	1237	1392	1546
$\delta_1 = 0.55$	202	253	303	303	354	404	404	455	505	396	495	594	594	693	792	792	891	990
$\delta_1 = 0.60$	155	194	232	232	271	310	310	348	387	275	344	413	413	481	550	550	619	687
$\delta_1 = 0.65$	123	153	184	184	214	245	245	275	306	202	253	303	303	354	404	404	455	505
$\delta_1 = 0.70$	99	124	149	149	174	198	198	223	248	155	194	232	232	271	310	310	348	387
Relative difference																		
$\delta_2 = 0.40$	310	464	619	310	464	619	310	464	619	1237	1855	2474	1237	1855	2474	1237	1855	2474
$\delta_2 = 0.50$	138	207	275	138	207	275	138	207	275	310	464	619	310	464	619	310	464	619
$\delta_2 = 0.60$	78	116	155	78	116	155	78	116	155	138	207	275	138	207	275	138	207	275

19.4.1 Absolute difference Versus Relative difference

In Table 19.2, the required sample sizes for the test of noninferiority based on the absolute difference (X_{ij}) and relative difference (Y_{ij}). In particular, the nominal power level ($1 - \beta$) is chosen to be 0.80 and α is 0.05. The corresponding sample sizes are calculated using the formulae in Equations 19.9 and 19.12. It is difficult to conduct any comparison because the corresponding noninferiority margins are based on different measurement scales. However, to provide some idea to assess the impact of switching from a clinical endpoint based on absolute difference to that based on relative difference, a numerical study on the power of the test was conducted. In particular, Table 19.3 presents the power of the test for noninferiority based on relative difference (Y) with the sample sizes determined by the power based on absolute difference (X). The power was calculated using the result given in Equation 19.11. The results demonstrate that the effect is, in general, very significant. In many cases, the power is much smaller than the nominal level 0.8.

19.4.2 Responders' Rate Based on Absolute Difference

Similar computation was conducted for the case when the hypotheses are defined in terms of the responders' rate based on the absolute difference; that is, hypotheses defined in Equations 19.3 and 19.4. Table 19.4 gives the required sample sizes, with the derived results given in Equations 19.15 and 19.19, for the corresponding hypotheses with noninferiority margins given both in terms of absolute difference and relative difference of the responders' rates. Similarly, Table 19.5 presents the power of the test for noninferiority based on relative difference of the responders' rate with the sample sizes determined by the power based on absolute difference of the responders' rate. The power was calculated using the result given in Equation 19.14. Again, the results demonstrate that the effect is, in general, very significant. In many cases, the power is much smaller than the nominal level 0.8.

19.4.3 Responders' Rate Based on Absolute Difference

Suppose that the responders' rate is defined based on the relative difference. Equations 19.5 and 19.6 give the hypotheses with non-inferiority margins given both in terms of absolute difference and relative difference of the responders' rate. The corresponding required sample sizes are given in Table 19.6. Following the similar steps, Table 19.7 presents the power of the test for noninferiority based on relative difference of the responders' rate with the sample sizes determined by the power based on absolute difference of the responders' rate. The similar pattern emerges and the results demonstrate that the power is usually much smaller than the nominal level 0.8.

19.5 Concluding Remarks

In clinical trials, it is not uncommon that a study is powered based on expected absolute change from baseline of a primary study endpoint but the collected data are analyzed based on relative change from baseline (e.g., percent change from baseline) of the primary study endpoint, or the collected data are analyzed based on the percentage of patients who show some improvement (i.e., responder analysis). The definition of a responder could be based on either absolute change from baseline or relative change from baseline of the primary study endpoint. It is very controversial in terms of the interpretation of the analysis results, especially when a significant result is observed based on a study endpoint (e.g., absolute change from baseline, relative change from baseline, or the responder analysis) but not on the other study endpoint (e.g., absolute change from baseline, relative change from baseline, or responder analysis). Based on the numerical results of this study, it is evident that the power of the test can be decreased drastically when the study endpoint is changed. However, when switching from a study endpoint based on absolute difference to the one based on relative difference,

TABLE 19.3 Power of the Test of Noninferiority Based on Relative Difference (× 10^{-2})

		$(\mu_R+\mu_{\Delta R})-(\mu_T+\mu_{\Delta T})=0.20$									$(\mu_R+\mu_{\Delta R})-(\mu_T+\mu_{\Delta T})=0.30$								
	$\sigma_T^2+\sigma_R^2$	1.0			2.0			3.0			1.0			2.0			3.0		
	$\sigma_{\Delta T}^2+\sigma_{\Delta R}^2$	1.0	1.5	2.0	1.0	1.5	2.0	1.0	1.5	2.0	1.0	1.5	2.0	1.0	1.5	2.0	1.0	1.5	2.0
$\delta_1=.50$	$\delta_2=0.40$	75.8	69.0	65.1	89.0	81.3	75.8	95.3	89.0	83.6	54.6	48.4	45.2	69.5	60.0	54.5	80.0	69.5	62.6
	$\delta_2=0.50$	96.9	94.2	92.0	99.6	98.4	96.9	100.0	99.6	98.9	97.0	94.1	91.9	99.6	98.4	96.9	100.0	99.6	98.9
	$\delta_2=0.60$	99.9	99.6	99.2	100.0	100.0	99.9	100.0	100.0	100.0	100.0	99.9	99.8	100.0	100.0	100.0	100.0	100.0	100.0
$\delta_1=.55$	$\delta_2=0.40$	64.2	57.6	53.8	79.3	70.1	64.2	88.4	79.3	72.7	40.6	35.9	33.5	53.1	45.0	40.6	63.5	53.1	47.1
	$\delta_2=0.50$	91.5	86.7	83.3	98.0	94.7	91.5	99.6	98.0	95.8	87.9	82.2	78.6	96.4	91.8	87.9	99.0	96.4	93.3
	$\delta_2=0.60$	99.1	97.9	96.7	99.9	99.7	99.1	100.0	99.9	99.8	99.5	98.6	97.8	100.0	99.8	99.5	100.0	100.0	99.9
$\delta_1=.60$	$\delta_2=0.40$	54.6	48.5	45.2	69.5	60.1	54.6	80.1	69.5	62.6	31.8	28.3	26.5	41.8	35.2	31.8	50.5	41.7	36.9
	$\delta_2=0.50$	84.0	77.9	73.9	94.4	88.6	84.0	98.2	94.4	90.4	75.8	69.0	65.1	89.0	81.3	75.8	95.3	89.0	83.6
	$\delta_2=0.60$	97.0	94.2	91.9	99.6	98.4	97.0	100.0	99.6	98.9	96.9	94.2	92.0	99.6	98.4	96.9	100.0	99.6	98.9
$\delta_1=.65$	$\delta_2=0.40$	47.0	41.4	38.7	60.8	51.8	46.8	71.5	60.6	54.2	26.1	23.4	21.9	33.9	28.8	26.1	41.2	34.0	30.1
	$\delta_2=0.50$	76.0	69.1	65.2	89.1	81.3	75.9	95.3	89.0	83.6	64.2	57.6	53.8	79.3	70.1	64.2	88.4	79.3	72.7
	$\delta_2=0.60$	93.2	88.7	85.7	98.6	95.8	93.1	99.7	98.6	96.8	91.5	86.7	83.3	98.0	94.7	91.5	99.6	98.0	95.8
$\delta_1=.70$	$\delta_2=0.40$	40.6	36.0	33.6	53.2	45.2	40.6	63.5	53.2	47.2	22.2	20.0	18.9	28.5	24.4	22.2	34.5	28.5	25.4
	$\delta_2=0.50$	67.9	61.2	57.4	82.8	73.9	67.9	91.0	82.7	76.3	54.6	48.5	45.2	69.5	60.1	54.6	80.1	69.5	62.6
	$\delta_2=0.60$	87.9	82.3	78.7	96.5	91.9	87.9	99.0	96.4	93.4	84.0	77.9	73.9	94.4	88.6	84.0	98.2	94.4	90.4

TABLE 19.4 Sample Sizes for Noninferiority Testing Based on Absolute Difference and Relative Difference of Response Rates Defined by the Absolute Difference (X_{ij}) ($\alpha = 0.05, \beta = 0.20, \rho = 1, c_1 - (\mu_T + \mu_{\Delta T}) = 0$)

	$c_1 - (\mu_R + \mu_{\Delta R}) = -0.60$									$c_1 - (\mu_R + \mu_{\Delta R}) = -0.80$								
$\sigma_R^2 + \sigma_T^2$	1.0			2.0			3.0			1.0			2.0			3.0		
$\sigma_{\Delta R}^2 + \sigma_{\Delta T}^2$	1.0	1.5	2.0	1.0	1.5	2.0	1.0	1.5	2.0	1.0	1.5	2.0	1.0	1.5	2.0	1.0	1.5	2.0
									Absolute difference									
$\delta_3 = 0.25$	399	284	228	228	195	173	173	157	146	2191	898	558	558	410	329	329	279	245
$\delta_3 = 0.30$	159	128	111	111	99	91	91	85	81	382	253	195	195	162	141	141	127	116
$\delta_3 = 0.35$	85	73	65	65	60	56	56	53	51	153	117	98	98	86	78	78	72	68
$\delta_3 = 0.40$	53	47	43	43	40	38	38	37	35	82	68	59	59	54	50	50	47	44
$\delta_3 = 0.45$	36	33	31	31	29	28	28	27	26	51	44	40	40	37	34	34	33	31
									Relative difference									
$\delta_4 = 0.35$	458	344	285	285	249	224	224	206	193	1625	869	601	601	469	391	391	340	304
$\delta_4 = 0.40$	199	166	147	147	134	124	124	117	112	392	288	234	234	202	180	180	165	153
$\delta_4 = 0.45$	109	96	88	88	82	78	78	75	72	168	139	121	121	110	102	102	95	91

TABLE 19.5 Power of the Test of Noninferiority Based on Relative Difference of Response Rates ($\times 10^{-2}$) ($\alpha = 0.05$, $\beta = 0.20$, $\rho = 1$, $c_1 - (\mu_T + \mu_{\Delta T}) = 0$)

		$c_1-(\mu_R+\mu_{\Delta R})=-0.60$									$c_1-(\mu_R+\mu_{\Delta R})=-0.80$								
	$\sigma_R^2+\sigma_T^2$	1.0			2.0			3.0			1.0			2.0			3.0		
	$\sigma_{\Delta R}^2+\sigma_{\Delta T}^2$	1.0	1.5	2.0	1.0	1.5	2.0	1.0	1.5	2.0	1.0	1.5	2.0	1.0	1.5	2.0	1.0	1.5	2.0
$\delta_3=0.25$	$\delta_4=0.35$	75.1	73.1	71.9	71.9	71.2	70.6	70.6	70.1	69.9	89.3	81.2	77.4	77.4	75.2	73.8	73.8	72.9	72.3
	$\delta_4=0.40$	97.0	94.6	92.8	92.8	91.4	90.2	90.2	89.2	88.5	100.0	99.7	98.6	98.6	97.1	95.7	95.7	94.5	93.4
	$\delta_4=0.45$	99.9	99.6	99.1	99.1	98.6	98.1	98.1	97.6	97.2	100.0	100.0	100.0	100.0	99.9	99.8	99.8	99.6	99.3
$\delta_3=0.30$	$\delta_4=0.35$	42.9	44.9	46.3	46.3	47.0	47.7	47.7	48.1	48.8	33.0	38.1	41.0	41.0	42.8	44.0	44.0	45.1	45.7
	$\delta_4=0.40$	71.9	70.5	69.9	69.9	69.1	68.6	68.6	68.3	68.3	79.1	75.5	73.5	73.5	72.1	71.1	71.1	70.6	70.0
	$\delta_4=0.45$	91.4	89.1	87.6	87.6	86.3	85.3	85.3	84.5	84.1	98.2	95.7	93.5	93.5	91.6	90.2	90.2	89.1	88.0
$\delta_3=0.35$	$\delta_4=0.35$	28.3	30.9	32.4	32.4	33.6	34.4	34.4	35.1	35.8	18.9	23.2	26.1	26.1	28.1	29.7	29.7	30.9	32.0
	$\delta_4=0.40$	49.3	50.2	50.5	50.5	50.9	51.0	51.0	51.2	51.5	46.4	47.7	48.6	48.6	49.2	49.7	49.7	50.1	50.6
	$\delta_4=0.45$	71.2	70.2	69.1	69.1	68.7	68.0	68.0	67.6	67.5	76.7	74.0	72.4	72.4	71.2	70.5	70.5	69.9	69.7
$\delta_3=0.40$	$\delta_4=0.35$	21.2	23.4	24.9	24.9	25.9	26.8	26.8	27.7	28.0	13.9	17.1	19.3	19.3	21.2	22.5	22.5	23.6	24.3
	$\delta_4=0.40$	35.9	37.4	38.3	38.3	38.9	39.4	39.4	40.3	40.1	30.6	33.2	34.6	34.6	36.0	36.9	36.9	37.6	37.8
	$\delta_4=0.45$	53.8	54.0	54.0	54.0	53.8	53.8	53.8	54.4	53.7	53.7	53.9	53.7	53.7	54.1	54.1	54.1	54.2	53.7
$\delta_3=0.45$	$\delta_4=0.35$	17.2	19.1	20.5	20.5	21.3	22.2	22.2	22.8	23.3	11.4	13.9	15.8	15.8	17.2	18.1	18.1	19.2	19.8
	$\delta_4=0.40$	27.9	29.6	30.8	30.8	31.4	32.2	32.2	32.6	32.9	22.7	25.1	26.9	26.9	28.1	28.7	28.7	29.8	30.0
	$\delta_4=0.45$	41.6	42.7	43.5	43.5	43.5	44.0	44.0	44.2	44.2	39.2	40.4	41.5	41.5	42.1	42.0	42.0	42.9	42.6

TABLE 19.6 Sample Sizes for Noninferiority Testing Based on Absolute Difference and Relative Difference of Response Rates Defined by the Relative Difference (Y_{ij}) (α 0.05, $\beta = 0.20$, $\rho = 1$, $c_2 - \mu_{\Delta T} = 0$)

	$c_2 - \mu_{\Delta R} = -0.30$				$c_2 - \mu_{\Delta R} = -0.40$				$c_2 - \mu_{\Delta R} = -0.50$				$c_2 - \mu_{\Delta R} = -0.60$			
$\sigma^2_{\Delta R} + \sigma^2_{\Delta T}$	1.0	1.5	2.0	2.5	1.0	1.5	2.0	2.5	1.0	1.5	2.0	2.5	1.0	1.5	2.0	2.5
Absolute difference																
$\delta_5 = 0.25$	173	130	111	101	329	201	157	135	836	351	238	189	4720	745	399	284
$\delta_5 = 0.30$	91	74	66	61	141	102	85	76	244	147	114	97	504	229	159	128
$\delta_5 = 0.35$	56	48	44	41	78	61	53	49	114	81	67	59	180	110	85	73
$\delta_5 = 0.40$	38	33	31	29	50	41	37	34	66	51	44	40	92	64	53	47
$\delta_5 = 0.45$	28	25	23	22	34	29	27	25	43	35	31	29	56	42	36	33
Relative difference																
$\delta_6 = 0.35$	224	173	151	138	391	256	206	180	823	412	297	243	2586	754	458	344
$\delta_6 = 0.40$	124	104	94	88	180	137	117	106	279	186	151	132	478	266	199	166
$\delta_6 = 0.45$	78	68	63	60	102	83	75	69	136	104	90	81	189	132	109	96

TABLE 19.7 Power of the Test of Noninferiority Based on Relative Difference of Response Rates ($\times 10^{-2}$) ($\alpha = 0.05$, $\beta = 0.20$, $\rho = 1$, $c_2 - \mu_{\Delta T} = 0$)

		$c_2 - \mu_{\Delta R} = -0.30$				$c_2 - \mu_{\Delta R} = -0.40$				$c_2 - \mu_{\Delta R} = -0.50$				$c_2 - \mu_{\Delta R} = -0.60$			
	$\sigma^2_{\Delta R} + \sigma^2_{\Delta T}$	1.0	1.5	2.0	2.5	1.0	1.5	2.0	2.5	1.0	1.5	2.0	2.5	1.0	1.5	2.0	2.5
$\delta_5 = 0.25$	$\delta_6 = 0.35$	70.6	69.5	68.8	68.7	73.8	71.2	70.1	69.6	80.5	74.3	72.1	70.9	95.7	79.6	75.1	73.1
	$\delta_6 = 0.40$	90.2	87.4	85.7	84.9	95.7	91.6	89.2	87.7	99.6	96.2	93.1	91.0	100.0	99.4	97.0	94.6
	$\delta_6 = 0.45$	98.1	96.4	95.2	94.5	99.8	98.7	97.6	96.7	100.0	99.8	99.2	98.5	100.0	100.0	99.9	99.6
$\delta_5 = 0.30$	$\delta_6 = 0.35$	47.7	49.3	50.1	50.5	44.0	47.0	48.1	49.0	38.6	43.7	45.9	47.1	29.2	39.2	42.9	44.9
	$\delta_6 = 0.40$	68.6	67.7	67.3	66.8	71.1	69.4	68.3	67.7	75.2	71.4	69.9	68.9	81.9	74.6	71.9	70.5
	$\delta_6 = 0.45$	85.3	83.1	81.8	80.9	90.2	86.7	84.5	83.3	95.4	90.6	87.9	86.0	99.2	94.9	91.4	89.1
$\delta_5 = 0.35$	$\delta_6 = 0.35$	34.4	36.9	38.2	38.7	29.7	33.3	35.1	36.5	23.6	29.4	32.2	33.8	16.1	24.4	28.3	30.9
	$\delta_6 = 0.40$	51.0	52.0	52.5	52.4	49.7	50.8	51.2	51.8	47.8	49.9	50.6	50.9	45.3	48.2	49.3	50.2
	$\delta_6 = 0.45$	68.0	67.4	67.0	66.3	70.5	68.7	67.6	67.4	73.7	71.1	69.6	68.5	78.4	73.5	71.2	70.2
$\delta_5 = 0.40$	$\delta_6 = 0.35$	26.8	28.8	30.3	30.8	22.5	25.8	27.7	28.7	17.3	22.1	24.6	26.3	12.0	17.9	21.2	23.4
	$\delta_6 = 0.40$	39.4	40.5	41.6	41.7	36.9	39.0	40.3	40.7	33.2	36.6	38.2	39.3	29.0	33.6	35.9	37.4
	$\delta_6 = 0.45$	53.8	53.7	54.2	53.7	54.1	54.1	54.4	54.0	53.5	54.0	54.1	54.2	53.7	53.6	53.8	54.0
$\delta_5 = 0.45$	$\delta_6 = 0.35$	22.2	24.2	25.1	25.8	18.1	21.0	22.8	23.7	14.1	17.9	20.0	21.6	10.0	14.5	17.2	19.1
	$\delta_6 = 0.40$	32.2	33.7	34.1	34.6	28.7	31.0	32.6	33.1	25.2	28.6	30.3	31.7	21.4	25.6	27.9	29.6
	$\delta_6 = 0.45$	44.0	44.7	44.5	44.8	42.0	43.1	44.2	44.1	40.3	42.1	42.9	43.8	38.6	40.5	41.6	42.7

one possible way to maintain the power level is to modify the corresponding noninferiority margin, as suggested by the results given in Section 19.3.2. More research effort, say, conducting an extensive simulation study, to explore the effects of switching between different clinical endpoints would help provide valuable insight to practitioners in selecting the suitable endpoint to assess the efficacy and safety of a test treatment.

References

Chow, S. C., and Liu, J. P. (2004). *Design and Analysis of Clinical Trials.* New York: John Wiley and Sons.

Chow, S. C., Shao, J., and Wang, H. (2008). *Sample Size Calculation in Clinical Research.* New York: Chapman & Hall/CRC Press, Taylor & Francis.

Chow, C. S., Tse, S. K., and Lin, M. (2008). Statistical methods in translational medicine. *Journal of the Formosan Medical Association*, 107 (12): S61–S73.

Johnson, N. L., and Kotz, S. (1970). *Distributions in Statistics—Continuous Univariate Distributions—I.* New York: John Wiley & Sons.

Paul, S. (2000). Clinical endpoint. In *Encyclopedia of Biopharmaceutical Statistics,* ed. S. C. Chow. New York: Marcel Dekker, Inc.

Serfling, R. (1980). *Approximation Theorems of Mathematical Statistics.* New York: John Wiley & Sons.

20

Adaptive Infrastructure

Bill Byrom, Damian McEntegart, and Graham Nicholls
Perceptive Informatics

This chapter focuses on some of the practical aspects of conducting adaptive trials, in particular the infrastructure required to operate these studies appropriately and smoothly. Although many of our recommendations and considerations apply to a range of types of adaptive trial, we concern ourselves primarily with those designs that include preplanned adjustments to the randomization procedure or to the number of treatment arms in play. Such designs bring with them unique challenges for those managing clinical trials, some of which require adjustments to processes and procedures, careful planning and consideration, and the implementation of technologies to ensure the study runs smoothly. These we consider as adaptive infrastructure—the elements that those putting in place an adaptive clinical trial should consider to ensure effective implementation and appropriate compliance with regulatory guidance and thinking.

As we consider implementation of adaptive clinical trials, and specifically those involving modifications to randomization or the treatments studied, we are faced with a number of challenges:

Challenge 1. How do we design the optimal study?
Challenge 2. How do we efficiently implement changes to the randomization during the study?
Challenge 3. How do we perform design adaptations in a way that is invisible to the site and possibly also the sponsor?
Challenge 4. How do we plan supplies requirements for an adaptive clinical trial?
Challenge 5. How do we ensure each site has sufficient supplies of the correct types following a design adaptation?

Challenge 6. How do we ensure timely access to quality data for rapid decision making?

Challenge 7. How do we operate a data monitoring committee (DMC) effectively and what sponsor involvement/participation is appropriate?

In considering Challenge 1, optimal study design, this may lead us to question, for example:

- Is my primary endpoint suitable for this kind of design? Can it be measured quickly enough relative to the anticipated recruitment rate? If not, we may need to consider staged recruitment strategies or use of a surrogate endpoint.
- How will I combine the consideration of both efficacy and safety endpoints? For example, is there a suitable utility index that would be valid and appropriate for my study?
- When would be the optimal point to assign a preplanned interim analysis?
- Should the study utilize a Bayesian response adaptive methodology or a frequentist approach using fixed interim analyses?

These questions are not the focus of this chapter, but the reader should refer to other chapters in this book and examples in the literature. For example, Krams et al. (2003) describe the development and validation of a surrogate endpoint for the ASTIN trial, and Jones's (2006) article considers the optimal design and operating characteristics for an adaptive trial in COPD. It should be noted that adaptive trials do not need to be very complicated. A study with a single interim analysis incorporating simple decision rules can still provide large benefits to researchers.

In the remainder of this chapter, we focus on providing a perspective on the remaining challenges listed above (Challenges 2–7) and the adaptive infrastructure recommended to effectively implement these types of studies.

20.1 Implementation of Randomization Changes

One of the critical components of an adaptive trial that involves changing the treatment groups studied or their allocation ratio is the ability to make modifications to the randomization scheme during the study recruitment period.

Conventionally in clinical trials, randomization is administered one of two ways—either by picking sequentially from predefined code list(s) or using a dynamic method that uses random number generation to essentially flick a coin at the point of randomization. Except for instances where treatment groups need to be balanced for a number of predefined patient variables, the most common approach is to use a prevalidated code list to deliver the randomization. This can be administered by the study site by simply selecting the next available entry in a list of patient numbers, each with the appropriate blinded treatment prepacked against the corresponding patient number, or by using a central randomization system such as an interactive voice response (IVR) system.

When it comes to a trial that requires mid-study modification to either the treatments in play, or the allocation ratio of the treatments, it becomes a requirement to deliver the randomization centrally. There are two reasons for this. The first is that it is desirable that study site personnel are not aware of the design adaptation as this may influence subject selection and introduce bias into the sample before and after the design adaptation is made. The rationale for this is that sites may be less reluctant to enter certain subjects into the trial if they are aware that suboptimal treatments have been eliminated as a result of an adaptation. The second reason is simply ensuring that randomization is applied correctly and without errors. Asking site personnel to skip patient numbers (these will correspond to the randomization list) after design adaptations have been made is prone to introducing human error into the randomization procedure. The skipping pattern may also enable the investigator to deduce the randomization block size and hence increase their ability to infer the treatment allocations of current and future subjects.

We discuss below a number of approaches to managing midstudy changes to randomization, and also describe one or two common pitfalls that should be avoided.

20.1.1 Approaches to Implementation of Randomization Changes

In this section we describe four common approaches to implementing preplanned changes to the randomization midstudy. As described above, these all require technology infrastructure, and specifically central computer-controlled randomization to implement effectively and without error-making within a clinical trial. This is typically administered using an IVR system in which study sites interact with a central computer to input subject details and receive blinded medication pack allocations in accordance with the in-built randomization method.

20.1.1.1 Method 1: Switching Code Lists

An adaptive study may have a specified number of potential scenarios, each of which can be accommodated by a unique randomization code list. When the number of scenarios is relatively low, holding a unique code list for each and enabling a defined study representative to action a switch to an alternative code list is a simple and practical approach. An example is illustrated in Figure 20.1. In this example, subjects are initially randomized to one of three treatments in a 1:1:1 ratio. After an interim analysis, the study design dictates that either Treatment A or B will be terminated, and the randomization ratio changed to 2:1 in favor of the remaining Treatment (A or B). In this case, the adjustment to the randomization can be simply achieved by switching to a new list—the system being preloaded with lists to cover both scenarios. The switch between lists can be prebuilt and validated within the IVR system, and triggered by an approved user making an IVR call to select the list from which to randomize new subjects. As described above, this is a suitable approach when the exact nature of all the possible adaptations is known up front, and the number of possible scenarios is relatively small.

20.1.1.2 Method 2: Modifying an Existing Code List

A second approach utilizes a single code list but applies a change to the randomization process by skipping entries to ensure the appropriate treatment allocation ratios are maintained. Figure 20.2 illustrates

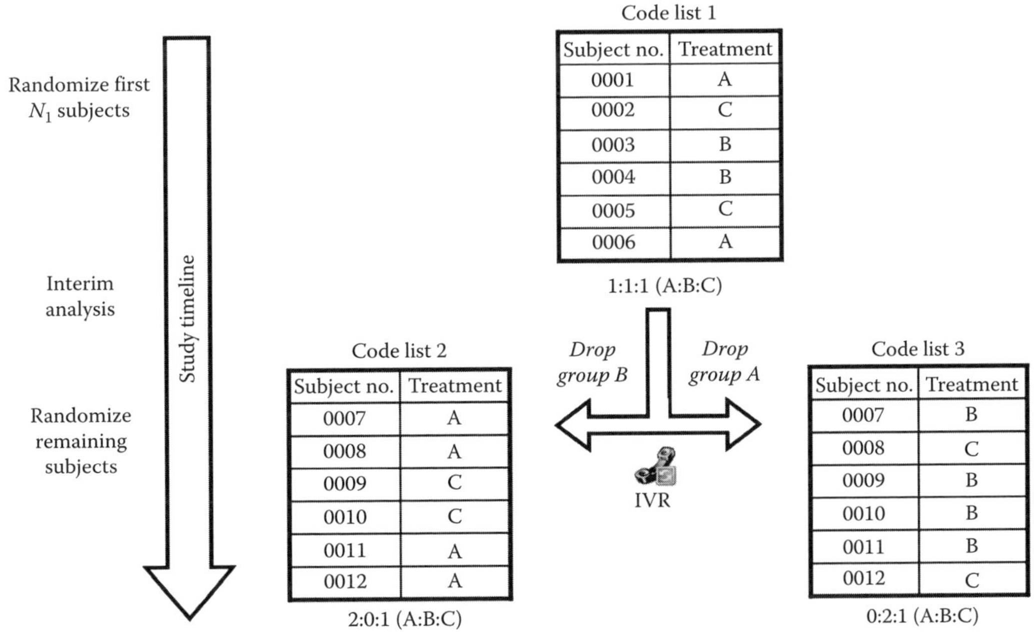

FIGURE 20.1 Applying a design adaptation by switching predefined code lists.

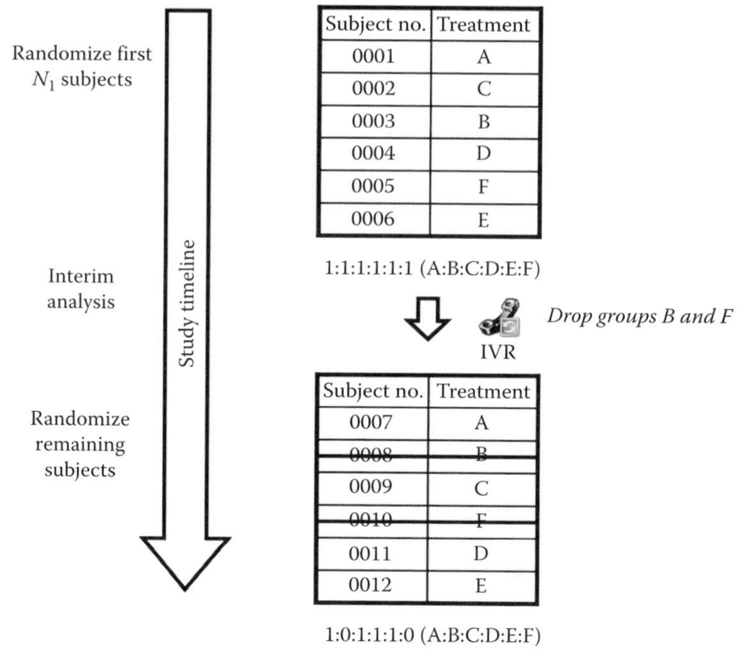

FIGURE 20.2 Applying a design adaptation by modifying a predefined code list.

this with a simple scenario. Initially, subjects are randomized to one of five treatments in a 1:1:1:1:1 ratio. After an interim analysis, it is determined that two treatments are to be terminated and the remainder to continue in a 1:1 allocation ratio. This is achieved by simply deactivating or skipping all entries in the remainder of the list that are associated with the terminated treatments. This is a simple method as it utilizes only a single list, but because of this it is limited in the nature of adaptations it can accommodate and may not be practical for all studies. In addition, there may be instances when removal of treatment groups results in an inappropriate block size being applied (see possible pitfalls and considerations later in this section).

When there are a high number of possible scenarios that a design adaptation could follow, and when these cannot be accommodated by modification of a single list, there are two other approaches possible: mid-study generation of a code-list, or using a dynamic allocation method (such as minimization with biased coin assignment).

20.1.1.3 Method 3: Mid-Study Generation of Code Lists

In this approach, following an interim analysis or the results of a new feed of subject data through a Bayesian response-adaptive algorithm, new treatment allocation ratios will be determined (Figure 20.3). Based upon these, a statistician will determine the appropriate block size and generate a new randomization code list for use for subsequent randomizations. As is normal practice with the generation of randomization codes, the statistician responsible will not be a member of the study team. This approach is resource intensive as it requires the rapid generation, inspection and QC of a new code list, and its importing into the IVR system with corresponding testing and QC activities. This needs to be performed rapidly so as not to delay the randomization of new subjects or to continue with the previous list (containing suboptimal treatments) for too long before the modification can be implemented.

An alternative would be to allow the IVR system to generate the required new code dynamically within the system according to instructions from an approved user via an IVR or web interface. The user could visualize the list and release it via the web interface. Such interfaces are available from vendors

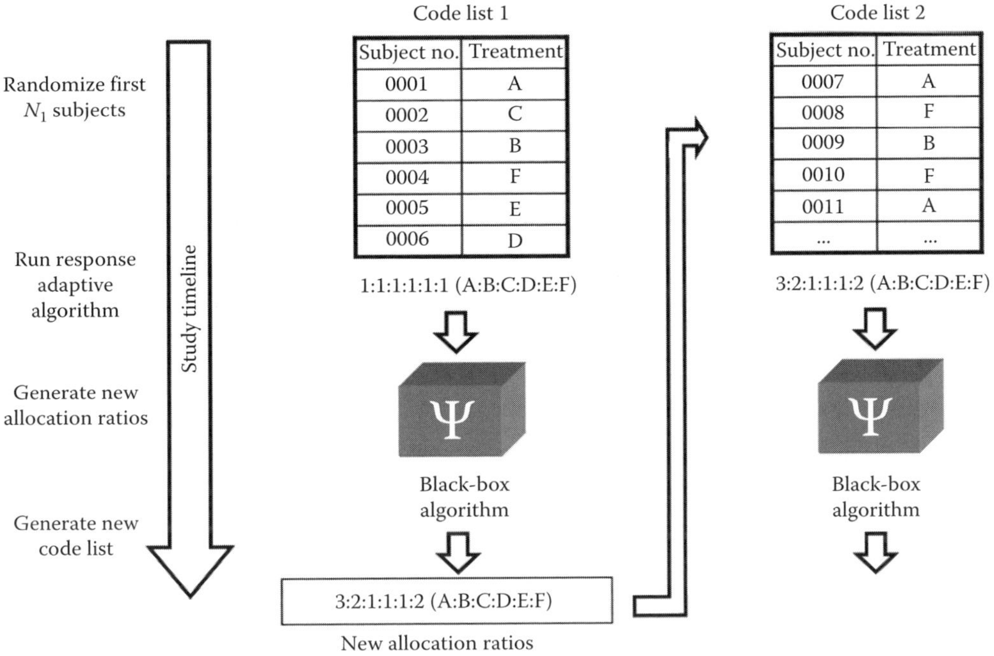

FIGURE 20.3 Applying a design adaptation by creation of a new code list.

as a Bespoke Solution at the moment. The challenge for vendors is to develop generic, validated, and configurable applications to meet the needs of all studies.

20.1.1.4 Method 4: Dynamic Allocation Methods

Dynamic allocation methods are attractive as they can very simply incorporate changes in the treatment allocation. In particular, when Bayesian response adaptive methods are in use, the output of these algorithms is usually the treatment allocation probabilities that should be applied moving forward. A dynamic allocation method uses a random number generator to determine the treatment to be assigned based upon the probabilities associated with each treatment group. Changes to the assignment probabilities can be incorporated simply by making changes to their values held in the IVR system. Often, the study will commence with an initial set of allocation probabilities, or an initial code list constructed according to the appropriate initial allocation ratios, as illustrated in Figure 20.4. After response data has been collected for a certain number of subjects, these are fed into the Bayesian algorithm that returns a new set of allocation probabilities. These can be input directly into the IVR randomization algorithm either via a web-interface or an IVR call, or directly through a secure automated file transfer between the algorithm and the IVR system. Dynamic allocation methods can be particularly appropriate when either the number of possible scenarios following an adaptation is very high and it is not desirable to manually create and implement new randomization lists midstudy, or when a Bayesian response adaptive methodology is employed that provides midstudy adjustments to allocation probabilities. It should be noted that code list methods can be used with Bayesian response adaptive designs by converting the allocation probabilities into approximate allocation ratios that can be accommodated by a predefined blocked randomization list. Some researchers are cautious over the use of dynamic allocation methods due to a perception that regulatory bodies have a negative view of such approaches. In fact, European (CPMP 2003) guidance states that these methods are acceptable if they can be justified on scientific grounds and in the case of response adaptive designs this should be quite justifiable.

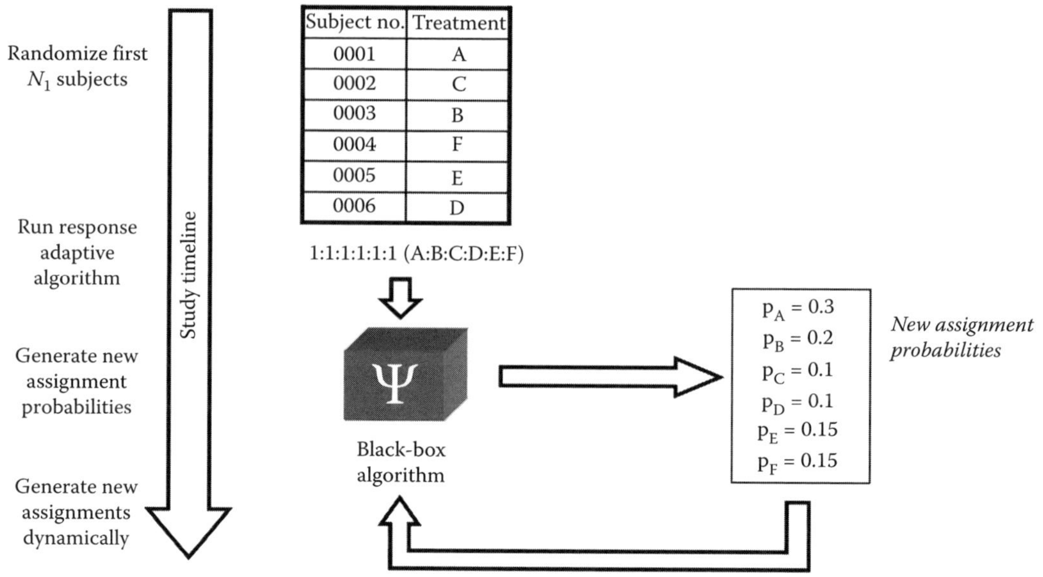

FIGURE 20.4 Applying a design adaptation by employing a dynamic allocation method.

20.1.2 Possible Pitfalls and Considerations

It is important to ensure that the methodology employed does not limit the randomness of the algorithm, increase the predictability of treatment allocations, or reveal that a design adaptation has taken place. Below we describe three instances where this could be the case. Although these are not an exhaustive list of possibilities, they serve to illustrate the kinds of issues that should be considered when determining the best approach for a specific study.

20.1.2.1 Example 1. Loss of Randomness of the Algorithm

One approach that we have seen presented at a conference utilizes an existing code list, and skips entries to accommodate changes in the randomization ratio. Initially, subjects may be allocated in a 1:1:1 ratio, across (say) three Treatments A, B, and C (Figure 20.5). This coded list is likely generated using a certain block size, but the same issue occurs if the list is not blocked, as in our example. At a certain decision point, or continually during the study, the randomization ratio is changed based upon the response data reported and decision criteria in place. If, as in the example, the randomization ratio is changed to 7:6:1, this method would simply go down the list counting the first seven new entries for Treatment A, the first six for Treatment B, and the first one for Treatment C. All other entries would be skipped, thus leaving a randomization list of the appropriate balance to accommodate the new randomization ratios. If more than 14 new patients are required, the process is repeated further down the list to create a further block of 14 patients and so on. The flaw in this approach is seen if we examine the properties of each block of 14 allocations created from this list. A fundamental property of an appropriate randomization approach is that the randomness is conserved. In this case, if we consider the one allocation of Treatment C within our block of 14, we would expect that treatment to be equally likely to occur at any position within the block of 14 if our code list is truly random. However, because the initial list was created with a 1:1:1 ratio (and not blocked in our example), the chance of the C treatment occurring in position 1 of the block is 1/3, and at position 14 is $(2/3)^{13} \times (1/3)$. In other words, the allocation of Treatment C is more likely higher up the block, which disturbs the true randomness of the allocation procedure. This property is even more pronounced if the initial code list is blocked. In theory, this draws into question

Subject no.	Treatment
001	A
002	C
003	B
004	A
005	B
006	C
007	C
008	B
009	A
010	C
011	A
012	B
013	A
014	C
015	B
016	C
017	A
018	A
019	B
020	C
021	B
022	A
023	C
024	A
025	C
026	B
027	C
028	A
029	C
030	B
031	A
032	B

1:1:1 ratio

Subject no.	Treatment
001	A
002	C
003	B
004	A
005	B
~~006~~	~~C~~
~~007~~	~~C~~
008	B
009	A
~~010~~	~~C~~
011	A
012	B
013	A
~~014~~	~~C~~
015	B
~~016~~	~~C~~
017	A
018	A
019	B
020	C
021	B
022	A
023	C
024	A
025	C
026	B
027	C
028	A
029	C
030	B
031	A
032	B

Next block of 14 subjects

7:6:1 ratio

FIGURE 20.5 Loss of randomness due to inappropriate entry skipping methodology.

the applicability of the statistical properties of the design and the associated inference tests, and it is recommended that this kind of approach is avoided. Instead, switching to predefined code lists of the appropriate properties, or using a dynamic allocation method might be the best approach.

20.1.2.2 Example 2. Increased Predictability of Treatment Assignments

In the event that a code list is modified to accommodate the removal of treatment arms, careful consideration must be given to the block size. As illustrated in Figure 20.6, a study of four Treatments (A to D) in 1:1 ratio could be modified to include only two Treatments (A and B). In this case, an initial four-treatment code list prepared in blocks of four, would reduce to a two-treatment list in blocks of two. This block size, if detected, provides increased predictability of treatment allocations, which is undesirable. Careful consideration of block size is important when utilizing an approach that involves skipping entries within a single predefined list. In this example, the problem could be avoided by employing an initial list with block size of eight, or if this was not desirable then using a list-switching method.

Subject no.	Treatment
001	A
002	C
003	B
004	D
005	B
006	C
007	A
008	D
009	A
010	C
011	D
012	B

1:1:1:1 ratio
block size 4

⇨

Subject no.	Treatment
001	A
~~002~~	~~C~~
003	B
~~004~~	~~D~~
005	B
~~006~~	~~C~~
007	A
~~008~~	~~D~~
009	A
~~010~~	~~C~~
~~011~~	~~D~~
012	B

1:1 ratio
block size 2

FIGURE 20.6 Modifying lists can affect the block size and increase predictability of treatment assignments.

20.1.2.3 Example 3. Revealing that a Design Adaptation has Taken Place

Somewhat related to Example 1 is the information that may be unwittingly revealed to site personnel if care is not taken with the planning of the trial supplies. Consider the following scenario that is typical of many adaptive designs:

- The trial commences with equal allocation ratios but at some point the randomization ratio has the potential to be altered.
- Separate packaging and randomization schedules are to be used as is standard practice in IVR trials. The system determines the treatment that is to be allocated at the point of randomization. It then selects at random a pack of the appropriate type from the inventory of supplies at the site. The pack number to be dispensed is read out to the investigator.
- The packaging list is constructed in a randomized manner in blocks defined according to the initial allocation ratio. The pack numbers are sequential and thus correlated with the sequence number of the packaging list.
- The system is programed to manage the flow of packs to sites by sending resupply consignments to sites as necessary. The packs for such consignments are selected in pack number order according to the sites' needs.

In this example, if the randomization ratio changes midstudy, for example, from 1:1:1 to 2:2:1 and the system continues to manage and dispense supplies according to the original packaging list in the 1:1:1 ratio, the same kind of phenomenon as seen in Example 1 can occur. In this case, because packs associated with treatments with a higher allocation ratio will be used more frequently, as new packs are sent to sites, the ranges of pack numbers associated with higher allocation ratio treatments will be higher, and may become numerically distinct from other treatment groups. It will then be possible for a site to deduce that certain patients are provided with packs that are consistently lower in pack ID number than other patients, giving some indication that certain patients are receiving the same or different treatments, and that a design adaptation has taken place. This phenomenon is known as pack separation. If site staff notice this then there is scope for unblinding, particularly if an emergency code break is performed.

The remedy to this situation is to scramble the pack numbers to break the link between the pack number and the sequence number. This involves a random reordering of the randomized pack list. This process has been termed double randomization by Lang, Wood, and McEntegart (2005).

If this process is employed, then there is no way that the site staff can deduce any patterns from the consignments they receive and the dispensations made. The use of double-randomized pack lists can be recommended for all trials managed via IVR but it is particularly important in trials where the randomization ratio has the scope to deviate from the packing ratio. Readers wishing to read further on this topic are referred to the publication by Lang, Wood, and McEntegart (2005), which is freely available online and includes pictorial examples that help visualize the phenomenon of pack separation if a double-randomized list is not employed.

20.1.2.4 Design Considerations

There are a number of other practical points that are relevant when considering how to implement a study design that includes the possibility of midstudy changes to the randomization method.

For example, what should the sponsor choose to do about patients that are scheduled to be randomized during the period of time taken to perform an interim analysis and apply the decision criteria? There is no hard and fast rule about this—some would prefer randomization not to be slowed down and so new patients would continue to be randomized using the existing code list until a new one is applied. Others would consider that a short halt in randomization is appropriate and would have the advantage in ensuring that new patients are allocated to optimal treatments. In either case, the approach taken should be documented in the study protocol.

In addition, when using a dynamic allocation method, it may be a requirement to always conserve the active: placebo allocation ratio, particularly while samples are small initially. This can be accomplished by using a combined approach where a blocked code list determines whether a subject will receive active or placebo, and if active is chosen a dynamic procedure is used to determine what active treatment is to be assigned.

20.2 Maintaining the Invisibility of Design Changes

We discuss later in this chapter whether the sponsor should be represented on the DMC, a related question is who needs to know what information when any adaptation does or does not occur?

20.2.1 Invisibility of Changes to Site Personnel

The regulatory guidance would imply that the site should be kept unaware of the changes if possible, at least in certain situations. For instance, the European Guidance (CHMP 2007) discusses the case of a confirmatory Phase III trial that contains both active and placebo controls. Should it be planned that the placebo control is dropped after the superiority of the experimental treatment (or the reference treatment, or both) over placebo has been demonstrated then sponsors are warned to plan carefully. The regulators surmise that different types of patients might be recruited into trials involving a placebo arm as opposed to those involving an active control; that is, placebo-controlled trials may tend to include a patient population with less severe disease. Thus, if site staff become aware that the placebo arm has been stopped after an interim analysis then the treatment effect from the different stages of the trial may then differ to an extent that combination of results from the different stages is not possible. The guidance thus states that:

> Consequently, all attempts would ideally be taken to maintain the blind and to restrict knowledge about whether, and at what time, recruitment to the placebo arm has been stopped. Concealing the decision as to whether or not the placebo-group has been stopped may complicate the practical running of the study and the implications should be carefully discussed. (p. 7)

Similarly, the guidance also discusses the case where sponsors may wish to investigate more than one dose of the experimental treatment in Phase III; this would be where some doubts remain about the most preferable dose. Early interim results may resolve some of the ambiguities with regard to efficacy or safety considerations, and recruitment may be stopped for some doses of the experimental treatment. The second stage of such a study would then be restricted to the control treatment and the chosen dose of the experimental treatment. The guidance states that again, potential implications regarding the patient population selected for inclusion should be discussed in the study protocol. If this meant that the dropping of the dose should be kept from investigators then this is a conservative position—would investigators really hold back certain types of patients until they know the less preferable effective dose has been dropped even though there is supporting information for this dose from Phase II results? There remains some uncertainty about this situation.

If the nature of the adaptation in a particular trial means it is advisable to keep the site unaware of any changes to treatment randomization including cessation or even addition of treatment arms, then an IVR system has to be used for randomization and dispensation of supplies (McEntegart, Nicholls, and Byrom 2007). To see why this is the case consider the example of a study involving four treatments using a simple randomization list.

Without an IVR system, kits of supplies are prelabeled with patient numbers and sites allocate the next available patient number to newly randomized patients. The contents of kits are dictated by a predefined randomization list, and so (for example) a study including four Treatments A, B, C, and D might be supplied in such a way that each subsequent group of four patients would contain one on each treatment group, the order of which is randomized. In this scenario, if a treatment arm is dropped midstudy, this would be immediately apparent to the investigators as they would be required to skip certain future patient numbers in their future allocations. It may also reveal the block size giving them more possibility of guessing the treatment groups that current patients belong to.

By employing an IVR system with a central distribution method, the knowledge of any change to the allocated treatments can be kept from investigators. Thus, there is no potential for bias and no reason to expect any observed differences between the before and after results (something the regulators will be specifically looking at). There are two aspects to the protection provided by IVR system.

The first is the separation of the randomization and dispensing steps in IVR system. By using pack labels that are not linked to the patient number in any way, the knowledge of any alteration in treatment allocation can be restricted. As previously described, by using a pack list with scrambled numbers, the supplies allocated by the investigator are completely disconnected, so there is no hint of the randomization block size and, importantly, no information about changes in treatments can be detected by the site staff. By leaving gaps in the pack list numbering system, it is even possible to add a new treatment to be randomized midstudy without the investigator knowing.

The other component of IVR's protection relates to the automated management of the supply chain and maintenance of stocks at site. Even if the investigator cannot deduce anything from the altered numbering in an IVR trial, he might deduce something is occurring if there is a sudden surge in supply deliveries to his site as might happen if the site inventories are adjusted to cope with the altered allocation. But IVR systems can be configured to maintain low stock levels at site with regular resupplies as needed and so he is unlikely to deduce anything related to the change. The adjustment of the stock levels to account for the changed situation is automatically handled by the IVR system, as discussed later in this chapter.

Even with IVR system, one question remains. That is, can the material relating to discontinued treatments be left on site or does it have to be withdrawn? In our experience most sponsors do arrange for the removal of packs relating to treatments that have been withdrawn. The argument is that this reduces the risk of incorrect pack assignment. But as the risk of an incorrect assignment is very low (circa 1% in our experience) then for many trials we regard it as acceptable not to remove the packs relating to withdrawn treatments. Clearly the circumstances for each individual trial will be an important consideration, most importantly are there any safety concerns, are the patients that have already been randomized to the dropped dose going to continue through to the end of the trial; that is, is it just new randomizations to that specific dose that are being ceased, is there likely to be an updating exercise to account for expiry, the length of the trial and so on?

20.2.2 Invisibility of Changes to Sponsor Personnel

The above deals with the situation at the site. While it may be possible to restrict knowledge of any adaptation from the site, for some studies it may not be practical to keep the knowledge of the adaptation from the study team. Indeed Maca et al. (2006) state that such masking is not usually feasible in seamless Phase II/III designs. Certainly the drug supply manager will need to know about any adaption. The clinical staff involved in monitoring at sites and the study leaders monitoring the study as a whole may deduce something about the need to withdraw stocks from site. Nevertheless in some studies as described below complete invisibility may be practical.

Quinlan and Krams (2006) point out that using doses of 0X, 1X, 3X, and 4X allow for equidistant dose progression from 0X to 8X in a blinded manner when two tablets are taken by each patient; the downside of this is potential reduced compliance as compared to the patient just taking single tablet. On the other hand patients regularly take two different tablets in clinical trials and we have not heard of differential compliance. Thus if this type of packaging is used any switch can take place in a masked manner. Another alternative may be to ask the site pharmacist to prepare the study medication as happens regularly in trials where the product is infused.

Our recommendation is where it is practical, the number of study personnel who are cognizant of any change is kept to a minimum. This is a conservative stance as we agree with Gallo (2006b) that the fact that an adaptation has occurred seems to provide no direct mechanism for noticeable bias in the trial if good statistical practice is employed, for example, statistical analysis plan for the *final* analysis with general rules for inclusion/exclusion of data outlined should be available at the study protocol stage and a version history is maintained. In that way more hypothetical and convoluted forms of bias in monitoring and analysis can be ruled out. We agree with Gaydos et al. in 2006 that it is a good idea to withhold full statistical details of the adaption criteria from the trial protocol and document them elsewhere in a document with controlled access. Of course the details presented need to be enough to satisfy the need for patients, investigators, and ethics committees to be sufficiently informed.

Gallo (2006b) goes further and argues that steps should be taken to minimize what can be inferred by observers but that the amount of information and its potential for bias should be balanced against the advantages that the designs offer. Consider the general case of a dose group of the experimental treatment being dropped; if appropriate care has been taken there would often be little information that could be inferred about the magnitude of treatment effects and thus minimal potential for introducing bias into the trial. In the case of a seamless Phase II/III trial, he contrasts the information available compared to the traditional path of a Phase II trial followed by a phase III trial. More information on the inefficacious treatments is available in the latter model and thus there is a sense that the seamless adaptive design controls information better than the traditional approach. He argues that it is unreasonable to require that no information should be conferred to observers of a midtrial adaptation.

In summary, this is a controversial area about which consensus is still to emerge and we recommend that sponsors give the issue careful consideration when planning their trial.

The case of sample size reestimation is somewhat more clear-cut. If the blind is broken and the treatment effect is used directly in the reestimation process, or indirectly in that it is accounted for in the statistical model to more precisely estimate the error variance, then observers may be able to back calculate some information about the size of the treatment effect. Clearly this is not appropriate and in common with others, our advice is to perform the sample size reestimation on blinded data. As explained in a later section there may be a role for minimization or other dynamic randomization technique (McEntegart 2003) to minimize the influence of nuisance factors.

20.3 Drug Supply Planning Considerations

As discussed earlier in this chapter, the planning for an adaptive design throws out new challenges. Not the least of these is faced by those responsible for ensuring sufficient supplies are formulated and packaged to meet the needs of the study. This is often a complex question for conventional study designs, how much more so for trials that have the possibility of adjusting the proportion of subjects allocated to each treatment in a variety of possible ways as the study progresses?

Simulation models are valuable tools to researchers in not only exploring the optimal design of the study as discussed earlier in this textbook, but also in understanding the possible and likely supply requirements of the trial. In our industry there are a small number of commercial Monte Carlo simulation models used to specifically explore and estimate clinical trial medication supply requirements (see Peterson et al. 2004, for example). Combining these models that simulate the medication supply chain and estimate study drug requirements with models that simulate the adaptive trial time-course, in particular the possible design adaptations, provides researchers with comprehensive information from which to plan study medication requirements. Simulation provides the means to obtain confidence intervals for the total study medication requirements, establish the minimum medication required to start the study (on the understanding that more supplies can be packaged and made available upstream), determine the timing and content of midstudy production runs, and optimize the packaging configuration so as to make the most use of the medication available (for example, making up doses from two medication packs in a flexible manner—20 mg being composed of 1 × 20 mg with 1 × placebo, or 2 × 10 mg packs). This is illustrated in the case study published by Nicholls, Patel, and Byrom (2009), which we review in the following section. It is our recommendation that researchers use simulation not only in exploring optimal study design and operating characteristics, but also in estimating medication requirements both pre- and midstudy to assist in effective supply planning.

20.3.1 Case Study

In this study, reported in full and freely available on line (Nicholls, Patel, and Byrom 2009), the value of simulation as a planning tool for adaptive clinical trials was demonstrated, and in particular in assessing medication supply requirements. The study was a dose finding study investigating six active dose levels (10 mg, 20 mg, 30 mg, 40 mg, 60 mg, and 80 mg) and placebo, with a total of 140 subjects to be enrolled. Subjects were allocated to treatment in a 1:1 ratio until a single interim analysis at which ineffective treatment arms were dropped. If all dose levels were considered ineffective then the study would be stopped at this point.

In terms of simulation, the time-course of the adaptive trial was simulated for a range of possible dose–response relationships (Figure 20.7). Dose–response relationships ranged from no effect across

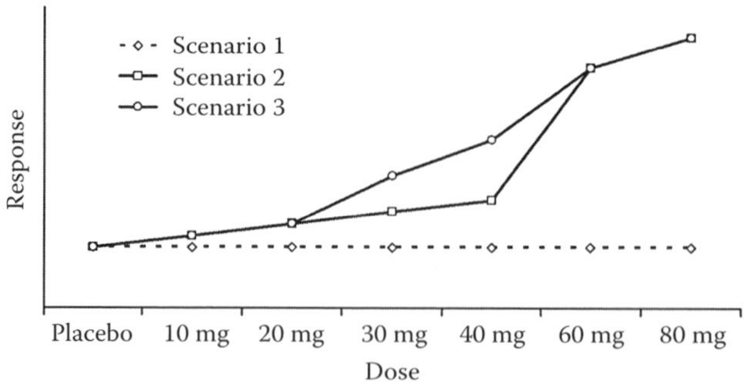

FIGURE 20.7 Dose–response scenarios in simulated adaptive dose-finding study. (From Nicholls, G., Patel, N., and Byrom, B., *Applied Clinical Trials*, 6, 76–82, 2009. With permission.)

the dose range (Scenario 1), to effective only at the high doses (Scenario 2), to increasing effect across the entire dose range (Scenario 3). Simulating the adaptive trial outcome based upon the different dose-response possibilities provided input for the supply chain simulation in terms of the sequence of treatment assignments and the outcome of the interim analysis.

Based upon these scenarios, 51% of simulations under the no-effect scenario (Scenario 1) indicated the study would stop for futility at the interim analysis whereas in the other scenarios the study would be erroneously stopped for futility only 1% of the time. The simulations also provided information about which dose levels were dropped at the interim analysis, and this information was used to feed the supply chain simulation model to calculate corresponding medication requirements. These simulations resulted in estimation of the maximum number of packs of each pack type required by the study (Figure 20.8). Interestingly, the case study showed that introducing flexibility into the use of medication packs could dramatically reduce the amount of medication required by the study. When dose levels were made up of a combination of four packs (e.g., 60 mg = 3 × 20 mg packs and 1 placebo pack) as opposed to manufacturing a single pack of the exact dose strength for each treatment group, the amount of active ingredient required by the study was reduced by over 37%. Although in this example allocating four packs per subject may be impractical when patients are required to self-medicate at home, large savings can also be observed when patients are asked to take medication from only two packs and this is quite acceptable in terms of medication compliance behavior when patients are responsible for taking medication at home.

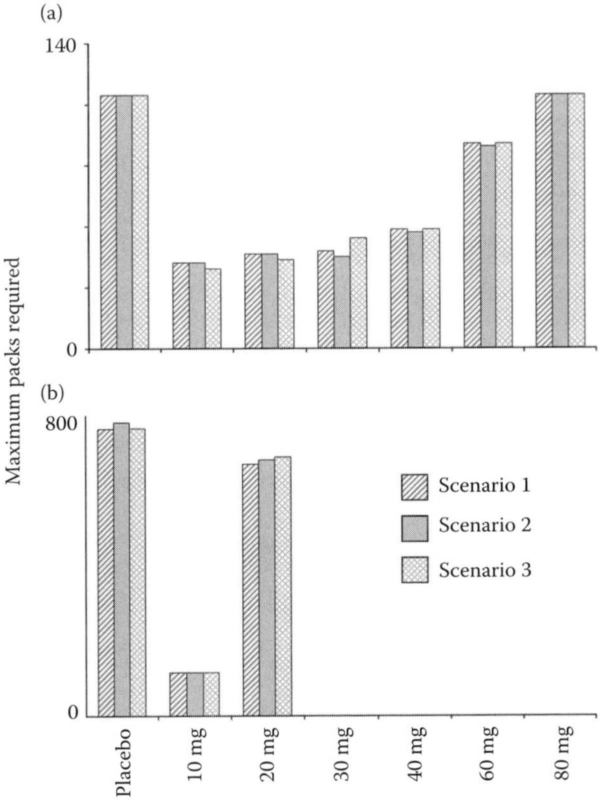

FIGURE 20.8 Simulated pack requirements for two packaging scenarios: (a) single unique pack per treatment group, and (b) flexible use of four packs (placebo, 10 mg or 20 mg) to make up each treatment group. (From Nicholls, G., Patel, N., and Byrom, B., *Applied Clinical Trials*, 6, 76–82, 2009. With permission.)

The purpose of describing this case study was to illustrate that simulation is an important tool to understanding and estimating medication requirements for adaptive clinical trials. To take advantage of this, simulation must be used early in the study design process so that supply forecasts can be used to inform production runs. In many studies it may be practical to estimate the amount of medication required to get a study started (e.g., to account for the first 6 months) and then simulate using study data the remainder of the trial to estimate the additional medication demand and use that to determine the timing and content of midstudy production runs. These midstudy simulations often use a snapshot of the IVR system database as an input as this contains a full picture of medication usage and location to date, the future demand of current subjects, and the recruitment rates observed to predict new subjects and their medication needs (Dowlman et al. 2004).

20.4 Drug Supply Management

When implementing a design adaptation that affects the allocation of future treatments, it is important not to simply consider the randomization implementation in isolation. When changing to a new allocation ratio, the changed proportion of subjects applied to each treatment has an impact on the future rate at which medication packs of the remaining treatments are required. A simple example is illustrated in Figure 20.9. In this case, the study is adjusted from a 1:1:1 ratio to a 2:0:1 ratio. This means that, assuming the site recruitment rate continues, there will be an increased demand for treatment group A medication moving forward, and it will be important to accommodate this effectively so as to avoid the possibility of having insufficient supplies at site.

As discussed previously in this chapter, IVR systems are an essential component of adaptive infrastructure in controlling both randomization and the medication supply chain. Typically, IVR systems automate the restocking of study sites by assigning trigger and stock levels for each pack type. When packs are allocated to subjects (or expire), stock eventually falls to the trigger level that causes the system to automate a request to resupply the site with the quantity of medication required to bring all pack types to their stock level. Trigger levels are estimated based upon the anticipated recruitment rate of the site and the time taken to deliver new stock, effectively a Poisson process where we seek to limit the possibility of more than the trigger level of arrivals within the delivery time. When applying a design adaptation, this effectively modifies our arrivals rate for various treatment types. In the example above (Figure 20.9) we now anticipate a doubling of recruitment into treatment group A, and hence we must increase the trigger level and stock level that the system uses to calculate stock requirements. This could be done automatically by the system on applying a change in the randomization method, or applied manually. What's important is that this is considered up

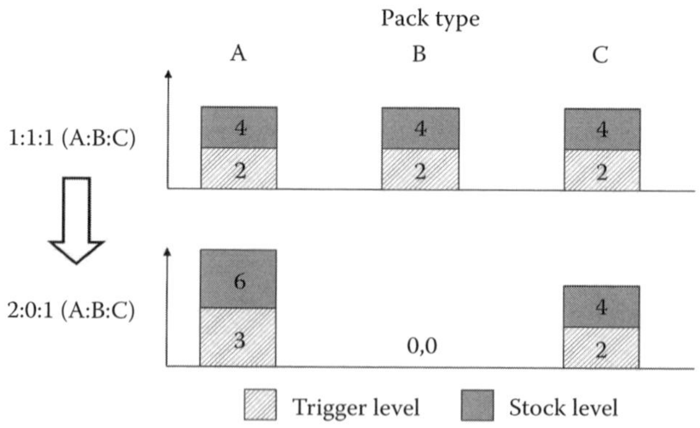

FIGURE 20.9 Adjustments to the site supply strategy following a design adaptation.

front and it is determined how the supply strategies for each site will be adjusted following a design adaptation.

It should be noted that, depending upon the study design methodology, adaptations may have a greater or lesser effect on the supply chain. A Bayesian response adaptive method that makes gradual adjustments on a regular basis is unlikely to result in a large change in the allocation ratios at any one instance. However, a design with fixed interim analyses where a number of dose groups may be terminated at a single point may have a much more sudden impact on the supply chain. In these cases it may be important to perform an assessment of current site supply adequacy before implementing the design change, and build in time to make site resupply shipments if required. Alternatively, it may be that ensuring that treatment groups are restocked to their stock levels prior to an adaptation would be optimal. In either case, flexible use of stock (as illustrated in the case study in the previous section) would be beneficial to prevent sudden urgent stock requirements.

20.5 Rapid Access to Response Data

Adaptive trials rely upon response data (efficacy and safety) from which to make rapid decisions regarding the future course of the study. Two questions arise as a consequence of this. First, how clean does the data need to be, and in particular, should interim analyses be conducted on only cleaned and verified data? Second, how should data be collected, given that there is a requirement to make data available electronically in a rapid manner to enable the independent statistician to conduct analyses, or to feed a Bayesian response adaptive algorithm?

20.5.1 How Clean Should the Data be?

It is clear that better data quality will lead to more reliable conclusions and decision making, so it is important that in all we do we strive to use the cleanest data possible in inference making. However, does this mean that all data we use need to be completely cleaned and verified before it is used to inform our design adaptations? The literature presents some compelling arguments to suggest that using more data is superior to using only completely cleaned data.

Reporting on the recommendations of the Pharmaceutical Research and Manufacturers of America (PhRMA) working party on adaptive trials, Quinlan and Krams (2006) state:

> The potential value of adaptive protocols is underpinned by timely data capture, interim analyses, and decision making. Timely data capture may be sufficient; real-time data capture would be ideal. Any discussions about data and interim analyses will raise questions about the level of data cleanliness. Ideally, we would aim for completely cleaned data sets for interims. Unfortunately, achieving this goal often introduces time delays that work against the potential benefits of adaptive designs. Given that only a small subset of "uncleaned" data will have to be changed eventually, we believe that "more data" are usually better than exclusively relying on "completely cleaned data. (p. 442)

Balancing the risks, Quinlan and Kram (2006) believe that more value can be obtained from a full data set rather than a reduced set of completely cleaned data. They also recommend that a sensitivity analysis would be useful in assessing the risk of uncleaned data:

> A simple way of assessing the risk of being misled by uncleaned data is to compare the results of analyses based on (1) the full data set (including uncleaned data points) and (2) the subset of completely cleaned data. (p. 442)

This is a position supported elsewhere in the literature. A good example was published by Simon Day and colleagues in 1998, in their examination of the importance of double data entry (Day et al. 1998). We summarized their simulation experiments in our own article (Byrom and McEntegart 2009). In essence, Day et al. (1998) explored the impact of increasing error rates in data on the conclusions made by inference tests. They considered tests on small samples with a range of error rates and a range of differences between simulated population means. They also explored the impact on test conclusions following the implementation of a simple range check on the data that corrected outliers. Their results can be summarized as follows:

- Data that were not corrected by a simple range check showed inflation of sample mean and variance, leading to significant loss of power and uncontrolled type 1 error.
- Data that had outliers corrected by employing a simple range check to detect them (still leaving around 50% of data errors, although these were of smaller magnitude not being detected by the range checks), showed little loss of power compared to the true data and good control of type 1 error.

In summary, they concluded that simple range checks enable us to detect and correct the main errors that impact the analysis results and conclusions, even among very small samples, and that those errors that cannot be easily detected in this way have little importance in drawing the correct conclusions from the statistical analyses. Similar conclusions were made by McEntegart, Jadhav, and Brown (1999) who provide analytical formula to estimate the loss of power in trials with range checks.

As we consider adaptive infrastructure, we believe it is important to consider methods to collect data that facilitate both rapid access to data but also the application of logic and range checking. As pointed out by Quinlan and Krams (2006) in the quotation above, real-time data capture would be an ideal approach:

> Real-time electronic data capture, accompanied by adequate resources and planning, can facilitate data quality as it allows for faster instream data cleaning. As a trial progresses, there will be relatively fewer unclean data at the time of any interim analysis. A pragmatic approach to this issue may involve prioritizing cleaning data that are most relevant to the decision making (e.g., the primary endpoint). (Quinlan and Krams 2006, pp. 442–443)

In the next section, we explore different data collection methods and their pros and cons, and make recommendations for adaptive trials.

20.5.2 Data Collection Methods

The need to facilitate rapid access and logic/range checking of data may influence our choice of data collection approach for an adaptive trial. Table 20.1 compares common approaches to clinical data collection, many of which have been used effectively in adaptive trials.

Paper data management suffers from speed of data access and checking, but there are strategies that can be used to mitigate this. For example, monitoring and data management can be scaled up when interim milestones are approached and data collection and cleaning focused primarily around endpoints used in the adaptive decision making. Intensive monitoring initially may increase the overall quality of data collected at site by early identification and elimination of issues. In addition, techniques such as direct mailing of CRFs can increase the speed at which data are received in-house.

Interestingly Fax/OCR (Krams et al. 2003) and IVR (Smith et al. 2006) have been used to speedily collect endpoint data in adaptive trials. Of the two, IVR (or its web-based equivalent—IWR) has the advantage of delivering range and logic checks directly to sites at the point of data entry, which facilitates quick data checking and cleaning. Both approaches are effective but require some additional data

TABLE 20.1 Comparison of Data Collection Methods for Adaptive Trials

	Paper	IVR/IWR	Fax/OCR	Digital pen	EDC	ePRO
Pro	Simple	Simple	Simple	Ease of data collection	Real-time error checks	Real-time error checks
	Inexpensive	Real-time error checks		Instant access to data	Full query management and data cleaning	True eSource data
		Combined with randomization				Instant access to data
Con	Slowest method	Simple endpoints only via phone interface (IVR)	Time consuming for sites	Data checks executed when data received in-house	Timeliness of data entry	Expense and support
	Data checks executed when data received in-house	Data reconciliation with clinical database required	Data checks executed when data received in-house	Not integrated with randomization	Expense and support	
			Not integrated with randomization	Hardware supply and support		
			Data reconciliation with clinical database required	Expense		

Source: Byrom, B., and McEntegart, D., *Good Clinical Practice Journal*, 16, 4, 12–15, 2009.

management activities in ensuring that the data collected is updated as the data originating on paper CRFs are cleaned and updated. This will require reconciliation of the adaptive analysis dataset with the clinical database at regular intervals.

The digital pen, aside from its use in cognitive testing, has little real value in clinical trials. Conceptually appealing as an early step into electronic data capture (EDC), it offers fast access to data but none of the other advantages inherent in other electronic data collection methods including important range checking at point of data entry. Using a digital pen, query logs are generated manually once data have been uploaded into a clinical database and may be as slow to resolve as with paper data collection.

EDC and ePRO (electronic Patient Reported Outcomes Solutions, used when the response is patient reported—such as pain severity recorded in a daily diary) have the advantage of real-time error and logic checking in addition to immediate data access. It is our recommendation that EDC and ePRO would be the solutions of choice although both have an implication on study budgets.

20.6 Data Monitoring Committees, the Independent Statistician and Sponsor Involvement

20.6.1 Data Monitoring

There is a long history of data monitoring in clinical trials for safety concerns, application of group sequential methods with the potential to cease a trial early if predefined efficacy criteria are reached and consideration of early cessation on the grounds of futility where a trial has little chance of establishing its objectives. Questions have included those trials that are appropriate for such monitoring, who should be knowledgeable of the data considered during the monitoring and who should input into any recommendations made and decisions taken. The answers to these questions are discussed in regulatory guidances and various textbooks, for example, Ellenberg, Fleming, and DeMets (2002). It seems reasonable that many of the practices established historically should also apply to modern adaptive trials, for example, clear establishment of charters and operating rules, documentation of meetings in a format suitable for subsequent regulatory inspection, and so on. But there are two areas in which adaptive trials are worthy of special consideration—these are the sponsor interface or participation with monitoring committees and the degree of extra expertise necessary. It can be argued that in adaptive trials the sponsor perspective may be more important than in traditional trials to fully provide the relevant knowledge for decision making, as would seem appropriate for learning trials, and also to factor in commercial considerations in certain situations. Before addressing the specific case of adaptive trials, it is instructive to review the historical context on the role of sponsor staff in trial monitoring.

20.6.1.1 Historical Context of Involvement of Sponsor Staff

Generally, it seems to have been accepted that major trials involving key safety endpoints should have DMCs that are independent of the sponsor. The concept of internal sponsor staff monitoring efficacy or safety comparisons is recognized by the ICH E9 Guidance but sponsors are cautioned to take particular care to protest the integrity of the trial and manage the sharing of information. The 2005 European Guideline on DMCs states that "it is obvious that, for example, employees of the sponsor who naturally have an interest in the trial outcome should not serve on a DMC" (p. 6). But it should be noted that this guidance is primarily aimed at safety monitoring in Phase III trials and thus maybe there is scope for internal DMCs for adaptive decision making in Phase IIb trials. Also this guidance was written in 2005 and much has transpired since then; thus the phrase that "major design modifications are considered exceptional" (p. 5) need not be taken too literally. If sponsor employees are involved in the analysis, the European guidance (CHMP 2007) requires that the documented working procedures clearly describe the measures to avoided dissemination of unblinded treatment information.

Similarly the 2006 FDA guidance on clinical trial data monitoring committees notes that when "the trial organizers are the ones reviewing the interim data, their awareness of interim comparative results cannot help but affect their determination as to whether such changes should be made. Changes made in such a setting would inevitably impair the credibility of the study results" (p. 5). There is a distinction made between trials monitoring major outcomes and those monitoring symptom relief in less critical conditions. The guidance notes that "the need for an outside group to monitor data regularly to consider questions of early stopping or protocol modification is usually not compelling in this situation" (p. 22).

While historically it seems accepted that sponsor staff should not be represented on independent DMCs, there has been less consensus about the interface between the sponsor and DMC. It is interesting to report on discussions following the issue of the ICH E9 guidance (Phillips et al. 2003). Specifically there was no consensus reached in a discussion group of European statisticians debating the practicality/desirability of an independent statistician/programmer generating the unblinding data reports for a DMC. Some delegates felt strongly that there should be no problem for the company statistician/programer to be involved in the generation of reports, others felt it should be done by someone external to the sponsor. Where there was consensus, however, was that the sponsor should recognize the burden of proof changes if an internal statistician/programer generates the unblinded reports. It was felt that ideally the internal statistician/programer generating the unblinding reports should not be on the project and ideally should be located at another site. It was agreed that reports should only be generated for the issues being considered by the DMC. Further, only the patients included in the reports should be unblinded.

20.6.2 Monitoring for Adaptive Designs

The topic has been extensively addressed by the PhRMA Working Group on Adaptive Designs and we draw heavily on their work. The logistical and operational considerations around monitoring were specifically addressed by Quinlan and Krams (2006). They proposed routinely to establish:

1. A DMC charged with the task of potentially looking at safety *and* efficacy data, evaluating risk-benefit, as well as assessing the functioning of algorithms that might be used in the conduct of the adaptive design. The traditional role of the DMC to monitor safety data in trials of serious conditions is thus being expanded to take over risk-benefit and the interpretation of results from any algorithms used in the adaptive component. Some specialist expertise might be needed to evaluate the aspects of the adaptive design, for example, a response adaptive Bayesian design. The expertise may relate to monitoring the adaptation algorithm or experience in making decisions that may be called for. Gallo (2006a) muses that it might be considered whether a separate monitoring group might be needed, one for safety and one for adaptation, especially if the trial will have a DMC in place for safety monitoring anyway. In our view this may be overly complex to coordinate unless there is a clear set of decision rules for the adaptation that can be mechanistically applied without regard to the overall risk-benefit, which is probably unlikely. Nevertheless this suggestion may be appropriate in certain situations as there is no one size fits all solution.
2. An independent statistical center (ISC) to prepare data, conduct interim analyses, and prepare a briefing document for discussion at the DMC. In our opinion quality control of the algorithms and programs used in performing interim analyses is primarily the function of the ISC but there should also be some involvement of the sponsor and DMC.
3. DMC charter and guidelines and appropriate standard operating procedures (SOPs) to ensure that the integrity and validity of the adaptive experiment can be maintained. We would expect that the DMC charter would detail clear guidelines for the DMC around decision making with as much planning for contingencies and "what ifs" as possible. SOPs should lay out the implementation in great detail. We envisage that adaptations occur by design, and therefore

it should be possible to clearly lay out the range of planned adaptations as well as the decision process leading to them. The charter should describe the remit of the DMC, ISC, and other bodies critical to the study infrastructure and which data are available for decision making, when, and to whom. Such a document not only makes the process of the information flow transparent, but also helps facilitate coordination and speed within the process. The charter should be finalized prior to study start, ideally at the time of finalization of the protocol. It should contain sufficient detail to explain the adaptive trial process to potential members of the DMC and ISC.

4. A contract formally establishing the need *not* to disclose unblinded information to parties other than the ones specified in the DMC guidelines. This would be signed by all members of the DMC, ISC, and other parties (including drug supply management) who are privy to unblinded information to reduce the risk of operational bias by building watertight firewalls between these unblinded bodies and everybody in the project team involved in the day-to-day running of the study.

Quinlan and Krams (2006) note that the DMC and ISC can be located either within the sponsor or external to the sponsor. There is more credibility if the DMC and ISC are external and independent from the sponsor, and this might be the appropriate approach in confirmatory trials. For internal decision-making projects in early development, it is more conceivable to set up these infrastructures internally to the sponsor as long as great care is given to establishing the firewall to the project team. One variant that may be appropriate in some cases is that the data preparation and statistical programing is done by the sponsor company using dummy treatment codes and that these materials are provided to the ISC who then merge on the real treatment code and run the official analyses. The advantage here is that the use of sponsor's standards creates efficiencies in that project rules, standards, and established code can be applied. The use of prevalidated code also allows/permits a degree of quality control by the sponsor—this may be more difficult logistically if an independent statistician/group is conducting the analyses.

It can be argued that in adaptive trials there is more motivation for some sponsor involvement than there is in nonadaptive confirmatory trials. As by definition less is known about the test treatments in adaptive trials, then the sponsor's knowledge could be a useful input into any decision making process. Similarly in larger, long-term trials with important commercial considerations, some sponsor input into the decision making process may be necessary. Again ideally such representation should be minimal and removed from the actual study team; Gallo (2006a) suggests just one or two senior managers will suffice and that these individuals will only have access to results at the time of adaptation decisions and will see only the results relevant to the decision with which they are assisting. Of course such involvement carries risks and confidentiality should be assured as far as possible with written procedures, SOPs, and firewalls. We would not expect sponsors to be usually represented on the DMC for confirmatory trials.

The literature provides examples of three models of operation. The ESCAMI trial (Zeymer et al. 2001) was a two-stage adaptive design in a life-threatening medical condition and thus had an independent advisory and safety committee and a separate independent ISC. The ASTIN trial in stroke (Grieve and Krams 2005) that used Bayesian response adaptive methods was run by an executive steering committee and an independent DMC with an expert Bayesian statistician who were responsible for all aspects of monitoring; that is, ensuring the safety of the patients, the integrity of the study, monitoring the performance of the algorithm, and confirming decisions to continue or stop the study according to the prespecified rules. In contrast the Smith et al. trial (2006) had a primarily internal committee for a dose finding trial in a less serious condition. In this trial the DMC consisted of two clinical experts in the therapeutic area (pain) and a statistician; two of the DMC were sponsor staff. A second internal statistician without voting rights on the panel prepared all the analyses.

20.7 Sample Size Reestimation

Within this chapter we concentrate primarily on those designs that alter the randomization mechanism including trials that drop or add doses or otherwise alter the randomization ratio on a regular or irregular basis. We do not include those trials where the only adaptive component is a sample size reestimation. This is because generally the preference is for blinded sample size reestimation as outlined in regulatory guidance (ICH E9 1998; CHMP guidance 2007) and the PhRMA working group (Chuang-Stein et al. 2006). Thus, such trials will not generally require much in the way of adaptive infrastructure as they can be carried out by sponsor personnel; of course such exercises should be planned and appropriately documented. But we note that the faster the data collection exercise the better the sample size reestimation process will be.

If a blinded exercise is undertaken then there is imprecision in the variance estimate from two sources:

1. Accidental bias caused by covariate imbalance if the covariates are not fitted in a model to estimate the variance—this will often be the case due to data not being clean or being conveniently located in a single database.
2. Inequality in the overall (study level) allocations to each treatment caused by incomplete blocks at each center/country/strata if a blocked randomized list is used.

A dynamic algorithm such as minimization could control both of these sources of noise by respectively balancing for the covariates/cofactors and an additional single level factor representing study level balance. Should this be considered desirable then clearly an electronic system of randomization will be needed to implement the dynamic algorithm. In passing we note that the use of such an algorithm could also help ensure that covariate imbalances do not affect the treatment effects over the course of the different phases of the trial. The European reflection paper on adaptive designs (CHMP 2007) notes that "studies with interim analyses where there are marked differences in estimated treatment effects between different study parts or stages will be difficult to interpret" (p. 6). This requirement has been challenged (Gallo and Chuang-Stein 2009) but nevertheless as a final regulatory guidance note it has to be carefully considered.

20.8 Case Study

Before concluding, we present a detailed case study that illustrates the planning required to meet many of the challenges we have described.

Eastham (2009) describes the operational aspects of a seamless adaptive Phase II to Phase III design currently being conducted. The Phase II trial is initiated with two active doses and a placebo comparator. The key features of the trial are described below.

At the end of Phase II, an independent DMC performs the analysis used prespecified criteria. The DMC makes recommendations about the further progression of the study. The possibilities are:

1. To stop the study and unblind all patients.
2. To stop the study but keep patients blinded. Effectively the study then becomes a standalone Phase II study.
3. To stop the study completely.
4. To drop one of the doses and continue the study with one active dose and placebo.
5. An extended review scenario where recruitment is halted and there is a pause for further endpoint incidence and then the DMC would reanalyze the study.

From the viewpoint of infrastructure and organization there are several interesting features of this trial.

A large amount of planning and detail was put into the DMC process. All decision criteria were prospectively agreed in advance including the stop/go rules for determining whether the trial should continue, the criteria for making the adaption and situations where the sponsor company would want to become unblinded. The principle was that there should be limited access to decision criteria in order to maintain the trial integrity. Thus there was limited access internally and no mention of the decision criteria in the protocol, statistical analysis plan, or at the investigator meeting. The Phase II analysis was to be performed by an independent statistician and the results were not to be shared with company personnel.

20.8.1 Operational Considerations

Operational aspects included the following.

- A 3-month period for decision making and implementation. Recruitment into the Phase II study was allowed to continue during this decision making period.
- A double dummy design for the supplies with patients in Phase II receiving two pack types (X + placebo Y, placebo X + Y, placebo X + placebo Y) and patients in Phase III receiving just one pack. So in this instance there was no attempt to hide the decision from the investigator and patients. The protocol design accounted for all possible outcomes in a "Go" scenario and described what will happen to patients from Phase II who are on the dose not progressed into Phase III. Detailed planning went into the communication with ethics committees. Detailed scenarios were documented for sending to the ethics committees at the end of Phase II; these included patient consent forms for new and ongoing patients according to the decision taken. The communications package included a letter to investigators, guidance document for investigators, ethics committee letter, a guidance document and cover letter for pharmacists, and a question and answer document. To maximize speed the packages for all scenarios were developed up front and translated—clearly this is a large amount of up-front planning.
- The study is implemented on an IVR system. The system was built flexibly so that all Phase II options are designed and tested at the beginning of Phase II. This includes planning for the investigational product kit changes that are necessary and the communication of the decision with the IVR system. In passing we note that generally options for the communication with the IVR system include written communication or a call from the data and safety monitoring board (DSMB) member—whichever form is chosen careful consideration needs to be given to the confirmation of the decision, for example, should independent calls be made by two DSMB members?

The topic of regulatory perspectives is covered elsewhere in this book, but it is interesting to view the questions received from health authorities that included questions on the appropriateness of combining an exploratory Phase II trial with a confirmatory Phase III trial, a desire to see the Phase II data before approving the progression to Phase III, and queries on the acceptability of continuing recruitment while the Phase II analysis is being conducted. But the study was accepted by health authorities.

20.9 Conclusions

Adaptive clinical trials provide enormous opportunity but also present new challenges to researchers. Our chapter describes the infrastructure required to conduct an effective adaptive clinical trial, and that has been effective in implementing such designs. Our final recommendation is not to be discouraged by these additional challenges, but to use the tools we describe in this chapter to ensure the value of these designs can be realized. We summarize below our recommendations in the form of an infrastructure checklist.

Adaptive Infrastructure Checklist

Challenge	Infrastructure Recommendation
Optimal study design	Use simulation techniques to explore different design alternatives and their operating characteristics.
Effective implementation of randomization changes	Utilize a central randomization solution such as an IVR system.
Maintain invisibility of design adaptations	Utilize IVR system.
	Employ double randomization techniques to ensure pack numbers dispensed and resupplied do not reveal that a treatment has been dropped or added.
	Consider using packaging and dispensing supplies in a way that kits can be allocated to more than a single treatment group.
Estimate drug supply requirements	Use supply chain simulation to estimate the quantity of supplies required under different trial outcomes.
Ensure all sites have sufficient medication supplies in place following a design change	Use IVR system and adjust site supply strategies based upon the revised allocation procedure.
Rapid access to response data	Where practically possible, use electronic data capture such as EDC and ePRO solutions (when key data are patient reported).
Ensuring data are as clean as possible when using adaptive decision making	Employ a data capture method that incorporates real-time data logic and range checks to enable erroneous data likely to impact decision conclusions to be reviewed and corrected.
Establish DMC and independent statistician roles	Establish with appropriate level of sponsor involvement and oversight, as described in Section 20.6 above.

References

Byrom, B., and McEntegart, D. (2009). Data without doubt: Considerations for running effective adaptive clinical trials. *Good Clinical Practice Journal,* 16 (4): 12–15. Available at http://www.perceptive.com/Library/Papers/Data_Without_Doubt.pdf. Accessed 1 February, 2010.

Chuang-Stein, C. (2006). Sample size reestimation: A review and recommendations. *Drug Information Journal,* 40: 475–84.

Committee for Medicinal Products for Human Use (CHMP). (2005). *Guideline on Data Monitoring Committees.* London: EMEA; Adopted July 27, 2005. Available at http://www.emea.europa.eu/pdfs/human/ewp/587203en.pdf. Accessed July 31, 2009.

Committee for Medicinal Products for Human Use (CHMP). (2007). Discussion of reflection paper on *Methodological Issues in Confirmatory Clinical Trials Planned with an Adaptive Design.* Adopted 18 October 2007. Available at http://www.emea.europa.eu/pdfs/human/ewp/245902enadopted.pdf. Accessed July 31, 2009.

Committee for Proprietary Medicinal Products. (2003). Points to consider on *Adjustment for Baseline Covariates.* CPMP/EWP/283/99. Available at http://www.emea.europa.eu/pdfs/human/ewp/286399en.pdf. Accessed July 31, 2009.

Day, S., Fayers, P., and Harvey, D. (1998) Double data entry. What value, what price? *Controlled Clinical Trials,* 19: 15–25.

Dowlman, N., Lang, M., McEntegart, D., Nicholls, G., Bacon, S., Star, J., and Byrom, B. (2004). Optimizing the supply chain through trial simulation. *Applied Clinical Trials,* 7: 40–46. Available at http://www.perceptive.com/Library/papers/Optimizing_the_Supply_Chain_Through_Trial_Simulation.pdf. Accessed July 31, 2009.

Eastham, H. (2009). Considering operational aspects of an adaptive design study. Talk at *SMI Adaptive Designs in Clinical Drug Development Conference,* February 4–5. Copthorne Tara Hotel, London, United Kingdom.

Ellenberg, S. S., Fleming, T. R., and DeMets, D. L. (2002). *Data Monitoring Committees in Clinical Trials.* Chichester: John Wiley & Sons.

FDA. (2006). *Guidance for Clinical Trial Sponsors on the Establishment and Operation of Clinical Trial Data Monitoring Committees.* Rockville, MD: U.S. Food and Drug Administration. Available at http://www.fda.gov/cber/gdlns/clintrialdmc.pdf. Accessed July 31, 2009.

Gallo, P. (2006a). Confidentiality and trial integrity issues for adaptive designs. *Drug Information Journal,* 40: 445–50.

Gallo, P. (2006b). Operational challenges in adaptive design implementation. *Pharmaceutical Statistics,* 5: 119–24.

Gallo P., and Chuang-Stein, C. (2009). What should be the role of homogeneity testing in adaptive trials? *Pharmaceutical Statistics,* 8 (1): 1–4.

Gaydos, B., Krams, M., Perevozskaya, I., Bretz, F., Liu, Q., Gallo, P., Berry, D., et al. (2006). Confidentiality and trial integrity issues for adaptive designs. *Drug Information Journal,* 40: 451–61.

Grieve, A. P., and Krams, M. (2005). ASTIN: A Bayesian adaptive dose–response trial in acute stroke. *Clinical Trials,* 2 (4): 340–51.

International Conference on Harmonisation (ICH). (1998). E-9 Document, Guidance on Statistical Principles for Clinical Trials. *Federal Register,* 63 (179): 49583–598. Available at http://www.fda.gov/cder/guidance/91698.pdf. Accessed July 31, 2009.

Jones, B., Atkinson, G., Ward, J., Tan, E., and Kerbusch, T. (2006). Planning for an adaptive design: A case study in COPD. *Pharmaceutical Statistics,* 5: 135–44.

Krams, M., Lees, K. R., Hacke, W., Grieve, A. P., Orgogozo, J-M., and Ford, G. A. (2003). Acute stroke therapy by inhibition of neutrophils (ASTIN). An adaptive dose–response study of UK-279,276 in acute ischemic stroke. *Stroke,* 34: 2543–48.

Lang, M., Wood, R., and McEntegart, D. (2005). Double-randomised packaging lists in trials managed by IVRS. *Good Clinical Practice Journal,* November: 10–13. Available at http://www.clinphone.com/files/item93.aspx. Accessed July 31, 2009.

Maca, J., Bhattacharya, S., Dragalin, V., Gallo, P., and Krams, M. (2006). Adaptive seamless phase II/III designs—Background, operational aspects, and examples. *Drug Information Journal,* 40: 463–73.

McEntegart, D. J. (2003). The pursuit of balance using stratified and dynamic randomisation techniques. *Drug Information Journal,* 37: 293–308. Available at http://www.clinphone.com/files/item81.aspx. Accessed July 31, 2009.

McEntegart, D. J., Jadhav, S. P., and Brown, T. (1999). Checks of case record forms versus the database for efficacy variables when validation programs exist. *Drug Information Journal,* 33: 101–7.

McEntegart, D., Nicholls, G., and Byrom, B. (2007). Blinded by science with adaptive designs. *Applied Clinical Trials,* 3: 56–64. Available at http://www.perceptive.com/files/pdf/item43.pdf. Accessed July 31, 2009.

Nicholls, G., Patel, N., and Byrom, B. (2009). Simulation: A critical tool in planning adaptive trials. *Applied Clinical Trials,* 6: 76–82. Available at http://www.perceptive.com/Library/papers/Simulation_A_Critical_Tool_in_Adaptive.pdf. Accessed July 31, 2009.

Peterson, M., Byrom, B., Dowlman, N., and McEntegart, D. (2004). Optimizing clinical trial supply requirements: Simulation of computer-controlled supply chain management. *Clinical Trials,* 1: 399–412.

Philips, A., Ebbutt, A., France, L., Morgan, D., Ireson, M., Struthers, L., and Heimann, G. (2003). Issues in applying recent CPMP "Points to Consider" and FDA guidance documents with biostatistical implications. *Pharmaceutical Statistics,* 2: 241–51.

Quinlan, J. A., and Krams, M. (2006). Implementing adaptive designs: Logistical and operational considerations. *Drug Information Journal,* 40: 437–44.

Smith, M. K., Jones, I., Morris, M. F., Grieve, A. P., and Tan, K. (2006). Implementation of a Bayesian adaptive design in a proof of concept study. *Pharmaceutical Statistics,* 5: 39–50.

Zeymer, U., Suryapranata, H., Monassier, J. P., Opolski, G., Davies, J., Rasmanis, G., Linssen, G., et al. (2001). The Na(+)/H(+) exchange inhibitor eniporide as an adjunct to early reperfusion therapy for acute myocardial infarction. Results of the evaluation of the safety and cardioprotective effects of eniporide in acute myocardial infarction (ESCAMI) trial. *Journal of the American College of Cardiology,* 38: 1644–51. Available at http://content.onlinejacc.org/cgi/reprint/38/6/1644.pdf. Accessed July 31, 2009.

21

Independent Data Monitoring Committees

Steven Snapinn
and Qi Jiang
Amgen, Inc.

21.1 Introduction

A data monitoring committee (DMC) is a group of individuals charged with monitoring the accumulating data of an ongoing clinical trial and taking actions based on their findings. The DMC's primary responsibility is typically to protect the safety of the trial participants by periodically reviewing the safety data, and, if they discover any unacceptable safety risks, recommending modifications to the study to alleviate that risk or termination of the study. The DMC can also go by a number of different names, such as data and safety monitoring board (DSMB) or ethical review committee (ERC), but the responsibilities are the same regardless of the name. DMCs have become relatively routine for many clinical trials, and there is a large literature on the topic, including several overview articles (e.g., Ellenberg 2001; Wilhelmsen 2002), two text books (Ellenberg, Fleming, and DeMets 2002; Herson 2009), and one book of case studies (DeMets, Furberg, and Friedman 2006). Pocock (2006) discussed some real-life challenges that can face a DMC. While many issues associated with DMCs apply equally to adaptive and nonadaptive trials, certain features of adaptive trials raise special issues with regard to the composition and functioning of a DMC.

In this chapter we describe DMCs and the general issues associated with them, with emphasis on the issues of most relevance to adaptive trials. These include the types of trials that require a DMC, the DMC's composition and responsibilities, and independence of the DMC. We focus on pharmaceutical industry-sponsored trials, since the industry is particularly interested in the use of adaptive trials. In addition, we discuss the special issues that DMCs face that are unique to adaptive trials, including special expertise required to make adaptive decisions, the potential for adaptive decisions to unblind study participants, and the need for sponsor involvement in the adaptive decision-making.

21.2 Overview of Data Monitoring Committees

21.2.1 History

The use of DMCs has been evolving over the past several decades. While some clinical trials have used some form of data monitoring since at least the 1960s, the modern notion of a DMC began to take shape after the National Heart Institute, which was part of the National Institutes of Health, commissioned the so-called Greenberg Report (1988), which was issued in 1967. Among the recommendations of this report were that the trial should be monitored by a group of experts independent from the individuals involved in conducting the trial, and that there should be a mechanism for early termination of the trial if the data warrant it.

One of the earliest trials to use an independent monitoring committee (known at the time as a policy board) was the Coronary Drug Project (The Coronary Drug Project Research Group 1973). Begun in 1965, this was a trial evaluating the efficacy of five lipid-lowering therapies in 8341 subjects. Responsibilities of the policy board included "to act in a senior advisory capacity to the [study investigators] in regard to policy questions on design, drug selection, ancillary studies, potential investigators and possible dropping of investigators whose performance is unsatisfactory" (DeMets, Furberg, and Friedman 2006, p.4).

DMCs were initially used primarily in government-sponsored trials, with little use by the pharmaceutical industry. However, more recently the pharmaceutical industry has been making greater and greater use of DMCs, and they are now relatively routine in industry-sponsored trials. Reasons for this shift may include the increasing number of industry-sponsored trials that address mortality or major morbidity endpoints, and the increasing collaboration between industry and government on major clinical trials (Ellenberg 2001). Two of the earliest industry-sponsored trials to use a DMC were the Cooperative North Scandinavian Enalapril Survival Study CONSENSUS (The CONSENSUS Trial Study Group 1987) and the cimetidine stress ulcer clinical trial (Herson et al. 1992) in 1988–1989.

21.2.2 Need for a DMC

While all trials require some form of monitoring, it is well accepted that not all trials require a formal DMC. Pharmaceutical companies run a large number of clinical trials, and it would not be practical or necessary for all of them to have a DMC. For example, Phase I and early Phase II trials are typically monitored by the study team, possibly to make dose escalation decisions. Later Phase II trials might be monitored for safety by a committee that is internal to the sponsor, but independent of the team directly responsible for the conduct of the study. In Phase III, however, fully independent DMCs are typical.

While there is no hard and fast rule, there are various factors that tend to determine whether or not a DMC is necessary. The most relevant factor is the seriousness of the medical condition; DMCs are most often used in trials in which the primary endpoint involves mortality or serious morbidity. According to Ellenberg (1996), DMCs tend to be used in trials where there is a lot at stake. The level of knowledge about the investigational agent is also important—clearly, it is more important to have a DMC early in the development program when less is known about the effects of the drug. Also, DMCs are more necessary in large trials of long duration than in small, short trials.

Another factor to consider is whether or not having a DMC is practical. If the trial is likely to be completed quickly there may not be an opportunity for the DMC to have any impact. However, if there are important safety concerns it may be preferable to have a DMC and build in pauses in the recruitment process to allow the DMC to adequately assess safety (FDA 2006).

There are many benefits to the pharmaceutical sponsor of having a DMC. They tend to give the trial credibility in the eyes of the medical community, and the DMC members can bring a great degree of experience and neutrality to the decision-making process. In addition, as we will discuss below, DMCs can play an important role in adaptive decision-making.

21.2.3 Composition

DMCs invariably include some number of clinicians with expertise in the specific therapeutic area under investigation, and most committees include a statistician as well. Among other disciplines sometimes included in a DMC are an ethicist, a patient advocate, or an epidemiologist. The typical size of a DMC ranges from three to seven members. One issue that will be discussed below is whether a DMC for an adaptive trial requires any special expertise.

21.2.4 Scope of Responsibilities

Clearly, all DMCs are involved in safety monitoring; in fact, that is usually the primary reason for their existence. However, they often have a variety of other responsibilities, and some of these can be somewhat controversial. DMCs often monitor efficacy data as well as safety, and many trials have boundaries the DMC can use as guidelines to recommend stopping the trial for overwhelming evidence of efficacy, or for futility. In order for a DMC to adequately protect patient safety they need to have access to accurate and timely data; therefore, it seems reasonable that the DMC should be able to assess how accurate and how timely the database is, and demand improvements if necessary. Another potential responsibility involves protocol adherence; for example, should the DMC check to see if all the sites are following the protocol, and recommend some action to the sponsor if one or more of the sites has a problem? One disadvantage of this is that, since the DMC is unblinded, every action they take can be influenced by knowledge of the interim results. Therefore, one could argue that any decisions that do not require knowledge of the interim results, like monitoring protocol adherence, should not be part of the DMC's responsibilities.

DMCs in industry-sponsored trials typically have a narrower scope than DMCs in government sponsored trials. For example, DMCs in government-sponsored trials are typically involved in trial design, evaluation of investigators, and publication policy, while this is less common in industry-sponsored trials (Herson 2009, p. 3). DeMets et al. (2004) discuss the issue of legal liability and indemnification for DMC members.

Of particular interest in this paper is the DMC's role in adaptive decision-making, which will be discussed below.

21.2.5 Independence of the DMC

As we will discuss below, the issue of independence is extremely important in the context of adaptive trials. In general, the purpose of having an independent DMC is to ensure that neither the decision-making nor the trial conduct is subject to inappropriate influences (Ellenberg 2001). Since a pharmaceutical sponsor has an important financial conflict pertaining to the conduct of a clinical trial, in a fully independent DMC no employees of the sponsor serve as members. DMC members are typically academic researchers who are not otherwise involved in the trial. The sponsor does usually have some involvement with the DMC: certain employees of the sponsor serve as liaisons to the DMC, and attend the DMC open session to keep the DMC up to date on issues they need to know, such as new information about the drug development program. However, the sponsor should remain blind to the study's results, and so the sponsor employees should not attend the closed session where those results are discussed. Califf et al. (2003) were not completely satisfied with this situation, mentioning that dependence on the sponsor for the data and for the meeting arrangements limits the DMC's independence. Lachin (2004) argues that conflicts of interest pose a low risk of threatening the integrity of a publicly financed trial, and, therefore, independence of the DMC is less important in this setting.

It is critical for the DMC to maintain confidentiality of the interim results. Fleming, Ellenberg, and DeMets (2002) discuss the potential damage to the trial if the results were to be disclosed. This includes prejudgment of the study's conclusions, resulting in an adverse impact on recruitment and adherence, and the potential for publication of the interim and final results to be inconsistent. Ellenberg (2001) also gives an example of a trial that suffered from this problem.

The DMC members should be free of substantial conflicts of interest. While it can be difficult to precisely define what constitutes a substantial conflict of interest, the concept is clear. For example, DMC members should not own a large amount of the sponsor's stock or of any of the sponsor's competitors.

One area of some controversy is who should prepare the interim reports. While DMCs almost always include a statistician as a member, the statistician is generally there because of that person's experience and insight, and the interim report is generally prepared by a separate statistician or statistical group. So, the question is whether the interim report should be prepared by the sponsor. While regulatory agencies do not prohibit this, they clearly frown upon it (Siegel et al. 2004; Committee for Medicinal Products in Human Use 2006; FDA 2006), and it is typical for the sponsor to hire an independent group, often a contract research organization (CRO), to prepare the report. However, not all of them do, and in fact one can make a reasonably strong case in favor of the sponsor preparing the report (Snapinn et al. 2004). Clearly, if the pharmaceutical sponsor is going to prepare the report, there needs to be a firewall, or clear separation between this individual or group and the study team involved with the conduct of the study. One clear advantage of this approach is that the sponsor is usually much more familiar with the study and the molecule than a CRO would be (Wittes 2004). In addition, Bryant (2004) argues that in the context of the National Cancer Institute Cooperative Group program, the Group study statistician should prepare the interim reports. However, DeMets and Fleming (2004) argue that the statistician preparing the interim report should be independent of the sponsor, and Pocock (2004) argues that major trials require three statisticians: the trial statistician, the DMC statistician, and the statistician who prepares the interim reports.

21.2.6 Setting Statistical Boundaries

DMCs are usually guided by prespecified stopping boundaries, although it is recognized that they are free to ignore those boundaries based on the totality of evidence in front of them. While efficacy boundaries based on the primary efficacy endpoint are usually prespecified, safety issues tend to be more unpredictable and so it is less common to have prespecified boundaries. This is usually more a judgment call by the DMC. However, if there are safety concerns that can be prespecified there is certainly an advantage to prespecifying the type of interim result that the DMC should act on; that will help avoid future disagreements between the DMC and the sponsor.

One tension faced when setting stopping boundaries for overwhelming efficacy is between making it fairly easy to stop (thus protecting the patients in the trial from an inferior treatment) or very difficult to stop (making it more likely that the trial will change medical practice and thus benefit future patients). This is the issue of individual versus collective ethics described by Ellenberg (1996). Either approach can be reasonable, as long as the protocol states the approach that will be followed so patients can be fully informed.

Some DMCs are chartered to monitor safety only, but find it difficult to do that without at least looking at the efficacy results, in order to help assess the risk-benefit ratio. That is, some interim safety findings might be important enough to stop the trial in the absence of an efficacy benefit, but not important enough in the presence of a huge efficacy benefit. In a situation like this it is usually best to include a very conservative stopping rule for overwhelming evidence of efficacy, such as a critical p-value of 0.0005. This protects the sponsor from a situation in which the DMC looks at the efficacy data without a stopping boundary but finds them so compelling that they recommend stopping the trial. Usually the stopping rule is based on a group sequential approach that provides the critical p-value necessary for the trial to stop. Another potential approach is to make the decision based on a conditional probability calculation; that is, the probability that the trial will ultimately be significantly positive, conditional on the results observed so far at the interim look.

21.3 Adaptive Trials and the Need for Data Monitoring

There are many different types of adaptation that can take place during the course of a clinical trial. Some of these types of adaptation do not involve unblinding the trial, such as certain sample size reestimation procedures or modification of the inclusion/exclusion criteria based on information external to the trial; as discussed above, these may or may not involve the DMC. Other types of adaptation that do involve unblinding, such as group sequential stopping rules, are generally handled by the DMC as part of their routine practice. However, there are several types of adaptation that do involve unblinding but fall outside of the DMC's usual responsibilities. This includes adaptive dose-finding decisions, seamless Phase II/III designs, and unblinded adaptive sample size reestimation procedures. These adaptations all require interim decisions to be made based on unblinded data, and therefore require data monitoring. Although the primary goal of a DMC is protection of patient safety, and these adaptations focus more on efficacy than on safety, the fact that the DMC is an independent and unblinding group monitoring the trial make this a natural venue for the adaptive decisions. In the next section we discuss some of the issues surrounding DMCs that are specific to adaptive trials.

21.4 DMC Issues Specific to Adaptive Trials

21.4.1 Composition of the Committee

As mentioned above, adaptive decision-making is outside of the usual set of DMC responsibilities. The specific skills required for adaptive decision-making may not be the same skills that are required for safety monitoring. Therefore, a typical DMC may not have the appropriate expertise to make adaptive decisions, and it may be necessary to include different or additional members on a DMC making adaptive decisions than would ordinarily be included. All members of the committee, particularly the statistician, must understand and be comfortable with the adaptive rules. It should be recognized that not all traditional DMC members will want to accept the responsibility of making adaptive decisions. Herson (2009, p. 124) recommends that before any review meeting where an adaptation is a possibility, the statistician should lead the clinicians through a decision matrix of steps that might take place contingent on the data. Gallo et al. (2006) also suggest that the DMC should review the adaptive algorithm's performance, and perhaps recommend changes to it. Another potential issue that seamless phase II/III adaptive designs can involve a very long-term commitment for DMC members that they may be unwilling to accept.

Gallo (2006a, 2006b) raises the issue of whether adaptive decisions should be made by a separate committee from the DMC. According to Gallo (2006b),

> Depending on the type of adaptation being addressed and the methodology being used, some additional expertise might be desirable that has not traditionally been represented on a DMC; thus, care should be taken to ensure that all relevant experience or expertise is represented on the monitoring committee. In an adaptive trial that would have a DMC in place regardless (say, for safety monitoring), it might be considered whether it is an optimal approach to have this DMC make adaptation decisions as well, or whether it is more appropriate for adaptation decisions to be made by a separate group of individuals. (p. 121)

As noted above, there is some controversy regarding who should perform the interim analysis; specifically, whether or not it should be performed by a statistician otherwise independent of the trial. While this is true for traditional interim designs, Coffey and Kairalla (2008) point out that the additional degree of complexity involved in adaptive calculations makes this debate even more important.

21.4.2 Need for Sponsor Involvement

One key advantage of DMCs is that they increase the credibility of the trial by allowing the sponsor to remain blinded to its results. However, some adaptive decisions, such as a decision to proceed from Phase II to Phase III, may be too important to a sponsor to allow them to be made in isolation by an external committee. According to Fleming (2006),

> Decisions about significant design changes ideally should be based on an understanding not only of the totality of the data regarding efficacy, safety, and quality of trial conduct, but also of other drug development considerations. If the complexity of this process leads to the need to provide such unblinded interim data to the investigators and sponsors, and not just the DMC, this would exacerbate the serious risks to trial integrity and credibility that result from the implementation of these adaptive monitoring procedures. (p. 3310)

Once unblinded to the interim results in order to make an adaptive decision, the sponsor would no longer have credibility to make other design changes based on information external to the trial. Even with special procedures in place to limit sponsor involvement, as we will discuss below, it is not clear that the scientific community would view that sponsor as sufficiently independent.

Hung et al. (2006) discuss the potential for operational bias that cannot be quantified statistically when interim results are known by the sponsor. They go on to propose having in place a standard operation procedure (SOP) that guides the conduct of all parties involved in the adaptive design. The SOP would cover issues such as who will see what data; how knowledge of the trial results will be protected from investigators, patients, and within the sponsor; and how to minimize any possible influence of the adaptive decisions on investigator and patient behavior.

Gallo (2006b) acknowledges that concerns about operational biases are equally relevant in the case of traditional interim decisions and adaptive interim decisions, and, therefore, the interim results should remain in the hands of a limited number of individuals in both cases. However, he also recognizes that the sponsor perspective may be important in some settings, to factor in the commercial implications of the potential decisions, for example. Recognizing that sponsor involvement in the adaptive decision-making process may be inevitable, he has four key recommendations: (1) the sponsor representatives should be a minimum number of individuals required to make the decision; (2) these individuals should not otherwise be involved in the trial; (3) these individuals should have access to results only at the times of adaptation decisions; and (4) appropriate firewalls should be in place to ensure that access to the results not be disseminated beyond those authorized to receive it (e.g., the trial team, investigators, steering committee). These recommendations were also discussed by Gallo (2006a), who also commented that sponsors must recognize the potential risks to the trial's integrity, and therefore should have all procedures and protections well-documented.

Gallo et al. (2006), representing a PhRMA working group, have similar recommendations. Specifically: (1) there should be a specific rationale provided for why sponsor ratification of a DMC recommendation is required (for example, business implications or the complex nature of the calculations); (2) there should be a firewall between sponsor personnel involved in the adaptive decision-making and other sponsor personnel; and (3) sponsor access to the interim results should be strictly limited to those required to make the decision.

Krams et al. (2007, p. 961), reporting on a 2006 PhRMA workshop on adaptive trials, recommend limited and controlled sponsor involvement in the DMC process if warranted by the nature of the adaptive decision. "This should involve a small number of designated individuals distanced from trial operations, receiving summary information on a limited basis particular to the need and according to a prespecified plan, and bound to confidentiality agreements and SOPs." This could involve a separate group within the sponsor to make adaptive decisions, separated by a firewall from other sponsor personnel. They contend that this approach will allow for better decision-making that benefits patients as well as sponsors, and that trial integrity can be adequately maintained. However, they acknowledge that more effort and experience are needed to define the appropriate operational models and processes.

It should also be recognized that not all pharmaceutical companies are alike, and firewalls and other procedures designed to protect the integrity of the trial may be feasible in larger companies, but not in smaller companies.

21.4.3 Potential for Adaptive Decisions to Unblind

All interim decision-making processes, including traditional processes, have the potential to convey information about the interim results to individuals involved in the trial, such as the sponsor, investigators, and subjects, who are meant to remain blinded. For example, the fact that a trial with a sequential stopping boundary is continuing suggests that the interim results are not extreme enough to cause the trial to terminate. However, there is concern that adaptive rules are particularly sensitive to this problem. As Fleming (2006) points out, adaptive decisions that are based on emerging information about treatment efficacy will tend to unblind the sponsor or others outside the DMC. For example, a particularly problematic approach would be a sample size reestimation procedure in which there is a one-to-one correspondence between the magnitude of the treatment effect observed at the interim analysis and the new sample size. In such a case, it would be a simple matter for the sponsor or an investigator to back-calculate the interim effect size from the sample size.

Gallo (2006a, 2006b) argues that similar standards should be applied to adaptive trials as are applied to traditional trials; that is, while steps should be taken to minimize the information that could be inferred by observers, the key question is whether the information conveyed by the adaptation is limited with regard to the magnitude of interim treatment effects. He also argues that any potential for the introduction of bias should be balanced against the advantages of the adaptive design, and points out that a seamless Phase II/III design can actually protect the confidentiality of the interim results better than a traditional design, since in a seamless Phase II/III design the Phase II results would not be broadly disseminated. Therefore, in this case, the adaptive approach is better at preserving equipoise than the traditional approach. To avoid the issue raised above, regarding the ability to invert a sample size reestimation rule in order to calculate the interim treatment effect size, he suggests basing the sample size changes on multiple considerations, perhaps including a nuisance parameter or incorporating new external information. He also suggests not providing full numerical details of action thresholds in protocols. While the protocol might describe the general approach, the precise details would be in a separate document with more limited circulation, such as the DMC charter.

This issue is also discussed by Gallo et al. (2006), representing a PhRMA working group. They point out that the potential for interim decisions to unblind study personnel to the interim results is not unique to adaptive trials, and that the same standard should be applied to traditional and adaptive trials. They also propose that steps should be considered in the protocol design stage to limit the potential for interim results to be inferred by observers. They feel that selection decisions (for example, the decision to select a dose or a patient population in a seamless Phase II/III design) or other adaptations that might provide information on the direction of the treatment effect, but not its magnitude, should be acceptable.

21.4.4 Other Issues

Herson (2008, 2009, pp. 120–124) discusses the potential conflict between an adaptive decision, typically based on efficacy data, and the accumulating safety data being reviewed by the DMC. While he seems to assume that there will be a committee separate from the DMC charged with adaptive decision-making, the same issues would apply if the DMC is responsible for the adaptive decision-making. One example he gives involves a three-arm trial (two experimental treatments plus a control) with an adaptive rule for dropping an experimental arm that appears to be ineffective. Suppose that the arm to be dropped appears to be safe, but the DMC has some concerns with the safety of the arm to remain; could this have any impact on whether or not the DMC should recommend termination of the trial? Another example is one in which the adaptive rule requires the allocation ratio to be changed (based on efficacy data) such that a greater fraction of patients will be assigned to the more toxic treatment. As another example, suppose the adaptive sample-size reestimation rule requires the size of the trial to be increased because the magnitude of the treatment benefit appears to be less than expected, but the safety profile of the treatment, while perhaps adequate for the larger treatment effect size, is not adequate for the smaller size.

Gallo et al. (2006) discuss an important logistical issue in the implementation of an adaptive trial: the requirement for rapid data collection, which is best achieved if the study endpoints have short follow-up time relative to the total study duration, and when an electronic data capture process is used. However, just as with traditional interim decision-making processes, they do not feel that adaptive decisions require fully cleaned data sets. Fleming (2006) raises the issue of the ethics of withholding interim results from subjects participating in the trial. In his view, if the sponsor feels that the interim results are informative enough to be the basis of an adaptive design change, then perhaps patients deserve this information as well. However, providing that information could undermine the trial by negatively impacting recruitment and adherence to study therapy. Coffey and Kairalla (2008) and Gallo et al. (2006) discuss the computational complexity of some adaptive procedures. The former also discuss the relative lack of well-documented, user-friendly software, but give some suggested packages.

21.5 Summary

Data monitoring committees play an important role in clinical trials, and their use in pharmaceutical industry trials has increased greatly over the past several years. These committees add a level of protection to trial participants, and their independence from the trial's sponsor helps protect the trial's integrity. Although there are certain issues associated with the use of DMCs in general, there are some issues specific to adaptive trials. These include the special expertise required to make adaptive decisions, the potential for adaptive decisions to unblind study participants, and the need for sponsor involvement in the adaptive decision-making. Increased experience with adaptive trials will be required in order for a consensus to form regarding these issues.

References

Bryant, J. (2004). What is the appropriate role of the trial statistician in preparing and presenting interim findings to an independent data monitoring committee in the U.S. cancer cooperative group setting? *Statistics in Medicine,* 23: 1507–11.

Califf, R. M., Morse, M. A., Wittes, J., Goodman, S. N., Nelson, D. K., DeMets, D. L., Iafrate, R. P., and Sugarman, J. (2003). Toward protecting the safety of participants in clinical trials. *Controlled Clinical Trials,* 24: 256–71.

Coffey, C. S., and Kairalla, J. A. (2008). Adaptive clinical trials: Progress and challenges. *Drugs in R&D,* 9: 229–42.

Committee for Medicinal Products for Human Use (CHMP). (2006). *Guideline on Data Monitoring Committees.* London: European Medicines Agency.

The CONSENSUS Trial Study Group. (1987). Effects of Enalapril on mortality in severe congestive heart failure: Results of the Cooperative North Scandinavian Enalapril Survival Study (CONSENSUS). *New England Journal of Medicine,* 316 (23): 1429–35.

The Coronary Drug Project Research Group. (1973). The Coronary Drug Project: Design, methods, and baseline results. *Circulation,* 47 (Supplement I): I1–I79.

DeMets, D. L., and Fleming, T. R. (2004). The independent statistician for data monitoring committees. *Statistics in Medicine,* 23: 1513–17.

DeMets, D. L., Fleming, T. R., Rockhold, F., Massie, B., Merchant, T., Meisel, A., Mishkin, B., Wittes, J., Stump, D., and Califf, R. (2004). Liability issues for data monitoring committee members. *Clinical Trials,* 1: 525–31.

DeMets, D. L., Furberg, C. D., and Friedman, L. M. (2006). *Data Monitoring in Clinical Trials: A Case Studies Approach*. New York: Springer.

Ellenberg, S. (1996). The use of data monitoring committees in clinical trials. *Drug Information Journal*, 30: 553–57.

Ellenberg, S. S. (2001). Independent data monitoring committees: Rationale, operations and controversies. *Statistics in Medicine*, 20: 2573–83.

Ellenberg, S. S., Fleming, T. R., and DeMets, D. L. (2002). *Data Monitoring in Clinical Trials: A Practical Perspective*. Chichester: John Wiley.

FDA. (2006). *Guideline for Clinical Trial Sponsors: Establishment and Operation of Clinical Trial Data Monitoring Committees*. Rockville, MD: U.S. Food and Drug Administration.

Fleming, T. R. (2006). Standard *versus* adaptive monitoring procedures: A commentary. *Statistics in Medicine*, 25: 3305–12.

Fleming, T. R., Ellenberg, S., and DeMets, D. L. (2002). Monitoring clinical trials: Issues and controversies regarding confidentiality. *Statistics in Medicine*, 21: 2843–51.

Gallo, P. (2006a). Confidentiality and trial integrity issues for adaptive trials. *Drug Information Journal*, 40: 445–50.

Gallo, P. (2006b). Operational challenges in adaptive design implementation. *Pharmaceutical Statistics*, 5: 119–24.

Gallo, P., Chuang-Stein, C., Dragalin, V., Gaydos, B., Krams, M., and Pinheiro, J. (2006). Adaptive designs in clinical drug development—An executive summary of the PhRMA Working Group. *Journal of Biopharmaceutical Statistics*, 16: 275–83.

Greenberg Report. (1988). A report from the heart special project committee to the National Advisory Heart Council, May 1967. *Controlled Clinical Trials*, 9: 137–48.

Herson, J. (2008). Coordinating data monitoring committees and adaptive clinical trial designs. *Drug Information Journal*, 42: 297–301.

Herson, J. (2009). *Data and Safety Monitoring Committees in Clinical Trials*. Boca Raton, FL: Chapman & Hall/CRC Press.

Herson, J., Ognibene, F. P., Peura, D. A., and Silen, W. (1992). The role of an independent data monitoring board in a clinical trial sponsored by a pharmaceutical firm. *Journal of Clinical Research and Pharmacoepidemiology*, 6: 285–92.

Hung, H. M. J., O'Neill, R. T., Wang, S.-J., and Lawrence, J. (2006). A regulatory view on adaptive/flexible clinical trial design. *Biometrical Journal*, 48: 565–73.

Krams, M., Burman, C.-F., Dragalin, V., Gaydos, B., Grieve, A. P., Pinheiro, J., and Maurer, W. (2007). Adaptive designs in clinical drug development: Opportunities, challenges and scope: Reflections following PhRMA's November 2006 workshop. *Journal of Biopharmaceutical Statistics*, 17: 957–64.

Lachin, J. M. (2004). Conflicts of interest in data monitoring of industry versus publicly financed clinical trials. *Statistics in Medicine*, 23: 1519–21.

Pocock, S. J. (2004). A major trial needs three statisticians: Why, how and who? *Statistics in Medicine*, 23: 1535–39.

Pocock, S. J. (2006). Current controversies in data monitoring for clinical trials. *Clinical Trials*, 3: 513–21.

Siegel, J. P., O'Neill, R. T., Temple, R., Campbell, G., and Foulkes, M. A. (2004). Independence of the statistician who analyses unblinded data. *Statistics in Medicine*, 23: 1527–29.

Snapinn, S., Cook, T., Shapiro, D., and Snavely, D. (2004). The role of the unblinded sponsor statistician. *Statistics in Medicine*, 23: 1531–33.

Wilhelmsen, L. (2002). Role of the Data and Safety Monitoring Committee (DSMC). *Statistics in Medicine*, 21: 2823–29.

Wittes, J. (2004). Playing safe and preserving integrity: Making the FDA model work. *Statistics in Medicine*, 23: 1523–25.

22

Targeted Clinical Trials

Jen-Pei Liu
National Taiwan University and Institute of Population Health Sciences

22.1 Introduction

For traditional clinical trials, the inclusion and exclusion criteria for the intended patient population include clinical endpoints and clinical-pathological signs or symptoms. However, despite the efforts to reduce the heterogeneity of patients, substantial variation exists in the responses to the new treatment even for the patients meeting the same inclusion and exclusion criteria. Because these endpoints and clinical signs or symptoms are not well correlated with the clinical benefits of the treatments in the patient population defined by clinical-based inclusion and exclusion criteria, the current paradigm for the development of a drug or a treatment uses a shot-gun approach that may not be beneficial for most patients. One of the reasons is that the potentially important genetic or genomic variability of the trial participants is not utilized by the traditional inclusion/exclusion criteria.

New breakthrough technology such as microarrays, mRNA transcript profiling, single nucleotide polymorphisms (SNP), and genome-wide association studies (GWAS) have emerged in a rapid speed since the completion of the human genome project. Molecular disease targets can be identified and treatments specific for the molecular targets can therefore be developed for the patients who are most likely to benefit. These treatments are referred to as targeted therapy or targeted modalities. Unlike the shot-gun blast approach, a precision guided-missile methodology is employed by the targeted therapy to reach the molecular disease targets. Hence, personalized medicine can finally become a reality (FDA 2007a, 2007b).

The development of targeted modalities requires: (a) the knowledge of the molecular targets involved in the disease pathogenesis; (b) a device for detecting the molecular targets; and (c) a treatment aimed at the molecular targets. Hence, the development of targeted therapies involves evaluation of the translational ability from molecular disease targets to the treatment modalities for the patient population with the targets. To address these new challenges in clinical research and development, the U.S. Food and Drug Administration (FDA) recently issued the draft "Drug-Diagnostic Co-development Concept Paper" (FDA 2005). The three designs in Figure 22.1 were introduced in the FDA draft concept paper. One of the three designs is the enrichment design given as Design A in Figure 22.1 (Chow and Liu 2004). For the targeted trials using an enrichment design, only those patients with a positive result for the disease molecular target by a validated diagnostic device are randomized to receive either the targeted treatment or the concurrent control.

However, in practice, no diagnostic test is perfect with 100% positive predicted value (PPV). For example, Mammaprint, a Class II device based on a microarray platform approved by the FDA in 2007

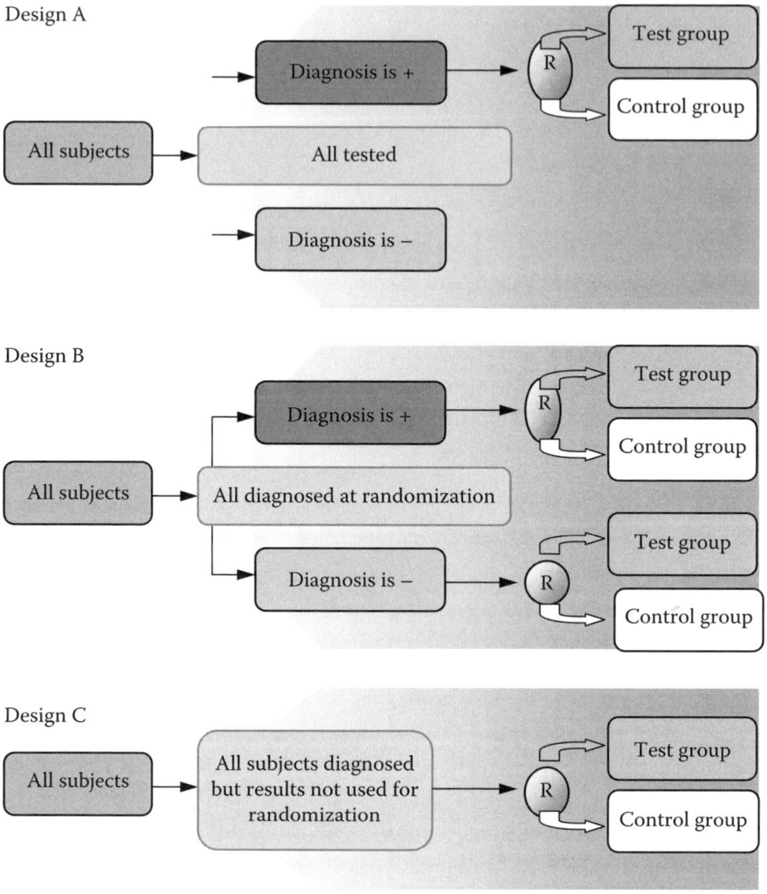

FIGURE 22.1 Designs for targeted trials in drug-diagnostic codevelopment concept paper. (From FDA. *The Draft Concept Paper on Drug-Diagnostic Co-Development.* Rockville, MD: U.S. Food and Drug Administration, 2005.)

for metastatic disease of breast cancer has a PPV only of 0.29 for 10-year metastatic disease. In addition, measures for diagnostic accuracy such as sensitivity, specificity, PPV, and a negative predicted value (NPV) are in fact estimators with variability. Therefore, some of the patients enrolled in targeted clinical trials under the enrichment design might not have the specific targets and hence the treatment effects of the drug for the molecular targets could be under-estimated (Chow and Liu 2004). In the next section, we will first provide some examples of targeted clinical trials on breast cancer that are being currently conducted. Next, examples of the inaccuracy of diagnostic devices for molecular disease targets are presented in Section 22.3. Under the enrichment design, in Section 22.4, we review the methods proposed by Liu and Lin (2008) and Liu, Lin, and Chow (2009) to incorporate the accuracy of the diagnostic device and its uncertainty in detecting the molecular targets for the inference of the treatment effects with binary and continuous endpoints. Simulation results of both continuous and binary data are given in this section. A discussion and concluding remarks are given in Section 22.5.

22.2 Examples of Targeted Clinical Trials

22.2.1 ALTTO Trial

The human epidermal growth factor receptor (*HER2*) is a growth factor receptor gene that encodes the *HER2* protein found on the surface of some normal cells that play an important role in the regulation of cell growth. Tumors with over expressed *HER2* are more likely to recur, and patients have a statistically significantly shorter progression-free survival (PFS) and overall survival (OS; Seshadri et al. 1993; Ravdin and Chamness 1995). Because the over-expression of the *HER2* gene is a prognostic and predictive marker for clinical outcomes, it provides a target to search for an inhibitor of the *HER2* protein as a treatment for patients with metastatic breast cancer. Herceptin is a recombinant DNA-derived humanized monoclonal antibody that selectively binds with high affinity in a cell-based assay to the extracellular domain of the *HER2* protein. Its effectiveness and safety in patients with metastatic breast cancer with an over-expressed *HER2* protein have been confirmed in several large-scale, randomized Phase III trials (Slamon et al. 2001).

Some patients do not respond or develop a resistance to the treatment of Herceptin despite the fact that it is efficacious for patients with an over-expression of the *HER2* gene. On the other hand, Lapatinib is a small molecule and a tyrosine kinase inhibitor that binds to part of the *HER2* protein beneath the surface of the cancer cell. It may have the ability to cross the blood–brain barrier to treat the spread of breast cancer to the brain and the central nervous system. Currently both Herceptin and Lapatinib are approved to treat these patients that have cancer with an over-expression of the *HER2* gene. However, the questions of which agent is more effective, which drug is safer, whether additional benefits can be obtained if two agents are administrated together, and in what order still remain unanswered. To address these issues, the U.S. National Cancer Institute and the Breast International Group (BIG) have launched a new study dubbed Adjuvant Lapatinib and/or Trastuzumab Treatment Optimization (ALTTO) trial. This is a randomized, open-label, active control, and parallel study conducted in 1300 centers of 50 countries with a preplanned enrollment of 8000 patients (ALTTO Trial 2009a, 2009b, 2009c). Since the *HER2* gene is a prognostic and predictive molecular target for clinical outcomes such as overall survival or progression-free survival, over-expression and/or amplification of the *HER2* gene in the invasive component of the primary tumor must be confirmed by a central laboratory prior to randomization. The immunohistochemical (IHC) assay is used to detect the over-expression, and fluorescent *in situ* hybridization (FISH) is employed to identify *HER2* gene amplification in the ALTTO Trial with the following criteria:

a. 3+ over-expression by IHC (> 30% of invasive tumor cells)
b. 2+ or 3+ (in 30% or less neoplastic cells) over-expression by IHC and FISH test demonstrating *HER2* gene amplification
c. HER2 gene amplification by FISH (> 6 *HER2* gene copies per nucleus or a FISH ratio of greater than 2.2)

The four treatments are

1. Standard treatment of Herceptin for 1 year
2. Lapatinib alone for 1 year
3. Herceptin for 12 weeks, followed by a washout period of 6 weeks and then Lapatinib for 34 weeks
4. Herceptin and Lapatinib together for 1 year

The primary endpoint of the ALTTO study is the disease-free survival and the secondary endpoints include overall survival, serious or severe adverse events, cardiovascular events such as heart attacks and strokes, and incidence of brain metastasis.

22.2.2 TAILORx Trial

Currently, reliable predictors for the clinical outcomes of the patients with breast cancer include the absolute expression levels of estrogen receptor (ER), those of the progesterone receptor (PR, an indicator of ER pathway), and involvement of the lymph nodes. ER positive and lymph node negative breast cancers occur is over half of newly diagnosed patients. The current standard treatment practice for 80–85%

of these patients is the surgical incision of the tumor followed by radiation and hormonal therapy. Chemotherapy is also recommended for most of these patients. However, the toxic chemotherapy benefits only a very small proportion of these patients. In addition, no accurate method exists for predicting the necessity of chemotherapy for individual patients. Therefore, the ability to accurately predict the outcome of chemotherapy for an individual patient should significantly advance the management of this group of patients and to achieve the goal of personalized medicine.

Oncotype DX is a reverse-transcriptase-polymerase-chain-reaction (RT-PCR) assay that transforms the levels of expression of 21 genes into a recurrence score (RS) with a range from 0 to 100; the higher the score, the higher the risk of recurrence of tumors in the patients receiving hormonal therapy (Paik et al. 2004). Based on the encouraging results provided by Paik et al. (2006), in 2006, the U.S. National Cancer Institute (NCI) launched the Trial Assigning Individualized Options for Treatment Rx (TAILORx) trial to investigate whether genes that are frequently associated with a risk of recurrence for patients of early-stage breast cancer can be employed to assign patients to the most appropriate and effective treatment (TAILORx, 2006). The TAILORx, trial intends to enroll around 10,000 patients with early stage breast cancer. Based on their RSs, the patients are classified into three groups with different treatments:

1. The patients with an RS greater than 25 will receive chemotherapy plus hormonal therapy.
2. The patients with an RS lower than 11 will be given hormonal therapy alone.
3. The patients with an RS between 11 and 25 inclusively will be randomly assigned to hormonal therapy alone or to chemotherapy plus hormonal therapy.

To address the issue of necessity of chemotherapy for the patients with ER positive and lymph node-negative breast cancer, one of the three primary objectives of the TAILORx trial is to compare the disease-free survival (DFS) of the patients with previously resected axillary-node negative breast cancer with an RS of 11–25 treated with adjuvant combination chemotherapy and hormonal therapy versus adjuvant therapy alone. The primary outcomes of the TAILORx trial consist of:

a. Disease-free survival
b. Distant recurrence-free survival
c. Recurrence-free survival
d. Overall survival

22.2.3 MINDACT Trial

For similar reasons as the TAILORx trial, the Microarray In Node negative Disease may Avoid ChemoTherapy (MINDACT) trial is a prospective, randomized study sponsored by the European Organization for Research and Treatment of Cancer (EORTC) to compare the 70 gene expression signatures with common clinical-pathological criteria in selecting for adjuvant chemotherapy in node negative breast cancer (The MINDACT Trial 2009). The MINDACT trial employs a device called MammaPrint, approved by the FDA in February 2007 as a Class II device. Based on the microarray platform, it is a qualitative in vitro diagnostic test that yields a correlation, denoted as a MammaPrint index, between the expression profiles of 70 genes from fresh frozen breast cancer tissue samples with that of the low risk template profile (van't Veer et al. 2002; Van de Vijver et al. 2002; Buyse et al. 2006). Tumor samples with a MammaPrint index equal to or less than +0.4 are classified as high risk of distant metastasis. Otherwise, tumor samples are classified as low risk.

One of the primary objectives for the MINDACT trial is to compare the clinical outcomes of treatment decisions selected for the patients with discordant results on the risk of distant metastasis between clinical-pathological evaluation and the 70 gene signatures (randomization-treatment decision component). The patients with discordant results on the risk of distant metastasis will then be randomized to a test arm or to a control arm. The test arm is to employ the results on the risk of distant metastasis based on the 70 gene signatures from the MammaPrint to determine whether the patients will receive the adjuvant chemotherapy or the less aggressive endocrine therapy. On the other hand, for the control arm, the traditional clinical-pathological evaluation will be used to select the treatments, either chemotherapy or endocrine therapy for the patients with discordant results. The primary endpoint for the randomization-treatment decision component is the distant metastasis free survival (DMFS).

22.3 Inaccuracy of Diagnostic Devices for Molecular Targets

Herceptin was approved by the FDA as a single agent with one or more chemotherapies or in combination with Paclitaxel for treatment of patients with metastatic breast cancer whose tumors over-express the *HER2* protein. In addition, in the U.S. package insert, Herceptin should be used when tumors have been evaluated with an assay validated to predict *HER2* protein over-expression. The clinical trial assay (CTA) was an investigational IHC assay used in the Herceptin clinical trials. The CTA uses a four-point ordinal score system (0, 1+, 2+, 3+) to measure the intensity of expression of the *HER2* gene. A score of 2+ is assigned to weak-to-moderate staining of the entire tumor-cell membrane for the *HER2* in more than 10% of tumor cells. Patients with more than moderate staining in 10% of tumor cells have a CTA score of 3+. Only those patients with a CTA score of 2+ or 3+ were eligible for the Herceptin clinical trials (Slamon et al. 2001). Summarized from results in Study 3 given in the U.S. package insert of Herceptin, Table 22.1 provides relative risks of mortality between the Herceptin plus chemotherapy arm and the chemotherapy arm alone as a function of *HER2* over-expression by CTA (FDA 2006). The relative risk of mortality for the 469 patients with a CTA +2 or above is 0.8 with a corresponding 95% confidence interval from 0.64 to 1.00. Therefore, the treatment effect of the Herceptin plus chemotherapy arm is barely statistically significant at the 0.05 level because the upper limit of the 95% confidence interval is 1. On the other hand, for the 329 patients with a CTA score of 3+ , the relative risk for mortality is 0.70 with the corresponding 95% confidence interval from 0.51 to 0.90. Therefore, Herceptin plus chemotherapy provides a superior clinical benefit in terms of survival over chemotherapy alone in this group of patients. However, for the 120 patients with a CTA score of 2+ , the relative risk for mortality is 1.26 with corresponding 95% confidence intervals from 0.82 to 1.94. These results imply that Herceptin plus chemotherapy may not provide additional survival benefit for patients with a CTA score of 2+.

Table 22.2 provides concordant results on the detection of over-expression of the *HER2* gene between CTA and the DAKO HercepTest (FDA 1998), one of the IHC assays approved by the FDA and cited in the package insert of Herceptin. DAKO HercepTest is also an IHC assay with the same four-point ordinal score system as the CTA. Because the results of these assays have significant impact on clinical outcomes such as death or serious adverse events, they are classified as Class III devices that require clinical trials as mandated by the premarket approval (PMA) of the FDA. From Table 22.2, considerable inconsistency in identification of over-expression of the *HER2* gene exists between CTA and DAKO HercepTest. For example, if a cut-off of > = 2+ is used for detection of over-expression of the *HER2* gene, then a total of 21.4% (117/548) of the samples have discordant results between CTA and the DAKO HercepTest. In other

TABLE 22.1 Treatment Effects as a Function of the *HER2* Over-expression

HER2 Assay Result	No. of Patients	RR for Mortality (95% CI)
CTA 2+ or 3+	469	0.80 (0.64, 1.00)
CTA 2+	120	1.26 (0.82, 1.94)
CTA 3+	329	0.70 (0.51, 0.90)

Source: Summarized from FDA. *Annotated Redlined Draft Package Insert for Herceptin®*. Rockville, MD: U.S. Food and Drug Administration, 2006.

TABLE 22.2 Concordant Result in Detection of *HER2* Gene

Comparison: DAKO HercepTest vs. Clinical Trial Assay					
HercerpTest	≤	1	2	3	Total
≤1	215	(39.2%)	50 (9.1%)	8 (1.5%)	273 (49.8%)
2	53	(9.7%)	57 (10.4%)	16 (2.9%)	126 (23.0%)
3	6	(1.1%)	36 (6.6%)	107 (19.5%)	149 (27.2%)
Total	274	(50.0%)	143 (26.1%)	131 (23.9%)	548

Sources: FDA. *Decision Summary P980018*. Rockville, MD: U.S. Food and Drug Administration, 1998.

words, due to different results in detection of over-expression of the *HER2* gene, an incorrect decision for selection of treatments will be made for at least one out of five patients with metastasis breast cancer. If a more stringent threshold of 3+ is used, discordant results still occur in 12.1% of the samples.

In addition, from the decision summary of HercepTest (P980018), the findings of inter-laboratory reproducibility studies showed that 12 of 120 samples (10%) had discrepancy results between 2+ and 3+ staining intensity. It follows that some patients tested with a score of 3+ may actually have a score of 2+ and the patients tested with a score of 2+ may in fact have a score of 3+ . As a result, the patient population defined by these assays are not exactly the same as those who truly have the molecular targets and will benefit from the treatments. As a result, because the patients with a CTA score of 3+ may in fact have a score of 2+ , the treatment effect of the Herceptin plus chemotherapy in terms of relative risk for mortality given in Table 22.1 is underestimated for the patients truly with over-expression of the *HER2* gene.

As mentioned above, MammaPrint is a Class II device approved by the FDA to assess a patient's risk of distant metastasis based on a 70 gene signatures. The PPV is computed based on the data of the TRANSBIG study (Buyse et al. 2006). In decision summary of MammaPrint, the PPV is the probability that metastatic disease occurs within a given time frame given the device output for that patient that is high risk (FDA 2007c). For the metastatic disease at 10 years, the TRANSBIG trial provides an estimate of 0.29 for the PPV with a 95% confidence interval from 0.22 to 0.35. In other words, the patients testing positive for high risk using the MammaPrint do in fact have a 71% probability that the metastatic disease will not occur within 10 years and may receive unnecessary chemotherapy from which these patients will not benefit. Therefore, a futile result from the component of chemotherapy randomization of the MINDACT trial does not mean that the chemotherapy is not effective for the patients truly with a high risk of metastasis. This is because 71% of the patients that tested positive for high risk of distant metastasis by the MammaPrint in fact are not at high risk at all, and the treatment effect of chemotherapy may be underestimated for patients truly at a high risk of distant metastasis.

22.4 Inference for Treatment Under Enrichment Design

For the purpose of illustration and simplicity, only the situation where a particular molecular target involved with the pathway in pathogenesis of the disease has been identified and there is a validated diagnostic device available for detection of the identified molecular target is considered here. Suppose that, a test drug for the particular molecular target is currently being developed. Under an enrichment design, one of the objectives of the targeted clinical trials is to evaluate the treatment effects of the molecular targeted test treatment in the patient population with the true molecular target. With respect to Figure 22.1 we consider a two-group parallel design in which patients with a positive result by the diagnostic device are randomized in a 1:1 ratio to receive the molecular targeted test treatment (T) or a control treatment (C). We further assume that the primary efficacy endpoint is an approximate

TABLE 22.3 Population Means by Treatment and Diagnosis

Positive Diagnosis	True Target Condition	Accuracy of Diagnosis	Test Group	Control Group	Difference
	+	γ	μ_{T+}	μ_{C+}	$\mu_{T+} - \mu_{C+}$
+	−	$1 - \gamma$	μ_{T-}	μ_{C-}	$\mu_{T-} - \mu_{C-}$

Source: Liu, J. P., Lin, J. R., and Chow, S. C., *Pharmaceutical Statistics*, 6, 356–70, 2009.
Note: γ is the PPV.

normally distributed variable, which is denoted by Y_{ij}, $j = 1, \ldots, n_i$; I = *T*, *C*. Table 22.3 gives the expected values of Y_{ij} by treatment and diagnostic result of the molecular target. In Table 22.1, μ_{T+}, μ_{C+} (μ_{T-}, μ_{C-}) are the means of test and control groups for the patients truly with (without) the molecular target. Our parameter of interest is the treatment effects for the patients truly having the molecular target $\theta = \mu_{T+} - \mu_{C+}$. The hypothesis for detection of treatment difference in the patient population with the true molecular target is the hypothesis of interest:

$$H_0: \mu_{T+} - \mu_{C+} = 0 \quad vs. \quad H_a: \mu_{T+} - \mu_{C+} \neq 0. \tag{22.1}$$

Let $\bar{y}_T$ and $\bar{y}_C$ be the sample means of test and control treatments, respectively. Liu and Chow (2004) showed that

$$E(\bar{y}_T - \bar{y}_C) = \gamma(\mu_{T+} - \mu_{C+}) + (1-\gamma)(\mu_{T-} - \mu_{C-}), \tag{22.2}$$

where γ is the PPV.

Liu and Chow (2008) indicated that the expected value of the difference in sample means consists of two parts. The first part is the treatment effects of the molecular target drug in patients with a positive diagnosis who truly have the molecular target of interest. The second part is the treatment effects of the patients with a positive diagnosis but in fact they do not have the molecular target. It follows that the difference in sample means obtained under the enrichment design for targeted clinical trials actually underestimates the true treatment effects of the molecular targeted drug in the patient population with the true molecular target of interest if $\mu_{T+} - \mu_C + > \mu_{T-} - \mu_{C-}$. As it can be seen from ALTTO Trial (2009b), the bias of the difference in the sample means decreases as the PPV increases. On the other hand, the PPV of a diagnostic test increases as the prevalence of the disease increases (Fleiss 2003). For a disease that is highly prevalent, say greater than 10%, even with a high-diagnostic accuracy of a 95% sensitivity and a 95% specificity for the diagnostic device, the PPV is only about 67.86%. It follows that the downward bias of the traditional difference in sample means could be substantial for estimation of treatment effects of the targeted drug in patients with the true target of interest. In addition, since $\bar{y}_T - \bar{y}_C$ underestimates $\mu_{T+} - \mu_{C+}$, the planned sample size may not be sufficient for achieving the desired power for detecting the true treatment effects in those patients with the true molecular target of interest.

Although all patients randomized under the enrichment design have a positive diagnosis, the true status of the molecular target for individual patients in the targeted clinical trials is, in fact, unknown. Liu, Lin, and Chow (2009) proposed applying the EM algorithm for the inference of the treatment effects for the patients with the true molecular targets. It follows that under the assumption of the homogeneity of variance, Y_{ij} are independently distributed as a mixture of two normal distributions with mean μ_{i+} and μ_{i-} respectively, and a common variance σ^2 (McLachlan and Peel 2000). Let X_{ij} be the latent variable indicting the true status of the molecular target of patient *j* in treatment *i*; $j = 1, \ldots, n_i$, $i = T, C$.

Under the assumption that X_{ij} are i.i.d. Bernoulli random variables with probability γ for the molecular target, the complete-data log-likelihood function for Ψ is given by:

$$\log L_c(\Psi) = \sum_{j=1}^{n_T} x_{Tj}\left[\log\gamma + \log\varphi(y_{Tj} \mid \mu_{T+}, \sigma^2)\right] + \sum_{j=1}^{n_T}(1-x_{Tj})\left[\log(1-\gamma) + \log\varphi(y_{Tj} \mid \mu_{T-}, \sigma^2)\right]$$
$$+\sum_{j=1}^{n_C} x_{Cj}\left[\log\gamma + \log\varphi(y_{Cj} \mid \mu_{C+}, \sigma^2)\right] + \sum_{j=1}^{n_C}(1-x_{Cj})\left[\log(1-\gamma) + \log\varphi(y_{Cj} \mid \mu_{C-}, \sigma^2)\right]. \quad (22.3)$$

Where $\Psi = (\gamma, \mu_{T+}, \mu_{T-}, \mu_{C+}, \mu_{C-}, \sigma^2)'$, and $\mathbf{y}_{obs} = (y_{T1}, \ldots, y_{Tn_T}, y_{C1}, \ldots, y_{Cn_C})'$, γ is an unknown PPV, and ϕ (.|.) denotes the density of a normal variable.

Liu, Lin, and Chow (2009) provide procedures for implementation of the EM algorithm in conjunction with the bootstrap procedure for inference of θ in the patient population with the true molecular target. They also pointed out that although the assumption that $\mu_{T+} - \mu_{C+}, > \mu_{T-} - \mu_{C-}$, is one of the reasons for developing the targeted treatment, this assumption is not used in the EM algorithm for estimation of θ. Hence, the inference for θ by the proposed procedure is not biased in favor of the targeted treatment. The procedure of application of the EM algorithm to the binary endpoints under the enrichment design can be found in Liu and Lin (2008).

Extensive simulation studies for comparing the performance of the EM procedures and traditional approach in statistical inference in terms of relative bias for estimation size, and power of hypothesis testing were conducted by Liu and Lin (2008) and Liu, Lin, and Chow (2009) for binary and continuous endpoints, respectively. Some of their results are summarized below.

First they empirically demonstrated that the standardized treatment effect follows a standard normal distribution. For continuous endpoints, the relative bias of the estimated treatment effect by the traditional method ranges from −8.5% to more than −50%. The bias increases as the PPV decreases. On the other hand, the absolute relative bias of the estimator by the EM algorithm does not exceed 4.6% while most of them are smaller than 2%. The variability has little impact on the bias of both methods. The empirical coverage probabilities of the 95% confidence interval of the traditional method can be as low as only 8.6% when the PPV is 50%. On the contrary, 96.87% of the coverage probabilities for the 95% confidence interval constructed by the EM algorithm are above 0.94. No coverage probability of the EM method is below 0.92. Similar conclusions can be reached for the binary data.

Figure 22.2 presents the power curves for a two-sided test based on the continuous endpoints when $n = 50$, $\sigma = 20$, and PPV is 0.8, while Figure 22.3 provides a comparison of the power curves for the one-sided hypothesis based on binary endpoints for PPV being 0.8. In general, the power of the current method is an increasing function of the PPV. For both methods, the power increases as the sample size increases. However, the simulation results demonstrate that the EM testing procedure for the treatment effects in the patient population with the true molecular target is uniformly more powerful than the current method as depicted in Figure 22.3. Additional simulation studies also show that the impact of the heterogeneity of variances and the value of $\mu_{T-} - \mu_{C-}$ on the bias, coverage probability, size, and power is inconsequential. Similar results can be found for the binary endpoints.

22.5 Discussion and Concluding Remarks

The ultimate goal of targeted clinical trials is to achieve personalized medicine by improving clinical outcome using individual genomic information or variability for the targeted therapy. The key to accomplishing this goal is to find a validated diagnostic device that can accurately measure the true magnitude of an individual genomic variation. As pointed out by Liu and Lin (2008), and Liu, Lin, and Chow (2009), the relative bias of the estimated treatment effect can be as high as −50% when the PPV

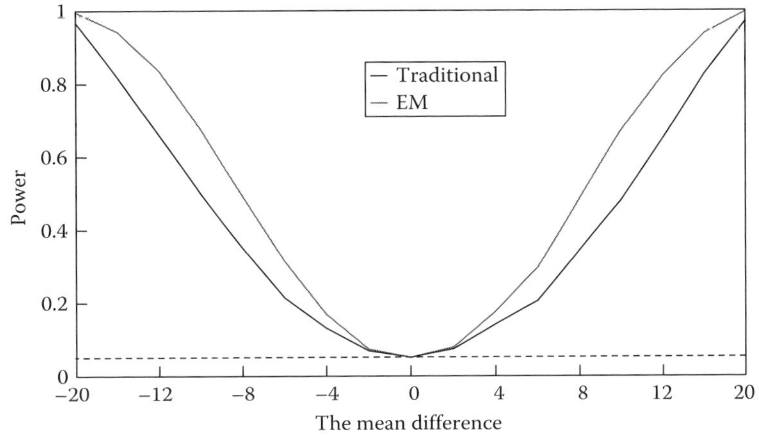

FIGURE 22.2 Empirical power curve when the positive predicted value is 0.8, n = 50 and SD = 20 for the continuous endpoint. (From Liu, J. P., Lin, J. R., and Chow, S. C., *Pharmaceutical Statistics*, 6, 356–70, 2009.)

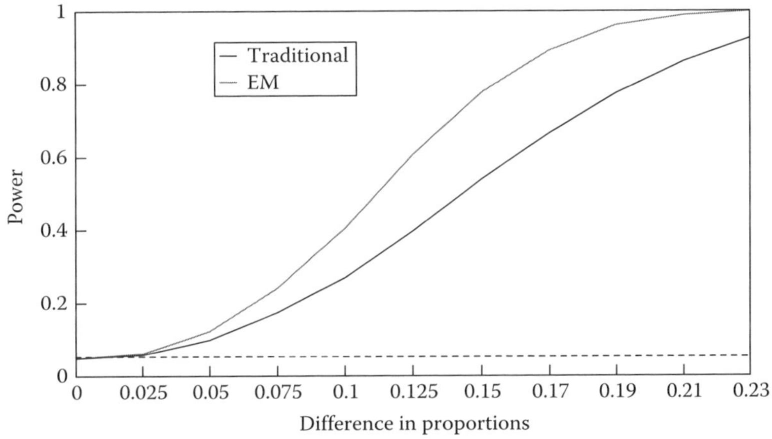

FIGURE 22.3 Empirical power curve when PPV is 0.8 for binary endpoints. (From Liu, J. P., Lin, J. R., and Chow, S. C., *Pharmaceutical Statistics*, 6, 356–70, 2009.)

is 50%. As mentioned above, the estimated PPV for the metastatic disease of breast cancer at 10 years for MammaPrint is only 0.29. Therefore, it is anticipated that the treatment effect of the component of chemotherapy randomization will be underestimated for more than 50%. In addition, an estimated PPV for the 10-year metastasis is not reliable because 10 years is a very long period during which many clinical advances or unexpected events may and will alter the status of metastasis of breast cancer. Therefore, we recommend that only diagnostic devices with a PPV greater than 0.75 for a clinical outcome within 5 years be used for screening of the molecular targets in targeted clinical trials.

Although amplification of gene numbers and over-expression of EGFR are associated with the response of the treatment of Erlotinib for patients with nonsmall cell lung cancer (NSCLC), objective responses were still observed in patients without increasing numbers of gene copies or over-expression of EGFR. On the other hand, the Iressa is effective in prolonging survival of NSCLC only in Asian female nonsmokers with adenocarcinoma. This may imply that some other unknown signing pathway may affect the effect of Erlotinib. Therefore, multiple pathological pathways and molecular targets are involved with the disease. As a result, treatments or drugs are being developed for multiple molecular targets. For example, Sorefenib is a multikinase inhibitor that inhibits Raf kinase, vascular endothelial growth factor receptors (VEGFR) 1, 2, and 3; RET receptor tyrosine kinase, c-kit protein, platelet-derived growth factor receptor β (PDGFRβ), and FMS-like tyrosine kinase. Sorefenib is an example of one drug for multiple targets (one too many). Should or could we have multiple drugs for multiple targets (many to many) or many drugs for just one target (many to one)? Mandrekar and Sargent (2009) provided a review of designs for targeted clinical trials including those in the FDA drug–device codevelopment draft concept paper. However, the issues associated with the design and analysis for the drug–device codevelopment for the multiple targets can be quite complex and require further research.

Acknowledgment

This research is partially supported by the Taiwan National Science Council Grants: 97 2118-M-002-002-MY2 to J. P. Liu.

References

The ALTTO Trial. (2009a). Available at http://www.cancer.gov/. Accessed on July 1, 2009.

The ALTTO Trial. (2009b). Available at http://www.clinicaltrial.gov. Accessed on July 1, 2009.

The ALTTO Trial, (2009c). Available at http://www.breastinternationalgroup.org. Accessed on July 1, 2009.

Buyse, M., Loi, S., Laura van't Veer, L., Viale, G., Delorenzi, M., Glas, A. M., d'Assignies, M. S., et al. (2006). Validation and clinical utility of a 70-gene prognostic signature for women with node-negative breast cancer. *Journal of the National Cancer Institute*, 98: 1183–92.

Chow, S. C., and Liu, J. P. (2004). *Design and Analysis of Clinical Trials*. 2nd ed. New York: John Wiley and Sons.

FDA. (1998). *Decision Summary P980018*. Rockville, MD: U.S. Food and Drug Administration.

FDA. (2005). *The Draft Concept Paper on Drug-Diagnostic Co-Development*. Rockville, MD: U.S. Food and Drug Administration.

FDA. (2006). *Annotated Redlined Draft Package Insert for Herceptin®*. Rockville, MD: U.S. Food and Drug Administration.

FDA. (2007a). *Guidance on Pharmacogenetic Tests and Genetic Tests for Heritable Marker*. Rockville, MD: U.S. Food and Drug Administration.

FDA. (2007b). *Draft Guidance on In Vitro Diagnostic Multivariate Index Assays*. Rockville, MD: U.S. Food and Drug Administration.

FDA. (2007c). *Decision Summary K062694*. Rockville, MD: U.S. Food and Drug Administration.

Fleiss, J. L., Levin, B., and Paik, M. C. (2003). *Statistical Methods for Rates and Proportions*, 3rd ed. New York: John Wiley and Sons.

Liu, J. P., and Chow, S. C. (2008). Issues on the diagnostic multivariate index assay and targeted clinical trials. *Journal of Biopharmaceutical Statistics*, 18: 167–82.

Liu, J. P., and Lin, J. R. (2008). Statistical methods for targeted clinical trials under enrichment design. *Journal of the Formosan Medical Association*, 107: S35–S42.

Liu, J. P., Lin, J. R., and Chow, S. C. (2009). Inference on treatment effects for targeted clinical trials under enrichment design. *Pharmaceutical Statistics*, 6, 356–70.

Mandrekar, S. J., and Sargent, D. J. (2009). Clinical trial designs for predictive biomarker validation: One size does not fit all. *Journal of Biopharmaceutical Statistics*, 19: 530–42.

McLachlan, G. J., and Peel, D. (2000). *Finite Mixture Models*. New York: Wiley.

MINDACT Design and MINDACT trial overview. (2009). Available at http://www.breast internationalgroup.org/transbig.html. Accessed on July 1, 2009.

Paik, S., Shak, S., Tang, G., Kim, C., Baker, J., Cronin, M., Baehner, F. L., et al. (2004). A multigene assay to predict recurrence of tamoxifen-treated, node-negative breast cancer. *New England Journal of Medicine*, 351: 2817–26.

Paik, S., Tang, G., Shak, S., Kim, C., Baker, J., Kim, W., Cronin, M., et al. (2006). Gene expression and benefit of chemotherapy in women with node-negative, estrogen receptor-positive breast cancer. *Journal of Clinical Oncology*, 24: 1–12.

Ravdin, P. M., and Chamness, G. C. (1995). The c-erbB-2 proto-oncogene as a prognostic and predictive marker in breast cancer: A paradigm for the development of other macromolecular markers—A review. *Gene*, 159: 19–27.

Seshadri, R., Figaira, F. A., Horsfall, D. J., McCaul, K., Setlur, V., and Kitchen, P. (1993). Clinical significance of HER-2/neu oncogene amplification in primary cancer. *Journal of Clinical Oncology*, 11: 1936–42.

Slamon, D. J., Leyand-Jones, B., Shak, S., Fuchs, H., Paton, V., Bajamonde, A., Fleming, T., et al. (2001). Use of chemotherapy plus a monoclonal antibody against HER2 for metastatic breast cancer that overexpresses HER2. *New England Journal of Medicine*, 344: 783–92.

TAILORX Trial Design and Overview. (2006). Available at http://www.cancer.gov/clinicaltrials/ECOG-PACCT-1. Accessed on July 1, 2009.

Van de Vijver, M. J., He, Y. D., van't Veer, L. J., Dai, H., Hart, A. A. M., Voskuil, D. W., Schreiber, G. J., et al. (2002). A gene-expression signature as a predictor of survival in breast cancer. *New England Journal of Medicine*, 347: 1999–2009.

van 't Veer, L. J., Dai, H., van de Vijver, M. J., He, Y. D., Hart, A. A. M., Mao, M., Peterse, H. L., et al. (2002). Gene expression profiling predicts clinical outcome of breast cancer. *Nature*, 415: 530–36.

Jiangtao Luo
Pennsylvania State College of Medicine
University of Florida

Arthur Berg
Pennsylvania State College of Medicine

Kwangmi Ahn
Pennsylvania State College of Medicine

Kiranmoy Das
Pennsylvania State University

Jiahan Li
Pennsylvania State University

Zhong Wang
Pennsylvania State College of Medicine

Yao Li
West Virginia University

Rongling Wu
Pennsylvania State College of Medicine, Pennsylvania State University, and Beijing Forestry University

23

Functional Genome-Wide Association Studies of Longitudinal Traits

23.1 Introduction

The completion of the human genome sequence in 2005 and its derivative, the HapMap Project, together with rapid improvements in genotyping analysis, have allowed a genome-wide scan of genes for complex traits or diseases (Altshuler, Daly, and Lander 2008; Ikram et al. 2009; Psychiatric GCCC 2009). Such genome-wide association studies (GWAS) have greatly stimulated our hope that detailed genetic control mechanisms for complex phenotypes can be understood at individual nucleotide levels or nucleotide combinations. In the past several years, more than 250 loci have been reproducibly identified for polygenic traits (Hirschhorn 2009). It is impressive that many genes detected affect the outcome of a trait or disease through its biochemical and metabolic pathways. For example, of the 23 loci detected for lipid levels, 11 trigger their effects by encoding apolipoproteins, lipases, and other key proteins in lipid biosynthesis (Mohlke, Boehnke, and Abecasis 2008). Genes associated with Crohn's disease encode autophagy and interleukin-23 related pathways (Lettre and Rioux 2008). The height loci detected regulate directly chromatin proteins and hedgehog signaling (Hirschhorn and Lettre 2009). GWAS have also identified genes that encode action sites of drugs approved by the U.S. Food and Drug Administration, including thiazolidinediones and sulfonylureas (in studies of type 2 diabetes; Mohlke, Boehnke, and Abecasis 2008), statins (lipid levels; Mohlke, Boehnke, and Abecasis 2008), and estrogens (bone density; Styrkarsdottir et al. 2009).

In the next few years, GWAS methods will detect an increasing number of significant genetic associations for complex traits and diseases, supposedly leading to new pathophysiological hypotheses. However, only small proportions of genetic variance have thus far been found, making it difficult to elucidate a comprehensive genetic atlas of complex phenotypes. Also, therapeutic applications of GWAS results will require substantial knowledge about the biological and biochemical functions of significant genetic variants. Previous studies of genetic mapping for complex traits indicate that statistical power for gene detection can increase if the trait is considered as a biological process (Ma, Casella, and Wu 2002; Wu and Lin 2006). In this chapter, we show that the integration of GWAS with the underlying biological principle of a trait, termed functional GWAS or *f*GWAS, will similarly improve the genetic relevance and statistical power of GWAS. We particularly show that *f*GWAS can address the limitations of classic GWAS methods.

23.2 Why *f*GWAS: A Must-Tell Story

23.2.1 A Biological Perspective

The formation of every trait or disease undergoes a developmental process. For example, in humans, there are distinct stages that children pass through from birth to adult (Thompson and Thompson 2009). These stages, including infancy, childhood, puberty, adolescence, and adulthood, are the same for boys and girls, although girls generally mature before boys. There are important changes in body size (Figure 23.1, upper) and proportions (Figure 23.1, lower) over the stages. At birth, infants are only about a quarter of their adult height. The age to reach the final adult height is usually about 20 years of age, although there is a substantial variability among individuals. Four characteristic stages provide a full description of growth from birth to adult:

- Rapid growth in infancy and early childhood
- Slow, steady growth in middle childhood
- Rapid growth during puberty
- Gradual slowing down of growth in adolescence until adult height is reached

In addition to size difference, children are not just smaller versions of adults. There are pronounced differences in the physical proportions of the body at birth and adulthood. Some body parts grow more than others during development to reach a particular body shape of the adult. In childhood, the head is proportionally large and the legs proportionally short. At birth the head is one-quarter of the length of the body, compared with about one-sixth for the adult. The legs are about one-third the length of the

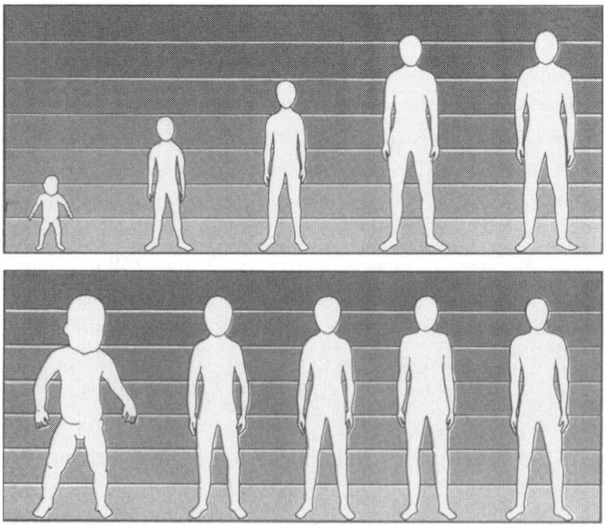

FIGURE 23.1 Changes in the size (upper) and proportion (lower) of human body from birth to adult. (Adapted from Thompson, P. and Thompson, P. J. L., *Introduction to Coaching Theory*, Meyer & Meyer Sport, U.K., 2009.)

body at birth and one-half in the adult. The body proportions change over time, because not all of the body segments grow by the same amount.

Given these developmental changes in size and shape, human body growth can typically be better described by multiple measures at different time points. One measure at any single time point fails to capture a picture of body growth and development in a time course.

23.2.2 A Genetic Perspective

The genetic and pathological mechanisms of complex traits can be better understood by incorporating the process of trait formation into an analytical model. Traditional quantitative genetics is integrated with developmental models to estimate the genetic variation of growth and development (Atchley and Zhu 1997). Meyer (2000) used random regression models to study the ontogenetic control of growth for animal breeding, whereas Kirkpatrick, Pletcher, and colleagues utilized the orthogonal, additive and universally practicable properties of Legendre polynomials to derive a series of genetic models for growth trajectories in the evolutionary context (Kirkpatrick, Lofsvold, and Bulmer 1990; Kirkpatrick, Hill, and Thompson 1994; Pletcher and Geyer 1999). These models have been instrumental in understanding the genetic control of growth by modeling the covariance matrix for growth traits measured at different time points. Ma, Casella, and Wu (2002) implemented a mixture-model based method to map quantitative trait loci (QTL) in a controlled cross.

Hence, the integration of a biological process into GWAS will not only identify genes that regulate the final form of the trait, but also characterize the dynamic pattern of genetic control in time. Using a growth trait as an example, the pattern of genetic effects on growth processes can be categorized into four different types (Figure 23.2):

a. **Faster–slower genes** control variation in the time at which growth is maximal. Although two genotypes have the same maximal growth, a faster genotype uses a shorter time to reach peak height than a slower genotype does. The former also displays a greater overall relative growth rate than the latter (Figure 23.2a).
b. **Earlier–later genes** are responsible for variation in the timing of maximal growth rate. Although two genotypes have no effect on the maximal growth, an earlier genotype is quicker to reach its maximal growth rate than a later genotype (Figure 23.2b).
c. **Taller–shorter genes** produce a taller genotype that exhibits consistently taller height over the shorter genotype. The taller and shorter genotypes have growth curves that do not crossover during growth (Figure 23.2c).
d. **Age–dependent taller-shorter genes** determine variation in growth curves by altering their effect direction in time. A taller genotype is not always taller, whereas a shorter genotype is not always shorter. The two genotypes crossover during growth, producing a maximal degree of variation of the growth trajectories (Figure 23.2d).

In practice, it is possible that a growth gene operates in a mix of all these four types, which will produce more variation in the growth curves. Also, the expression of a typical gene can be age-specific. For example, the taller–shorter gene may be activated after a particular time point, whereas the earlier–later gene may be active only before a particular time point prior to adult age. The use of *f*GWAS models that incorporate the dynamic features of trait formation can identify these types of growth genes and their biological functions.

23.2.3 A Statistical Perspective

Traditional GWAS analyze the association between single nucleotide polymorphism (SNP) genotypes and phenotypic values at a single time point. Whereas GWAS can only detect differences among genotypes for phenotype measurements at a single point in time, *f*GWAS can capture genotypic differences

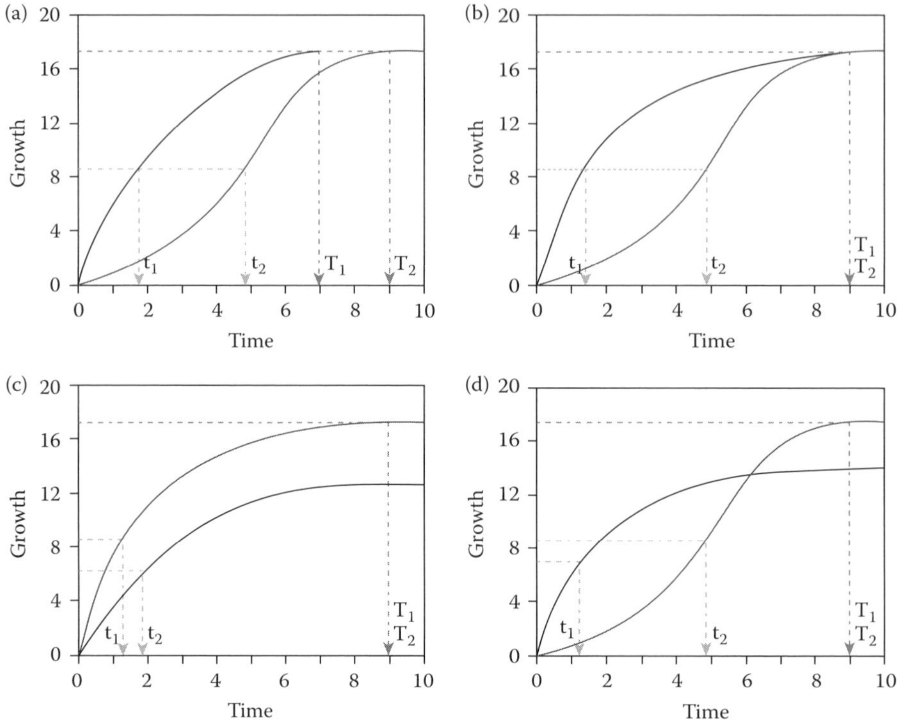

FIGURE 23.2 Four different types of a QTL that triggers its effect on growth in time. (a) Faster–slower genes, (b) Earlier–later genes, (c) Taller–shorter genes, and (d) Age-dependent taller–shorter genes. For each QTL type, there are two genotypes each displayed by growth curves. We use T to denote the time when growth reaches a maximal value and t to denote the time at which growth rate is maximal (inflection point). Times T and t, subscripted by a QTL genotype, can be used to describe the developmental characteristic of a growth curve.

at the level of phenotypic curves accumulated in the entire process of growth, thereby increasing the statistical power of gene detection.

Statistical merits of *f*GWAS will be exemplified in the case where longitudinal data are measured irregularly, leading to data sparsity. This phenomenon is common in clinical trials. For example, AIDS patients are periodically scheduled to measure viral loads in their bodies after a particular drug is administrated. As patients visit the clinic on different dates, there may be no single time point that includes all patients. Table 23.1 shows a toy example of 12 subjects for such a data structure; here, each subject is genotyped for m genome-wide SNPs and phenotyped at different time points (t_1–t_{10}), with intervals and number depending on subjects. Such sparse longitudinal data cannot be well analyzed by traditional GWAS for two fundamental reasons.

First, because only a small fraction of the subjects has measurements at a given time point, traditional GWAS based on the association analysis between SNP genotypes and phenotypes at a single time is unable to capitalize on all subjects, thus leading to biased parameter estimation and reduced gene detection ability. For example, at time t_1, only subjects 1 and 2 are measured phenotypically, with no phenotypic information available for the other 10 subjects at this particular time after administration of the drug. Therefore, an analysis of phenotypic data measured at a single time point like t_1 severely limits the data and does not reflect the whole picture of all 12 subjects.

Second, individual subjects are measured at a few number of time points, limiting the fit of an informative curve. For example, subject 1 was measured at times t_1 and t_3, subject 2 measured at times t_1 and t_7, and together these two subjects have three time points t_1, t_3, and t_7. If these two subjects are analyzed separately, only a straight line can be fit. But, when analyzed jointly, three time points allow the fit of a curve that

TABLE 23.1 Structure of Sparse Longitudinal Data for GWAS for a Toy Example of 12 Subjects

	SNP Data				Viral Load at Different Time Points										
Subject	1	2	...	m	t_1	t_2	t_3	t_4	t_5	t_6	t_7	t_8	t_9	t_{10}	Total
1	1	1	...	1	x		x								2
2	1	2	...	2	x						x				2
3	1	3	...	1		x			x						2
4	1	1	...	3				x		x			x		3
5	2	2	...	2								x			1
6	2	3	...	2						x					1
7	2	3	...	3		x									1
8	2	1	...	1				x			x				2
9	3	1	...	2							x			x	2
10	3	2	...	1									x	x	3
11	3	3	...	1			x								1
12	2	1	...	3				x				x		x	3
Projected					x	x	x	x	x	x	x	x	x	x	10

Note: Each subject is genotyped for m SNP markers and phenotyped for a complex trait at uneven-spaced time points. At each marker, three genotypes are *AA*, *Aa*, and *aa*, symbolized by 1, 2, and 3, respectively.

is more informative than a line. This is exemplified further when all 12 subjects combine to yield 10 distinct time points whereas each individual subject only consists of 1–3 time points (Table 23.1).

23.3 A Statistical Framework for *f*GWAS

23.3.1 Model for *f*GWAS

Let $\mathbf{y}_i = (y_i(t_{i1}), \cdots, y_i(t_{iT_i}))$ denote the vector of trait values for subject i measured at age $\mathbf{t}_i = (t_{i1}, \cdots, t_{iT_i})$. These denotations allow subject-specific differences in the number and interval of time points. Consider a SNP **A** with two alleles A and a, generating three genotypes AA (coded by 1) with n_1 observations, Aa (coded by 2) with n_2 observations, and aa (coded by 3) with n_3 observations. The phenotypic value of subject i at time $t_{i\tau}$ ($\tau = 1, \ldots, T_i$) for this SNP is expressed as:

$$y_i(t_{i\tau}) = \mu(t_{i\tau}) + a(t_{i\tau})\xi_i + d(t_{i\tau})\zeta_i + \beta(t_{i\tau})\mathbf{x}_i(t_{i\tau}) + e_i(t_{i\tau}) + \varepsilon_i(t_{i\tau}), \tag{23.1}$$

where $\mu(t_{i\tau})$ is the overall mean at time $t_{i\tau}$, $a(t_{i\tau})$ and $d(t_{i\tau})$ are the additive and dominant effects of the SNP on the trait at time $t_{i\tau}$, respectively, ξ_i and ζ_I are the indicator variables for subject i, defined as:

$$\xi_i = \begin{cases} 1 & \text{if the genotype of subject } i \text{ is } AA \\ 0 & \text{if the genotype of subject } i \text{ is } Aa \\ -1 & \text{if the genotype of subject } i \text{ is } aa \end{cases} \tag{23.2a}$$

$$\zeta_i = \begin{cases} 1 & \text{if the genotype of subject } i \text{ is } Aa \\ 0 & \text{if the genotype of subject } i \text{ is } AA \text{ or } aa, \end{cases} \tag{23.2b}$$

$\mathbf{x}_i(t_{i\tau})$ is the $p \times 1$ covariate vector for subject i at time $t_{i\tau}$, $\beta(t_{i\tau})$ is a vector of unknown regression coefficients, $e_i(t_{i\tau})$ and $\varepsilon_i(t_{i\tau})$ are the permanent and random errors at time $t_{i\tau}$, respectively, together called the residual errors.

Averaging effects that determine the residuals allows $\mathbf{y}_i$ to follow a multivariate normal distribution. Under the natural assumption that the residual errors of any two subjects are independent, we have the likelihood:

$$L(\mathbf{y}) = \prod_{i-1}^{n_1} f_1(\mathbf{y}_i) \prod_{i-1}^{n_2} f_2(\mathbf{y}_i) \prod_{i-1}^{n_3} f_3(\mathbf{y}_i), \tag{23.3}$$

where $f_j(\mathbf{y}_i)$ is a multivariate normal distribution of the trait for subject i who carries SNP genotype j ($j = 1, 2, 3$), with subject-specific mean vectors:

$$\mathbf{u}_{ij} = \begin{cases} (\mu(t_{i1}) + a(t_{i1}) + \beta^T \mathbf{x}_i(t_{i1}), \ldots, \mu(t_{iT_i}) + a(t_{iT_i}) + \beta^T \mathbf{x}_i(t_{iT_i})) & \text{for SNP genotype } AA \\ (\mu(t_{i1}) + d(t_{i1}) + \beta^T \mathbf{x}_i(t_{i1}), \ldots, \mu(t_{iT_i}) + a(t_{iT_i}) + \beta^T \mathbf{x}_i(t_{iT_i})) & \text{for SNP genotype } Aa, \\ (\mu(t_{i1}) - a(t_{i1}) + \beta^T \mathbf{x}_i(t_{i1}), \ldots, \mu(t_{iT_i}) - a(t_{iT_i}) + \beta^T \mathbf{x}_i(t_{iT_i})) & \text{for SNP genotype } aa \end{cases} \tag{23.4}$$

and subject-specific covariance matrix:

$$\sum_i = \phi \begin{bmatrix} \sigma^2_{t_{i1}} & L & \sigma_{t_{i1}t_{iT_i}} \\ M & O & M \\ \sigma_{t_{iT_i}t_{i1}} & L & \sigma^2_{t_{iT_i}} \end{bmatrix} + (1-\phi) \begin{bmatrix} \sigma^2_{t_{i1}} & L & 0 \\ M & O & M \\ 0 & L & \sigma^2_{t_{iT_i}} \end{bmatrix} \equiv \phi \sum_{iP} + (1-\phi) \sum_{iR}. \tag{23.5}$$

In Matrix 23.5, the residual variance $\sigma^2_{t_{i\tau}}$ is composed of the permanent error variance due to the temporal pattern of longitudinal variables and the random error variance (also called the innovative variance) arising from random independent unpredictable errors. The relative magnitude of the permanent and innovative components is described by parameter φ. The covariance matrix (Σ_{iP}) due to the permanent errors contains autocorrelation structure that can be modeled, whereas the random errors are often assumed to be independent among different time points so that the random covariance matrix Σ_{iR} is diagonal.

23.3.2 Modeling the Mean Vectors

The first task for *f*GWAS involves modeling the mean Vector 23.4 for different SNP genotypes in a biologically and statistically meaningful way and modeling the longitudinal structure of covariance Matrix 23.5 in a statistically efficient and robust manner. Below is a list of concrete tasks for modeling the mean and covariance structures within the *f*GWAS framework:

23.3.2.1 Parametric Modeling

The biological mean for modeling the mean Vector 23.4 implies that time-specific genotypic values should be modeled, reflecting the biological principles of trait development. For example, if a growth trait is studied, the logistic curve that explains growth law (West, Brown, and Enquist 2001) can be fit by mathematical parameters. There are many biologically well-justified curves such as:

1. Sigmoid equations for biological growth (von Bertalanffy 1957; Richards 1959; Guiot et al. 2003, 2006)
2. Triple-logistic equations for human body growth (Bock and Thissen 1976)

3. Bi-exponential equations for HIV dynamics (Perelson et al. 1996)
4. Sigmoid E_{max} models for pharmacodynamic response (Giraldo 2003)
5. Fourier series approximations for biological clock (Brown et al. 2000)
6. Biological thermal dynamics (Kingsolver and Woods 1997)
7. Aerodynamic power curves for bird flight (Tobalske et al. 2003; Lin, Zhao, and Wu 2006)
8. Hyperbolic curves for photosynthetic reaction (Wu et al. 2007)

23.3.2.2 Nonparametric and Semiparametric Modeling

The statistical mean implies that such a fit should meet a required statistical test. If no exact mathematical equation exists, nonparametric approaches, such as B-spline or Legendre orthogonal polynomial, should be used. These approaches have displayed some success in modeling age-specific genotypic values for traits that do not fit a specific mathematical curve (Cui et al. 2009; Yang, Wu, and Casella 2009). If trait formation includes multiple distinct stages, at some of which the trait can be modeled parametrically but at others of which cannot, it is crucial to derive a semiparametric model that combines the precision and biological relevance of parametric approaches and the flexibility of nonparametric approaches. Such a semiparametric model was derived in Cui, Zhu, and Wu (2006) and can be well implemented in the *f*GWAS framework.

In general, parametric approaches are more parsimonious by keeping the dimension of the parameter space down to a reasonable size, whereas nonparametric approaches possess a better flexibility for fitting the model to the data. The choice of parametric or nonparametric approaches can be made on the basis of biological knowledge and model selection criteria.

23.3.2.3 Wavelet-Based Dimension Reduction

If the dimension of time points is too high to be handled, a wavelet-based approach can be derived to reduce high-dimensional data into its low-dimensional representative (Zhao et al. 2007; Zhao and Wu 2008). This approach shows a high flexibility and can be derived in either a parametric or nonparametric way. The idea of wavelet-based dimension reduction was also used for functional clustering of dynamic gene expression profiles (Kim et al. 2008). The incorporation of wavelet-based approach will help *f*GWAS to analyze dynamic data of high dimensions.

23.3.3 Modeling the Covariance Structure

Robust modeling of longitudinal covariance structure (Matrix 23.5) is a prerequisite for appropriate statistical inference of genetic effects on longitudinal traits. Several different approaches are available for covariance modeling, including parametric, nonparametric, and semiparametric.

23.3.3.1 Parametric Modeling

The advantage of parametric approaches includes the existence of closed forms for the determinant and inverse of a longitudinal matrix. This will greatly help to enhance computational efficiency. Below is a list of existing parametric approaches used to model functional mapping:

1. Stationary parametric model—assuming the stationarity of variance and correlation (e.g., autoregressive (AR) model; Ma, Casella, and Wu 2002)
2. Nonstationary parametric model—variance and correlation may not be stationary [e.g., structured antedependence (SAD) model; Zimmerman et al. 2001; Zhao et al. 2005]
3. General parametric model (autoregressive moving average model ARMA(p,q); Li, Berg, and Wu, unpublished results)

For each model above, it is important to determine its optimal order to model covariance structure. A model selection procedure will be established to determine the most parsimonious approach. We will implement these approaches into the *f*GWAS model, allowing geneticists to select an optimal approach for covariance structure for their longitudinal data.

23.3.3.2 Nonparametric Modeling

Relative to nonparametric modeling of the mean structure, nonparametric covariance modeling has received little attention. Many authors have considered only the stationary case (e.g., Glasbey 1988; Hall, Fisher, and Hoffmann 1994). However, some papers have considered the possibility of estimating the nonstationary case (Diggle and Verbyla 1998; Wang 2003). Diggle and Verbyla (1998) used kernel-weighted local linear regression smoothing of sample variograms ordinates and of squared residuals to provide a nonparametric estimator for the covariance structure without assuming stationarity. In addition, they used the value of the estimator as a diagnostic tool but did not study the use of the estimator in more formal statistical inference concerning the mean profiles. Wang (2003) used kernel estimators to estimate covariance functions in a nonparametric way. His only assumption was to have a fully unstructured smooth covariance structure, together with a fixed effects model. The proposed kernel estimator was consistent with complete but irregularly spaced follow-ups, or when the missing mechanism is strongly ignorable MAR (Rosenbaum and Rubin 1983).

23.3.3.3 Semiparametric Modeling

Zeger and Diggle (1994) and Moyeed and Diggle (1994) studied a semiparametric model for longitudinal data in which the covariates entered parametrically and only the time effect entered nonparametrically. To fit the model, they extended to longitudinal data the backfitting algorithm of Hastie and Tibshirani (1990) for semiparametric regression.

23.3.3.4 Special Emphasis on Modeling Sparse Longitudinal Data

In many longitudinal trials, data are often collected at irregularly spaced time points and with measurement schedules specific to different subjects (see Table 23.1). The efficient estimation of covariance structure in this situation will be a significant concern for detecting the genes that control dynamic traits. Although there are many challenges in modeling the covariance structure of subject-specific irregular longitudinal data, many workers have considered this issue using different approaches. These include nonparametric analysis derived from a two-step estimation procedure (Fan and Zhang 2000; Wu and Pourahmadi 2003), a semiparametric approach (Fan and Li 2004), a penalized likelihood approach (Huang et al. 2006), and functional data analysis (Yao, Müller, and Wang 2005a, 2005b). More recently, Fan, Huang, and Li (2007) proposed a semiparametric model for the covariance structure of irregular longitudinal data, in which they approached the time-dependent correlation by a parametric function and the time-dependent variance by a nonparametric kernel function. The Fan, Huang, and Li (2007) model's advantage lies in the combination between the flexibility of nonparametric modeling and parsimony of parametric modeling. The establishment of a robust estimation procedure and asymptotic properties of the estimators will make this semiparametric model useful in the practical estimation of covariance function.

The data structure in Table 23.1 shows subjects are measured at a few number of time points (1–3), with intervals and number depending subjects. But all subjects are projected in a space with a full measure schedule (10). In this project, we will incorporate Fan, Huang, and Li's (2007) and Fan and Wu's (2008) semiparametric model into the mixture model-based framework for *f*GAWS of longitudinal traits.

23.3.4 Hypothesis Tests

The significance test of the genetic effect of a SNP is key for detecting significant genetic variants. This can be done by formulating the hypotheses as follows:

$$H_0\text{: } a(t_{i\tau}) = d(t_{i\tau}) \equiv 0 \text{ versus } H_1\text{: At least one equality in the } H_0 \text{ does not hold.} \quad (23.6)$$

The likelihoods under the null and alternative hypotheses are calculated, from which the log-likelihood ratio (LR) is computed. The LR value is supposed to be asymptotically χ^2-distributed with the degree of freedom equal to the difference in the numbers of unknown parameters under the H_1 and H_0. The significance of individual SNPs will be adjusted for multiple comparisons with a standard approach such as the false discovery rate (FDR).

We can also test the additive (H_0: $a(t_{i\tau}) = 0$) and dominant effects (H_0: $a(t_{i\tau}) = 0$) of a SNP after it is detected to be significant. Similarly, the LR values are calculated separately for each test and compared with critical values determined from the χ^2-distribution.

23.4 High-Dimensional Models for *f*GWAS

23.4.1 Multiple Longitudinal Variables and Time-to-Events

In medical research, a number of different response variables (including longitudinal and event processes) are often measured over time because an underlying outcome of interest cannot be captured by any single response variable. For example, HIV viral loads and CD$^+$4 lymphocyte counts are two criteria that evaluate the effect of antiviral drugs for AIDS patients. After antiviral drugs are administrated, viral loads decay, while CD$^+$4 cell counts increase in time course. In this case, viral and CD$^+$4 cell trajectories are used as two different response variables that define HIV pathogenesis and the time to progress into AIDS. AIDS alone does not cause death; the opportunistic infections weakening the immune system of an AIDS patient eventually cause AIDS-related death. Thus, in addition to the study of longitudinal variables, HIV and CD$^+$4 dynamics indicate censored variables such as time-to-death should also be adapted into the analysis.

In a GWAS, it is of paramount interest to jointly model the genetic control of different response variables and time-to-events, to provide a deep understanding of the genetic and developmental mechanisms of complex traits or diseases. In the example mentioned above for AIDS research, some fundamental questions that can be addressed include:

- What kind of genes control HIV trajectories?
- What kind of genes control CD$^+$4 cell count changes?
- What kind of genes control death due to AIDS?
- Are there (pleiotropic) genes that control these three types of traits jointly?
- How do genes for HIV and CD$^+$4 cell count trajectories interact with those for AIDS-related death to determine the death of AIDS patients?

In biostatistics, models and algorithms have been proposed to study multidimensional longitudinal and event responses (Henderson, Diggle, and Dobson 2000; Brown, Ibrahim, and DeGruttola 2005). Tsiatis and Davidian (2004) provide a detailed overview of statistical methodologies for joint modeling of multiple longitudinal and survival variables. Such joint modeling has two objectives: (1) model the trends of longitudinal processes in time, and (2) model the association between time-dependent variables and time-to-events. Many of these previous results can be organized into the *f*GWAS model.

The *f*GWAS model allows the testing of whether the gene affecting a longitudinal process can also be responsible for time-to-event phenotypes, such as survival and age-at-onset. Age-at-onset traits can be related to pathogenesis including age at first stroke occurrence and time to cancer invasion and metastasis. Figure 23.3 is an illustration that explains the mechanisms of how the same gene or different genes affect longitudinal and event processes. As shown in Figure 23.3, a gene that determines age-specific change in body mass index (BMI) may or may not trigger an effect on the age at first stroke occurrence. In Figure 23.3a, the age at first stroke occurrence displays a pronounced difference between three SNP genotypes each with a discrepant BMI trajectory, suggesting that this SNP affects both BMI and age at first stroke occurrence. But the SNP for BMI trajectories in Figure 23.3b does not affect pleiotropically the age at first stroke occurrence.

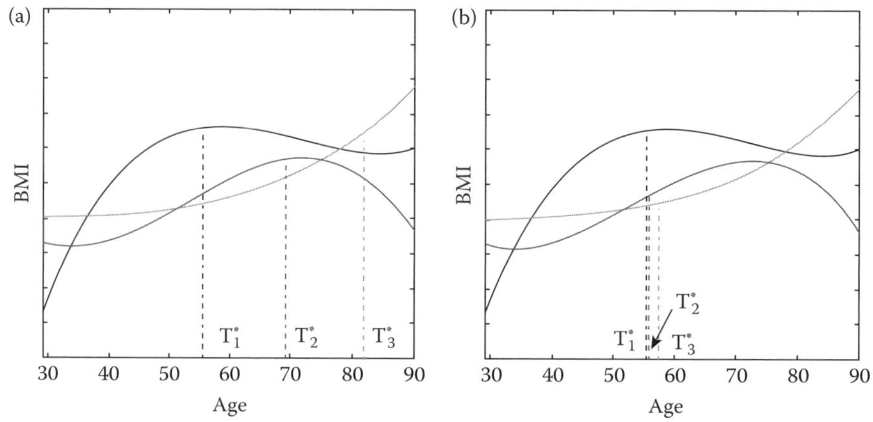

FIGURE 23.3 Model that illustrates how a SNP pleiotropically affects age-specific BMI change and age to get stroke (*T*). In (a), the SNP affects both features because there are significant differences in age to get stroke between three BMI-associated SNP genotypes, whereas, in (b), the BMI SNP does not govern age to get stroke because such a difference is small. On the left, the change of BMI over age can be used as a phenotypic biomarker for the diagnosis of age to get stroke.

23.4.2 Multiple Genetic Control Mechanisms

In the past decades, some phenomena related to genetic architecture have been re-recognized. For example, epistasis has been long thought to be an important force for evolution and speciation (Whitlock et al. 1995; Wolf 2000), but recent genetic studies from vast quantities of molecular data have increasingly indicated that epistasis critically affects the pathogenesis of most common human diseases, such as cancer or cardiovascular disease (Combarros et al. 2009; Moore and Williams 2009). The expression of an interconnected network of genes is contingent upon environmental conditions, often with the elements and connections of the network displaying nonlinear relationships with environmental factors.

Imprinting effects, also called parent-of-origin effects, are defined as the differential expression of the same allele with different parental origins. In diploid organisms, there are two copies at every autosomal gene, one inherited from the maternal parent and the other from the paternal parent. Both copies are expressed to affect a trait for a majority of these genes. Yet, there is also a small subset of genes for which one copy from a particular parent is turned off. These genes, whose expression depends on the parent-of-origin due to the epigenetic or imprinted mark of one copy in either the egg or the sperm, have been thought to play an important role in complex diseases and traits, although imprinted expression can also vary between tissues, developmental stages, and species (Reik and Walter 2001). Anomalies derived from imprinted genes are often manifested as developmental and neurological disorders during early development and as cancer later in life (Luedi, Hartemink, and Jirtle 2005; Waterland et al. 2006; Wen et al. 2009). With the availability of more GWAS data sets, a complete understanding of the genetic architecture of complex traits has become feasible.

23.5 Discussion

The GWAS with SNPs have proven to be a powerful tool for deciphering the role genetics plays in human health and disease. By analyzing hundreds of thousands of genetic variants in a particular population, this approach can identify the chromosomal distribution and function of multiple genetic changes that are associated with polygenic traits and diseases. Indeed, in the last two years, we have witnessed the successful applications of GWAS in the study of complex traits and diseases of major medical importance such as human height, obesity, diabetes, coronary artery disease, and cancer.

The successes and potentials of GWAS have not been explored when complex phenotypes arise as a curve. In any regard, a curve is more informative than a point in describing the biological or clinical feature of a trait. By integrating GWAS and functional aspects of dynamic traits, a new analytical model, called functional GWAS (*f*GWAS), can be naturally derived, which provides an unprecedented opportunity to study the genetic control of developmental traits. *f*GWAS is not only able to identify genes that determine the final form of the trait, but also displays power to study the temporal pattern of genetic control in a time course. From a statistical standpoint, *f*GWAS capitalizes on the full information of trait growth and development culminating in a time course and, therefore, increases the power of gene identification. In particular, *f*GWAS is robust for handling longitudinal sparse data in which no single time point has the phenotypic data for all subjects, facilitating the application of GWAS to study the genetic architecture of hard-to-measure traits.

With the completion of the human genome project, it has been possible to draw a comprehensive picture of genetic control mechanisms of complex traits and processes and, ultimately, integrate genetic information into routine clinical therapies for disease treatment and prevention. To achieve this goal, there is a pressing need to develop powerful statistical and computational algorithms for detecting genes that determine dynamic traits. Unlike static traits, dynamic traits are described by a series of developmental processes composed of a large number of variables. *f*GWAS, derived by integrating mathematical models for the molecular mechanisms and functions of biological processes into a likelihood framework, will allow a number of hypothesis tests to be made at the interplay between genetics and developmental disorders.

Acknowledgment

This work is partially supported by joint grant DMS/NIGMS-0540745 and the Changjiang Scholar Award.

References

Altshuler, D., Daly, M. J., and Lander, E. S. (2008). Genetic mapping in human disease. *Science,* 322: 881–88.

Atchley, W. R., and Zhu, J. (1997). Developmental quantitative genetics, conditional epigenetic variability and growth in mice. *Genetics,* 147: 765–76.

Bock, R. D., and Thissen, D. (1976). Fitting multi-component models for growth in stature. *Proceedings of the 9th International Biometrics Conference,* 1: 431–42.

Brown, E. N., Choe, Y., Luithardt, H., and Czeisler, C. A. (2000). A statistical model of the human core-temperature circadian rhythm. *American Journal of Physiology: Endocrinology and Metabolism,* 279: E669–E683.

Brown, E. R., Ibrahim, J. G., and DeGruttola, V. (2005). A flexible B-spline model for multiple longitudinal biomarkers and survival. *Biometrics,* 61: 64–73.

Combarros, O., Cortina-Borja, M., Smith, A. D., and Lehmann, D. J. (2009). Epistasis in sporadic Alzheimer's disease. *Neurobiology of Aging,* 30: 1333–49

Cui, Y., Zhu, J., and Wu, R. L. (2006). Functional mapping for genetic control of programmed cell death. *Physiological Genomics,* 25: 458–69.

Cui, Y. H., Wu, R. L., Casella, G., and Zhu, J. (2008). Nonparametric functional mapping quantitative trait loci underlying programmed cell death. *Statistical Applications in Genetics and Molecular Biology,* 7, 1, Article 4.

Diggle, P. J., and Verbyla, A. P. (1998). Nonparametric estimation of covariance structure in longitudinal data. *Biometrics,* 54: 401–15.

Fan, J., Huang, T., and Li, R. (2007). Analysis of longitudinal data with semiparametric estimation of covariance function. *Journal of the American Statistical Association,* 102: 632–41.

Fan, J., and Li, R. (2004). New estimation and model selection procedures for semiparametric modeling in longitudinal data analysis. *Journal of the American Statistical Association,* 99: 710–23.

Fan, J., and Wu, Y. (2008). Semiparametric estimation of covariance matrixes for longitudinal data. *Journal of the American Statistical Association,* 103: 1520–33.

Fan, J., and Zhang, J. T. (2000). Two-step estimation of functional linear models with applications to longitudinal data. Journal *of the Royal* Statistical Society, 62: 303–22.

Giraldo, J. (2003). Empirical models and Hill coefficients. *Trends in Pharmacological Sciences,* 24: 63–65.

Glasbey, C. A. (1988). Standard errors resilient to error variance misspecification. *Biometrika,* 75: 201–6.

Guiot, C., Degiorgis, P. G., Delsanto, P. P., Gabriele, P., and Deisboeck, T. S. (2003). Does tumor growth follow a "universal law"? *Journal of Theoretical* Biology, 225: 147–51.

Guiot, C., Delsanto, P. P., Carpinteri, A., Pugno, N., Mansury, Y., and Deisboeck, T. S. (2006). The dynamic evolution of the power exponent in a universal growth model of tumors. *Journal of Theoretical* Biology, 240: 459–63.

Hall, P., Fisher N. I., and Hoffmann, B. (1994). On the nonparametric estimation of covariance functions. *Annals of Statistics,* 22: 2115–34.

Hastie, T., and Tibshirani, R. (1990). *Generalized Additive Models.* London: Chapman & Hall.

Henderson, R., Diggle, P., and Dobson, A. (2000). Joint modelling of longitudinal measurements and event time data. *Biostatistics,* 1: 465–80.

Hirschhorn, J. N. (2009). Genomewide association studies—Illuminating biologic pathways. *New England Journal of Medicine,* 360: 1699–1701.

Hirschhorn J. N., Lettre G. (2009). Progress in Genome-Wide Association Studies of Human Height. *Hormone Research,* 71: 5–13.

Huang, J. Z., Liu, N., Pourahmadi, M., Liu, L. (2006). Covariance matrix selection and estimation via penalised normal likelihood. *Biometrika,* 93: 85–98.

Ikram, M. A., Seshadri, S., Bis, J. C., Fornage, M., DeStefano, A. L., Aulchenko, Y. S., Debette, S., et al. (2009). Genomewide association studies of stroke. *New England Journal of Medicine,* 360: 1718–28.

Kim, B. R., Zhang, L., Berg, A., Fan, J., and Wu, R. (2008). A computational approach to the functional clustering of periodic gene-expression profiles. *Genetics,* 180: 821–34.

Kingsolver, J. G., and Woods, H. A. (1997). Thermal sensitivity of growth and feeding in Manduca sexta caterpillars. *Physiological Zoology,* 70: 631–38.

Kirkpatrick, M., Hill, W., and Thompson, R. (1994). Estimating the covariance structure of traits during growth and ageing, illustrated with lactation in dairy cattle. *Genetical Research,* 64: 57–69.

Kirkpatrick, M., Lofsvold, D., and Bulmer, M. (1990). Analysis of the inheritance, selection and evolution of growth trajectories. *Genetics,* 124: 979–93.

Lettre, G., and Rioux, J. D. (2008). Autoimmune diseases: Insights from genome-wide association studies. *Human Molecular Genetics,* 17: R116–R121.

Li, N., McMurry, T., Berg, A., Wang, Z., Berceli, S. A., and Wu, R. L. (2010). Functional clustering of periodic transcriptional profiles through ARMA(p,q). *PLoS ONE,* 5(4): e9894.

Lin, M., Zhao, W., and Wu, R. L. (2006). A statistical framework for genetic association studies of power curves in bird flight. *Biological Procedures Online,* 8: 164–74.

Luedi, P. P., Hartemink, A. J., and Jirtle, R. L. (2005). Genome-wide prediction of imprinted murine genes. *Genome Research,* 15: 875–84.

Ma, C. X., Casella, G., and Wu, R. (2002). Functional mapping of quantitative trait loci underlying the character process: A theoretical framework. *Genetics,* 161: 1751–62.

Meyer, K. (2000). Random regressions to model phenotypic variation in monthly weights of Australian beef cows. *Livestock Production Science,* 65: 19–38.

Mohlke, K. L., Boehnke, M., and Abecasis, G. R. (2008). Metabolic and cardiovascular traits: An abundance of recently identified common genetic variants. *Human Molecular Genetics,* 17: R102–R108.

Moore, J. H., and Williams, S. M. (2009). Epistasis and its implications for personal genetics. *American Journal of Human Genetics,* 85 (3): 309–20.

Moyeed, R. A., and Diggle, P. J. (1994). Rates of convergence in semi-parametric modelling of longitudinal data. *Australian Journal of Statistics,* 36: 75–93.

Perelson, A. S., Neumann, A. U., Markowitz, M., Leonard, J. M., and Ho, D. D. (1996). HIV-1 dynamics in vivo: Virion clearance rate, infected cell life-span, and viral generation time. *Science,* 271: 1582–86.

Pletcher, S. D., and Geyer, C. J. (1999). The genetic analysis of age-titative genetics of natural populations. *Genetics,* 151: 825–35.

Psychiatric GCCC. (2009). Genomewide association studies: History, rationale, and prospects for psychiatric disorders. *American Journal of Psychiatry,* 166: 540–56.

Reik, W., and Walter, J. (2001). Genomic imprinting: Parental influence on the genome. *Nature Reviews Genetics,* 2: 21–32.

Richards, F. J. (1959). A flexible growth function for empirical use. *Journal of Experimental Botany,* 10: 290–300.

Rosenbaum, P. R., and Rubin, D. B. (1983). The central role of the propensity score in observation studies for causal effects. *Biometrika,* 70: 41–55.

Styrkarsdottir, U., Halldorsson, B. V., Gretarsdottir, S., Gudbjartsson, D. F., Walters, G. B., Ingvarsson, T., Jonsdottir, T., et al. (2009). New sequence variants associated with bone mineral density. *Nature Genetics,* 41: 15–17.

Thompson, P., and Thompson, P. J. L. (2009). *Introduction to Coaching Theory.* Fachverlag Und Buchhandel Gmbh. UK: Meyer & Meyer Sport.

Tobalske, B. W., Hedrick, T. L., Dial, K. P., and Biewener, A. A. (2003). Comparative power curves in bird flight. *Nature,* 421: 363–66.

Tsiatis, A. A., and Davidian, M. (2004). Joint modeling of longitudinal and time-to-event data: An overview. *Statistica Sinica,* 14: 793–818.

von Bertalanffy, L. (1957). Quantitative laws for metabolism and growth. *Quarterly Review of Biology,* 32: 217–31.

Wang, N. (2003). Marginal nonparametric kernel regression accounting for within-subject correlation. *Biometrika,* 90: 43–52.

Waterland, R. A., Lin, J. R., Smith, C. A., and Jirtle, R. J. (2006). Post-weaning diet affects genomic imprinting at the insulin-like growth factor 2 (Igf2) locus. *Human Molecular Genetics,* 15: 705–16.

Wen, S., Wang, C., Berg, A., Li, Y., Chang, M., Fillingim, R., Wallace, M., Staud, R., Kaplan, L., and Wu, R. (2009). Modeling genetic imprinting effects of DNA sequences with multilocus polymorphism data. *Algorithms for Molecular Biology,* 4: 11.

West, G. B., Brown, J. H., and Enquist, B. J. (2001). A general model for ontogenetic growth. *Nature,* 413: 628–31.

Whitlock, M. C., Phillips, P. C., Moore, F. B., and Tonsor, S. J. (1995). Multiple fitness peaks and epistasis. *Annual Reviews of Ecology and Systematics,* 26: 601–29.

Wolf, J. B. (2000). Gene interactions from maternal effects. *Evolution,* 54: 1882–98.

Wu, J. S., Zhang, B., Cui, Y. H., Zhao, W., Huang, M. R., Zeng, Y. R., Zhu, J., and Wu, R. L. (2007). Genetic mapping of developmental instability: Design, model and algorithm. *Genetics,* 176: 1187–96.

Wu, R. L., and Lin, M. (2006). Functional mapping—how to map and study the genetic architecture of dynamic complex traits. *Nature Reviews Genetics,* 7: 229–37.

Wu, W. B., and Pourahmadi, M. (2003). Nonparametric estimation of large covariance matrices of longitudinal data. *Biometrika,* 90: 831–44.

Yang, J., Wu, R. L., and Casella, G. (2009). Nonparametric functional mapping of quantitative trait loci. *Biometrics,* 65: 30–39.

Yao, F., Müller, H. G., and Wang, J. L. (2005a). Functional data analysis for sparse longitudinal data. *Journal of the American Statistical Association,* 100: 577–90.

Yao, F., Müller, H. G., and Wang, J. L. (2005b). Functional linear regression analysis for longitudinal data. *Annals of Statistics,* 33: 2873–2903.

Zeger, S. L., and Diggle, P. J. (1994). Semiparametric models for longitudinal data with application to CD4 cell numbers in HIV seroconverters. *Biometrics,* 50: 689–99.

Zhao, W, Chen, Y. Q., Casella, G., Cheverud, J. M., and Wu, R. (2005). A non-stationary model for functional mapping of complex traits. *Bioinformatics,* 21: 2469–77.

Zhao, W., Li, H. Y., Hou, W., and Wu, R. L. (2007). Wavelet-based parametric functional mapping of developmental trajectories. *Genetics,* 176: 1811–21.

Zhao, W., and Wu, R. L. (2008). Wavelet-based nonparametric functional mapping of longitudinal curves. *Journal of the American Statistical Association,* 103: 714–25.

Zimmerman, D., Núñez-Antón, V., Gregoire, T., Schabenberger, O., Hart, J., Kenward, M., Molenberghs, G., et al. (2001). Parametric modelling of growth curve data: An overview (with discussions). *Test,* 10: 1–73.

24

Adaptive Trial Simulation

Mark Chang
AMAG Pharmaceuticals Inc.

24.1 Clinical Trial Simulation

Clinical trial simulation (CTS) is a process that mimics clinical trials using computer programs. CTS is particularly important in adaptive designs for several reasons: (1) the statistical theory of adaptive design is complicated with limited analytical solutions available under certain assumptions; (2) the concept of CTS is very intuitive and easy to implement; (3) CTS can be used to model very complicated situations with minimum assumptions, and Type-I error can be strongly controlled; (4) using CTS, we cannot only calculate the power of an adaptive design, but we can also generate many other important operating characteristics such as expected sample-size, conditional power, and repeated confidence interval—ultimately this leads to the selection of an optimal trial design or clinical development plan; (5) CTS can be used to study the validity and robustness of an adaptive design in different hypothetical clinical settings, or with protocol deviations; (6) CTS can be used to monitor trials, project outcomes, anticipate problems, and suggest remedies before it is too late; (7) CTS can be used to visualize the dynamic trial process from patient recruitment, drug distribution, treatment administration, and pharmacokinetic processes to biomarkers and clinical responses; and (8) CTS has minimal cost associated with it and can be done in a short time.

CTS was started in the early 1970s and became popular in the mid 1990s due to increased computing power. CTS components include: (1) a trial design mode, which includes design type (parallel, crossover, traditional, adaptive), dosing regimens or algorithms, subject selection criteria, and time, financial, and other constraints; (2) a response model, which includes disease models that imitate the drug behavior (Pharmacokinetics (PK) and Pharmodynamics (PD) models) or intervention mechanism, and an infrastructure model (e.g., timing and validity of the assessment, diagnosis tool); (3) an execution model, which models the human behaviors that affect trial execution (e.g., protocol compliance, cooperation culture, decision cycle, regulatory authority, inference of opinion leaders); and (4) an evaluation model, which includes criteria for evaluating design models, such as utility models and Bayesian decision theory. In this chapter, we will focus on the adaptive trial simulations only.

24.2 A Unified Approach

There are many different methods for hypothesis-driven adaptive designs, for which we are going to present a unified approach using combinations of stage-wise p-values. There are four major components of adaptive designs in the frequentis paradigm: (1) Type-I error rate or α-control: determination of stopping boundaries; (2) Type-II error rate β: calculation of power or sample-size; (3) trial monitoring: calculation of conditional power or futility index; and (4) analysis after the completion of a trial: calculations of adjusted p-values, unbiased point estimates, and confidence intervals. The mathematical formulation for these components will be discussed and simulation algorithms for calculating the operating characteristics of adaptive designs will be developed.

24.2.1 Stopping Boundary

Consider a clinical trial with K stages and at each stage a hypothesis test is performed followed by some actions that are dependent on the analysis results. Such actions can be early futility or efficacy stopping, sample-size reestimation (SSR), modification of randomization, or other adaptations. The objective of the trial (e.g., testing the efficacy of the experimental drug) can be formulated using a hypothesis test:

$$H_o \text{ versus } \bar{H}_o. \tag{24.1}$$

Generally, the test statistics T_k at the kth stage can be a function η $(P_1,P_2,\ldots,P_k)$,where P_i is the one-sided p-value from the ith stage subsample and $\eta(P_1,P_2,\ldots,P_k)$ is strictly increasing function of all P_i $(i = 1,2,\ldots k)$.

The stopping rules are given by:

$$\begin{cases} \text{Stop for efficacy} & \text{if } T_k \le \alpha_k, \\ \text{Stop for futility} & \text{if } T_k > \beta_k, \\ \text{Continue with adaptations} & \text{if } \alpha_k < T_k \le \beta_k, \end{cases} \tag{24.2}$$

where $\alpha_k < \beta_k$ $(k = 1,\ldots,K - 1)$, and $\alpha_K = \beta_K$. For convenience, α_k and β_k are called the efficacy and futility boundaries, respectively.

To reach the kth stage, a trial has to pass the 1th to $(k - 1)$th stages. Therefore the c.d.f. of T_k is given by:

$$\begin{aligned} \psi_k(t) &= \Pr(\alpha_1 < T_1 < \beta_1,\ldots,\alpha_{k-1} < T_{k-1} < \beta_{k-1}, T_k < t) \\ &= \int_{\alpha_1}^{\beta_1} \cdots \int_{\alpha_{k-1}}^{\beta_{k-1}} \int_{-\infty}^{t} f_{T_1\ldots T_k}\, dt_k\, dt_{k-1} \ldots dt_1, \end{aligned} \tag{24.3}$$

where $f_{T_1\ldots T_k}$ is the joint p.d.f. of $T_1,\ldots,$ and T_k.

24.2.2 Type-I Error Control, p-Value and Power

When H_0 (or $\delta = 0$) is true, $\psi_k(t)$ is the stagewise p-value p_c if the trial stopped at the kth stage; that is,

$$p_c(t;k) = \psi_k(t \mid H_0). \tag{24.4}$$

The stagewise error rate (α spent) π_k at the kth stage is given by:

$$\pi_k = \psi_k(\alpha_k \mid H_0). \tag{24.5}$$

The stagewise power of rejecting H_0 at the kth stage is given by:

$$\varpi_k = \psi_k(\alpha_k \mid H_a). \tag{24.6}$$

When efficacy is claimed at a certain stage, the trial is stopped. Therefore, the Type-I errors at different stages are mutually exclusive. Hence the experiment-wise Type-I error rate can be written as:

$$\alpha = \sum_{k=1}^{K} \pi_k. \tag{24.7}$$

Similarly, the power can be written as:

$$power = \sum_{k=1}^{K} \varpi_k. \tag{24.8}$$

Equation 24.5 is the key to determining the stopping boundaries adaptive designs as illustrated in the next several chapters.

There are several possible definitions of (adjusted) p-values. Here we are most interested in the so-called stagewise-ordering p-values, defined as:

$$p(t;k) = \sum_{i=1}^{k-1} \pi_i + p_c(t;k). \tag{24.9}$$

The adjusted p-value is a measure of overall statistical strength against H_0. The later the H_0 is rejected, the larger the adjusted p-value is, and the weaker the statistical evidence (against H_0) is. A late rejection leading to a larger p-value is reasonable because the alpha at earlier stages has been spent. An important characteristic of the adjusted p-value is that when the test statistic t is on stopping boundary $a_{k,}$ P_k must be equal to alpha spent so far.

24.2.3 Selection of Test Statistics

To form the test statistic $\eta(P_1,P_2,\ldots,P_k)$, there are many possible combinations of the p-values such as:

1. Linear combination

$$T_k = \Sigma_{i=1}^{k} w_{ki} p_i, k = 1,\ldots,K, \tag{24.10}$$

where $W_{ki} > 0$ are constants.

2. Product of stagewise p-values (Fisher combination, Bauer and Kohne 1994),

$$T_k = \prod_{i=1}^{k} p_i, k = 1,\ldots,K, \tag{24.11}$$

and

3. Linear combination of inverse-normal stagewise p-values (Lan and DeMets 1983; Cui, Hung, and Wang 1999; Lehmacher and Wassmer 1999)

$$T_k = \sum_{i=1}^{k} w_{ki} \Phi^{-1}(1 - p_i), k = 1,\ldots,K, \tag{24.12}$$

where weight, $w_{ki} > 0, \Sigma_{i=1}^{k} w_{ki}^2 = 1$, can be constant or a function of data from previous stages, and K is the number of analyses planned in the trial.

Note that P_k is the naive p-value from the subsample at the kth stage, while $P_c(t; k)$ and $P(t; k)$ are stagewise and stagewise-ordering p-values, respectively.

24.2.4 Method for Stopping Boundary Determination

After selecting the type of test statistic, we can determine the stopping boundaries α_k and β_k by using Equations 24.3, 24.5, and 24.7 under the null Hypothesis 24.1. Once the stopping boundaries are determined, the power and sample-size under a particular H_a can be obtained using Equations 24.3, 24.6, and 24.8 in conjunction with the Monte Carlo method.

After selecting the test statistic, we can choose one of the following approaches to fully determine the stopping boundaries:

1. Classical Method: Choose certain types of functions for α_k and β_k. The advantage of using a stopping boundary function is that there are only limited parameters in the function to be determined. After the parameters are determined, the stopping boundaries are then fully determined using Equations 24.3, 24.5, and 24.7, regardless of the number of stages. The commonly used boundaries are OB–F (O'Brien and Fleming 1979), Pocock's (1977), and Wang-Tsiatis's boundaries (1987).
2. Error-Spending Method: Choose certain forms of functions for π_k such that $\Sigma_{k=1}^{K} \pi_k = \alpha$. Traditionally, the cumulative quantity $\pi_k^* = \Sigma_{i=1}^{k} \pi_i$ is called the error-spending function, which can be either a function of stage K or the so-called information time based on sample-size fraction. After determining the function π_k or equivalently π_k^*, the stopping boundaries α_k, and β_k ($k = 1,\ldots,K$) can be determined using Equations 24.3, 24.5, and 24.7.
3. Nonparametric Method: Choose nonparametric stopping boundaries; that is, no function is assumed, instead, use computer simulations to determine the stopping boundaries via a trial–error method. The nonparametric method does not allow for the changes to the number and timing of the interim analyses.
4. Conditional Error Function Method: One can rewrite the stagewise error rate for a two-stage design as:

$$\pi_2 = \psi_2(\alpha_2 \mid H_o) = \int_{\alpha_1}^{\beta_1} A(p_1) dp_1, \tag{24.13}$$

where $A(p_1)$ is called the conditional error function. For a given α_1 and β_1, by carefully selecting $A(p_1)$, the overall α control can be met (Proschan and Hunsberger 1995). However, $A(p_1)$ cannot be an arbitrary monotonic function of P_1. In fact, when the test statistic (e.g., sum of p-values, Fisher's combination of p-values, or inverse-normal p-values) and constant stopping boundaries are determined, the conditional error function $A(p_1)$ is determined. For example,

$$A(p_1) = \alpha_2 - p_1 \text{ for MSP,}$$

$$A(p_1) = \alpha_2 / p_1 \text{ for MPP,} \tag{24.14}$$

$$A(p_1) = (\alpha_2 - \sqrt{n_1}\, p_1)/\sqrt{n_2} \text{ for MINP,}$$

where n_i are subsample size for the ith stage.

On the other hand, if an arbitrary (monotonic) $A(p_1)$ is chosen for a test statistic (e.g., sum of p-values or inverse-normal p-values), the stopping boundaries α_2 and β_2 may not be constant anymore. Instead, they are usually functions of P_1.

5. Conditional Error Method: In this method, for a given α_1 and β_1 $A(p_1)$ is calculated on-the-fly or in real-time, and only for the observed p_1 under H_0. Adaptations can be made under the condition that keep $A(p_1|H_0)$ unchanged.

   Note that α_k and β_k are usually only functions of stage k or information time, but they can be functions of response data from previous stages; that is, $\alpha_k = \alpha_k(t_1,\ldots,t_{k-1})$ and $\beta_k = \beta_k(t_1,\ldots,t_{k-1})$. In fact, using variable transformation of the test statistic to another test statistic, the stopping boundaries often change from response-independent to response-dependent. For example, in MSP (see next sections), we use stopping boundary $p_1 + p_2 \le \alpha_2$, which implies that $p_1 p_2 \le \alpha_2 p_2 - p_2^2$. In other words, MSP stopping boundary at the second stage, $p_1 + p_2 \le \alpha_2$ is equivalent to the MPP boundary at the second stage, $p_1 p_2 \le \alpha_2 p_2 - p_2^2$—a response-dependent stopping boundary.
6. Recursive Design Method: Based on Müller–Shäfer's conditional error principle, this method recursively constructs two-stage designs at the time of interim analyses, making the method a simple but very flexible approach to a general K-stage design (Müller and Shäfer 2004; Chang 2007).

24.3 Method Based on the Sum of *p*-Values

Chang (2007) proposed an adaptive design method, in which the test statistic is defined as the sum of the stagewise p-values (MSP):

$$T_k = \Sigma_{i=1}^{k} p_i,\ k = 1,\ldots,K. \tag{24.15}$$

The Type-I error rate at stage k can be expressed as (assume $\beta_i \le \alpha_{i+1}$, $i = 1,\ldots$):

$$\pi_k = \int_{\alpha_1}^{\beta_1}\int_{\alpha_2-p_1}^{\beta_2}\int_{\alpha_3-p_2-p_1}^{\beta_3}\cdots\int_{\alpha_{k-1}-\sum_{i=1}^{k-2}p_i}^{\beta_{k-1}}\int_0^{\alpha_k-\sum_{i=1}^{k-1}p_i} dp_k\cdots dp_3\,dp_2\,dp_1, \tag{24.16}$$

where for nonfutility binding rule, let $\beta_i = \alpha_k$, $i = 1,\ldots$; that is,

$$\pi_k = \int_{\alpha_1}^{\alpha_k}\int_{\max(0,\alpha_2-p_1)}^{\alpha_k}\int_{\max(0,\alpha_3-p_2-p_1)}^{\alpha_k}\cdots$$

$$\int_{\max(0,\alpha_{k-1}-\sum_{i=1}^{k-2}p_i)}^{\alpha_K}\int_0^{\max(0,\alpha_k-\sum_{i=1}^{k-1}p_i)} dp_k\cdots dp_3\,dp_2\,dp_1. \tag{24.17}$$

We setup $\alpha_k > \alpha_{k-1}$ and if $p_i > \alpha_k$, then no interim efficacy analysis is necessary for stage $i+1$ to k because there is no chance to reject H_0 at these stages.

To control over Type-I error, it is required that:

$$\sum_{i=1}^{K} \pi_i = \alpha. \tag{24.18}$$

Theoretically, Equation 24.17 can be carried out for any k. Here, we provide the analytical forms for $k = 1–3$, which should satisfy most practical needs.

$$\pi_1 = \alpha_1 \tag{24.19}$$

$$\pi_2 = \frac{1}{2}(\alpha_2 - \alpha_1)^2 \tag{24.20}$$

$$\pi_3 = \alpha_1\alpha_2\alpha_3 + \frac{1}{3}\alpha_2^3 + \frac{1}{6}\alpha_3^3 - \frac{1}{2}\alpha_1\alpha_2^2 - \frac{1}{2}\alpha_1\alpha_3^2 - \frac{1}{2}\alpha_2^2\alpha_3. \tag{24.21}$$

π_i is error spent at the ith stage, which can be predetermined or specified as error spending function $\pi_k = f(k)$. The stopping boundary can be solved through numerical iterations. Specifically, (1) determine π_i ($i = 1,2,\ldots,K$); and (2) from $\pi_1 = \alpha_1$, solve for α_1; from $\pi_2 = 1/2(\alpha_2 - \alpha_1)^2$, obtain $\alpha_2,\ldots$, from $\pi_K = \pi_K(\alpha_1,\ldots,\alpha_{K-1})$, obtain α_K.

For two-stage designs, using Equations 24.18 through 24.20, we have the following formulation for determining the stopping boundaries:

$$\alpha = \alpha_1 + \frac{1}{2}(\alpha_2 - \alpha_1)^2. \tag{24.22}$$

To calculate the stopping boundaries for given α and α_1, solve Equation 24.22 for α_2.Various stopping boundaries can be chosen from Equation 24.22. See Table 24.1 for numerical examples of the stopping boundaries.

The stagewise-ordering p-value can be obtained by replacing α_1 with t in Equation 24.22 if the trial stops at Stage 2. That is:

$$p(t;k) = \begin{cases} t, & k = 1, \\ \alpha_1 + \frac{1}{2}(t - \alpha_1)^2, & k = 2, \end{cases} \tag{24.23}$$

where $t = p_1$ if trial stops at Stage 1 and $t = p_1 + p_2$ if it stops at Stage 2.

It is interesting to know that when $p_1 > \alpha_2$, there is no point in continuing the trial because $p_1 + p_2 > p_1 > \alpha_2$, and futility should be claimed. Therefore, statistically it is always a good idea to choose $\beta_l \le \alpha_2$. However, because the nonbinding futility rule is adopted currently by the regulatory bodies, it is better to use the stopping boundaries with $\beta_1 = \alpha_2$.

The condition power is given by (Chang 2007):

$$cP = 1 - \Phi\left(z_{1-\alpha_2+p_1} - \frac{\hat{\delta}}{\hat{\sigma}}\sqrt{\frac{n_2}{2}}\right), \quad \alpha_1 < p_1 \le \beta_1, \tag{24.24}$$

where n_2 = sample size per group at Stage 2; $\hat{\delta}$ and $\hat{\sigma}$ are observed treatment difference and standard deviation, respectively.

TABLE 24.1 Stopping Boundaries with MSP

α_1	0.000	0.0025	0.005	0.010	0.015	0.020
α_2	0.2236	0.2146	0.2050	0.1832	0.1564	0.1200

Note: One-sided $\alpha = 0.025$, $\alpha_2 = \beta_1 = \beta_2$.

To obtain power for group sequential design using MSP, Monte Carlo simulation can be used. Algorithm 24.1 is developed for this purpose. To obtain efficacy stopping boundaries, one can let $\delta = 0$, then the power from the simulation output is numerically equal to α. Using trial-and-error method, to adjust $\{\alpha_i\}$ until the output power = α. The final set of $\{\alpha_i\}$ is the efficacy stopping boundary.

Algorithm 24.1: *K*-Stage Group Sequential with MSP (large n)

Objective: return power for a two-group *K*-stage adaptive design

Input treatment difference δ and common σ, one-sided α, δ_{min}, stopping boundaries $\{\alpha_i\}$ and $\{\beta_i\}$, stagewise sample size $\{n_i\}$, number of stages *K*, nRuns.

```
power:=0
For iRun:=1 To nRuns
  T:=0
  For i:=1 To K
      Generate u from N(0,1)
    z_i = δ√(n_i/2)/σ+u
    p_i :=1-Φ(z_i)
    T :=T+p_i
    If T>β_i Then Exitfor
    If T≤α_i Then power := power+1/nRuns
  Endfor
Endfor
Return power
§
```

24.4 Method Based on Product of *p*-Values

This method is referred to as MPP. The test statistic in this method is based on the product (Fisher's combination) of the stagewise *p*-values from the subsamples (Bauer and Kohne 1994; Bauer and Rohmel 1995), defined as:

$$T_k = \Pi_{i=1}^{k} p_i, k = 1, \cdots, K. \tag{24.25}$$

$$\pi_k = \int_{\alpha_1}^{\beta_1} \int_{\alpha_2/p_1}^{\beta_2} \int_{\alpha_3/(p_1 p_2)}^{\beta_3} \cdots \int_{\alpha_{k-1}/(p_1 \cdots p_{k-2})}^{\beta_{k-1}} \int_0^{\alpha_k/(p_1 \cdots p_{k-1})} dp_k \cdots dp_1. \tag{24.26}$$

For nonfutility boundary, choose $\beta_1 = 1$. It is interesting to know that when $p_1 < \alpha_2$, there is no point in continuing the trial because $p_1 p_2 < p_1 < \alpha_2$ and efficacy should be claimed. Therefore it is suggested that we should choose $\beta_1 > \alpha_2$ and $\alpha_1 > \alpha_2$. In general, if $p_k \leq \max(\alpha_k, \ldots \alpha_n)$, stop the trial. In other words, α_k should monotonically decrease in *k*. The relationships between error-spent π_i and stopping boundary α_i at the *i*th stage are given up to three stages:

$$\pi_1 = \alpha_1, \tag{24.27}$$

$$\pi_2 = \alpha_2 \ln \frac{1}{\alpha_1}, \tag{24.28}$$

TABLE 24.2 Stopping Boundaries with MPP

α_1	0.001	0.0025	0.005	0.010	0.015	0.020
α_2	0.0035	0.0038	0.0038	0.0033	0.0024	0.0013

Note: One-sided $\alpha = 0.025$.

$$\pi_3 = \alpha_3 \left(\ln\alpha_2 - \frac{1}{2}\ln\alpha_1 \right) \ln\alpha_1, \tag{24.29}$$

Numerical examples of stopping boundaries for two-stage adaptive designs with MPP are presented in Table 24.2.

The stagewise-ordering p-value for a two-stage design can be obtained using:

$$p(t;k) = \begin{cases} t, & k=1, \\ \alpha_1 - t\ln\alpha_1, & k=2, \end{cases} \tag{24.30}$$

where $t = p_1$ if the trial stops at stage 1 (k = 1) and $t = p_1 p_2$ if the trial stops at Stage 2 (k = 2).

The condition power is given by (Chang 2007):

$$cP = 1 - \Phi\left(z_{1-\frac{\alpha_2}{p_1}} - \frac{\hat{\delta}}{\hat{\sigma}}\sqrt{\frac{n_2}{2}} \right), \quad \alpha_1 < p_1 \le \beta_1. \tag{24.31}$$

Algorithm 24.2 is a Monte Carlo simulation algorithm for K-stage group sequential design. To obtain efficacy stopping boundaries, one can let $\delta = 0$, then the power from the simulation output is numerically equal to α. Using trial-and-error method, to adjust $\{\alpha_i\}$ until the output power = α. Then the final set of $\{\alpha_i\}$ is the efficacy stopping boundary.

Algorithm 24.2: *K*-Stage Group Sequential with MPP (large sample)

Objective: return power for a two-group K-stage adaptive design.

Input treatment difference δ and common σ, one-sided α, δ_{min}, stopping boundaries $\{\alpha_i\}$ and $\{\beta_i\}$, stagewise sample-size $\{n_i\}$, number of stages K, nRuns.

```
power:=0
For iRun:=1 To nRuns
  T:=1
  For i :=1 To K
      Generate u from N(0,1)
    z_i = δ√(n_i/2)/σ+u
    p_i:=1-Φ(z_i)
    T:=T .p_i
    If T>β_i Then Exitfor
    If T≤α_i Then power := power+1/nRuns
  Endfor
Endfor
Return power
§
```

TABLE 24.3 Stopping Boundaries with MINP

α_1	0.0010	0.0025	0.0050	0.0100	0.0150	0.0200
α_2	0.0247	0.0240	0.0226	0.0189	0.0143	0.0087

Note: One-sided $\alpha = 0.025$, $w_1 = w_2$.

24.5 Method with Inverse-Normal *p*-Values

This method is based on inverse-normal *p*-values (MINP), in which the test statistic at the *k*th stage T_k is a linear combination of the inverse-normal of stagewise *p*-values. The weights can be fixed constants. MINP (Lecherman and Wassmer 1999) can be viewed as a general method, which includes the standard group sequential design and Cui–Hung–Wang method for SSR (Cui, Hung, and Wang 1999) as special cases.

Let z_k be the stagewise normal test statistic at the *k*th stage. In general, $z_i = \Phi^{-1}(1 - p_i)$, where p_i is the stagewise *p*-value from the *i*th stage subsample.

In a group sequential design, the test statistic can be expressed as:

$$T_k^* = \sum_{i=1}^{k} w_{ki} z_i, \tag{24.32}$$

where the prefixed weights satisfy the equality $\sum_{i=1}^{k} w_{ki}^2 = 1$ and the stagewise statistic z_i is based on the subsample for the *i*th stage.

Note that when w_{ki} is fixed, the standard multivariate normal distribution of $\{T_1^*,\ldots,T_k^*\}$ will not change regardless of adaptations as long as z_i $(i = 1,\ldots,k)$ has the standard normal distribution. To be consistent with the unified formations, in which the test statistic is on *p*-scale, we use the transformation $T_k = 1 - \Phi(T_k^*)$ such that:

$$T_k = 1 - \Phi\left(\sum_{i=1}^{k} w_{ki} z_i\right), \tag{24.33}$$

where Φ = the standard normal c.d.f.

The stopping boundary and power for MINP can be calculated using only numerical integration or computer simulation using Algorithm 24.

Table 24.3 shows numerical examples of stopping boundaries for two-stage adaptive designs, generated using ExpDesign Studio 5.0.

The conditional power for a two-stage design with MINP is given by:

$$cP = 1 - \Phi\left(\frac{z_{1-\alpha_2} - w_1 z_{1-p_1}}{w_2} - \frac{\hat{\delta}}{\hat{\sigma}}\sqrt{\frac{n_2}{2}}\right), \quad \alpha_1 < p_1 \le \beta_1, \tag{24.34}$$

where weights satisfy $w_1^2 + w_2^2 = 1$.

The stopping boundary and power can be obtained using Algorithm 24.3.

Algorithm 24.3: *K*-Stage Group Sequential with MINP (large *n*)

Objective: Return power for *K*-stage adaptive design.

Input treatment difference δ and common σ, one-sided α, $\delta_{\min}$, stopping boundaries $\{\alpha_i\}$ and $\{\beta_i\}$, stagewise sample-size $\{n_i\}$, weights $\{w_{ki}\}$, number of stages *K*, nRuns.

```
power:=0
For iRun :=1 To nRuns
  T :=1
  For i :=1 To K
      Generate δ̂_i from N (δ,2σ²/n_I)
      z_i = δ_i √(n_i/2) / σ
  Endfor
  For k:= 1 To K
      T*_k :=0
  For i :=1 To k
      T*_k := T*_k + w_ki z_i
  Endfor
    T_k:=1−Φ(T*_k)
    If T_k > β_k Then Exitfor
    If T_k ≤ α_k Then power := power + 1/nRuns
  Endfor
Endfor
Return power
§
```

Chang (2007) has implemented Algorithms 24.1 through 24.3 using SAS and R for normal, binary, and survival endpoints.

24.6 Probability of Efficacy

In practice, to have the drug benefit to patients, statistical significance is not enough, the drug must demonstrate its clinical significance and commercial viability. Statistical and clinical significance are requirements for FDA approval for marketing the drug. The requirement of being commercially viable is to ensure the financial incentive to the sponsor such that they are willing to invest in drug development. Both clinical significance and commercial viability can be expressed in terms of the observed treatment effect exceeding over the control with a certain amount δ_{min}:

$$\hat{\delta} > \delta_{min}, \tag{24.35}$$

where δ_{min} is usually an estimation.

It is a better measure for the trial success using the probability of having both statistical significance and $\hat{\delta} > \delta_{min}$ then power alone. For convenience, we define the probability as probability of efficacy (PE), given by:

$$PE = \Pr\left(p < \alpha \text{ and } \hat{\delta} > \delta_{min}\right). \tag{24.36}$$

We will implement PE in Algorithms 24.4 and 24.5 for adaptive designs. But let us first discuss the operating characteristics of an adaptive design.

24.7 Design Evaluation: Operating Characteristics

24.7.1 Stopping Probabilities

The stopping probability at each stage is an important property of an adaptive design, because it provides the time-to-market and the associated probability of success. It also provides information on the cost (sample-size) of the trial and the associated probability. In fact, the stopping probabilities are used to calculate the expected samples that represent the average cost or efficiency of the trial design and the duration of the trial.

There are two types of stopping probabilities: unconditional probability of stopping to claim efficacy (reject H_0) and unconditional probability of futility (accept H_0). The former refers to the efficacy stopping probability (ESP), and the latter refers to the futility stopping probability (FSP). From Equation 24.3, it is obvious that the ESP at the kth stage is given by:

$$ESP_k = \psi_k(\alpha_k), \tag{24.37}$$

and the FSP at the kth stage is given by:

$$FSP_k = 1 - \psi_k(\beta_k). \tag{24.38}$$

24.7.2 Expected Duration of an Adaptive Trial

The stopping probabilities can be used to calculate the expected trial duration, which is definitely an important feature of an adaptive design. The conditionally (on the efficacy claim) expected trial duration is given by:

$$\bar{t}_e = \sum_{k=1}^{K} ESP_k t_k, \tag{24.39}$$

where t_k is the time from the first-patient-in to the kth interim analysis.

The conditionally (on the futility claim) expected trial duration is given by:

$$\bar{t}_f = \sum_{k=1}^{K} FSP_k t_k. \tag{24.40}$$

The unconditionally expected trial duration is given by:

$$\bar{t} = \sum_{k=1}^{K} \left(ESP_k + FSP_k\right) t_k. \tag{24.41}$$

24.7.3 Expected Sample-Sizes

The expected sample-size is a commonly used measure of the efficiency (cost and timing of the trial) of the design. The expected sample-size is a function of the treatment difference and its variability, which are unknowns. Therefore, expected sample-size is really based on hypothetical values of the parameters. For this reason, it is beneficial and important to calculate the expected sample-size under various critical or possible values of the parameters. The total expected sample-size per group can be expressed as:

$$N_{\exp} = \sum_{k=1}^{K} n_k \left(ESP_k + FSP_k\right) = \sum_{k=1}^{K} n_k \left(1 + \psi_k(\alpha_k) - \psi_k(\beta_k)\right). \tag{24.42}$$

It can also be written as:

$$N_{\exp} = N_{\max} - \sum_{k=1}^{K} n_k\left(\psi_k(\beta_k) - \psi_k(\alpha_k)\right), \tag{24.43}$$

where $N_{\max} = \sum_{k=1}^{K} n_k$ is the maximum sample-size per group.

24.7.4 Conditional Power and Futility Index

The conditional power is the conditional probability of rejecting the null hypothesis during the rest of the trial based on the observed interim data. The conditional power is commonly used for monitoring an on-going trial. Similar to the ESP and FSP, conditional power is dependent on the population parameters or treatment effect and its variability. The conditional power at the kth stage is the sum of the probability of rejecting the null hypothesis at stage $k+1$ to K (K does not have to be predetermined), given the observed data from Stages 1 through k.

$$cP_k = \sum_{j=k+1}^{K} \Pr\left(\cap_{i=k+1}^{j-1}\left(a_i < T_i < \beta_i\right) \cap T_j \le \alpha_j \mid \cap_{i=1}^{k} T_i = t_i\right), \tag{24.44}$$

where t_i is the observed test statistic T_i at the ith stage. For a two-stage design, the conditional power can be expressed as:

$$cP_1 = \Pr\left(T_2 \le \alpha_2 \mid t_1\right). \tag{24.45}$$

Specific formulations of conditional power for two-stage designs with MSP, MPP, and MINP were provided in earlier sections.

The futility index is defined as the conditional probability of accepting the null hypothesis:

$$FI_k = 1 - cP_k. \tag{24.46}$$

Algorithm 24.4 can be used to obtain operating characteristics of a group sequential design, which can be modified for other adaptive designs and other adaptive design methods (e.g., MPP, MINP).

Algorithm 24.4: Operating Characteristics of Group Sequential Design

Objective: return power, average sample-size per group (AveN), FSP_i, and ESP_i for a two-group K-stage adaptive design with MSP.

Input treatment difference δ and common σ, one-sided α, stopping boundaries $\{\alpha_i\}$ and $\{\beta_i\}$, stage-wise sample size $\{n_i\}$, number of stages K, nRuns.

```
Power:=0
For iRun := 1 To nRuns
  T := 0
For i := 1 To K
  FSP_i := 0
  ESP_i := 0
Endfor
```

```
    For i := 1 To K
      Generate u from N (0,1)
      z_i = δ√(n_i/2)/σ+u
      p_i := 1-Φ(z_I)
      T := T+p_i
      If T>β_i Then
        FSP_i := FSP_i + 1/nRuns
        Exitfor
      Endif
      If T≤α_i Then
        ESP_i := ESP_i + 1/nRuns
        power := power + 1/nRuns
        Exitfor
      Endif
    Endfor
  Endfor
  aveN := 0
  For i := 1 To K
    aveN := aveN+ (FSP_i + ESP_i) n_i
  Endfor
  Return {power, aveN, {FSP_i},{ESP_i}}
  §
```

24.8 Sample-Size Reestimation

Sample size determination is critical in clinical trial designs. It is estimated about 5000 patients per NDA on average. The average cost per patient ranges from \$20,000 to \$50,000. Small but adequate sample size will allow sponsor to use their resources efficiently, shorten the trial duration, and deliver the drug to the patients earlier.

From efficacy point of view, sample size is often determined by the power for the hypothesis test of the primary endpoint. However, the challenge is the difficulty in getting precise estimates of the treatment effect and its variability at the time of protocol design. If the effect size of the new molecular entity (NME) is overestimated or its variability is underestimated, the sample size will be underestimated and consequently the power is to low to have reasonable probability of detecting the clinical meaningful difference. On the other hand, if the effect size of the NME is underestimated or its variability is overestimated, the sample size will be overestimated and consequently the power is higher than necessary, which could lead to unnecessary exposure of many patients to a potentially harmful compound when the drug, in fact, is not effective. The commonly used adaptive design, called sample-size reestimation (SSR), emerged for this purpose.

A SSR design refers to an adaptive design that allows for sample-size adjustment or reestimation based on the review of interim analysis results. There are two types of SSR procedures, namely, SSR based on blinded and unblinded data. In the first scenario, the sample adjustment is based on the (observed) pooled variance at the interim analysis to recalculate the required sample-size, which does not require unblinding the data. In this scenario, the Type-I error adjustment is practically negligible. In the second scenario, the effect size and its variability are reassessed, and sample-size is adjusted based on the unblinded information. The statistical method for the adjustment can be based on observed effect size or the conditional power.

For a two-stage SSR, the sample size for the second stage can be calculated based on the target conditional power:

$$\begin{cases} n_2 = \dfrac{2\hat{\sigma}^2}{\hat{\delta}^2}\left(z_{1-\alpha_2+p_1} - z_{1-cP}\right)^2, & \text{for MSP} \\ n_2 = \dfrac{2\hat{\sigma}^2}{\hat{\delta}^2}\left(z_{1-\alpha_2/p_1} - z_{1-cP}\right)^2, & \text{for MPP,} \\ n_2 = \dfrac{2\hat{\sigma}^2}{\hat{\delta}^2}\left(\dfrac{z_{1-\alpha_2}}{w_2} - \dfrac{w_1}{w_2} z_{1-p_1} - z_{1-cP}\right)^2, & \text{for MINP} \end{cases} \quad (24.47)$$

where, for the purpose of calculation, $\hat{\delta}$ and $\hat{\sigma}$ are taken to be the observed treatment effect and standard deviation at Stage 1; cP is the target conditional power.

For a general K-stage design, the sample-size rule at the kth stage can be based on the observed treatment effect in comparison with the initial assessment:

$$n_j = \min\left(n_{j,\max}, \left(\frac{\delta}{\bar{\delta}}\right)^2 n_j^0\right), j = k, k+1, \ldots, K, \quad (24.48)$$

where n_j^0 is original sample size for the jth stage, δ is the initial assessment for the treatment effect, $\bar{\delta}$ is the updated assessment after interim analyses, given by:

$$\bar{\delta} = \frac{\sum_{i=1}^{k} n_i \hat{\delta}_i}{\sum_{i=1}^{k} n_i} \text{ for MSP and MPP,} \quad (24.49)$$

$$\bar{\delta} = \sum_{i=1}^{k} w_{ki}^2 \hat{\delta}_i \text{ for MINP.} \quad (24.50)$$

We now can develop algorithms for sample-size reestimation using MSP, MPP, and MINP. As samples, Algorithm 24.5 is implemented for two-stage SSR based on conditional power using MSP and Algorithm 24.6 is provided for K-stage SSR using MINP. Both algorithms return power and PE as simulation outputs.

Algorithm 24.5: Two-Stage Sample-Size Reestimation with MSP

Objective: Return power and PE for two-stage adaptive design.

Input treatment difference δ and common σ, stopping boundaries α_1, α_2, β_1, n_1, n_2, target conditional power for SSR, sample size limits $n_{\max}$, clinical meaningful and commercial viable $\delta_{\min}$, and nRuns.

```
power := 0
PE := 0
For iRun := 1 To nRuns
   T := 0
   Generate u from N (0,1)
```
$z_1 = \delta\sqrt{n_1/2}/\sigma + u$

```
    p₁ := 1-Φ(z₁)
    If p₁ > β₁ Then Exitfor
    If p₁ ≤ α₁ Then power := power + 1/nRuns
  If p₁ ≤ α₁ And δ̂₁ ≥ δ_min Then PE := PE + 1/nRuns
  If α₁ < p₁ ≤ β₁ Then
```

$$n_2 := \frac{2\sigma^2}{\hat{\delta}_1^2}\left(z_{1-\alpha_2+p_1} - z_{1-cP}\right)^2$$

```
    Generate u from N (0,1)
```

$$z_2 = \delta\sqrt{n_2/2}/\sigma + u$$

```
    p₂ :=1-Φ(z₂)
    T :=p₁ + p₂
    If T ≤ α₂ Then power := power + 1/nRuns
```

$$\hat{\delta} = (\hat{\delta}_1 n_1 + \hat{\delta}_1 n_2)/(n_1 + n_2)$$

```
    If T ≤ α₂ And δ̂ ≥ δ_min Then PE := PE + 1/nRuns
    Endif
  Endfor
  Return {power, PE}
  §
```

Algorithm 24.5 can be easily modified using MPP.

Algorithm 24.6: *K*-Stage Sample-Size Reestimation with MINP (large sample size)

Objective: Return power and PE for *K*-stage adaptive design.

Note: sample-size reestimation will potentially increase the overall sample size only by the subsample size for the last stage n_K.

Input treatment difference δ and common σ, one-sided α, δ_{min}, stopping boundaries $\{\alpha_i\}$ and $\{\beta_i\}$, stagewise sample size $\{n_i\}$, sample size limits $\{n_{i,max}\}$ number of stages K, weights $\{w_{ki}\}$, nRuns.

```
  Power:= 0
  PE := 0
  For iRun := 1 To nRuns
    For i := 1 To K
      Generate u from N (0,1)
```

$$z_i = \delta\sqrt{n_i/2}/\sigma + u$$

```
    Endfor
    For k :=1 To K
```

$$T_k^* := 0$$

```
      For i := 1 To k
```

$$T_k^* := T_k^* + w_{ki} z_i$$

$$\bar{\delta} = \bar{\delta} + w_{ki}^2 \hat{\delta}_i$$

```
    Endfor
```

$$T_k; = 1 - \Phi(T_k^*)$$

```
    If T_k > β_k Then Exitfor
    If T_k ≤ α_k Then power := power + 1/nRuns
    If T_k ≤ α_k And δ̄ ≥ δ_min Then PE := PE + 1/nRuns
```

```
    If α_k < T_k ≤ β_k Then
      For j := k To K
        n_j := min(n_{j,max}, (δ/δ̄)^2 n_j^0)
          Endfor
        Endif
      Endfor
    Endfor
  Return {power, PE}
  §
```

The stagewise adjusted p-value can be calculated using the Monte Carlo method. Specifically, if the trial is stopped at the $\tilde{k}$th stage with $T_{\tilde{k}} = t_{\tilde{k}}$, we replace $\alpha_{\tilde{k}}$ with $t_{\tilde{k}}$, the probability conditional probability $P(T_{\tilde{k}} > t_{\tilde{k}})$ is the stagewise p-value and stagewise-ordering p-value is given by:

$$p = \sum_{i=1}^{\tilde{k}-1} \pi_i + P(T_{\tilde{k}} > t_{\tilde{k}}). \tag{24.51}$$

As an example, Algorithm 24.7 is developed for obtaining stagewise ordering p-value using the Monte Carlo simulation.

Algorithm 24.7: Stagewise p-value of Adaptive Design SSR

Objective: Return stagewise ordering p-value.

Note: sample-size reestimation will potentially increase the overall sample size only by the subsample size for the last stage n_k.

Input treatment difference δ and common σ, one-sided α, δ_{min}, stopping boundaries $\{\alpha_i\}$ and $\{\beta_i\}$, where $\alpha_{\tilde{k}}$ is replaced with $t_{\tilde{k}}$, stagewise sample size $\{n_i\}$, sample size limits $\{n_{i,max}\}$ number of stages K, weights $\{w_{ki}\}$, nRuns.

```
Power:= 0
For iRun := 1 To nRuns
  For i :=1 To k̃
    Generate u from N (0,1)
    z_i = δ√(n_i/2)/σ + u
  Endfor
  For k :=1 To k̃
    T_k^* := 0
    For i := 1 To k
    T_k^* := T_k^* + w_ki z_i
    δ̄ = δ̄ + w_ki^2 δ̂_i
  Endfor
  T_k := 1 − Φ(T_k^*)
  If T_k > β_k Then Exitfor
  If T_k ≤ α_k And k = k̃ Then power := power + 1/nRuns
  If α_k < T_k ≤ β_k Then
      For j := k To k̃
```

```
            n_j := min(n_{j,max}, (δ/δ)^2 n_j^0)
        Endfor
      Endif
    Endfor
  Endfor
  Return power
  §
```

24.9 Examples

We are going to discuss adaptive trial simulations for a phase III asthma study and a phase III oncology trial.

Example 1: An Asthma Adaptive Trial Simulation

In a Phase III asthma study with two dose groups (control and active), the primary efficacy endpoint is the percent change from baseline in FEV1. The estimated FEV1 improvement from baseline is 5–12% for the control and active groups, respectively, with a common standard deviation of $\sigma = 22\%$. Based on a large sample assumption, the sample-size for a fixed design is 208 per group with 95% power and a one-sided $\alpha = 0.025$. Using MSP, an interim analysis is planned based on the response assessments of 50% of the patients. The interim analysis is used for SSR and also for futility stopping. We follow the steps below to design the adaptive trial.

The simulation results are presented in Table 24.4. From Table 24.3, we can see that the adaptive design has a smaller expected sample-size ($\bar{N}$) under H_0 than the classic design (208). When using the n-reestimation mechanism, the power is protected to a certain degree (72.2% for the classic versus 73.3% for adaptive design without SSR and 80.4% with SSR). Of course, this power protection is at the cost of sample-size. Note the average $n = 285$/group with sample-size adjustment when the effect is 5% versus 10.5%. If this sample-size is used in a classic design, the power would be 84.7%. The SSR has lost its efficiency in this sense, though there is a saving in sample-size under H_0.

Example 2: An Oncology Adaptive Trial Simulation

Suppose in a two-arm comparative oncology trial, the primary efficacy endpoint is time to progression (TTP). The median TTP is estimated to be 8 months (hazard rate = 0.08664) for the control group, and 10.5 months (hazard rate = 0.06601) for the test group. Assume uniform enrollment with an accrual period

TABLE 24.4 Operating Characteristics of a GSD with MSP

Simulation Condition	Method	FSP	$\bar{N}$	N_{max}	Power
H_0	classic	0	208	208	0.025
	without SSR	0.750	151	242	0.025
	with SSR	0.750	177	350	0.025
H_a	classic	0	208	208	0.900
	without SSR	0.036	238	242	0.900
	with SSR	0.036	278	350	0.928
H_s	classic	0	208	208	0.722
	without SSR	0.102	230	242	0.733
	with SSR	0.102	285	350	0.804

TABLE 24.5 Operating Characteristics of Adaptive Methods (MPP)

Median Time		Expected			
Test	Control	ESP	FSP	N	Power (%)
8	8	0.010	0.750	248	2.5
10.5	8	0.512	0.046	288	88.8

Note: 1,000,000 simulation runs.

of 9 months and a total study duration of 24 months. The log-rank test will be used for the analysis. An exponential survival distribution is assumed for the purpose of sample-size calculation.

When there is a 10.5-month median time for the test group, the classic design requires a sample-size of 323 per group with 85% power at a level of significance (one-sided) $\alpha = 0.025$. To increase efficiency, an adaptive design with an interim sample-size of 200 patients per group is used. The maximum sample-size allowed for adjustment is 400. The simulation results are presented in Table 24.5, where the abbreviations ESP and FSP stand for early efficacy stopping probability and early futility stopping probability, respectively.

24.10 Summary

In this chapter, we have introduced the uniform formulations for hypothesis based adaptive design, and provided sample algorithms for adaptive designs. Readers can develop algorithms for obtaining other adaptive design operating characteristics in a similar way using various adaptive design methods. Implementation of these algorithms are straightforward using any computer language such as C#, Visual Basic.net, Java, PHP, SAS, R, and so on.

References

Bauer, P., and Kohne, K. (1994). Evaluation of experiments with adaptive interim analyses. *Biometrics,* 50: 1029–41.

Bauer, P., and Rohmel, J. (1995). An adaptive method for establishing a dose–response relationship, *Statistics in Medicine,* 14: 1595–1607.

Chang, M. (2007). Adaptive design method based on sum of *p*-values. *Statistics in Medicine,* 26: 2772–84.

Cui, L., Hung, H. M. J., and Wang, S. J. (1999). Modification of sample-size in group sequential trials. *Biometrics*, 55: 853–57.

Lan, K. K. G., and DeMets, D. L. (1983). Discrete sequential boundaries for clinical trials. *Biometrika,* 70: 659–63.

Lehmacher, W., and Wassmer, G. (1999). Adaptive sample-size calculations in group sequential trials. *Biometrics,* 55: 1286–90.

Müller, H. H., and Shäfer, H. (2004). A general statistical principle of changing a design any time during the course of a trial. *Statistics in Medicine,* 23: 2497–2508.

O'Brien, P. C., and Fleming, T. R. (1979). A multiple testing procedure for clinical trials. *Biometrika,* 35: 549–56.

Pocock, S. J. (1977). Group sequential methods in the design and analysis of clinical trials. *Biometrika,* 64: 191–99.

Proschan, M. A., and Hunsberger, S. A. (1995). Designed extension of studies based on conditional power. *Biometrics,* 51: 1315–24.

Wang, S. K., and Tsiatis, A. A. (1987). Approximately optimal one-parameter boundaries for a sequential trials. *Biometrics,* 43: 193–200.

25

Efficiency of Adaptive Designs

Nigel Stallard
The University of Warwick

Tim Friede
Universitätsmedizin Göttingen

25.1 Introduction

The U.S. Food and Drug Administration (FDA) recognizes in their critical path initiative that drug development is increasingly expensive with successful development of a single drug costing around $2 billion (FDA 2004). The initiative aims to make drug development more efficient and was described as a "serious attempt to bring attention and focus to the need for more scientific effort and for more publicly available information about the evaluation tools used in product development" (O'Neill 2006, p. 559). The initial white paper was followed up by an opportunity list that mentions adaptive designs as one potential remedy to make drug development more efficient (FDA 2006).

What are *adaptive designs*? Definitions of adaptive designs are given in the white paper of the Working Group on Adaptive Designs of the Pharmaceutical Research and Manufacturers of America (PhRMA) and also in the EMEA Reflection Paper on Adaptive Designs. In the PhRMA white paper an adaptive design is defined as "a clinical study design that uses accumulating data to decide how to modify aspects of the study as it continues, without undermining the validity and integrity of the trial" (Gallo et al. 2006, p. 276), whereas the EMEA reflection paper states more specifically: "A study design is called 'adaptive' if statistical methodology allows the modification of a design element (e.g., sample-size, randomisation ratio, number of treatment arms) at an interim analysis with full control of the type I error" (CHMP 2007, p. 10).

Adaptations of interest in clinical trials include early termination for futility or because of a positive effect, sample size reestimation, treatment or dose selection, subgroup selection, changing objectives, and adapting the primary endpoint or analysis method. In this chapter we focus on the most commonly used adaptations of early termination, sample size reestimation and treatment, dose or subgroup selection. Sample size reestimation can aim either at assuring a certain power at a specified alternative independent of nuisance parameters or to achieve a certain minimum power over a range of alternatives. The former is covered in Section 25.2 whereas the latter is considered in Section 25.3 along with designs that allow early stopping based on the estimated effect size. Designs with adaptive treatment or dose selection combine essentially the Phases IIb and III and are often referred to as adaptive seamless designs (ASD), which are described in more detail in Section 25.4 alongside designs with adaptive subgroup selection.

Switching between noninferiority and superiority is an example of an adaptation of trial objectives. We refer here to the literature (see for example, Brannath et al. 2003 and Koyama, Sampson, and Gleser 2005), but do not discuss these designs any further. Designs with adaptive choice of primary endpoints were investigated by, for example, Hommel (2001), Hommel and Kropf (2001), and Kieser (2005), and designs allowing change of the primary analysis by Lang, Auterith, and Bauer (2000), Kieser, Schneider, and Friede (2002), and Friede et al. (2003). Again, these are not discussed in detail below.

Another class of adaptive designs are designs with so-called response-adaptive randomization. In these designs the randomization ratio is not fixed, but changes as the trial progresses biasing the randomization toward the superior treatment(s) as evidence of superiority emerges. In this chapter we do not discuss this class of adaptive designs, but refer to Hu and Rosenberger (2006) for an overview.

In evaluating adaptive designs we use various criteria and the choice will depend on the specific design or adaptation at hand. Group-sequential and sample size reestimation designs are often assessed in terms of power and expected sample sizes under a specific alternative and/or null hypothesis. Other summaries describing sample size distributions such as minimum, maximum, or specific quantiles are not uncommon, however. In an ASD or response-adaptive design we might be interested in selection probabilities of the best treatment. To assess the validity of a design one might look at type I error rates or coverage probabilities for confidence intervals. Finally, criteria can be defined based on costs and utilities.

Although this chapter will focus on the efficiency of adaptive designs, what we mean by efficiency will vary with the application at hand. For instance, nuisance-parameter-based sample size reestimation designs are efficient if they provide robustness against nuisance parameter misspecification in the planning phase of a trial by allocating patients efficiently to those situations where higher sample sizes are required. In contrast a design with effect-based sample size reestimation might be considered efficient if the expected sample size for a specific alternative is minimized under a given power constraint.

25.2 Efficiency of Nuisance Parameter-Based Sample Size Reestimation Methods

In this section we consider methods for adaptation of clinical trials based on the use of interim analysis data to estimate nuisance parameters. In particular, we consider methods that aim to maintain the power of the trial over a range of nuisance parameter values.

Sample size calculation is a key task in the planning of any trial since the sample size has immediate consequences for the budget, the duration of the study, and decisions of ethics committee and institutional review boards. In the setting of a trial aiming to demonstrate superiority of an experimental treatment over a control treatment (e.g., placebo) in terms of a continuous primary outcome the total sample size is given by:

$$N(\alpha,1-\beta,\Delta^{*},\sigma^{2})=4\frac{(\Phi^{-1}(\alpha)+\Phi^{-1}(\beta))^{2}}{\Delta^{*2}}\sigma^{2} \tag{25.1}$$

with significance level α, target power $1 - \beta$, clinically relevant mean difference Δ^*, within-group variance σ^2, and Φ^{-1} denoting the inverse of the cumulative distribution function of the standard normal distribution.

The sample size given by $N(\alpha, 1 - \beta, \Delta^*, \sigma^2)$ depends on the assumed value of σ^2. In reality, however, this is unknown at the planning stage for a clinical trial. This can have important consequences.

For example, suppose that we are planning a randomized, placebo-controlled trial to demonstrate the efficacy of a new antidepressant in mild to moderate depression. The primary endpoint is the change in Hamilton Rating Scale for Depression (HAM-D) from baseline to week 6. A power of $1 - \beta = 0.80$ is targeted for a mean difference $\Delta^* = 4$ points on the HAM-D, which is considered clinically relevant (Montgomery 1994). Assuming a standard deviation $\sigma = 8$ points on the HAM-D, the required total sample size is 126 patients (i.e., 63 patients per group) according to Equation 25.1. However, a systematic review of 11 studies (Linde and Mulrow 2000) suggests that there is considerable uncertainty with regard to the size of the standard deviation. The observed standard deviations of HAM-D at end of therapy reported in the review range from 4 to 14.5. Assuming a standard deviation of 4 leads to a total sample size of 32 whereas a standard deviation of 14.5 would require a total sample size of 414. If the study would be conducted with 126 patients as initially calculated based on the assumption $\sigma = 8$, then the power would be nearly 100% if σ was in fact 4 or drop to 34% if σ was 14.5.

Wittes and Brittain (1990) proposed the use of so-called *internal pilot studies* in clinical trials. Here we describe the procedure for a single nuisance parameter, namely the within-group variance σ^2, but the procedure applies more generally for multiple nuisance parameters and different types of data. An initial sample size $n_0 = N(\alpha, 1-\beta, \Delta^*, \hat{\sigma}_0^2)$ is calculated based on an initial estimate $\hat{\sigma}_0^2$ of the variance σ^2. This initial estimate might be obtained from previous studies. After recruiting a prespecified number of patients into the study, say $n_1 = \pi n_0$ patients with, for example, $\pi = 1/2$, the sample size review is carried out by estimating the nuisance parameters from the data of the first n_1 patients and recalculating the sample size based on the new variance estimate $\hat{\sigma}^2$ resulting in $\hat{N} = N(\alpha, 1-\beta, \Delta^*, \hat{\sigma}^2)$ with the function N being defined as in Equation 25.1. The sample size n_2 for the second stage is then determined either by $n_2 = \max(n_0, \hat{N}) - n_1$ ("restricted" design) or by $n_2 = \max(n_1, \hat{N}) - n_1$ ("unrestricted" design; Birkett and Day 1994). Finally, the analysis is carried out based on the data from all $n_1 + n_2$ patients.

Using the usual, unbiased estimator of σ^2 in the sample size review it can be shown that the type I error rate is inflated above the nominal level α and suggestions have been made on how to adjust the critical value of the final analysis to achieve control of the type I error rate at the prespecified level α (Coffey and Muller 1999, 2001; Denne and Jennison 1999; Kieser and Friede 2000; Miller 2005; Timmesfeld, Schäfer, and Müller 2007). Kieser and Friede (2000) give adjusted significance levels α_{adj} for the final analysis that ensure control of the type I error rate at level α. The adjusted levels α_{adj} only depend on α and the total sample size n_1 of the internal pilot study with larger n_1 requiring smaller adjustments. For instance, α_{adj} is 0.0210 for $n_1 = 20$ and 0.0241 for $n_1 = 100$ achieving control at $\alpha = 0.025$. Whereas the procedure by Kieser and Friede (2000) requires prespecification of the sample size reestimation rule, the approach by Timmesfeld, Schäfer, and Müller (2007), which is based on the conditional rejection probability principle (Müller and Schäfer 2004), allows increase of the sample size without prespecification of the adaptation rule while controlling the type I error rate.

International guidelines such as the ICH Guideline E9 (1998) and the CHMP Reflection Paper on Adaptive Designs (2007) highlight two requirements for sample size adjustment procedures, namely maintaining the blinding and control of the type I error rate. We will come back to these points when discussing various procedures in the following. The CHMP Reflection Paper on Adaptive Designs (2007) is more explicit in that it favors blinded procedures; that is, procedures that do not require breaking the treatment code at interim (see Section 4.2.2 in CHMP 2007).

The first requirement—that of type I error rate control—can be achieved as described above. The use of the usual unbiased estimator of σ^2 as described above, however, requires the treatment code to be broken. To maintain blinding of patients and trial personnel an independent body such as a data monitoring committee (DMC) would be required. Alternative blinded procedures would, however, be clearly easier to implement since they do not require any DMC or such like. Though various procedures for blinded sample size reestimation have been suggested and disputed (Gould and Shih 1992; Zucker et al. 1999; Friede and Kieser 2002; Kieser and Friede 2003; Xing and Ganju 2005; Waksman 2007), we focus our discussion on a simple, yet very effective procedure. The total variance is the sum of the within-group variance and the between-group variance with the latter being the squared treatment difference. Typically the between-group variance is much smaller than the within-group variance in clinical trials since treatment effects are usually only a fraction of the standard deviation σ. Hence, the total variance should provide a reasonable, though biased estimate of the within-group variance. The total variance of course can be estimated without unblinding. In the context of sample size reestimation the total variance is also referred to as the one-sample variance since it is ignored that the observations come from two treatment groups and are considered together as one sample. Kieser and Friede (2003) investigated the type I error rate of the blinded reestimation procedure based on the one-sample variance and found that no practically relevant inflation could be observed. To illustrate that this procedure can be very efficient in making the trial robust against misspecification of the variance in the planning phase, we consider again the example of the study in depression introduced above. Figure 25.1 shows power and sample size distribution of the blinded sample size reestimation procedure (given by the solid line) with a size of the internal pilot study of $n_1 = 66$; that is, just over half of the initially planned sample size based on an assumed standard deviation of 8. In practice, sample sizes are usually constrained and therefore we limited the total sample size to a maximum of 300 patients in this example. As can be seen from Figure 25.1 the power of the blinded sample size reestimation procedure is close to the target of 80% over a wide range of standard deviations σ whereas the power of the fixed design with a total sample size of 126 patients (given by the dotted line for comparison) deviates quite substantially from the target power when the standard deviation was misspecified in the planning phase. From the boxplots showing the sample size distribution it is apparent that the blinded sample size reestimation design leads to efficient use of patients, with a larger or smaller sample size as needed given the true value of the unknown standard deviation. If the standard deviation is correctly specified in the planning phase, both designs give a similar power of about 80% but the expected sample size of the blinded sample size reestimation design, at 134 patients, is in this case, eight patients higher than the sample size of the fixed design. Though this comparison is unfair in that it assumes that the standard deviation is known in the fixed design but not in the reestimation design, it gives some idea of the cost of using a design with blinded sample size reestimation.

As mentioned above the internal pilot study design is not restricted to normal data or superiority testing. Designs for various types of endpoints and hypotheses (e.g., noninferiority) have been developed over the past years. The interested reader is referred to some recent reviews on this topic (Proschan 2005, 2009; Chuang-Stein et al. 2006; Friede and Kieser 2006).

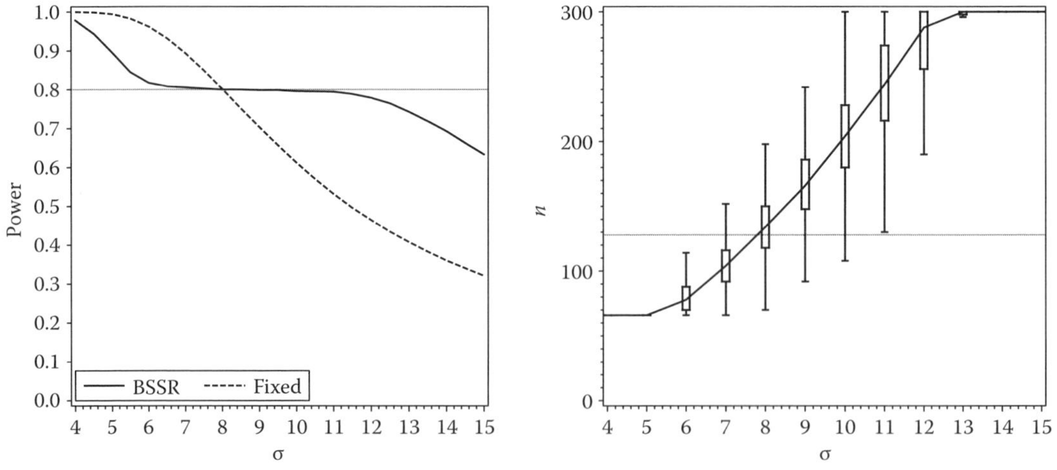

FIGURE 25.1 Power and sample size distribution of the blinded sample size reestimation procedure (BSSR) depending on the standard deviation σ for the example study in depression. For comparison the power and sample size of the fixed design (Fixed) are also given.

25.3 Efficiency of Group-Sequential Designs and Effect-Based Sample Size Reestimation

In this section we consider methods for the monitoring of clinical trial data based on estimation of the treatment effect on the primary efficacy outcome. As above, we continue to focus on clinical trials in which two treatments, typically an experimental treatment and a control, are compared. The comparison of the treatment groups at a number of interim looks obviously gives considerable potential, with the possibility of modifying the trial design in the light of the observed treatment effect estimates.

The estimation of the effect estimate at interim analyses enables two important adaptations to the trial design. The first is the ability to modify the sample size to detect an effect consistent with that observed up to that point in the trial, for example, to reflect the value of a nuisance parameter. Such an approach is known as *effect-based sample size reestimation*. This can lead to power being maintained over a wide range of alternative hypotheses. The second adaptation is to stop the trial entirely as soon as a treatment difference is sufficiently apparent, or for futility if treatments appear similar or if an experimental treatment appears to be inferior to a control treatment. Such adaptations are usually called *sequential designs*. Such monitoring can reduce the sample size of clinical trials by leading to termination once a result has been obtained, and can thus serve an important ethical or economic function.

Whilst, for the reasons just outlined, interim monitoring of efficacy data can be appealing, it should be conducted with some care in order to ensure that the scientific and statistical integrity of the clinical trial is maintained. There are two important reasons why care must be taken.

The first reason concerns the release of information on the treatment effect during the course of the trial. A knowledge by investigating clinicians of the treatment effect might lead to a reduction in recruitment or to the absence of equipoise. In an open-label or single-blinded trial it might also lead to bias due to an emerging belief that one treatment is superior to the other. For this reason, details of the interim analysis are not usually made generally available, with the results typically being known only to data monitoring and trial steering committees responsible for making decisions regarding the trial conduct.

The second reason why interim analyses should be conducted with care is the risk of type I error rate inflation. In conventional statistical analysis the probability of making a type I error; that is, of erroneously concluding that the treatments differ when in fact they do not, is controlled to be no larger than some specified level α, where usually $\alpha = 0.05$. If the sample size of later stages in the trial are modified based on the observed effect size, this can lead to type I error rate inflation if positive effects early in the trial lead to smaller sample sizes for later stages and the two stages are combined in the conventional way with weights proportional to the sample sizes (see Cui, Hung, and Wang 1999). Similarly, if a conventional statistical test comparing the two treatment groups is repeated at more than one interim analyses, with the trial stopped as soon as a significant result is obtained, the overall probability of making a type I error at any of the interim analyses is necessarily increased above the nominal 0.05 level (Armitage, McPherson, and Rowe 1969). In order to maintain the overall type I error rate at the 5% level, and hence to maintain statistical integrity, it is therefore necessary to adjust the statistical methods to allow for the interim analyses. There are a number of ways in which this can be done, as described in more detail in the remainder of this section. We consider first the situation of a clinical trial in which interim analyses are used to decide whether or not to stop the study but in which no sample size recalculation is performed.

25.3.1 Methodology for Sequential Designs

The use of interim analyses for the comparison of efficacy in two groups to allow a clinical trial to be stopped when sufficient evidence was available was first widely proposed by Armitage (1960). The methods proposed assumed that patients were treated in pairs, one receiving each of the two treatments to be compared, with the accumulating data monitored after observation of each pair. This work built on methodology for sequential analysis developed by Barnard (1946) and Wald (1947) in the context of industrial experimentation during the second world war. The theoretical underpinning of this work comes from consideration of a continuously monitored sample path that is modeled as a Brownian motion process. This work has been developed by, among others, Siegmund (1985) and Whitehead (1997).

In the specific context of clinical trials, following specification of a parameter of interest, which he denotes θ, Whitehead proposes monitoring the efficient score test statistic, which we will denote by S_j at interim analysis j, at each interim analysis, plotting this against the observed Fisher's information, which we will denote by I_j. The observed test statistic values form a sample path, which is compared with a stopping boundary. If the test statistic exceeds the stopping boundary, the clinical trial is terminated and the null hypothesis rejected. As the boundary is specified in advance by a small number of parameters, Whitehead has called this the boundaries approach. Although based on a model of continuous monitoring, approximations have been proposed to allow for monitoring after groups of patients (Whitehead 1997).

In the special case of a single sample of normal data with known variance, S_j is the sample sum at interim analysis j and I_j is the sample size. In this case, $S_1,\ldots,S_J$ are distributed with multivariate normal form with:

$$S_1 \sim N(\theta I_1, I_1) \tag{25.2}$$

and

$$S_j - S_{j-1} \sim N(\theta(I_j - I_{j-1}), (I_j - I_{j-1})), \tag{25.3}$$

with $S_j - S_{j-1}$ independent of S_j, $1 < j \leq J$, where J is the maximum number of interim analyses.

In a wide variety of cases, the efficient score statistics has asymptotic distribution of the form given by Equations 25.2 and 25.3 (see Scharfstein, Tsiatis, and Robins 1997 for further details). In these cases, S_j is a sufficient statistic for the parameter θ given the data available at interim analysis j. It is on the basis of the distribution assumption in Equations 25.2 and 25.3 that the stopping boundaries are constructed so as to maintain the overall type I error rate (see also Jennison and Turnbull 1997, for a discussion of the use of standardized test statistics).

Pocock (1977) and O'Brien and Fleming (1979) built on the work of Armitage and others to provide sequential analysis plans that did not require patients to be treated in pairs or monitoring after every observation. Since this allowed interim analyses to be taken after larger groups or patients, their work formed the basis of what is now usually called the group sequential approach. The approaches proposed by Pocock and O'Brien and Fleming required specification in advance of the number of interim analyses and the number of patients to be included in each. In practice, this prespecification can be restrictive. An alternative, more flexible, method was introduced by Lan and DeMets (1983) and Kim and DeMets (1987). They proposed that the form of the stopping boundary could be specified in advance by a spending function that describes the rate at which the total type I error rate, α, is spent through the course of the trial. In detail, the test is constructed in such a way that:

$$pr(\text{Reject } H_0 \text{ at or before interim analysis } j \,|\, H_0) = \alpha^*(t_j), \tag{25.4}$$

where t_j is the *information time* at interim analysis j, increasing from 0 at the start of the trial to 1 at the maximum sample size proportionally to the information available at the interim analysis, I_j, and α^* is the specified *spending function*, increasing in t with $\alpha^*(0) = 0$ and $\alpha^*(1) = \alpha$.

Given $t_1,\ldots,t_J$, or equivalently, $I_1,\ldots,I_J$, the distributional assumptions given by Equations 25.2 and 25.3 can be used to obtain a stopping boundary as a series of critical values, $c_1,\ldots,c_J$, so that Equation 25.4 is satisfied if the trial is stopped and the null hypothesis rejected if $S_j \geq c_j$ using a recursive numerical integration technique. Further details are given by Jennison and Turnbull (2000). A two-sided boundary can also be constructed, either to allow rejection of the null hypothesis versus a two-sided alternative or to allow stopping for futility without rejection of the null hypothesis, as described by Kim and DeMets (1987), Stallard and Facey (1990), and Pampallona, Tsiatis, and Kim (2001). Provided the form of the spending function is specified, the critical values obtained depend only on the values of t_j observed up to that point. This means that the stopping boundary is not specified entirely in advance, but can depend on the observed number and timing of interim analyses, introducing considerable flexibility into the designs available.

It is sometimes desirable to have tests with upper and lower stopping boundaries given by $u_1,\ldots,u_J$ and $l_1,\ldots,l_J$ respectively in which the trial is stopped as soon $S_j \notin (l_j, u_j)$ with H_0 rejected if $S_j \geq u_j$ and not rejected if $S_j \leq l_j$. Such a test can be constructed using two spending functions, one of which, α_U^*, increases from 0 to α, and the other, α_L^*, increases from 0 to $1 - \alpha$, with:

$$pr(\text{Stop and reject } H_0 \text{ at or before interim analysis } j \mid H_0) = \alpha_U^*(t_j), \tag{25.5}$$

and

$$pr(\text{Stop and do not reject } H_0 \text{ at or before interim analysis } j \mid H_0) = \alpha_L^*(t_j). \tag{25.6}$$

Sequential designs obtained using the spending function approach are obtained conditionally given the observed values of t_j, or equivalently I_j, $j = 1,\ldots,J$. The type I error rate is thus maintained provided the choice of I_j is independent of the observed values of $S_1,\ldots,S_{j-1}$, $j = 2,\ldots,J$. If the timing of the interim analyses, and hence the values of I_j are chosen dependent on the previously observed test statistic values, as is the case, for example, if effect-based sample size reestimation is performed, the type I error rate can be inflated above the nominal level, α, as shown by Cui, Hung, and Wang (1999). Althernative methods that can maintain the type I error rate when $I_1,\ldots,I_J$ depend on $S_1,\ldots,S_J$ are described below.

The boundaries and group-sequential approaches require specification in advance of the form of the stopping boundaries, either directly or via choice of the spending function. An extension that provides some additional flexibility is the *conditional error approach* proposed by Müller and Schäfer (2001). In their method the trial is designed using a group-sequential method with a spending function specified. If, at an interim analysis, it is desired to change the form of the stopping rule for future inspections, this is possible provided the probability under H_0 of rejecting H_0 conditional on the data observed up to that point in the trial is the same as that for the original design.

25.3.2 Methodology for Adaptive Designs with Effect-Based Sample Size Reestimation

We consider next the methodology for interim analyses, the purpose of which is not primarily to lead to termination of the trial but to modify the sample size of later stages of the trial according to the estimated treatment effect. Such methods have been proposed by, among others, Cui, Hung, and Wang (1999), Denne and Jennison (2000), and Denne (2001) to lead to designs that maintain a specified level of power over a range of alternative hypothesis values. As explained above, such effect-based sample size reestimation cannot be accommodated in the boundaries or group-sequential frameworks since in these approaches it is required that the sample size be chosen independently of the observed data.

The efficient score statistics $S_1,\ldots,S_J$ define a method for the combination of evidence from the different stages of a trial conducted with interim analyses. As described above, a number of methods exist for the construction of stopping rules that maintain the overall type I error rate at the nominal level given that the test statistics satisfy the distributional assumptions of Equations 25.2 and 25.3 with $I_1,\ldots,I_J$ independent of $S_1,\ldots,S_J$. An alternative method of combining the evidence from the different stages of a clinical trial was proposed by Bauer and Köhne (1994). They consider a clinical trial conducted in two or three stages, though the methodology they propose was extended by Wassmer (1999) to trials with more than three stages. Consider the evidence from stage j is summarized by the one-sided p-value for the test of H_0 based on the data from that stage alone, which will be denoted p_j, $j = 1, 2$. Bauer and Köhne propose combining the evidence from the two stages by forming the product p_1p_2. Under H_0, $p_j \sim U[0, 1]$, $j = 1, 2$. If p_1 and p_2 are independent, a result due to Fisher states that, under H_0, $-\log(p_1p_2)/2$ has χ_4^2 distribution. A critical value can thus be obtained for a test of H_0 based on the value of p_1p_2 if there is no possibility of stopping the trial at the first interim analysis. If, at the first interim analysis, the trial is stopped with rejection of H_0 if $p_1 \le \alpha_1$ and without rejection of H_0 if $p_1 \ge \alpha_0$, Bauer and Köhne show that the test maintains the overall type I error rate at level α if at the second interim analysis H_0 is rejected if $p_1p_2 \le (\alpha - \alpha_1)/(\log\alpha_0 - \log\alpha_1)$.

The product p_1p_2 is just one of a number of functions of p_1 and p_2 that have been proposed to combine the evidence from the stages in a two-stage design. Such functions are usually called combination functions, and tests based on this approach are called combination tests. A combination function proposed by Lehmacher and Wassmer (1999) is the inverse normal combination function given by:

$$1-\Phi\left(w_1\Phi^{-1}(1-p_1)+w_2\Phi^{-1}(1-p_2)\right),$$

where Φ^{-1} is the inverse of the cumulative normal distribution function and w_1 and w_2 are predefined weights with $w_1^2+w_2^2=1$.

If p_1 and p_2 are one-sided p-values from a normal test based on the score statistic increments S_1 and $S_2 - S_1$, these are given by $1-\Phi(S_1/\sqrt{I_1})$ and $1-\Phi((S_2-S_1)/\sqrt{(I_2-I_1)})$, respectively, so that the combination test statistic is equal to:

$$1-\Phi(w_1S_1/\sqrt{I_1}+w_2(S_2-S_1)/\sqrt{(I_2-I_1)}). \qquad (25.7)$$

The combination test method relies only on the assumptions that, under H_0, the distribution of the p-value p_1 and the conditional distribution of p_2 given p_1 are uniform on [0, 1] or stochastically larger (Brannath, Posch, and Bauer 2002). These requirements are often satisfied since tests are used that control the type I error rates at prespecified levels and the data on which p_1 and p_2 are based come from different patients.

The method thus gives great flexibility, with the opportunity to modify the trial in many ways, including, for example, changing the sample size for the second stage depending on the treatment difference observed in the first stage, without inflation of the type I error rate. This flexibility has led to the combination test approach being called the *adaptive design approach*, though this term might more reasonably be used for any method that allows for the adaptation of a trial based on analysis of data at interim analyses.

If w_1 and w_2 in the Expression 25.7 are taken such that w_1^2 and w_2^2 proportional to the variances I_1 and $I_2 - I_1$, the test statistic is equal to $1-\Phi(S_2/\sqrt{I_2})$; that is, to the p-value corresponding to a normal test based on S_2, so that inference at the final analysis depends on the value of S_2. In this case, therefore, if the information at each interim analysis is as planned, so that the observed values of I_1 and $I_2 - I_1$ are proportional to the prespecified w_1 and w_2, the test based on the combination test is asymptotically equivalent to a two-stage group-sequential test in which inference is also based on S_2 at the second stage.

More generally, however, the test statistic arising from the combination test cannot be related directly to that used in the group-sequential approach. In particular, the combination test is not, except in the special case just described, based on a sufficient statistic for θ.

The fact that the combination test method depends on a nonsufficient statistic has led to criticism by some authors. For example, Burman and Sonesson (2006) give the example of a trial initially planned in 10 stages with 100 patients recruited in each stage and with $w_1^2 = \cdots = w_{10}^2 = 0.1$ in which, at the end of the first stage, it is decided to redesign the remainder of the trial so as to conduct just one more interim analysis including only a single patient. As we require $w_1^2 + \cdots + w_J^2 = 1$, $w_2^2 = 0.9$ so that the single patient in second stage has greater weight in the final analysis than the total information from the 100 patients in the first stage. Although the type I error rate is maintained, the unduly large influence of the single Stage 2 patient on the final analysis does seem unsatisfactory. In particular, if the response from the single second stage patient is sufficiently positive, H_0 can therefore be rejected, although the mean response from all 101 patients may be less than 0. In discussion of the paper by Burman and Sonesson (2006), Bauer (2006) argued that such a sample size modification, from the planned value of 900–1, is an abuse of the combination test method. It is certainly true that such an extreme deviation from the planned sample size would not be anticipated in practice.

25.3.3 Efficiency of Group-Sequential and Adaptive Designs Compared to Fixed Sample Size Tests

It is naturally desirable to compare different adaptive design methodologies with each other and with conventional clinical trial designs in terms of their efficiency and we will discuss some practical issues in Section 25.5. As described in the introduction, designs may be evaluated in a number of different ways, based on for example, power, expected sample size, and number of interim analyses. Even if it is agreed that designs should be compared in terms of power, or equivalently in terms of sample size if the power is fixed in advance, this may not be straightforward. The opportunities to stop a trial that uses an adaptive design on the basis of interim analysis data, or to modify the sample size for later stage(s) in the trial, mean that the total sample size is no longer fixed in advance, but is a random variable depending on the data observed. Direct comparison with a conventional, fixed sample size design, in which the sample size is specified in advance, are thus not possible. The distribution of the sample size for an adaptive trial depends on the stopping rules or sample size reestimation rules used. This means that the question of which design leads to the smaller sample size does not have a simple answer and it is necessary to compare the distributions of the sample sizes from different designs.

In the boundaries and group-sequential approaches described above, the stopping rules must be specified in advance, though this need not be the case if using the conditional error approach. It is not necessary to specify the sample size for each interim analysis in advance, but it is common to do so, at least approximately. In this case the distribution of the total sample size for the trial can be calculated in advance. The combination test approach, as described above, offers more flexibility. In this case again, the sample size for each stage is often calculated using a prespecified approach (e.g., Friede and Kieser 2001), and the distribution of the sample size can be calculated. In each case the distribution of the sample size also depends on the unknown true parameters of the distribution of the data that are being monitored at the interim analyses. The parameters include the true effect size, denoted θ above, but may also include nuisance parameters such as the variance for normally distributed data, or the control success rate for binary responses, though in many cases the effects of the latter can be ignored by considering the required information level; that is, the expected value of I for the interim analysis at which the trial is terminated.

Once the distribution of the sample size for a particular design has been obtained, this can be compared with that for other possible designs or with the (fixed) sample size for a conventional design with the same power requirement. A common approach, justified by a comparison of resources required for a long sequence of trials, is to compare the fixed sample size of the conventional design with the expected value for the adaptive design for various values of the effect size. In many cases the expected sample size of the adaptive design is less than the sample size of a conventional design with equal power for all effect size values, and can lead to considerable savings in sample size relative to the conventional design.

Generally the saving in sample size increases as the number of interim analyses increases, so that a maximal value is given under the model of a continuously monitored sample path as used in the derivation of stopping rules using the boundaries approach. A number of such designs have been shown to have optimal properties. Examples include the sequential probability ratio test (SPRT) of Wald (1947), which among all tests of specified size and power, $1 - \beta$, under a specified simple alternative hypothesis H_1: $\theta = \theta_1$, minimizes the expected sample size under H_0 and H_1 (Wald and Wolfowitz 1948), and the triangular test of Anderson (1960) that minimizes the maximum expected sample size for any value of θ for specific choices of α and β. The saving in expected sample size is, however, at the expense of an increase relative to the fixed sample size of the maximum sample size for the adaptive design. An extreme example is Wald's SPRT, which, although it can be shown to terminate with probability 1, does not have an upper bound for the sample size.

25.3.4 Comparison of Different Adaptive Design Approaches

Comparisons of the efficiency of different adaptive design approaches also rely on an agreed measure of efficiency. As in the comparison of adaptive designs with fixed sample size methods, it is common either to compare expected sample sizes for designs constructed so as to have the same power, or to compare the power of different designs with the same sample size.

Tsiatis and Mehta (2003) compare designs based on different test statistics. They obtain a result that reflects the Neymann-Pearson lemma for fixed sample size hypothesis tests and show that, among all tests that satisfy spending function requirements in Equations 25.5 and 25.6, the power is maximized for tests in which likelihood ratio test statistics that compare upper and lower critical values are used. Since, in the single sample normal case, and asymptotically in a wide variety of other settings, the efficient score statistic is monotonically related to the likelihood ratio test statistic, this means that, for given spending functions, tests that stop and reject H_0 if $S_j \geq u_j$ and stop without rejection of H_0 if $S_j \leq l_j$ are most powerful.

The comparison conducted by Tsiatis and Mehta (2003) is valid for all tests in which the values of $I_1,\ldots,I_J$ and the spending function form is specified in advance. The flexibility of the combination test approach is such that here $I_1,\ldots,I_J$ need not be specified in advance. In their comparison, Tsiatis and Mehta replicate this in the spending function framework by considering a larger number of interim analyses conducted at all possible values I. In their comparison, they thus ignore the cost of conducting the interim analyses and also ignore the possibility of choosing the form of the spending function in a data-dependent manner, as pointed out by Brannath, Bauer, and Posch (2006).

Jennison and Turnbull (2006a) also compare adaptive designs based on the efficient score statistic with those using the combination test. They consider the derivation of stopping rules that are admissible in that there is no other rule with higher probability of rejecting H_0 for all $\theta > 0$ and lower probability of rejecting H_0 for all $\theta < 0$. They show that these admissible rules are all Bayes rules that can be obtained as the optimal stopping rule explicitly considering the cost of interim analyses and of type I and type II errors in the construction of Bayes optimal designs, building on the optimal sequential design theory described by Schmitz (1993). As Bayes rules are based on sufficient statistics, these stopping rules necessarily dominate the inadmissible stopping rules, such as those obtained using the combination test method, which do not depend on sufficient statistics. Although the admissible rules depend on sufficient statistics, they are not necessarily of the form given by the spending function approach, though the examples given by Jennison and Turnbull (2006a) illustrate that the spending function designs can be obtained that dominate the combination test stopping rules in terms of power, though in some cases the gain in power can be quite small (see also Kelly et al. 2005). The conclusion reached by Jennison and Turnbull is that while the combination test method does allow increased flexibility over the group-sequential approach, if this flexibility is not used, this is necessarily at the cost of a loss of power compared to the optimal procedure, so that it is preferable to consider the form of the design carefully at the outset to avoid the need for the increased flexibility, though this could still be utilized in the event of unforeseen circumstances.

25.4 Efficiency of Methods for Treatment and Subgroup Selection

An area of considerable recent interest has been the development of *adaptive seamless designs*. These attempt to combine elements of Phases II and III clinical trials in a single trial that combines the selection of most promising treatments, doses, or patient subgroups common in Phase II clinical trials with the definitive analysis associated with Phase III clinical trials.

In an adaptive seamless design that allows dose selection, for example, a trial might start with patients randomized between a number of different dose groups and a control. At an interim analysis, the data observed to that point in the trial will be analyzed and a decision made as to which dose group(s) are sufficiently promising that they should continue. Randomization in the second stage is then to the selected dose group(s) and the control. The aim is then to perform a final analysis that compares the chosen dose group(s) and the control using data from both stages while maintaining the type I error rate.

In a trial with a number, say k, experimental treatments or doses, which we will denote $T_1,\ldots,T_k$, together with a control, T_0, type I error rate control is less straightforward than when two treatments are compared. Let H_j denote the null hypothesis that T_j and T_0 are of equal efficacy. It is desirable to control the familywise error rate in the strong sense; that is, to ensure that the probability of rejecting any true null hypothesis is at most α. In some settings, for example, when a single experimental treatment group is selected, this follows from control of the familywise error rate in the weak sense; that is, by ensuring that the probability of rejecting any H_j is at most α when all H_j are true (see Jennison and Turnbull 2006b). More generally, strong control of the familywise error rate can be achieved using a closed testing procedure (Marcus, Peritz, and Gabriel 1976).

A general approach to ASD that include treatment or dose selection was described by Bauer and Kieser (1999). They propose the use of the combination function approach of Bauer and Köhne (1994) with a closed testing procedure to control the type I error rate given both the multiple testing arising from comparison of several experimental treatment groups and the combination of data from two or more stages in the trial. A similar approach is advocated by Bretz et al. (2006). The choice of dose(s) to continue to the second stage can be made in any way that is independent of the data from the second and any subsequent stages while still maintaining strong control of the familywise error rate. ASD can also be obtained based on the group-sequential approach as proposed by Stallard and Todd (2003), in this case selecting a single experimental dose to continue with the control beyond the first interim analysis, or a prespecified number of doses as described by Stallard and Friede (2008) and Friede and Stallard (2008).

Todd and Stallard (2005) present an example comparing the sample size required for an adaptive seamless design with that for a more conventional program including separate Phases II and III clinical trials. In their example, the saving in sample size using the adaptive seamless design is approximately one-third of that required for a Phase II trial followed by a Phase III trial using a standard fixed sample size design with the same power. In comparison to a Phase II trial followed by a sequential Phase III trial the saving in patient numbers is more modest, though the use of the Phase II data in the final analysis means that the number of patients required is reduced by an amount similar to the size of the Phase II arms for the selected dose(s) and the control. Bretz et al. (2006) also evaluate the saving in sample size due to the use of an adaptive seamless design, concluding that the saving depends on the number of treatment groups included at the first stage, but is about one-quarter if three or four active treatments or doses are initially compared with the control group.

Adaptive methods for subgroup selection have also been proposed by a number of authors (see for example, Wang, O'Neill, and Hung 2007; Brannath et al. 2009). This work is motivated by the acknowledgment of the heterogeneity of treatment effects in different patients, particularly due to genetic variation, though others consider other prognostic factors or biomarkers. In such a study, the variation of treatment responses across previously specified patient subgroups is assessed at an interim analysis. If no patient heterogeneity is indicated, the patient population remains unchanged. If, however, there is an indication of heterogeneity, patient subgroups for whom the treatment does not appear to be effective can then be excluded from the trial, with further investigation focusing on subgroups for whom the treatment does appear effective. In the simplest setting of a prognostic factor that divides the patient population into two groups, three hypothesis tests can be considered; testing the null hypothesis that the treatment is ineffective in subgroup i, $i = 1, 2$ and that the treatment is ineffective in the entire population, with multiple testing procedures used to control the familywise error rate.

Both the treatment and subgroup selection methods lead to an increase in efficiency by focusing the resources of the second (and any subsequent) stage(s) of the clinical trial in an area in which a treatment effect is indicated by the results from the interim analysis. In the case of treatment selection, this is achieved by dropping ineffective treatments, and in the subgroup selection designs by restricting the entry criteria to those subpopulations in which the treatment appears to be effective. In both cases the power of the test can be increased if true heterogeneity in treatment effects between treatments or patient subgroups exists though, as described by Kimani, Stallard, and Hutton (2009) and Brannath et al. (2009) the decision as to which dose groups or patient subgroups should be dropped to maximize this gain in efficiency may not be straightforward.

25.5 Efficiency Evaluation in Practice

As indicated above, the use of a well-chosen adaptive design can lead to increased efficiency over a conventional fixed sample size design. The gain can be in terms of the ability of a clinical trial to have greater power to detect a truly effective treatment or the ability to maintain the robustness of the power of the test to unknown nuisance parameters. The use of adaptive designs does, however, come at the cost of increased complexity in both the design and analysis stages for the clinical trial. In particular, there are challenges associated with the choice of appropriate adaptive design parameters, such as the timing and conduct of interim analyses.

Benda et al. (2009, 2010) proposed a framework for the evaluation of competing drug development strategies that they called clinical scenario evaluation (CSE). The framework also applies to other settings such as studies or development programs of nonpharmacological treatments or diagnostics. The key components of the CSE framework are assumptions, options, clinical scenarios, and metrics. The assumptions describe the statistical model for the data generation process and include model parameters such as response rates and treatment effects. The alternative strategies for conducting the trial or series of trials at hand are called the options in the CSE framework. The combinations of all assumptions and options are referred to as the clinical scenarios. The metrics are the efficiency criteria that are used to decide what option to go for. As discussed in the introduction such criteria include for example power of hypothesis tests and summary statistics describing sample size distributions.

In practice, computer simulations to compare the efficiency of different design options under a range of assumptions are often at the heart of CSE exercises and Benda et al. (2009, 2010) give various examples with simulations on program, trial, and analysis level. These simulations can be used to estimate the power of a range of options or to explore the conservatism of a test that is known from theoretical results to control the type I error rate. The simulations required can at times be very intensive that makes an efficient implementation of such simulations necessary. So software packages for the design of adaptive trials such as ADDPLAN or EAST have been updated over the past few years and developments are still continuing to incorporate simulation capabilities into the software packages. Wassmer and Vandemeulebroecke (2006) review software for the design and conduct of adaptive trials, and Chow and Chang (2007) describe a simulation framework for clinical trials and discuss the application of the ExpDesign Studio software.

The development of such software that enable the use of adaptive designs and facilitate decision-making regarding the choice of appropriate designs to maximize the gains in efficiency continue to lead to increased practical use of adaptive designs of the types that we have described in this chapter.

References

Anderson, T. W. (1960). A modification of the sequential probability ratio test to reduce sample size. *Annals of Mathematical Statistics,* 31: 165–97.

Armitage, P. (1960). *Sequential Medical Trials.* Oxford: Blackwell.

Armitage, P., McPherson, C. K., and Rowe, B. C. (1969). Repeated significance test on accumulating data. *Journal of the Royal Statistical Society, Series A,* 132: 235–44.

Barnard, G. A. (1946). Sequential tests in industrial statistics. *Journal of the Royal Statistical Society, Supplement,* 8: 1–26.

Bauer, P. (2006). Discussion on "Are flexible designs sound?" *Biometrics,* 62: 676–77.

Bauer, P., and Kieser, M. (1999). Combining different phases in the development of medical treatments within a single trial. *Statistics in Medicine,* 18: 1833–48.

Bauer, P., and Köhne, K. (1994). Evaluation of experiments with adaptive interim analyses. *Biometrics,* 50: 1029–41.

Benda, N., Branson, M., Maurer, W., and Friede, T. (2009). Clinical scenario evaluation: A framework for the evaluation of competing development strategies. *Drug Development,* 4: 84–88.

Benda, N., Branson, M., Maurer, W., and Friede, T. (2010). Aspects of modernizing drug development using scenario planning and evaluation. *Drug Information Journal,* 44: 299–315.

Birkett, M. A., and Day, S. J. (1994). Internal pilot studies for estimating sample size. *Statistics in Medicine,* 13: 2455–63.

Brannath, W., Bauer, P., Maurer, W., and Posch, M. (2003). Sequential tests for noninferiority and superiority. *Biometrics,* 59: 106–14.

Brannath, W., Bauer, P., and Posch, M. (2006). On the efficiency of adaptive designs for flexible interim decisions in clinical trials. *Journal of Statistical Planning and Inference,* 136: 1956–61.

Brannath, W., Posch, M., and Bauer, P. (2002). Recursive combination tests. *Journal of the American Statistical Association,* 97: 236–44.

Brannath, W., Zuber, E., Branson, M., Bretz, F., Gallo, P., Posch, M., and Racine-Poon, A. (2009). Confirmatory adaptive designs with Bayesian decision tools for a targeted therapy in oncology. *Statistics in Medicine,* 28: 1445–63.

Bretz, F., Schmidli, H., König, F., Racine, A., and Maurer, W. (2006). Confirmatory seamless Phase II/III clinical trials with hypotheses selection at interim: General concepts. *Biometrical Journal,* 48: 623–34.

Burman, C.-F., and Sonesson, C. (2006). Are flexible designs sound? *Biometrics,* 62: 664–69.

Chow, S.-C., and Chang, M. (2007). *Adaptive Design Methods in Clinical Trials.* Boca Raton, FL: Chapman & Hall/CRC.

Chuang-Stein, C., Anderson, K., Gallo, P., and Collins, S. (2006). Sample size reestimation: A review and recommendations. *Drug Information Journal,* 40: 475–84.

Coffey, C. S., and Muller, K. E. (1999). Exact test size and power of a gaussian error linear model for an internal pilot study. *Statistics in Medicine,* 18: 1199–1214.

Coffey, C. S., and Muller, K. E. (2001). Controlling test size while gaining the benefits of an internal pilot design. *Biometrics,* 57: 625–31.

Committee for Medicinal Products for Human Use (CHMP) (2007). Reflection paper on *Methodological Issues in Confirmatory Clinical Trials with Flexible Design and Analysis Plan.* London, October 18, 2007, Doc. Ref. CHMP/EWP/2459/02.

Cui, L., Hung, H. M. J., and Wang, S.-J. (1999). Modification of sample size in group sequential clinical trials. *Biometrics,* 55: 853–57.

Denne, J. S. (2001). Sample size recalculation using conditional power. *Statistics in Medicine,* 20: 2645–60.

Denne, J. S., and Jennison, C. (1999). Estimating the sample size for a t-test using an internal pilot. *Statistics in Medicine,* 18: 1575–85.

Denne, J. S., and Jennison, C. (2000). A group sequential t-test with updating of sample size. *Biometrika,* 87: 125–34.

FDA. (2004). *Innovation/ Stagnation: Challenge and Opportunity on the Critical Path to New Medical Products FDA Report, March 2004*. Rockville, MD: U.S. Food and Drug Administration. Available at http://www.fda.gov/downloads/ScienceResearch/SpecialTopics/CriticalPathInitiative/CriticalPathOpportunitiesReports/ucm113411.pdf

FDA. (2006). *Innovation/Stagnation: Critical Path Opportunity List FDA Report, March 2006*, Rockville, MD: U.S. Food and Drug Administration. Available at http://www.fda.gov/downloads/ScienceResearch/SpecialTopics/CriticalPathInitiative/CriticalPathOpportunitiesReports/UCM077254.pdf

Friede, T., and Kieser, M. (2001). A comparison of methods for adaptive sample size adjustment. *Statistics in Medicine*, 20: 3861–73.

Friede, T., and Kieser, M. (2002). On the inappropriateness of an EM algorithm based procedure for blinded sample size re-estimation. *Statistics in Medicine*, 21: 165–76.

Friede, T., and Kieser, M. (2006). Sample size recalculation in internal pilot study designs: A review. *Biometrical Journal*, 48: 537–55.

Friede, T., Kieser, M., Neuhäuser, M., and Büning, H. (2003). A comparison of procedures for adaptive choice of location tests in flexible two-stage designs. *Biometrical Journal*, 45: 292–310.

Friede, T., and Stallard, N. (2008). A comparison of methods for adaptive treatment selection. *Biometrical Journal*, 50: 767–81.

Gallo, P., Chuang-Stein, C., Dragalin, V., Gaydos, B., Krams, M., and Pinheiro, J. (2006). Adaptive designs in clinical drug development: An executive summary of the PhRMA working group. *Journal of Biopharmaceutical Statistics*, 16: 275–83.

Gould, A. L., and Shih, W. J. (1992). Sample size re-estimation without unblinding for normally distributed outcomes with unknown variance. *Communications in Statistics—Theory and Methods*, 21: 2833–53.

Hommel, G. (2001). Adaptive modifications of hypotheses after an interim analysis. *Biometrical Journal*, 43: 581–89.

Hommel, G., and Kropf, S. (2001). Clinical trials with an adaptive choice of hypotheses. *Drug Information Journal*, 35: 1423–29.

Hu, F., and Rosenberg, W. F. (2006). *The Theory of Response-Adaptive Randomization in Clinical Trials*. Hoboken: Wiley.

ICH Harmonized Tripartite Guideline E9 (ICH) (1999). Statistical principles for clinical trials. *Statistics in Medicine*, 18: 1905–42.

Jennison, C., and Turnbull, B. W. (1997). Group-sequential analysis incorporating covariate information. *Journal of the American Statistical Association*, 92: 1330–41.

Jennison, C., and Turnbull, B. W. (2000). *Group Sequential Methods with Applications to Clinical Trials*. London: Chapman & Hall.

Jennison, C., and Turnbull, B. W. (2006a). Adaptive and nonadaptive group sequential tests. *Biometrika*, 93: 1–21.

Jennison, C., and Turnbull, B. W. (2006b). Confirmatory seamless Phase II/III clinical trials with hypothesis selection at interim: Opportunities and limitations. *Biometrical Journal*, 48: 650–55.

Kelly, P. J., Sooriyarachchi, R. M., Stallard, N., and Todd, S. (2005). A practical comparison of group-sequential and adaptive designs. *Journal of Biopharmaceutical Statistics*, 15: 719–38.

Kieser, M. (2005). A note on adaptively changing the hierarchy of hypotheses in clinical trials with flexible design. *Drug Information Journal*, 39: 215–22.

Kieser, M., and Friede, T. (2000). Re-calculating the sample size in internal pilot study designs with control of the type I error rate. *Statistics in Medicine*, 19: 901–11.

Kieser, M., and Friede, T. (2003). Simple procedures for blinded sample size adjustment that do not affect the type I error rate. *Statistics in Medicine*, 22: 3571–81.

Kieser, M., Schneider, B., and Friede, T. (2002). A bootstrap procedure for adaptive selection of the test statistic in flexible two-stage designs. *Biometrical Journal*, 44: 641–52.

Kim, K., and DeMets, D. L. (1987). Design and analysis of group sequential tests based on the type I error spending rate function. *Biometrika*, 74: 149–54.

Kimani, P., Stallard, N., and Hutton, J. (2009). Dose selection in seamless Phase II/III clinical trials. *Statistics in Medicine,* 28: 917–36.

Koyama, T., Sampson, A. R., and Gleser, L. J. (2005). A framework for two-stage adaptive procedures to simultaneously test non-inferiority and superiority. *Statistics in Medicine,* 24: 2439–56.

Lan, K. K. G., and DeMets, D. L. (1983). Discrete sequential boundaries for clinical trials. *Biometrika,* 70: 659–63.

Lang, T., Auterith, A., and Bauer, P. (2000). Trendtests with adaptive scoring. *Biometrical Journal,* 42: 1007–20.

Lehmacher, W., and Wassmer, G. (1999). Adaptive sample size calculations in group sequential tests. *Biometrics,* 55: 1286–90.

Linde, K., and Mulrow, C. D. (2000). St John's wort for depression (Cochrane Review). In *The Cochrane Library*, Issue 3. Oxford: Update Software.

Marcus, R., Peritz, E., and Gabriel, K. R. (1976). On closed testing procedures with special reference to ordered analysis of variance. *Biometrika,* 63: 655–60.

Miller, F. (2005). Variance estimation in clinical studies with interim sample size reestimation. *Biometrics,* 61: 355–61.

Montgomery, S. A. (1994). Clinically relevant effect sizes in depression. *European Neuropsychopharmacology,* 4: 283–84.

Müller, H.-H., and Schäfer, H. (2001). Adaptive group sequential designs for clinical trials: Combining the advantages of the adaptive and of classical group sequential approaches. *Biometrics,* 57: 886–91.

Müller, H.-H., and Schäfer, H. (2004). A general statistical principle for changing a design any time during the course of a trial. *Statistics in Medicine,* 23: 2497–2508.

O'Brien, P. C., and Fleming, T. R. (1979). A multiple testing procedure for clinical trials. *Biometrics,* 35: 549–56.

O'Neill, R. T. (2006). FDA's critical path initiative: A Perspective on contributions of biostatistics. *Biometrical Journal,* 48: 559–64.

Pampallona, S., Tsiatis, A. A., and Kim, K. (2001). Interim monitoring of group sequential trials using spending functions for the type I and type II error probabilities. *Drug Information Journal,* 35: 1113–21.

Pocock, S. J. (1977). Group sequential methods in the design and analysis of clinical trials. *Biometrika,* 64: 191–99.

Proschan, M. (2005). Two-stage sample size re-estimation based on a nuisance parameter: A review. *Journal of Biopharmaceutical Statistics,* 15: 559–74.

Proschan, M. A. (2009). Sample size re-estimation in clinical trials. *Biometrical Journal,* 51: 348–57.

Scharfstein, D. O., Tsiatis, A. A., and Robins, J. M. (1997). Semiparametric efficiency and its implications on the design and analysis of group-sequential studies. *Journal of the American Statistical Association,* 92: 1342–50.

Schmitz, N. (1993). *Optimal Sequentially Planned Decision Procedures, Lecture Notes in Statistics, 79.* New York: Springer-Verlag.

Siegmund, D. (1985). *Sequential Analysis.* New York: Springer.

Stallard, N., and Facey, K. M. (1990). Comparison of the spending function method and the Christmas tree correction for group sequential trials. *Journal of Biopharmaceutical Statistics,* 6: 361–73.

Stallard, N., and Friede, T. (2008). Flexible group-sequential designs for clinical trials with treatment selection. *Statistics in Medicine,* 27: 6209–27.

Stallard, N., and Todd, S. (2003). Sequential designs for Phase III clinical trials incorporating treatment selection. *Statistics in Medicine,* 22: 689–703.

Timmesfeld, N., Schäfer, H., and Müller, H.-H. (2007). Increasing the sample size during clinical trials with t-distributed test statistics without inflating the type I error rate. *Statistics in Medicine,* 26: 2449–64.

Todd, S., and Stallard, N. (2005). A new clinical trial design combining Phases II and III: Sequential designs with treatment selection and a change of endpoint. *Drug Information Journal,* 39: 109–18.

Tsiatis, A. A., and Mehta, C. (2003). On the efficiency of the adaptive design for monitoring clinical trials. *Biometrika,* 90: 367–78.

Waksman, J. A. (2007). Assessment of the Gould-Shih procedure for sample size reestimation. *Pharmaceutical Statistics,* 6: 53–65.

Wald, A. (1947). *Sequential Analysis.* New York: Wiley.

Wald, A., and Wolfowitz, J. (1948). Optimum character of the sequential probability ratio test. *Annals of Mathematical Statistics,* 19: 326–39.

Wang, S.-J., O'Neill, R. T., and Hung, H. M. J. (2007). Approaches to evaluation of treatment effect in randomized clinical trials with genomic subset. *Pharmaceutical Statistics,* 6: 227–44.

Wassmer, G. (1999). Multistage adaptive test procedures based on Fisher's product criterion. *Biometrical Journal,* 41: 279–93.

Wassmer, G., and Vandemeulebroecke, M. (2006). A brief review of software developments for group sequential and adaptive designs. *Biometrical Journal,* 48: 732–37.

Whitehead, J. (1997). *The Design and Analysis of Sequential Clinical Trials.* Chichester: Wiley.

Wittes, J., and Brittain, E. (1990). The role of internal pilot studies in increasing the efficiency of clinical trials. *Statistics in Medicine,* 9: 65–72.

Xing, B., and Ganju, J. (2005). A method to estimate the variance of an endpoint from an on-going blinded trial. *Statistics in Medicine,* 24: 1807–14.

Zucker, D. M., Wittes, J. T., Schabenberger, O., and Brittain, E. (1999). Internal pilot studies II: Comparison of various procedures. *Statistics in Medicine,* 18: 3493–3509.

26

Case Studies in Adaptive Design*

Ning Li, Yonghong Gao, Shiowjen Lee
U.S. Food and Drug Administration

26.1 Introduction

To support regulatory standards for evidence in a medical product application, statistical inferences in larger-scale, confirmative trials are generally performed. One of the critical issues is whether results generated from the trials are interpretable with respect to the safety and effectiveness of the proposed medical product in the seeking indication.

The United States Food and Drug Administration (FDA) in March 2004 issued a report titled "Innovation or Stagnation?—Challenge and Opportunity on the Critical Path to New Medical Products" (FDA 2004). One of the issues was that the medical product development path has become increasingly challenging, inefficient, and costly. The critical path initiative covers three major dimensions of the medical product development process, namely, safety, medical utility (efficacy/benefits), and industrialization (production). The ultimate attempt of the critical path initiative is to call attention and focus to the need for more scientific efforts and efficient evaluation tools used in product development. Adaptive trial design is one of the topics focused in medical utility areas.

For a clinical trial with adaptive design, interim analyses are needed. It however, should be recognized that not all clinical trials require an interim analysis plan since patient recruitment in some trials can be fairly easy, the treatment duration is short, and response can be obtained immediately. On the other hand, interim analyses may be planned for trials that require months and even years of patient enrollment, require longer treatment duration, and treatment response is not immediately derived. For trials with the conventional study design, planning parameters are derived based on previous trials and other relevant sources prior to the initiation of confirmatory trials. As opposed to the conventional study design, one significant aspect of adaptive design is to use data from inside or outside the on-going trials to decide study modification without undermining the validity and integrity of the trial while the

* **Disclaimer:** The views expressed are those of the authors and do not represent the official position of the U.S. Food and Drug Administration.

type I error rate is properly controlled. Such a design is thought to maximize the chance of study success and reduce the burden of medical product development process by industry.

One strong argument for the use of adaptive design is that it allows those engaged in development to respond to what they learn about the safety and potential benefits of new medical products during the process. Study modifications during a phase of testing can help focus on the optimal form of an experimental treatment more rapidly. The methodology of adaptive design may help to arrive at a positive conclusion about an effective treatment with exposure of fewer patients in the testing process, or alternatively patients can be protected from harm if interim results show a clear detrimental tendency of the experimental treatment. Study modification that is achieved with adaptive design fits the early phase of product development. Their use in late Phase II or confirmatory Phase III trials however should be carefully examined. The modification of an on-going Phase III trial on one hand could be viewed as a contradiction to the confirmatory nature in the medical product development process. On the other hand, it may be necessary because uncertainty still exists when conducting confirmatory trials. Post hoc study modification of a trial however is rarely acceptable without adequate justification in regulatory submissions.

Although statistical methods in a broader context of adaptive design have been investigated for decades, the application of adaptive design strategies to clinical trials, however, has just been increasing recently in regulatory submissions over different centers in the FDA. For a clinical trial with adaptive design, the central issues of concern are the clinical interpretation of overall trial results, operational logistics, trial conduct, and integrity of study results. Our experience indicates that only a small proportion of the applications involving adaptive design strategies have been acceptable for regulatory decision making; while quite a few applications were discouraged at the protocol stage for numerous reasons. The following gives a summary of design adaptations regulatory submissions proposed:

- Sample size reestimation—the sample size planned originally was not appropriate. This could be due to incorrect assumptions, variation in the current on-going trial is greater than expected, or external information indicates different estimates of treatment effect.
- Change of study objective—the superiority objective originally planned may be to ambitious after interim results are available, or vice versa that benefit of the experimental product based on interim results turns out to be greater than expected.
- Change of the primary endpoint—the primary endpoint was chosen inappropriately at the planning stage, for example, the choice of components in a composite endpoint may be suboptimal, or external information may indicate noninformative components.
- Termination/addition of treatment arms—interim results may suggest that some treatment arms are not efficacious or harmful and therefore should be dropped from the study, or treatment arms or schedule are not optimal and should be modified.
- Change of statistical tests—interim results may suggest that more optimal statistical methods could be chosen for the primary analysis. For example, the distribution of some baseline covariates are different between groups and therefore analysis of covariance (ANCOVA) or propensity score method is more appropriate than the originally planned t-test.
- Change of study population—results from internal or external studies may suggest benefits of a subgroup, or may want to expand the inclusion criteria due to slow patient recruitment.
- Study adaptation is supported by simulations only that indicate type I error of the study under controlled conditions.

The layout of the chapter is as follows: a discussion of some issues and concerns regarding the above referred design adaptations is included in Section 26.2. Section 26.3 provides case studies to illustrate the issues associated with study adaptations; some are from premarket applications (PMAs), while others are investigational applications. For product proprietary purposes, the names of products and sponsors are masked and numerical results are modified for investigational applications. Section 26.4 gives some concluding remarks. The discussion in this chapter is restricted to the considerations when late Phase II/III trials or pivotal trials are planned based on adaptive designs.

26.2 Some Concerns on Types of Design Adaptation

The following lays out concerns on design adaptation in regulatory submissions.

26.2.1 Sample Size Reestimation

Sample size reestimation is a design adaptation that occurs most frequently in regulatory submissions, some are prespecified and some are post hoc. For sample size reestimation that was not prespecified at the protocol stage, there is a serious concern that the adaptation is due to knowing study results post hoc. Such a study adaptation is usually not acceptable by regulatory agencies. On the other hand, even though a study is planned to allow a sample size modification based on the prespecified interim analyses, such a design adaptation sometimes may not be justifiable. The need to resize an on-going clinical trial may indicate that the original assumptions of the study design are not met in the current study. Such a problem could be serious and could indicate inadequate product development process.

The following lists a few concerns regarding sample size reestimation:

a. The effect size initially assumed in the study size determination may be to optimistic and may not be realistic. It was chosen in order to determine a study size.
b. Suppose a smaller effect size is observed at an interim analysis and therefore the study adaptation is to increase sample size to detect the smaller treatment effect statistically. Such a smaller effect size however may not be clinically meaningful to warrant the approval of the product.
c. Even though the smaller effect size in (b) may be clinically meaningful, the implication of ruling out zero effect planned in most studies (i.e., superiority) is that the effect size at the completion of the study would be much lower than the effect observed at the interim look and shows statistically significant. In fact, Hung and O'Neill (2003) pointed out that when the study is planned to detect a treatment effect of size δ at two-sided $\alpha = 0.05$ and 90% power the estimated effect size would be only approximately 60% of δ at a p-value of 0.05.
d. Conditional power strategy is a commonly used criterion for sample size reestimation. However, Bauer and Koenig (2006) indicated that the conditional power computed based on the effect size estimate at the midcourse of the study can be unreliable to provide useful guidance for sample size reestimation.
e. The need of multiple sample size reestimations is a serious concern as this raises an issue that data generated from the study fluctuate and that the effect of the proposed product is not understood to a degree of conducting confirmatory trials.

In summary, the sample size reestimation changes the initially planned study size and may not be justifiable. In regulatory submissions, adequate justification, both clinical and statistical, should be provided in protocols with prespecified approach for sample size reestimation.

26.2.2 Withdrawal of Treatment/Dose Arms

Some regulatory submissions have proposed dropping dose arms that show lack of therapeutic effect or have substantial side effects. In many product developments, there may be still some doubts about the optimal dose of the experimental product for Phase III even after a carefully conducted Phase II program. One of the reasons is that patients exposed to the product in the Phase II program may be limited and therefore questions about the estimates of treatment effect still remain. As a result, several possible doses of the product may be investigated further in Phase III. An adaptive design combined with multiple doses of the experimental product in confirmatory trials is thought to offer the opportunity to select the optimal dose of the product by sponsors. Another example is the noninferiority trials that include the experimental product, active-control, and placebo arms. An adaptive design in the above-mentioned three-arm noninferiority trial may provide the opportunity to stop recruitment to the placebo group after an interim analysis that demonstrates the superiority of the experimental product to placebo. The trial then continues to establish the noninferiority of the experimental product to the active-control. Careful planning and prespecification of the procedure in both cases are needed.

From a statistical perspective, the first issue is whether or not the type I error is controlled for this type of study adaptation. In fact, simulation results in Tsong et al. (1997) have shown that the type I error rate can be inflated if the withdrawal of an arm is based on the internal data of the trial. Such an inflation of type I error rate can be great in the case of the redistribution of the unused significance level to the remaining arms for comparisons after the withdrawal of a treatment arm, unless the group-withdrawal is independent of the study results of the primary outcome variable. However, in practice, it is rarely possible to justify that the withdrawal of a treatment arm is not related to the study results.

For the withdrawal of placebo arm in noninferiority three-arm trials, there is a concern that the treatment effect may be different before and after dropping the placebo arm since patient populations enrolled could be different as pointed out by Koch (2006). As a result, the pooling of outcomes from stages before and after dropping the placebo arm can be problematic.

26.2.3 Change of the Primary Endpoint

The primary endpoint is the variable that is most relevant to the product indication and best reflect the disease progression and the effect of treatment. To establish the efficacy of an experimental treatment for a specified indication, study results would need to show benefit of the experimental treatment to the control (can be placebo) statistically and clinically with respect to the primary efficacy endpoint that is prespecified in the study. For many applications, primary endpoints are well-established within the regulatory agencies and clinical societies; some are not due to the complexity of multifaceted diseases. For example, in a heart failure clinical trial, the primary efficacy endpoint is usually a composite endpoint that consists of several components, such as deaths, myocardial infarction (MI), stroke, and so on. Death or MI alone is not adequate to capture the progression of heart failure. It is possible in a heart failure clinical trial that an experimental treatment does not show effect statistically for the specified composite endpoint. It, however, may show a statistically significant effect for a different composite endpoint that consists of different components. Therefore, changing the primary endpoint during the course of clinical trials may seem attractive to some sponsors.

From statistical points of view, changing the primary endpoint alters the intended fundamental clinical/statistical questions, which are the originally planned hypotheses, and therefore contradict the confirmatory nature of pivotal trials. Changing the primary endpoint based on results from on-going pivotal trials may not be justifiable. Changing the primary endpoint based on results of external studies can be risky because study populations, clinical practice, and whether studies are controlled, for example, may be factors attributed to the treatment effect size. Searching of appropriate primary endpoints that are sensitive to an experimental treatment should be done in the earlier phase of exploratory studies. The selection of an endpoint should also better reflect patient benefit.

26.2.4 Changes Between Superiority and Noninferiority

The use of active-control trials has been increasing in regulatory submissions. Most of them do not incorporate a placebo arm due to ethical reasons in some disease areas. The effectiveness of the experimental product in active-control trials in the absence of the placebo arm can be established via two strategies—the superiority of the experimental product to the active control product (or standard of care), or the noninferiority that the experimental product is not much worse than the active control product and therefore it would have been superior to placebo if the placebo had been in the trials. For the later strategy, the effectiveness of the control group must have been established previously as compared to placebo in well-controlled clinical trial setting, as the noninferiority margin would rely on such information.

The statistical literatures have concluded that the alpha adjustment is not needed for the testing of superiority and noninferiority simultaneously or in sequence of any order with the same confidence interval of the treatment effect (Morikawa and Yoshida 1995; Wang et al. 2001). Such an assertion however is no longer true if the determination of the noninferiority margin depends on data derived from the current on-going trial (Huang and Wang 2004). The noninferiority margin in a noninferiority trial would need to be prespecified in regulatory submissions. The change of the noninferiority margin based on data observed during the course of the trial is not justifiable and the study results may not be interpretable. In contrast, if a trial is planned to demonstrate noninferiority and this is achieved based on interim results, there may be a motivation to complete the study enrollment to demonstrate the superiority of the experimental treatment to the active control in efficacy and to generate more safety data. This possibility however, should be planned in advance and should be prespecified in the protocol.

26.2.5 Selection of Patient Subgroups Based on Interim Results

In some clinical trials, there will be differential responses to the experimental treatment for subgroups or strata of patients. For example, patients having diabetes tend to have a higher rate of death, stroke, MI, and so on, when they are implanted with a drug eluting stent (DES). Although it is desirable that results derived from a clinical trial can be generalized to a wider patient population, sometimes interest may focus on the identification of patient subgroups that are most beneficial from the experimental treatment. On the other hand, when a substantial difference in responses between subgroups (or strata) is apparent, one is tempted to drop the patient stratum that is not responsive to the treatment and randomize the treatment in the responsive patient strata. This consequently may increase study power. Another reason for dropping a stratum is that the experimental treatment shows detrimental effect (Coronary Drug Project Group 1981).

Adaptive selection of patient subgroups based on interim results has been proposed in regulatory submissions. Some even proposed to use results of point estimates to drop a patient stratum midway through the trial. The first concern is that it is not clear how to quantify the operating characteristics. Simulated type I error rate may no longer correspond to the proper hypotheses to be tested. In other words, the assumptions made at the beginning of the simulation apply to global hypotheses (wider patient population) that may no longer be considered for rejection after the study adaptation or at the end of the trial (narrower patient population). Further, the decision to drop a patient stratum based on a point estimate can be detrimental to the study since point estimates carry with uncertainty. Additionally, the pooling of study results for the remaining patient strata may not be justifiable after the study adaptation. This is because that if there is a reason to test the patient strata and to drop a patient stratum at an interim analysis, there could be an issue of heterogeneous results over the remaining patient strata. The pooling of results at the end of the trial can be problematic.

Such study adaptation trials are similar in spirit to enrichment designs, for which prior to randomization, patients who are likely responders are identified. Temple (1994) had argued that enrichment designs can be useful in the early phases of product development when the first task is to identify subgroup in which the drug might be working. In addition, he also has a concern about the generalizability of early studies. Therefore, the study adaptation of selecting patient subgroups should be appealing in the early phases of experimental treatment evaluation when relatively little information is available about which groups of patients would benefit. However, there should be good ideas about the target patient population to be treated with the experimental treatment at the stage of confirmatory trials. It is of a great concern if the purpose of such study adaptation is to salvage trials that would otherwise be compromised due to low study powers or heterogeneous response across patient strata.

26.2.6 Issues on Simulations

Some regulatory submissions proposed study adaptation of sample size reestimation using solely simulations to support the control of type I error rate. There are concerns about such an approach since it has limitations and does not cover different clinical trial scenarios that are not included in the simulations. Most often, the submitted results cannot be replicated and validated. It therefore is difficult to evaluate whether the sample size reestimation controls the study-wise type I error rate and whether the worst type I error rate is attainable based on simulations. To illustrate the referred issues about simulations, a hypothetical and simple example from Zhen (2008) is given as one of the case studies in the next section.

26.3 Case Studies

Four case studies with features of adaptive design are presented in this section.

26.3.1 Case Study 1

Coronary artery disease occurs when plaque build-up narrows the arteries and reduces blood flow to the heart, which can lead to chest pain or heart attack. Drug eluted stent (DES) is often used to treat coronary artery disease by propping open a narrowed or blocked artery and releasing the drug in a controlled manner to prevent the artery from becoming blocked again following a stent procedure. To establish the safety and effectiveness of DES X, a prospective, multicenter, randomized, patient-blinded, controlled clinical trial comparing DES X to a marketed DES, say DES Y, in 1002 patients with either one or two de novo native coronary artery lesions was conducted. Patients were randomized to DES X and DES Y in a ratio of 2:1 in the trial. The trial was conducted in the United States during 2005 and 2006.

The primary endpoint of the pivotal study was in-segment late loss at eight months postprocedure and the coprimary endpoint was target vessel failure (TVF) at 9 months postprocedure. The 8-months in-segment late loss is a surrogate endpoint that measures the renarrowing of the vessel for which smaller late loss indicates better treatment effect. The clinical endpoint TVF is a composite endpoint comprised of cardiac death, MI, ischemia-driven target lesion revascularization, and ischemia-driven target vessel revascularization. The primary hypotheses for both the primary and coprimary endpoints were noninferiority testing. The superiority testing follows if the noninferiority objective is met for both endpoints.

The hypotheses for the primary endpoint are:

$$H_0: \mu_e \geq \mu_c + \delta_1$$

$$H_a: \mu_e < \mu_c + \delta_{1,}$$

where μ_e and μ_c are the means in-segment late loss at 8-months for DES X and DES Y arm, respectively, and δ_1 is the noninferiority margin that was prespecified as 0.195 mm in the protocol. A sample size of 338 in DES X and 169 in DES Y would have a power of 99% at one-sided alpha level of 0.025 based on t-test. The in-segment late loss is an angiographic measure using cardiac catheterization. The procedure to derive angiographic measure is considerably costly and some risk is involved. Since this endpoint requires smaller sample sizes, and since the cost and risk associated with getting angiographic measure are not ignorable, only a subgroup of the enrolled patients had the scheduled angiographic follow-up. This was prespecified in the protocol.

The hypotheses for the coprimary endpoint are:

$$H_0: P_e \geq P_c + \delta_2$$

$$H_a: P_e < P_c + \delta_2$$

where P_e and P_c are the 9-months TVF rates for DES X and DES Y arm, respectively, and δ_2 is the non-inferiority margin that was prespecified as 5.5% in the protocol. Sample size calculation indicated 660 subjects in DES X group and 330 subjects in DES Y group would have a power of 89% at one-sided alpha level of 0.05 based on two-sample proportion test. The pivotal study was sized based on this endpoint.

The success of the pivotal trial requires that both the primary and coprimary endpoints were statistically significant. The sponsor had high confidence in meeting the primary endpoint based on information from a feasibility study but had some concerns for the coprimary endpoint of TVF. During the planning stage, sample size was calculated under some assumptions of the performance of DES X. Due to the uncertainty of the TVF event rates for DES X (especially for the dual vessel treated patients), the sponsor proposed adaptive sample size reestimation so that the trial could be sized appropriately. One interim analysis was proposed at 80% information time (when 792 subjects had 270 day information) and the conditional power would be calculated. If the conditional power is lower than 80%, the required new sample size to reach 80% conditional power would be estimated. The maximum increase in sample size was 900 subjects. The total 5% type I error rate alpha was allocated as .0101 for Stage I and .0492 for Stage II using Gamma family alpha spending function proposed by Huang, Shih, and DeCani (1990). To combine the information from Stage I and Stage II for the final analysis, the down-weighting stage II information approach proposed by Cui, Hung, and Wang (1999) was used to control the overall type I error rate.

During the protocol review stage, simulations according to the trial design were conducted by FDA and the sponsor to evaluate the validity of the trial design. The findings under several possible scenarios are:

a. The overall type I error rate is controlled under the nominal 5%.
b. The unconditional power is adequate for the proposed adaptive design.
c. The average size of the proposed design is reasonable under several assumptions of the event rates. Results of a–c are presented in Tables 26.1 through 26.3, respectively.

It is recognized that operational bias incurred by interim looks of data is a complex and multifaceted issue. To minimize possible operational bias, the sponsor proposed that an independent statistician performs sample size reestimation based on two sets of TVF rate estimates: the observed rates for each arm, the average of the observed rate, and the assumed rate for each arm. A range of the new sample size based on these rates would be conveyed back to the sponsor by the independent statistician. In addition,

TABLE 26.1 Simulated Type I Error Rate

P_c	9.4%	9.9%	10.4%	10.9%
$P_e = P_c + 5.5\%$	4.92%	4.94%	4.84%	4.69%

TABLE 26.2 Empirical Unconditional Power of the Proposed Adaptive Design

P_c	$P_e = P_c$	$P_e = P_c + 0.5\%$	$P_e = P_c + 1\%$	$P_e = P_c + 1.5\%$	$P_e = P_c + 2\%$
9.4%	96.5%	93.4%	87.8%	79.2%	67.9%
11.4%	93.8%	89.2%	82.5%	73.1%	63.1%

TABLE 26.3 Average Sample Size of the Proposed Design

P_c	$P_e = P_c$	$P_e = P_c + 0.5\%$	$P_e = P_c + 1\%$	$P_e = P_c + 1.5\%$	$P_e = P_c + 2\%$
9.4%	1107	1155	1217	1282	1350
11.4%	1145	1199	1267	1326	1384

TABLE 26.4 Analysis of the Endpoint—TVF at 9-Months

	DES X	DES Y	p-value for noninferiority testing
Overall TVF	7.61% (50/657)	9.69% (31/320)	< 0.0001

most individuals involved in the trial were not informed about the adaptive strategy. The blinded parties included data safety monitoring board (DSMB), CEC, sponsor statisticians and programmers, data management personnel, investigational site personnel, patients, and primary investigators. FDA granted the approval of the investigational device exemption (IDE).

At the planned interim analysis, DES X was shown to be noninferior to DES Y with respect to the coprimary endpoint (TVF rate) with a p-value less than 0.0001 (Table 26.4). After the database was locked for the coprimary endpoint analysis, the recommendation was that no additional patients were needed to sustain conditional power of 80%.

Since the sample size was not changed, the accumulated data collected from the pivotal trial were analyzed with the traditional group sequential approach (equal weight for data from Stages I and II) at the end of the study. The observed TVF rates for DES X and DES Y were 7.61 and 9.69%, respectively, out of 657 DES X patients and 320 DES Y patients. The p-value for the noninferiority testing was < 0.0001. The observed average and the standard deviation of the late loss at 8-month postprocedure for DES X and DES Y were 0.14 ± 0.41 and 0.28 ± 0.48, respectively, out of 301 DES X patients and 134 DES Y patients. The p-value for the noninferiority testing was < 0.0001. Since the noninferiority claim was established for both the primary and coprimary endpoints, superiority testing was conducted. The p-value of the superiority testing for TVF at 9-month postprocedure was 0.27; while the p-value for late loss at 8-months postprocedure was .0037. As a summary, DES X is superior to DES Y with respect to 8-months late loss; and is noninferior to DES Y with respect to 9-months TVF. This application went to a panel meeting and later gained FDA's approval.

Note that the test statistic proposed and presented in this case study was calculated based on Farrington and Manning (1990) in the following:

$$z = \frac{\hat{p}_e - \hat{p}_c - \delta}{Se},$$

where *Se* is the maximum likelihood estimate of the standard error under the null hypothesis:

$$Se = \sqrt{\frac{p_{eml}(1 - p_{eml})}{n_e} + \frac{p_{cml}(1 - p_{cml})}{n_c}}$$

$$p_{eml} = p_{cml} + \delta .$$

Here p_{eml} and p_{cml} are the maximum likelihood estimates of DES X arm event rate and DES Y arm event rate under the null hypothesis.

26.3.2 Case Study 2

This case study discusses a study with Bayesian adaptive design that was implemented with interim monitoring for the purpose of recruiting and trial success. Due to the evolving nature of medical devices, several medical devices have been evaluated through PMA submissions based on data collected via Bayesian adaptive trial design, and numerous IDE applications with Bayesian adaptive design have been submitted for regulatory review.

The device was an ablation catheter that has been approved for other indications. The newly proposed indication was for drug refractory symptomatic paroxysmal atrial fibrillation (AF) through radiofrequency ablation. The pivotal study was a randomized, unblinded controlled evaluation of symptomatic, paroxysmal AF patients who were refractory to at least one antiarrhythmic drug (AAD) and had at least three episodes of AF in the 6 months prior to randomization. Eligible subjects from 19 worldwide centers were randomized to catheter ablation (test arm) and medical therapy (control arm) in a 2:1 ratio. The primary effectiveness endpoint was success rate at 9-month postprocedure, where a patient was considered to be a success if he/she was free from documented symptomatic paroxysmal AF episodes and from changes in drug therapy after the blanking period (i.e., within 3-month postprocedure) during which continued drug therapy was allowed. The study objective was the superiority of catheter ablation to medical therapy with respect to the success rate at 9-month postprocedure.

Due to significant difficulty in recruiting patients, Bayesian adaptive design approach was proposed. Based on the proposed Bayesian approach, the trial would be considered to be successful with respect to effectiveness if the posterior probability that the device success rate is larger than the control success rate is greater than 0.98. In symbols,

$$P(P_T \geq P_c|\text{data}) \geq 0.98,$$

where P_T and P_c are the probability of success in effectiveness for the device and the control arm, respectively. The prior distributions of P_T and P_c are assumed both noninformative (uniform distribution).

A maximum of 230 subjects were proposed, and two monitoring mechanisms, one for accrual and one for claim of study success after accrual stops, were planned. They are summarized in the following:

- Monitoring for accrual:
  Interim analyses would be performed when sample size reaches 150, 175, and 200. If predictive probability of trial success for all enrolled patients so far, based on knowing only the information at the time of the interim look, is at least 0.90 at the 150-patient look or 0.80 at the 175-patient and 200-patient looks, then the accrual would be stopped and the interim look sample size would be the final sample size. On the other hand, the trial would be stopped for futility if the predictive probability of success for the current sample size and the maximum sample size (230 subjects) are less than 0.01 for the 150-subject, 175-subject, or 200-subject look. Otherwise, the sponsor would continue to enroll patients. The calculation of the predictive probability for the unknown results (enrolled-but-not-observed and the yet-to-be-enrolled) involves modeling of the patient response.
- Monitoring for trial success in effectiveness:
  When accrual stops, an analysis for an early claim of success was planned when either 4.5 months have passed or at least 50% of the enrolled subjects have completed effectiveness outcome measures. If predictive probability of trial success is at least 0.99, effectiveness would be claimed.

Simulations were performed to capture the frequentist operating characteristics, such as the distribution of the final sample size, power, and the type I error rate based on 10,000 simulated trials. The estimated type I error rate of the design was two-sided 5%. Sensitivity analyses were performed to evaluate the sensitivity of the priors and the predictive models.

When accrual reached 160 subjects (of which 148 were deemed eligible, 96 were in the device arm), the first interim analysis was performed. The status of the 148 subjects at the time of the interim

TABLE 26.5 Summary of the Current Status of Eligible Subjects

Treatment Group	Success	Failure	Censored	Total
Test	16	25	55	96
Control	6	38	8	52

analysis is given in Table 26.5. The censored subjects (55 in test group and eight in control group) are those subjects whose 9-month information was not available when the first interim analysis was conducted. A statistical model was built to predict the 9-month outcome of those censored subjects. It used the predictive distribution of the times to event, assuming a piecewise exponential model for time to event. Multiple imputation was performed using the predictive distribution, and averaging over the predictive distribution.

The predictive probability of concluding superiority when all 160 subjects reached 9 months of follow-up was calculated as greater than 0.999 (exceeding the threshold of 0.90). Therefore the conclusion of the interim analysis was to stop enrollment at 160 subjects. At the first interim look, the proportion of subjects having completed 9-month effectiveness determination exceeded 50%, therefore the sponsor performed a trial success evaluation. Early claim of success was made because the predictive probability exceeded 0.99.

Through the use of the Bayesian adaptive design, the sponsor made early claim of trial success in addition to the sample size saving at the first interim look. As mentioned previously, the trial was originally designed with a fixed sample size frequentist approach, Bayesian adaptive design was proposed to handle enrollment problems at U.S. sites when 106 patients had been enrolled. FDA had significant reservation regarding the change of the approach. The sponsor's justification was that the change of the methodology was data independent, as they were blinded to the chronic result of any patient and the majority of the 106 patients had not yet completed the 9-month follow-up. An agreement was reached between the FDA and the sponsor. That is, treating the first set of 106 enrolled patients as an interim look with high threshold value for stopping accrual and a statistical penalty was applied. This resulted in an increased posterior criterion for effectiveness, in order to maintain the type I error rate at the nominal level. This was incorporated into the simulations that characterized the operating characteristics of the trial design.

One should note that the maximal study size was specified up front with Bayesian adaptive design that has similarity to the conventional group sequential design. So that study can declare an early success when adequate safety and effectiveness of the device are established at the interim analyses. Because of the feature of medical devices (e.g., different generations) and because the aspect of Bayesian approach differs from the conventional frequentist approach, extensive simulations are the main tool to support the validity of Bayesian adaptive trial design with respect to the type I error rate in frequentist paradigm. Bayesian approach, including Bayesian adaptive design, has been employed in medical device studies to establish the safety and effectiveness of medical device applications [see the FDA guidance (2006) for more information].

26.3.3 Case Study 3

This case study concerns the change of the primary endpoint during the course of a clinical trial. The study was designed as multinational, double-blind, parallel-group, and randomized. The objective was to study the effects of Carvedilol on mortality and morbidity in patients with left ventricular dysfunction, with or without clinical evidence of heart failure, or postmyocardial infarction (MI). The test medication in the study was Carvedilol (6.25 mg bid, titrated if necessary, to 12.5 mg bid at 3–10 days and then to 25 mg bid for 5–10 days) compared against placebo. The trial was conducted during

1997 and 2002. A total of 975 and 984 patients were randomized to receive Carvedilol and placebo, respectively.

At the study design stage, the primary endpoint was specified as all-cause mortality; and the secondary endpoint was a composite of mortality and cardiovascular (CV) hospitalization. One interim analysis of all-cause mortality at 125 deaths was planned in the original protocol. On the basis of evidence from outside of the trial (e.g., MERIT-HF), DSMB in March 1999 recommended subjects who developed heart failure be permitted with the use of open-labeled beta blocker. Because such a recommendation was likely to reduce the effect of overall mortality, DSMB recommended an unplanned change in the primary endpoint to enhance study power. Recommendation was made prior to having carried out any efficacy analyses of the trial.

After careful consideration of the DSMB's recommendations, the steering committee added another primary endpoint, the composite of mortality and CV hospitalization that was originally prespecified as the secondary endpoint, in addition to the primary endpoint, all-cause mortality. The study would be declared as a success if Carvedilol is superior to placebo in either one of the primary endpoints. To ensure that the study had adequate power, the number of endpoint events remained as 633 in the revised study protocol. Consequently, the expected total enrollment fell from 2600 to 1850 since the estimated composite event rate would be relatively larger as compared to the all-cause mortality rate. For testing purpose, the revised protocol assigned the primary endpoint, composite of all-cause mortality and CV hospitalization, with a significance level of $\alpha = 0.045$; and the primary endpoint of all-cause mortality with a significance level of $\alpha = 0.005$, where $\alpha = 0.001$ for the interim analysis of mortality at 125 deaths; and $\alpha = 0.004$ for final analysis. The protocol was amended and submitted to FDA after implementation.

The final study results are presented in Table 26.6. As can be observed from Table 26.6, the study clearly failed the two primary endpoints. On the other hand, the study would have shown the statistical superiority of Carvedilol to placebo if the changing of endpoints at midcourse of the trial had not been proposed and implemented. One would argue that Carvedilol shows statistically significant effect on the all-cause mortality endpoint as the p-value of 0.031 is less than a significance level of 0.05. However, with the change of endpoints during the course of the trial, the comparison of $p = 0.031$ for the endpoint of all-cause mortality to 0.05 is no longer valid.

The change of endpoints in this case study was based on external evidence. As indicated in Section 26.2, it can be risky to change the primary endpoint based on external results. This is because that the patient populations observed, and clinical practice, and so on, may be factors attributed to, and resulted in, different treatment effect sizes.

26.3.4 Case Study 4

This case study concerns design adaptation using solely simulations to control the study-wise type I error rate without analytical approaches. The proposal was submitted to the regulatory agency as an investigational new drug (IND) application.

TABLE 26.6 Results of the Final Analysis—Carvedilol vs. Placebo

	Number of Events				
Endpoints	Carvedilol ($n = 975$)	Placebo ($n = 984$)	Hazard Ratio and 95% CI	p-value	Prespecified α Level
Death/CV hospitalization	340	367	0.92 (0.80, 1.07)	0.30	0.045
Death	116	151	0.77 (0.60, 0.98)	0.031	0.004

To illustrate the example, we assume the proposed study is a paired design (pre- and postscore). Each study subject serves as his/her own control. The objective was the superiority of the postscore to the prescore following a course of the proposed experimental treatment. The primary endpoint was the difference of post- and prescores, $d_{post-pre}$; and was assumed to have a normal distribution with a variance of 1. The hypotheses to be tested are:

$$H_O:\mu_d \leq 0$$

$$H_A:\mu_d \leq 0.33,$$

where μ_d is the population mean in difference of post- and prescores.

It was determined in the protocol that sample size 100 would have a power of 90% at one-sided significance level of 0.025 based on paired t-test. The study planned for one interim analysis. A study adaptation of sample size reestimation was proposed when data for the first 50 subjects were available. If the observed treatment effect of $d_{post-pre}$ at the interim look was between 0 and 0.25, the sample size would be increased by an additional 200 subjects that results in a total of 300 subjects in the final analysis. The proposal claimed that simulations showed no need for alpha adjustment in the final analysis. The study however proposed that the final analysis would be performed at a level of 0.024.

To evaluate the validity of the proposal, simulations were conducted using SAS. The general framework of the simulation procedure is as follows:

1. At a given random seed, a set of observations is generated from normal with mean 0 and variance 1 (under null hypothesis).
2. If the observed mean for the first 50 observations is between 0 and 0.25, then 300 observations will be tested using paired t-test. Otherwise, paired t-test applies to 100 observations.
3. Steps 1 and 2 are repeated for M times.
4. The percentage of M simulated data sets that are significant at a prespecified significance level is obtained.

As a result, a random seed of 13,017 and M = 10,000 given in SAS appear to yield reasonable outcomes. That is, at a significance level of 0.025, 0.024, and 0.023, the simulated type I error rates are 2.48%, 2.39%, and 2.27%, respectively. However, the use of different random seeds in data generation may result in different outcomes. Simulation results using 100 different random seeds are tabulated in Table 26.7 over various significance levels and M = 10,000 and 100,000 per simulation.

For example, among 100 different random seeds used for data generation and M = 10,000 per simulation, only eight of them with simulated type I error rate were ≤ 0.025. In contrast, none of them has

TABLE 26.7 Simulations Using 100 Different Random Seeds

	Number of Simulations ≤ α among 100 Simulations	
Prespecified α Level	M = 10,000/ per Simulation	M = 100,000/ per Simulation
0.025	8	0
0.024	25	1
0.023	51	23
0.022	71	87
0.021	90	100
0.020	97	100

simulated type I error rate ≤ 0.025 when $M = 100{,}000$/per simulation is used. More interestingly, the number of simulations with simulated type I error rate $\leq \alpha$ appears to have an increasing trend as the prespecified significance level α decreases. This raises issues about the use of random seeds for data generation, the number of replicates (M) per simulation, and, consequently, the distribution of simulated type I error rates due to different random seeds.

Study adaptation that is justified with analytical approach is preferred for regulatory review. Study design supported by simulations only may not easily be verified unless all parameters used in the simulations are prespecified, and may not be valid since simulations usually cannot cover all trial scenarios. Consequently, the worst type I error rate may not be attainable. For regulatory applications with simulations, an in-depth investigation regarding the impact on the simulated outcomes due to different random seeds, the number of replicates per simulation, and different clinical trial setting should be conducted. Obviously, submissions with simulations conducted under only limited and/or unrealistic clinical trial scenarios are inadequate.

26.4 Concluding Remarks

Adaptive designs have become recognized in clinical trials and other areas of public health research. Although statistical methodologies in a broader context of adaptive design have been investigated for decades, the application of adaptive design strategies to clinical trials has been increasing recently in regulatory submissions.

As the main focus in this chapter is on the adaptive designs for the confirmatory Phase III trials, one must keep in mind that the ultimate objectives of confirmatory Phase III studies are to confirm hypotheses generated in earlier studies regarding the treatment effect and to assess whether or not the treatment effect is reproducible in the targeted patient population after regulatory approval. Therefore, for a Phase III clinical trial with adaptive study design, one important goal is to confirm the treatment effect under the assumption of the prespecified design parameters and to allow minor correction of those design parameters. Issues, such as the operational biases and characteristics due to interim looks of data, pooling data before and after design adaptations, and so on, make the regulatory evaluation of outcomes generated from adaptive design trials more complex and challenge. The major concerns are the clinical interpretation of overall trial results, operational logistics, trial conduct, and whether the integrity of study results is maintained. Methods that simply gain control over the type I error rate are not good enough. As numerous information may be needed at the interim analyses to reach good decision making, the proper control of the information flow is critical. It is important to lay out a detailed plan for interim analyses when adaptive designs are considered, aside from statistical methods that control the type I error rate and appropriate statistical testing. For example, who decides when and what data to look at, who has access to unblinded data and information, who has the authority to suggest or to execute the study adaptations? How can confidentiality be maintained sufficiently due to the potential leakage of analyses of unblinded data and information? How are decisions and recommendations conveyed? How are the people outside the trial or the regulatory agencies convinced that the clinical trial is conducted properly and bias caused by such an adaptive design approach is minimized? All these issues need to be laid out in detail at the protocol design stage and prespecification is the key element in developing adaptive design trial protocols. As the experience of regulatory agencies is limited to date, considerable work and practical experience are needed to characterize how best to use adaptive designs in the clinical trial setting.

Finally, it should be emphasized that the added flexibility of adaptation is not without potential pitfalls. Study adaptation should never be used as a way to salvage study results and should never be used to avoid careful planning and thorough research and development of medical products during the development process. Adaptive design is adaptive by design, which requires careful planning in the trial development stage.

References

Bauer, P., and Koenig, F. (2006). The reassessment of trial perspectives from interim data—A critical view. *Statistics in Medicine,* 25: 23–36.

Coronary Drug Project Research Group. (1981). Practical aspects of decision making in clinical trials: The Coronary drug project as a case study. *Controlled Clinical Trials,* 1: 363–76.

Cui, L., Hung, H. M. J., and Wang, S. J. (1999). Modification of sample size in group sequential clinical trials. *Biometrics,* 55: 853–57.

Farrington, C. P., and Manning, G. (1990). Test statistics and sample size formulae for comparative binomial trials with null hypothesis of non-zero risk difference or non-unity relative risk. *Statistics in Medicine,* 9: 1447–54.

FDA. (2004). *Innovation or Stagnation?—Challenge and Opportunity on the Critical Path to New Medical Products.* Rockville, MD: U.S. Food and Drug Administration. Available at http://www.fda.gov/oc/initiatives/criticalpath/

FDA. (2006). *Draft FDA Guidance on the Use of Bayesian Statistics for Medical Device Trials.* Rockville, MD: U.S. Food and Drug Administration. Available at http://www.fda.gov/cdrh/osb/guidance/1601.pdf

Huang, H. M. J., and Wang, S. J. (2004). Multiple testing of noninferiority hypotheses in active controlled trials. *Journal of Biopharmaceutical Statistics,* 14: 327–35.

Huang, I. K., Shih, W. J., and DeCani, J. S. (1990). Group sequential designs using a family of type I error probability spending functions. *Statistics in Medicine,* 9: 1439–45.

Hung, H. M. J., and O'Neill, R. (2003). Utilities of the P-value distribution associated with effect size in clinical trials. *Biometrical Journal,* 45: 659–69.

Koch, A. (2006). Confirmatory clinical trials with an adaptive design. *Biomedical Journal,* 48: 574–85.

Morikawa, T., and Yoshida, M. (1995). A useful testing strategy in Phase III trials: Combined test of superiority and test of equivalence. *Journal of Biopharmaceutical Statistics,* 5: 297–306.

Temple, R. J. (1994). Special study designs: Early escape, enrichment, studies in non-responders. *Communications in Statistics-Theory and Methods,* 23: 499–531.

Tsong, Y., Hung, H. M. J., Wang, S. J., Cui, L., and Nuri, W. A. (1997). Dropping a treatment arm in clinical trial with multiple arms. *Proceedings of the Biopharmaceutical Section, American Statistical Association,* 1997: 58–63.

Wang, S. J., Hung, H. M. J., Tsong, Y., and Cui, L. (2001). Group sequential test strategies for superiority and non-inferiority hypotheses in active controlled clinical trials. *Statistics in Medicine,* 20: 1903–12.

Zhen, B. (2008). A statistical reviewer's perspective on sample size re-estimation. *Presented at 2008 FDA/Industry Statistics Workshop.* Available at http://www.amstat.org/meetings/fdaworkshop/index.cfm?fuseaction = EnterPass&file = 300431.ppt

27

Good Practices for Adaptive Clinical Trials

Paul Gallo
Novartis Pharmaceuticals

27.1 Introduction

The use of adaptive clinical trial designs is a topic that has received a substantial amount of interest in recent years. This has been reflected in numerous publications, special journal issues, workshops, and other scientific forums.

The interest is understandable, as there may be potential to improve the practice of drug development, and to perform it in a more efficient and ethical manner, especially in a challenging time for drug development as described by the U.S. Food and Drug Administration (FDA 2004). Adaptive trial designs may provide opportunities to better account for uncertainties in design assumptions, to decrease the chance that a trial will produce inconclusive results, or to proceed more quickly through the development process by avoiding or decreasing some of the discrete steps in a traditional sequential series of trials. The hope is that such designs can provide better answers to research questions faster and with smaller resource commitments, and subjecting fewer patients to therapies that may be suboptimal for them or carry unknown safety risks. From a theoretical statistical standpoint, much is at least possible in terms of adaptation. The challenge is to see whether and to what extent theory can match up with the very specific practical needs in drug development, and satisfy the varied concerns of sponsors, regulators, and the scientific community.

While the interest in adaptive trials is understandable, skepticism and criticism is understandable as well. This is in fact desirable, and if adaptive designs are to play an important role in clinical research, the expressing of challenges should play a necessary and constructive role in their evolution. For this larger role to become reality and provide real advantages, proponents of adaptive designs will need to provide convincing answers to challenging questions that are based on legitimate concerns; perhaps this may result in beneficial refinement or improvement in adaptive design technology or practice.

Resistance should not be based solely on a sense of unease because adaptive trials or programs differ from familiar practice and present challenges that are new or different from those we are used to. Conventional practice is certainly not free of difficulties. Clinical programs with adaptive aspects may differ from a traditional Phase I, II, III approach, and it has been stated that using adaptive designs can "blur the distinction between phases." Why it should be assumed from the start that this is a major disadvantage is by no means clear, however; why should it be written in stone for all time that the manner in which clinical research has been performed in recent decades must stand unchanged regardless of improvements in related technologies? Many recent technology changes, for example, developments in statistical methodology, computing capabilities, internet communications, real-time data capture, and so on, may well have some potential to be capitalized upon so that a development paradigm that has been effective in the recent past may now have opportunity for changes or improvements.

An illustrative comparison to evolution in the practice of performing group sequential trials may be instructive. Methods that allow a trial to be stopped prior to the initial planned maximum duration with a valid claim of having demonstrated an effect elicited interest and gained popularity following the work of Pocock (1977) and O'Brien and Fleming (1979). Methodology extensions such as the spending function approach (Lan and DeMets 1983) allowed flexibility in the number and timing of analyses that were much more in keeping with practical realities of clinical trials. Practical implementation of such methods and the development of standards and conventions presented challenges, and this was not completely free of controversy at that time. These designs would of course require some party to have access to unblinded trial data, so there was potential for introducing biasing influences into the trial if this process were not properly managed. Also, when such trials continue beyond an evaluation point, this may unavoidably convey some information about the trial results, as observers assume that known action thresholds have not been reached (depending on details of the methodology used, the information conveyed may be more than commonly believed). Additionally, when using a spending function approach, if analysis times are not chosen independently of results, the underlying theory is violated so that the false positive rate might not be protected.

Valid concerns such as these did not prevent interim analyses and group sequential designs from becoming the important and accepted aspect of clinical trials that they are today. Challenges were articulated and methods and practices evolved, supported by actual experiences, to overcome the challenges where possible, or to limit their impact; it thus became a consensus judgment that the advantages conferred by such designs could outweigh the challenges in particular applications where they were implemented in a quality manner.

While the analogy is imperfect because of the potentially broad scope of adaptive designs, this example illustrates the standard by which we feel adaptive approaches should be evaluated and may continue to evolve, so that it can be determined whether their promise might be achieved. They are not free of risks and challenges; but no paradigm for clinical development can be. It is a question of recognizing and quantifying the advantages and the challenges and downsides, improving aspects of this technology where possible, and setting up frameworks whereby adaptive approaches can be compared to conventional or alternate approaches on a case-by-case basis to see if and when they add value.

In this chapter, we provide a broad overview for a number of general issues of good practice that should be addressed when adaptive trial designs are considered or utilized, so that the decision to use an adaptive design (or not), and the manner in which it is implemented, are more sound and likely to be beneficial. Of course in particular situations it is the very specific details of the situation that will drive the decisions and implementation, in a manner not possible to fully address here; indeed some of the issues we raise in a general manner are in fact treated in more specific detail elsewhere within this handbook, but here we restrict ourselves to general principles and tendencies.

In the majority of this discussion, there is at the very least an implicit emphasis on *confirmatory* studies; that is, trials conducted in later stages of development that aim to obtain definitive evidence to be used as the basis for regulatory claims and to influence medical practice. While sound practices that follow from the relevant concerns may not be so critical to adhere to in trials of a more exploratory nature, it might still be useful to implement similar practices wherever feasible to enhance the impact of trials for any audience or purpose.

Among the types of questions we address here are: How in general should one go about considering whether an adaptive trial is a viable option within a program? What attributes of a trial lend themselves to considering an adaptive approach? What particular types of adaptations might be permissible and beneficial in confirmatory trials and what practices are advisable to follow when doing so? What kinds of biases might arise in adaptive trials, and what actions can we take to minimize this risk? What variations of current interim monitoring practices should be implemented for adaptive trials? and Should we retrospectively examine final trial data for signs that different parts of a trial yielded dissimilar results? Again, answers to questions such as these are clearly situation dependent, but we nevertheless attempt to give some general guidance on issues that need to be considered and good practices for implementation.

27.2 General Considerations and Motivation for Using an Adaptive Design

We start with some broad statements of overall principles and general practices. Recurring themes here will involve the necessity of having sound rationale, preidentifying challenges, and expending the necessary advance planning efforts. Adaptive trials should not be viewed as a remedy for poor planning, or as a device to rescue a trial that was not planned well, or as a way to undertake a trial when the research objectives have not been thoroughly decided upon and described. Certainly they should not be used simply for the sake of doing something perceived as novel and "cutting edge." Rather, an adaptive approach should be implemented as part of a rational strategy to address a research question when it is believed to offer quantifiable advantages within its particular placement in the development program. Sources of potential bias must be considered, and whether the aggregate results from the trial will be adequately interpretable and meet the needs of the intended audiences, whether that includes regulatory authorities, the scientific community, the study sponsor making strategic development decisions, and so on. Alternate design possibilities, both adaptive and nonadaptive, should be considered, and it should be demonstrable that the selected adaptive approach is expected to yield tangible advantages over other design options, whether in ethical treatment of patients, resource or time savings, or better quality of information. Logistic issues related to drug supply, resource allocation, data flow, and communication may well be more challenging than in conventional trials.

Aspects of the trial that are candidates for adaptation should be clearly understood and described in advance. It is not a matter of exploring, as the trial proceeds, what could be changed, but rather of having a sensible plan addressing those aspects that should be considered for change, and designing the trial based on that understanding, with the adaptation strategy embedded within a valid statistical plan. Correspondingly, there should be an understanding of how the accruing results will translate into adaptation decisions, perhaps following a rigid algorithm, but in some cases perhaps allowing some flexibility if appropriate to the decision and allowed by the analysis plan.

The design and adaptive algorithm should be robust in the sense of having good performance and behavior under varied underlying scenarios. A thorough evaluation of the design through simulation is usually called for. As well as satisfying the sponsor that the design is sound, a thorough simulation report in confirmatory trials will often be a critical aspect of demonstrating to regulatory authorities that the design has merit. The simulations will also help address the robustness concerns of all parties.

The following list contains brief descriptions of issues that may arise in deciding when adaptive designs are likely to be feasible and advantageous, and how they should be implemented:

- Generally, studies lend themselves to adaptive designs when the readout time to the endpoint used for adaptation is short relative to the enrollment rate. Information thus accrues more quickly, so adaptation decisions can be made earlier and/or based upon more dependable data, adding to the efficiency of the design. On the other hand, longer readout and faster enrollment tends to argue against the use of adaptive designs.

- The endpoint used for adaptation does not need to be the same as the primary study endpoint. A good surrogate may be considered, or some combination of the surrogate and primary endpoint, particularly in studies where the readout time to the primary endpoint is long. The predictive ability of the surrogate becomes an important factor; robustness against a weaker relationship between the surrogate and main endpoint is one of the issues that should be addressed in the prestudy simulation.
- Decisions should be made in advance about the quality of data to be used for the adaptation interim analyses. While resources should be allocated and applied sensibly (e.g., focus should be on the variables most important for decision making), it is not a requirement that all data used for an adaptation decision needs to be cleaned or adjudicated to final database quality. As in more conventional interim analysis settings, there is a tradeoff between the quality of the data and the amount and currentness of the data. It may be the case that a larger set of data not yet fully cleaned yields more precise information about a parameter than a smaller, cleaner set, especially early in a trial. Simulations that evaluate different scenarios regarding data quality and timeliness and strategies for determining analysis datasets can be helpful here as well.
- Infrastructure should be in place so that data flow and decision making can occur without undue delays, as delay will impact the potential efficiency and feasibility of the design. Details of efficient data collection, database preparation, analysis and review, necessary communication of decisions, and implementation of adaptations must all be addressed in advance.
- Drug supply issues must be considered fully in advance, particularly in studies that may utilize many dosage strengths, such as adaptive dose ranging studies.
- Resources of all relevant types must be available to accommodate any changes that could potentially occur within the trial.
- For planned adaptive trials in a confirmatory setting, early discussions with relevant regulatory authorities are very important, with sufficient details provided to allow them to judge whether they feel the plan is sound and can provide dependable and meaningful information. Details of the interim monitoring and decision making processes that will be followed and a thorough set of simulation results can be expected to play an important role in discussions.
- The statistical concepts of main concern are protection of the Type I error (false positive rate) and estimation of main study parameters, particularly in confirmatory studies. A broad base of statistical theory is available so that Type I error protection usually is not challenging to achieve using a well thought out analysis plan. The estimation issue is less settled; median unbiased estimates of treatment effects are available for some adaptive designs (see Brannath, König, and Bauer 2005; Posch et al. 2005). Research continues on mean unbiased estimation for adaptive designs, though bounds on the mean bias are available.

27.3 Scope of Adaptations in Confirmatory Trials

In many ways, adaptive designs lend themselves quite naturally to early development or exploratory trials. There tends to be a higher degree of uncertainty, and more aspects of trial conduct may be candidates for adaptation. There is often not the same need to strictly control error rates, nor perhaps to totally avoid bias, as would be the case in confirmatory trials.

Nevertheless, the question of what types of trial adaptations are appropriate in confirmatory settings has generated much interest. Confirmatory trials are in general larger and longer, so that the benefits of any gains in efficiency can be large; conversely, the negative implications of a trial that yields biased or misleading information, or that did not meet its objectives but might have done so if conducted differently, can be much more serious.

By the time a confirmatory trial is to be run, most uncertainties should have been resolved in trials from earlier development stages (though no trial can be designed fully free from uncertainty, nor can it be guaranteed that some design assumptions will not turn out to be inaccurate). What then can we say in general about the potential role of adaptive designs in confirmatory trials, and what type of situations might lend themselves better to this possible approach?

Answers of course will be highly situation-dependent, but as a general rule, the number of trial aspects adapted in a confirmatory study would be expected to be small, perhaps just one or two. If this were not the case, and multiple aspects of a study were subject to adaptation, it would be difficult to envision and justify that enough is known about the investigational treatment so that the trial can be viewed as able to provide confirmatory evidence. We cite a CHMP reflection paper (EMEA 2007): "The need to modify a number of design aspects ... may change the emphasis from a confirmatory trial to an hypothesis generating, or exploratory, trial" (p. 5). Adaptation in a confirmatory trial should aim to resolve only minor amounts of design uncertainty, generally from within a small number of prespecified possibilities.

As an additional general rule, hypotheses to be confirmed in a study need to be well understood and stated clearly in advance (i.e., in the study protocol), and embedded within a valid statistical plan. Multiple hypotheses can be addressed in a trial, just as in some nonadaptive confirmatory studies (e.g., think of a three-arm trial in which success can be claimed if either of two doses of an experimental treatment beats control), as long as the analysis methodology properly controls the overall false positive rate for the trial. On the other hand, for a hypothesis that arises from an examination of accruing data within a trial, we cannot expect that the data that generated the hypothesis can play a formal role in confirming that hypothesis. Thus, for example, it would not be appropriate to examine an interim set of data to identify on an exploratory basis a favorable endpoint or subgroup and use the entire body of data obtained from the trial for confirmatory purposes—because the hypothesis was not prestated, we cannot retrospectively embed it within a valid statistical plan.

A simple example of an adaptation that can be acceptable in a confirmatory trial (if conducted properly) would involve the group sequential designs mentioned previously. According to most proposed definitions of adaptive designs (e.g., Gallo et al. 2006), these would be viewed as adaptive because the trial can potentially stop at one of a number of points if the data support that a valid standard of evidence has been achieved. These designs are of course common in practice, and there are accepted associated statistical methods (see Jennison and Turnbull 2000) and conventions governing the operational aspects (Ellenberg, Fleming, and DeMets 2002; FDA 2006).

In the following two subsections, we more specifically discuss two study aspects that could lend themselves to adaptation in confirmatory trials: sample size and selection decisions as might be made in so-called "seamless" trials. We consider issues that should be kept in mind when considering implementing a plan allowing such modifications.

27.3.1 Sample Size Reestimation

Sample size would seem to be an aspect that could potentially be adapted in a confirmatory study, as this should be independent of most other trial details such as the nature of treatment administration or endpoints, and this does not change data structures. A straightforward application would involve sample size change based on within-trial information about a "nuisance parameter," such as a measure of variability. Even at the stage of running a confirmatory trial, there might well be uncertainty about such a parameter; for example, a broader setting of sites and patients used in a large Phase III study might yield more variable outcomes than were seen in Phase II data. Sample size reestimation (SSR) based on within-trial information on a nuisance parameter can be particularly noncontroversial, as it can often be done well using only blinded data (Kieser and Friede 2003). In fact, it might be argued that this should be considered on a fairly routine basis where applicable, as this will often be an easily correctable assumption with minimal downside.

Sample size change based upon unblinded data on the primary study endpoint can be more problematic. Statistical methods exist for changing sample size based on interim estimates of the primary efficacy endpoint (see Proschan and Hunsberger 1995; Cui, Hung, and Wang 1999; Posch, Bauer, and Brannath 2003; Bauer and König 2006; and a discussion in Chuang-Stein et al. 2006). In different manners, such methods seek to maintain power based on an observed interim value of the primary efficacy endpoint. Statistical criteria used for the final analysis must be modified to account for the reestimation procedure in order to protect the Type I error; that is, naively computing analysis criteria ignoring the reestimation would inflate the false positive rate. Generally, the change in sample size is inversely related to the size of the effect seen; that is, a smaller than hoped for effect observed at interim (perhaps within some prespecified range of effects) would lead to a sample size increase, and vice versa.

In a confirmatory study, the effect size of interest to detect should have an objective meaning that can be clearly justified in advance, for example, a particular effect size has importance to patients clinically, possibly taking risk-benefit or compliance considerations into account, it is sensible commercially, and so on. It should also be feasible given the state of knowledge about the treatment, perhaps obtained from Phase II trials or from related indications or populations. For the most part, the effect size we desire to detect when designing a confirmatory trial should be somewhat of a fixed quantity. See EMEA (2007): "In general, consideration of what magnitude of treatment effect might be of clinical importance should not be influenced by trial results (interim or final)" (p. 6). There may be some occasions in which the relevant effect size legitimately changes from the pretrial belief. For example, an effective competing treatment coming onto the market may affect the level of benefit that we would want a new experimental treatment to show; or an unexpected safety profile, whether positive or negative, may affect the judgment of risk/benefit.

In considering implementation of SSR methods based on the interim treatment effect, it is critical that full consideration has been given to a broad range of potential effect sizes, their value (to patients, perhaps to the sponsor), and the willingness to expend resources to demonstrate them. This is a sound approach for designing any trial, and with regard to SSR it will help decide whether such an approach is feasible, which method seems to be the best fit, and what are the numerical parameters of its implementation. It would be far from ideal, for example, to design a study casually to give a desired power for a particular effect size delta thought to be achievable, perhaps corresponding to sample size allowable within budget constraints; and then to reconsider based on weak interim data that the effect size seen there is one that we are really interested in after all. Such an approach should not be expected to yield as good a performance as an approach based on full consideration of the importance of different effect sizes, consideration of different methods that might be employed, quantifying the relevant tradeoffs, and evaluating operating characteristics under different scenarios.

When considering the use of SSR procedures, it will often be helpful to include more conventional group sequential plans as an option. For example, envision a situation where we believe it is feasible that the true effect size is some particular large value, but we would be willing to fully power the trial for a value noticeably smaller because that smaller level of benefit was still felt to be clinically relevant. The trial could be designed with a large maximum sample size corresponding to the smaller effect size judged to be relevant, and use a group sequential plan that is likely to allow stopping substantially earlier if the larger hoped-for effect is true. Useful perspectives for evaluating trade-offs between adaptive SSR and group sequential strategies are provided by Jennison and Turnbull (2003, 2006).

Operational aspects of SSR procedures and concerns about bias are discussed later in this chapter.

27.3.2 Seamless Trials

Another type of confirmatory adaptive design that has received attention and been conducted in actual practice relates to so-called inferentially seamless Phase II/III designs (Maca et al. 2006). In the most typical illustration, a study starts with a control group and two or more treatment arms, often different doses of an experimental treatment. At an interim analysis, some dose group(s) are selected to continue into a second stage of the trial, along with the control group, and some may be dropped. The final analysis of the continuing treatment arms uses data generated during both stages of the trial. Appropriate statistical methodology must be used to account for the number of hypotheses investigated in the trial (usually, the number of starting doses) and the nature of the selection.

Conceptually, this is quite similar to some conventional studies, which might, for example, include two active arms and a control, and use a statistical multiplicity adjustment such as the Bonferroni method. In the adaptive approach, we simply aim to increase efficiency and better utilize resources by allowing the interim selection decision. Also, if an alternative were to first run a separate Phase II trial to make the selection decision followed by a Phase III trial with the selected dose, then the seamless adaptive design can gain substantially by including patients from the "Phase II" part in the confirmatory analysis (though the amount of advantage depends on design details such as the number of treatment arms; a large number of arms may entail a multiplicity adjustment that largely negates this advantage). Additional benefits of the seamless design can include avoiding the "white space" between trials (if this is not needed for more in-depth examination of the selection data) and obtaining more long-term follow-up data. There are specific feasibility concerns that must be considered in deciding whether such a design is a good fit in a particular situation, discussed in Maca et al. (2006), such as the relationship between enrollment speed and the length of follow-up time to the endpoint used for the selection decision. Also, there may be important operational issues that must be handled properly with regard to how the interim analysis is conducted and acted upon, as discussed in the next section. Nevertheless, there seems no fundamental intrinsic reason why this approach cannot, if properly implemented, provide confirmatory evidence.

Also, while such proposals usually have involved multiple doses or treatment regimens, seamless trials making a selection among other study aspects would seem in particular instances to be possible. For example, a trial with a very small number of prespecified potential primary endpoints or primary patient populations, again with a selection decision made at interim, might be considered; the justifying rationale might be similar to conventional trials that have been performed with coprimary endpoints, either of which alone can be the basis for a positive claim, or allowing success in either of two patient populations, using an appropriate multiplicity adjustment.

27.4 Interim Monitoring Practices in Adaptive Trials

Adaptive trials raise new challenges with regard to monitoring of accruing interim data. Beyond the more familiar monitoring motivations, such as safety monitoring or the implementation of group sequential schemes, adaptive trials will certainly require examination of interim data, and for an additional purpose, namely, to consider or make adaptation to some aspect of the trial as it continues. A recent perspective on interim monitoring specific to adaptive trials is provided in Herson (2008).

In conventional interim monitoring practice, especially in confirmatory settings, there is an understanding that direct participation in the monitoring and access to unblinded data or comparative interim results by personnel directly involved in trial operations, or associated with the sponsoring organization, is not advisable. The underlying rationale is well described in an FDA guidance document (FDA 2006), and we briefly summarize the main concerns here:

- Trial management personnel may need to make decisions or take actions midtrial that can affect the conduct or ultimate outcome of the trial, for example, new external information obtained during a long-term trial may lead to protocol amendments or modification of the trial analysis plan. If trial personnel were to have access to unblinded data or accruing interim results, this would raise concerns about objectivity in making such decisions. It can only be assured that actions had been taken objectively, and not in an advantageous manner advised by access to unblinded results, if those individuals did not have such access (the guidance document refers to "diminution of the sponsor's ability to manage the trial without introducing bias").
- Knowledge of how results within a trial are trending can introduce subtle biases into the study by altering the behavior of trial participants. For instance, investigators might slightly change tendencies with regard to the types of subjects enrolled, or some aspect of patient treatment administration or outcome assessment, and so on.

On the basis of these concerns, a common operating model in confirmatory studies involves achieving the interim monitoring objectives through the use of an independent Data Monitoring Committee (DMC), a set of individuals with the necessary expertise and experience to perform the monitoring tasks, and who are external to the sponsoring organization and reasonably free of conflicts of interest. Unblinded data and results would be restricted within the DMC until such time as they were prepared to make a major recommendation regarding the trial (e.g., early termination). Similarly restricting access to interim results within an expert independent board in adaptive trials should thus have the same type of advantages for integrity of trial results.

In some adaptive studies, the types of adaptation decisions being made might in conventional development programs be viewed as primarily a sponsor responsibility, or at least are such that sponsor perspective may be considered relevant for making the best decision. As an illustrative example, we again consider a seamless Phase II/III trial in which selection of the continuing treatment arms is made based upon interim results. In a conventional separate-phase program, the decision to choose treatment arms for a Phase III trial based on Phase II results would normally be ultimately the sponsor's responsibility; the optimal decision may be complex and reflect different types of considerations for which sponsor perspective can be highly relevant. Thus, a type of conflict exists between the desire that interim data be shielded from the sponsor versus the potential relevance of sponsor perspective to the decision (or perhaps, the sponsor's perceived need to assure that a decision, even if made by an external board, is acceptable from its perspective). The challenge is to find operational models that resolve this conflict and maintain trial integrity while enabling optimal decisions reflecting all relevant perspectives and adequately addressing sponsor interests.

As elucidated in the FDA DMC guidance document (FDA 2006), the key principles are associated with restricting knowledge from personnel directly involved with the trial; that is, trial operations team, steering committee, investigators, and so on. The restriction against sponsor involvement is an added layer of protection against influence on the trial. If there were to be an opportunity for sponsor involvement in the adaptation decision process that does not provide major risks to the trial, it would seem to be through controlled limited involvement of sponsor personnel, who are clearly separated from trial activities, and with procedures, firewalls, and documentation in place to restrict information. The following model was proposed by the PhRMA Adaptive Designs Working Group (Gallo 2006):

- It should not be viewed that there is uniformly a need for sponsor involvement in the interim data review and decision making process in adaptive trials. If the nature of the adaptation decision can be made satisfactorily by an appropriately constituted external board, then it is advantageous for the integrity of the trial results to do so.
- If it is felt that sponsor input is called for, there should be a convincing rationale described and documented as to why this is the case, or why not having the ability to at least ratify a decision could put the sponsor in an untenable position.
- Sponsor personnel who receive access to interim results should be completely distanced from trial activities. All parties involved should understand the risks to the trial if confidentiality is not maintained. All activities should be governed by strict processes, with appropriate firewalls in place, and clear documentation and evidence should later be provided as to how those processes were followed.
- The smallest number of sponsor personnel who can supply the necessary perspectives should be involved (often, this may be just one or two management representatives who would typically not be involved in trial activities); they would receive the minimum amount of information necessary to meet the needs, and only at the relevant decision times.

As an example of how this process might play out in a given situation, an independent external DMC might be constituted, having more typical monitoring responsibilities (e.g., safety) in addition to those involving the adaptation, and with an ongoing role in the trial. At the adaptation point this board might initially deliberate in confidence among themselves; afterward, the sponsor representative(s) might be brought in as an adjunct to the board, and exposed only to the information necessary for their input into the adaptation decision, and with no further involvement as the trial proceeds.

Whether there is any such sponsor involvement or not, the overriding principle should always remain to insulate the information so that it cannot be accessed by anyone participating in the trial.

As a final note regarding distinctions between confirmatory and nonconfirmatory studies: the FDA guidance (FDA 2006) does distinguish between "late Phase II or Phase III studies" as opposed to "early phase studies," and for the latter case states that "issues regarding statistical interpretation of interim data, or confidentiality of interim data, are therefore generally less relevant"; and also "the need for *independent* DMCs in early phase studies will be infrequent." However this should not preclude employing confidentiality procedures similar to those used for confirmatory trials in earlier stages of development, in cases where this is feasible given the nature of the trial, and where this could strengthen the impact and interpretability of the results for any purpose or audience.

27.5 Other Trial Integrity Concerns for Adaptive Trials

Even if interim results are carefully restricted within a decision making board fully separated from trial operations, this does not totally eliminate the issue of possible biases based on interim results. The concern is that even if data remains confidential, adaptations implemented based on the interim results can convey information by which observers of the changes made may infer knowledge about the results that led to them.

As a typical example, consider a SSR in which a revised total sample size is computed in an algorithmic manner based upon the observed interim effect size. Someone who knows the method or algorithm (perhaps stated in the protocol, and very likely known by trial operations personnel) and sees the sample size modification can "back calculate" and have a pretty good idea of the interim effect size. For example, a large increase in sample size would likely correspond to a weak interim effect estimate. Adaptations such as changes to randomization allocation may similarly convey information about the relative benefits of different treatment arms. Knowledge of this type may have potential to change attitudes of trial participants in the manner discussed in the FDA guidance.

This issue may not be totally avoidable. As part of the process of deciding whether to use an adaptive design and how it should be implemented, advance thought must be given in particular situations as to whether the adaptations have potential to convey a precise level of information about the interim results. If some details of an adaptation decision do not need to be disseminated, they should not be; for example, in some seamless Phase II/III trials, perhaps it may not be necessary to broadly announce what treatment arms are continuing (although knowledge of selected treatment arms alone, with the numerical results remaining confidential, would probably not be considered to be serious in terms of the information conveyed).

Steps should always be considered to try to limit the information that might be conveyed by adaptations. Perhaps a protocol might not contain full numerical details of action thresholds, as long as the information withheld did not rise to a level of importance that was felt necessary for review boards, investigators, or patients to be aware of in order to be sufficiently informed about the trial. For example, suppose that selection of a treatment arm in a seamless design will be made using predictive probability criteria. The general approach and operating characteristics might be described in the study protocol, but without explicitly presenting the exact probability thresholds. These might be described in a document of more limited circulation, available to health authorities and the DMC. This information may not be unknown to all trial personnel, but at least this approach might limit what other parties (e.g., investigators) could infer from the actions eventually taken.

Returning to SSR, this concern might be a further point favoring the use of a group sequential design rather than a reestimation method to achieve sample size objectives: while a group sequential approach also conveys information (i.e., continuation of the trial generally means that a known stopping criterion has not been reached), it will generally be the case that far less information is conveyed compared to an SSR approach; the group sequential approach should also be more straightforward to implement operationally.

27.6 Consistency of Results Within Adaptive Trials

As we have described, adaptive trials can raise challenges with regard to interpretability of trial results since some aspect(s) of the trial may be explicitly changed as it proceeds. A main question of concern is: is the setting and conduct of the trial sufficiently stable so that the results can be viewed as a whole and interpreted as fully relevant to the initial research questions and able to be extrapolated to the envisioned target setting?

In different settings, within-trial changes may arise from different mechanisms. We have previously discussed possible operational bias due to knowledge of interim results, either directly or through observation of an adaptation. More subtly, just the existence of a structural difference across stages may induce a change in recruitment or behavior (Koch 2006); for example, in a seamless design the fact that first stage may contain a far lower proportion of placebo patients than the second stage may subtly change some aspect of behavior in an unknown manner. It is thus prudent to take whatever steps can be envisioned to minimize the chance for potential changes in trial conduct, and some of these have been described elsewhere in this article. This also suggests, though, it may be advisable to examine the final trial data to see whether there is numerical evidence that change or bias has occurred, so that the results can most correctly and meaningfully be interpreted.

It must be kept in mind that this investigation will tend to be limited numerically because of the lesser precision of results within subsets of trial data. Similar challenges arise here as in other types of subgroup evaluations. Trials are generally designed under some assumption of a reasonably homogeneous underlying setting, so that the totality of data is needed to have good ability (i.e., high power) to broadly distinguish between very different hypotheses, for example, a null hypothesis of no treatment effect versus an alternative hypothesis corresponding to a meaningful clinical benefit. If one attempts to detect treatment effects within subgroups or subsets of trial data, or to distinguish between different magnitudes of effects in subgroups, the operating characteristics will often be quite limited. For example, power may be low for determining if there are meaningful effect differences across subsets of the data, or false positive signals of differences may arise.

In addition, it should by no means be assumed that trial results do not drift in current conventional (i.e., nonadaptive) clinical trial practice, though there is often not particular focus on this question. Changes may occur for a number of reasons; some of these may be accounted for by other measurable covariates, for example as a trial expands to a broader setting of sites and locations, or the balance across other patient subgroups (perhaps defined by demographics or medical history) changes. Perhaps effects may change as investigators gain experience with administration of therapies and patient response to them as the trial proceeds ("learning curve"). Time-to-event analyses may present particular challenges in trying to evaluate whether there are within-study changes, since such changes may be confounded with nonconstant relative risk. One of the challenges in deciding how much evidence of change is a concern for proper interpretation of results in adaptive trials is that there are not common standards for how much change is acceptable in nonadaptive trials: if in an adaptive trial a signal of within-study change is seen that would not have been a concern in a nonadaptive trial, does it necessarily make sense to question the results because of the extra focus on this issue in adaptive trials?

The difficulties in evaluating subset effect differences and the lack of standards for this issue in general practice do not mean that this issue should be ignored; rather, it is simply an acknowledgement of the limitations of trying to address the question on a rigid and purely statistical basis. It is a responsible approach to investigate this issue during a thorough examination of the final data from an adaptive trial, much as might be done for other important factors defining subgroups, despite the numerical limitations. Large signals of within-trial change should be relevant to the overall interpretation. Statistical tools will be relevant in any investigation of this issue, but should be supported by operational and scientific considerations.

In a study with a small number of adaptation points, those points would often naturally define stages for which results can be compared to each other, whether descriptively or formally (even this may not be as easy as it sounds; for example, in studies in which there is long patient follow-up: What factor divides data into stages? When patients were randomized, or when most of their treatment occurred and they were evaluated?). In studies with more numerous or ongoing adaptations (e.g., response-adaptive randomization changes), cutpoints may be determined to divide the data more artificially into stages, which then might be handled in a similar manner.

Certainly, it should be very important, as described previously, to limit the potential for operational bias to have arisen in the first place, by implementing strict procedures to control access to the interim results used for the adaptation decisions. Strict documented procedures may not entirely resolve this issue, of course, because of the aforementioned possibilities of bias due solely to knowledge of adaptations made during the trial. Strong consideration should be given during trial planning to whether the adaptation plan is felt to have potential to introduce serious bias, and if so, what changes to the plan might be made to alleviate this, or how some of the problematic information might be masked. Where possible, specific mechanisms by which bias might be introduced should be hypothesized in advance, and descriptions of how we might expect this to be reflected in the trial results should be described: balancing numerical signals against scientific plausibility, an eventual signal of interaction might sensibly be viewed as a higher cause of concern or more likely to be real if the type of change seen makes sense scientifically based on a prespecified mechanism.

27.7 Conclusion

We are currently at a quite early point in the evolution of the practice of adaptive clinical trials. The main methodologic foundation that has spurred the recent interest dates back only to the last decade (e.g., Bauer and Köhne 1994). Due to the complexity and importance of clinical research, the long duration of clinical programs, and the varied interests and perspectives of all the different parties involved, it is only in recent years that we are beginning to gain a meaningful body of experience with important applications of adaptive trial designs. Thus, we probably do not yet have a clear sense of what their eventual role and importance will be. Perhaps the usage of adaptive designs will develop in ways that are not yet envisioned and demonstrate additional advantages, or perhaps they may not deliver as broadly as hoped on their theoretical promise and will play a more limited role. Input and interaction among industry sponsors, regulators, and the medical and academic communities will help evaluate the experiences, clarify the potential role, and guide further development. As the body of experiences grows and perhaps as practices continue to evolve, it will be very important that practitioners consider, implement, and evaluate such designs on a sound basis and in a quality manner based on current states of knowledge, with regard to practices such as those we have attempted to illustrate in a very general manner here.

References

Bauer, P., and Köhne, K. (1994). Evaluation of experiments with adaptive interim analyses. *Biometrics,* 50: 1029–41.

Bauer, P., and König, F. (2006). The reassessment of trial perspectives from interim data—A critical view. *Statistics in Medicine,* 25: 23–36.

Brannath, W., König, F., and Bauer, P. (2005). Estimation in flexible two-stage designs. *Statistics in Medicine,* 25: 3366–81.

Chuang-Stein, C., Anderson, K., Gallo, P., and Collins, S. (2006). Sample size reestimation: A review and recommendations. *Drug Information Journal,* 40: 475–84.

Cui, L., Hung, H. M. J., and Wang, S. J. (1999). Modification of sample size in group sequential clinical trials. *Biometrics,* 55: 853–57.

Ellenberg, S. S., Fleming, T. R., and DeMets, D. L. (2002). *Data Monitoring Committees in Clinical Trials: A Practical Perspective.* Chichester, UK: Wiley.

European Medicines Agency (EMEA). (2007). Reflection paper on *Methodological Issues in Confirmatory Clinical Trials Planned with an Adaptive Design. EMEA Doc. Ref. CHMP/EWP/2459/02.* Available at http://www.emea.europa.eu/pdfs/human/ewp/245902enadopted.pdf

FDA. (2004). Innovation or stagnation: Challenges and opportunities on the critical path to new medicinal products. *FDA Report.* Rockville, MD: U.S. Food and Drug Administration. Available at http://www.fda.gov/ScienceResearch/SpecialTopics/CriticalPathInitiative/default.htm

FDA. (2006). *Guidance for Clinical Trial Sponsors on the Establishment and Operation of Clinical Trial Data Monitoring Committees.* Rockville, MD: U.S. Food and Drug Administration. Available at http://www.fda.gov/cber/gdlns/clintrialdmc.pdf

Gallo, P. (2006). Confidentiality and trial integrity issues for adaptive designs. *Drug Information Journal,* 40: 445–49.

Gallo, P., Chuang-Stein, C., Dragalin, V., Gaydos, B., Krams, M., and Pinheiro, J. (2006). Adaptive designs in clinical drug development—An executive summary of the PhRMA working group. *Journal of Biopharmaceutical Statistics,* 16: 275–83.

Herson, J. (2008). Coordinating data monitoring committees and adaptive clinical trial designs. *Drug Information Journal,* 42: 297–301.

Jennison, C., and Turnbull, B. W. (2000). *Group Sequential Methods with Applications to Clinical Trials.* Boca Raton, FL: Chapman & Hall/CRC.

Jennison, C., and Turnbull, B. W. (2003). Mid-course sample size modification in clinical trials based on the observed treatment effect. *Statistics in Medicine,* 22: 971–93.

Jennison, C., and Turnbull, B. W. (2006). Efficient group sequential designs when there are several effect sizes under consideration. *Statistics in Medicine,* 25: 917–32.

Kieser, M., and Friede, T. (2003). Simple procedures for blinded sample size adjustment that do not affect the type I error rate. *Statistics in Medicine,* 22: 3571–81.

Koch, A. (2006). Confirmatory clinical trials with an adaptive design. *Biometrical Journal,* 48 (4): 574–85.

Lan, K. K. G., and DeMets, D. L. (1983). Discrete sequential boundaries for clinical trials. *Biometrika,* 70: 659–63.

Maca, J., Battacharya, S., Dragalin, V., Gallo, P., and Krams, M. (2006). Adaptive seamless Phase II/III designs—Background, operational aspects, and examples. *Drug Information Journal,* 40: 463–73.

O'Brien, P. C., and Fleming, T. F. (1979). A multiple testing procedure for clinical trials. *Biometrics,* 5: 549–56.

Pocock, S. J. (1977). Group sequential methods in the design and analysis of clinical trials. *Biometrika,* 64: 191–99.

Posch, M., Bauer, P., and Brannath, W. (2003). Issues in designing flexible trials. *Statistics in Medicine,* 22: 953–69.

Posch, M., König, F., Branson, M., Brannath, W., Dunger-Baldauf, C., and Bauer, P. (2005). Testing and estimation in flexible group sequential designs with adaptive treatment selection. *Statistics in Medicine,* 24: 3697–3714.

Proschan, M. A., and Hunsberger, S. A. (1995). Designed extension of studies based on conditional power. *Biometrics,* 51: 1315–24.

Index

A

C

D

E

F

G

H

N

Q

R

T

U

W

Z